Community-Based Nursing An Introduction

GET CONNECTED to the World

An ON-LINE resource created just for this book!

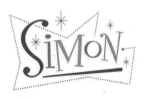 Sign on at: www.wbsaunders.com/SIMON/McEwen

A website just for you as you learn community-based

nursing with the new edition of *Community-Based*

Nursing: An Introduction.

What you will receive:

• Case Management Module

• WebLinks

• Frequently Asked Questions

• Content Updates

• Glossary

Simply register at the above URL to access this information.

SECOND EDITION

Community-Based Nursing
An Introduction

Melanie McEwen, PhD, RN

Associate Professor
Louise Herrington School of Nursing
Baylor University
Dallas, Texas

SAUNDERS
An Imprint of Elsevier Science
Philadelphia London New York St. Louis Sydney Tokyo

SAUNDERS

An Imprint of Elsevier Science

11830 Westline Industrial Drive
St. Louis, Missouri 63146

Vice President and Publishing Director, Nursing: Sally Schrefer
Executive Director: Darlene Como
Managing Editor: Linda Caldwell
Publishing Services Manager: Catherine Jackson
Project Manager: Jamie Lyn Thornton
Design Manager: Amy Buxton

Previous edition copyrighted 1998

Library of Congress Cataloging-in-Publication Data

McEwen, Melanie.
   Community-based nursing : an introduction / Melanie McEwen.–2nd ed.
     p. ; cm.
   Includes bibliographical references and index.
   ISBN 0-7216-9443-8
    1. Community health nursing. I. Title.
   [DNLM: 1. Community Health Nursing. WY 106 M478c 2002]
   RT98 .M3 2002
   610.73′43–dc21   2002066884

COMMUNITY-BASED NURSING: AN INTRODUCTION SECOND EDITION
ISBN 0-7216-9443-8
Printed in the United States of America.

Last digit is the print number: 9 8 7 6 5 4 3 2 1

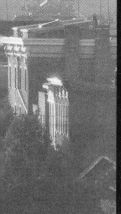

About the Author

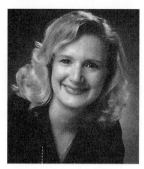

Melanie McEwen

Melanie McEwen, PhD, RN, is an Associate Professor at Louise Herrington School of Nursing, Baylor University. Dr. McEwen received her BSN from the University of Texas School of Nursing in Austin, her Master's in Community and Public Health Nursing from Louisiana State University Medical Center in New Orleans, and her PhD in Nursing at Texas Woman's University. Dr. McEwen is coauthor of *Theoretical Basis for Nursing*, which is targeted to graduate students, and a W.B. Saunders publication, *Community Health Nursing: Promoting the Health of Populations*.

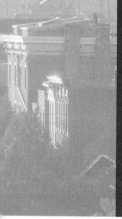

Preface

At the beginning of the twenty-first century, health care in the United States is still undergoing many changes. Cost consciousness among insurers, technology, and political decisions have altered *how* health care is provided, *who* is responsible for care delivery, *what* care is provided, and *when* clients are seen. One of the most significant changes, however, has been *where* care is given.

No longer is the hospital the central site for health care. Health care today is being provided in community-based settings such as homes, schools, clinics, offices, churches, and work sites, and even over the telephone or via e-mail. Correspondingly, there is a need for nurses prepared to practice in those settings. Therefore nursing education must include course content and clinical experiences that address community-based health care. *Community-Based Nursing: An Introduction* was written to be both a core and a supplemental textbook for nursing students who have an opportunity to deliver nursing care to clients in community-based settings.

ORGANIZATION

Community-Based Nursing: An Introduction, second edition, brings together the essential information necessary for nurses practicing in community settings. It includes content "hidden" in the major nursing textbooks that cover related material, information that may not be included in other resources, and content found in other books, but presented from a different perspective.

For example, Chapter 2 discusses roles and interventions emphasized in community-based nursing care and describes how they differ from roles and interventions in acute care settings. Chapter 5 gives an overview of the health care delivery system designed to help the reader understand why health care is becoming increasingly community based. Chapter 8 explores cultural influences on health and health care–seeking behaviors.

The chapters that focus on health care of major aggregates are presented from a different perspective from other major textbooks. In this textbook, the focus is on health promotion and illness prevention. For example, Chapter 9 discusses the care of infants, children, and adolescents. Information for community-based nursing care includes nutrition needs, growth, and development guidelines; immunization schedules; and suggested screenings. This chapter also discusses care of children with minor acute episodic illnesses, such as gastroenteritis, chicken pox, strep throat, and pediculosis (head lice), which are usually managed at home. In pediatric nursing textbooks, these topics are discussed largely from an acute care perspective and the information may be difficult to apply in community settings. This book presents the material in a format that emphasizes health teaching and care of the family.

The content of the book is organized into four units. Each unit covers different aspects of community-based nursing.

Unit 1, Foundations of Community-Based Nursing Practice, provides an overview of the many changes in the health care delivery system and corresponding opportunities for nurses to practice within the changing system. The unit also describes the roles and interventions used by nurses in community-based practice and gives an overview of the settings in which they practice (e.g., home health, clinics, ambulatory surgery centers, parish health programs).

Unit 2, Factors That Influence Health and Health Care, presents data about the factors that influence health and health care. Separate chapters describe the health care delivery system, epidemiology, environmental health issues, and culture.

Unit 3, Community-Based Nursing Care Across the Life Span, gives detailed information on health promotion activities and interventions appropriate for nursing care in community settings. Individual chapters cover the care of infants, children, adolescents, and adults. In addition, separate chapters describe the unique health needs of women, elders, and families.

Unit 4, Nursing Care of Clients with Special Needs in Community Settings, addresses nursing care for clients with special needs. In this unit, attention is given to vulnerable clients (i.e., those in poverty, the homeless, migrant farmworkers, disabled persons, and victims of disasters). This unit also has separate chapters on mental health care in the community and communicable disease prevention and intervention.

Community-Based Nursing: An Introduction includes material that will help direct nursing students in community-based practice, wherever the setting and whoever the population being served. For example, if the student is working with a home health care nurse providing skilled nursing services for older adults, helpful content would be found in Chapters 4 and 12. If the student is working in an elementary school, the section in Chapter 3 describing school nursing and information from Chapter 9 would be beneficial. Or, if the student is working in a women's clinic, appropriate information is found in Chapters 10, 11, and 16 (sexually transmitted diseases).

Much of the content of this text focuses on material that should be an integral part of client education (e.g., smoking cessation guidelines, how to bathe a newborn, fall prevention measures for elders). It includes guidelines for health promotion and illness prevention for all age groups (e.g., immunizations, screenings, risk identification); how to identify, intervene in, and refer various health problems and health threats in a variety of settings; and description, elaboration, and simplification of content the student needs to become community focused (e.g., cultural issues, the health care delivery system, and epidemiology).

KEY FEATURES

The following features are presented to enhance student learning:

New—Each chapter begins with **Learning Objectives** to explain the focus of the chapter.

New—Each chapter includes a list of **Key Terms** that are discussed in the chapter.

Each chapter is introduced by a **Case Study** illustrating how nurses in community-based practice use specific content covered within the chapter.

New—Goals, objectives, and information from *Healthy People 2010* are presented in *Healthy People 2010* boxes.

New—**Research Highlight** boxes present findings from research that is applicable to community-based practice.

New—**Health Teaching** boxes present specific information that the nurse can use for client education.

New—**Community Application** boxes give specific examples of how the content is relevant to nurses in community-based practice.

All chapters conclude with **Learning Activities & Application to Practice** exercises that students can use to gain more in-depth understanding of the content.

New—**Resources** boxes at the end of chapters contain a list of related community resources with instructions on accessing electronic information through the book's dedicated website.

New—A **Glossary** at the end of the book presents the definitions of the Key Terms in every chapter.

NEW CONTENT IN THIS EDITION

Chapter 13 focuses on nursing care for **families**, a large part of which is done in community settings.

Chapter 14 describes nursing care for **vulnerable groups**, specifically the homeless, migrant farmworkers, disabled persons, and victims of disasters.

TEACHING AND LEARNING WEBSITE*

New to this edition is a website with materials for both faculty and students. Visit the website at **www.wbsaunders.com/SIMON/McEwen** ṢiMoN

MATERIALS AVAILABLE FOR THE INSTRUCTOR:

- Annotated Learning Objectives
- Chapter Outlines, which can be used to create PowerPoint presentations
- Additional Learning Activities
- Test Bank with 400 multiple choice questions
- Cross-Curriculum Guide that explains how this content can be used in other courses, such as pediatrics and women's health

MATERIALS AVAILABLE FOR THE INSTRUCTOR AND STUDENT:

- Case Management Module
- WebLinks
- Glossary
- Content Updates
- Frequently Asked Questions

* Instructor material is also available in print format. Contact your sales representative for details.

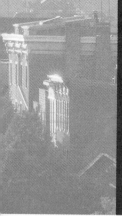

Acknowledgements

I would like to thank Linda Caldwell, Managing Editor, Nursing Division, Elsevier Science, for her eagerness in pursuing this project, her creativity in its development, and her untiring help in seeing it to completion.

I would also like to thank the manuscript reviewers for their help in developing this text: Debra Gartman Spring, RN, MS, Instructor, Division of Associate Degree Nursing, Hinds Community College, Jackson, Mississippi; and Deborah Huntley, MS, RN, CS, Assistant Professor, Department of Nursing, Georgia Perimeter College, Atlanta, Georgia.

Finally, a great deal of appreciation, gratitude, respect, and love go to my husband, Scott, for his many hours of help, for keeping me supplied with the latest computer gadgetry and fast Internet connections, and for putting up with the mess I made of his office.

Melanie McEwen

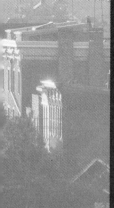

Contents

Unit TWO

Factors That Influence Health and Health Care, 85

Unit Three

Foundations of Community-Based Nursing Practice

Opportunities in Community-Based Nursing Practice

objectives

Upon completion of this chapter, the reader will be able to:

1. Define and discuss the focus of community-based nursing practice.

2. Discuss trends in employment for registered nurses and identify opportunities for their employment in community-based settings.

3. Describe the purpose of *Healthy People 2010* and give examples of the focus areas that encompass the national health objectives.

4. Explain the difference between primary, secondary, and tertiary care and give examples of how each may be provided in community-based settings.

key terms

Community-based nursing
Community health nursing
Healthy People 2010

Primary health care
Secondary health care
Tertiary health care

See Glossary for definitions.

case study

Martha McDonald will complete her nursing program and take the National Council Licensure Examination (NCLEX) in 3 months. Although she has enjoyed nursing school, Martha cannot wait to graduate and begin her new career. Anticipating graduation, she has begun the process of looking for employment and has been somewhat surprised by the variety of options available to her.

For the past year, Martha has worked two or three evenings each week as a "student nurse tech" on a general medical floor of a large, nonprofit hospital. Although she really enjoys working in the hospital, during the course of her studies, she became interested in the health promotion and illness prevention aspects of health care. Martha was particularly attracted to working with older adults and helping them achieve and maintain maximum wellness. She thought that a job in a community setting would be better suited to her.

Martha began her job search by reviewing the employment classified advertisements in the local Sunday paper. Surprisingly, many of the ads for registered nurses (RNs) were in the areas of home health nursing, case management, and managed care groups, such as health maintenance organizations (HMOs). In addition, there were opportunities for RNs to work in nursing homes and a variety of outpatient settings, such as day surgery centers and minor emergency or primary care clinics.

Martha discussed employment opportunities with the job placement office and several of her nursing instructors. After a month of interviews and weighing options, Martha chose a position as a staff nurse in a geriatric clinic affiliated with one of the large nonprofit health care organizations in her city.

Over the past decade, the health care delivery system has changed dramatically. Cost-consciousness among insurers at all levels has mandated massive alterations in health care delivery. This has resulted in a phenomenal decrease in the average length of hospital stays for virtually all illnesses and procedures. No one argues that patients are being discharged "sicker and quicker" now than in the past. Additionally, emphasis on health promotion and illness prevention is increasing throughout society, with recognition of the impact of lifestyle choices and behavior on individual and population health. Table 1-1 lists some of the trends that have been observed in the health care delivery system in recent years.

There is little doubt that health care delivery is moving from an acute care focus and hospital-based delivery of care to illness prevention and management and community-based delivery of care. As a result, hospitals are reducing capacity and downsizing, becoming specialized, or closing altogether.

In the United States, a significant shortage of nurses exists in virtually all areas and this short-age is expected to continue and even expand over the next decade. With a growing number of jobs in acute care facilities, there are many opportunities for nurses in community-based settings, whether in home care, HMOs, clinics, or other services.

In a position statement on the future of nursing education in the early 1990s, the National League for Nursing (NLN) (1993) discussed the importance of moving much of the content and clinical focus in nursing education from acute care settings into community settings. Indeed, nursing educators in both associate and baccalaureate degree programs recognize the trends in health care and understand the need to incorporate community-based nursing (CBN) concepts and clinical experiences into curricula. In baccalaureate programs, this often means expansion or integration of community content and clinical experiences throughout programs rather than confining them to the study of "community health nursing" (CHN) near the end of the program, as has been the traditional practice.

Associate degree nursing programs have also acknowledged the need to include community-based experiences and related content. In October

TABLE **1-1** Trends in Health Care Delivery Systems

FROM	TO
Acute inpatient care	Life-span care
Treating illness	Maintaining health
Focus on the individual	Focus on the aggregate/population
Product of care orientation	Value of care orientation
Number of admissions to hospital	Number of lives covered (capitation)
Managing organizations	Managing networks
Managing departments	Managing markets
Coordinating services	Documenting quality and outcomes

From Mengel, A., & Donnelly, G. (1999). Associate degree and baccalaureate nursing education. In M. E. Tagliareni & B. B. Marckx (Eds.), *Teaching in the community: Preparing nurses for the 21st century*. Sudbury, MA: Jones & Bartlett Publishers. www.jbpub.com. Reprinted with permission.

1994, the NLN Council of Associate Degree Programs (NLN/CADP) held a national video conference to discuss the "examination of opportunities for clinical learning available in community-based settings and the potential role of the associate degree nurse in these settings" (1994, p. 1). The discussions from this conference underscored the need to promote community-based clinical opportunities and offered a number of suggestions for settings and learning experiences for students pursuing an associate degree of nursing (ADN). Tagliareni and Murray (1995) agreed, stating that the "next step in curricular reform [is to include] community-based experiences in the AD curriculum" (p. 366) (Box 1-1).

COMMUNITY-BASED HEALTH CARE AND NURSING PRACTICE

For more than a decade, the nursing discipline has advocated an increasing emphasis on health promotion and illness prevention in all areas of the health care delivery system (American Nurses' Association [ANA], 1991; Hamner, 1999). Indeed, the ANA and many other organizations have recognized that homes, work sites, schools, churches, and neighborhood clinics are among the settings suggested to serve as "convenient familiar places" to enhance the delivery of preventive, systematic, and comprehensive health care. The emphasis on health care delivery in community-based settings has moved beyond **primary health care** (i.e., prevention activities, such as well-child check-ups, routine physical examinations, prenatal care, and diagnosis and treatment of common acute or episodic illnesses) and now encompasses secondary and tertiary care.

Secondary health care typically refers to relatively serious or complicated care that has historically been provided to patients in hospitals. However, recent changes in techniques, procedures, and medical practice have moved much of secondary health care into community settings. Examples of community-based secondary health care include the following:

- Outpatient surgery for complex procedures that would have required hospitalization just a few years ago (e.g., cholecystectomy, hysterectomy, appendectomy, herniorrhaphy)
- Treatment of serious illnesses (e.g., chemotherapy, radiotherapy)
- A wide variety of diagnostic testing procedures (e.g., computed tomography, magnetic resonance imaging, angiography)

BOX 1-1 Addressing the Nursing Shortage

The Tri-Council (2001), an organization comprised of representatives from the American Association of Colleges of Nursing, ANA, American Organization of Nurse Executives, and NLN, has stated that the current nursing workforce shortage is complex and very different from any in the past. They explained that the problem is difficult to quantify and not simply an issue of there being too few RNs. Furthermore, concern that the shortage will grow more serious over the next 20 years is significant.

The Tri-Council cited the following reasons for the nursing shortage: fewer nurses are entering the workforce; nursing shortages in certain geographic areas are acute; and a shortage of nurses prepared to meet certain areas of client need in the changing health care environment exists. In addition, they explained that although low pay rates continue to be cited by nurses as a professional drawback, the leading factor for nurse turnover is "increased market demand" exacerbated by "dissatisfaction with the job, the supervisor or career prospects" (Tri-Council, 2001, p. 1). The second most cited reason for turnover is workload and staffing. They also reported serious concerns over the increased need for more nurses because of the increasing age of the general population and the growing need for management of chronic disease conditions.

Recommendations from the Tri-Council are that health care environments must recognize and reward educational and practice competencies by defining nurses' roles and by utilizing and compensating nurses according to their educational preparation and competencies. They suggested that health care organizations need to implement specific strategies to retain experienced nurses in the provision of direct client care, create a partnership environment that advances the practice of nursing by establishing appropriate management structures within the health care system, and ensure adequate nurse staffing. Finally, they should provide nurses with sufficient autonomy over their practice in all settings.

Similarly, **tertiary health care** (management of chronic, complicated, long-term health problems) is now frequently delivered in community settings. Rehabilitation centers for clients with neurological conditions (e.g., spinal cord injuries, multiple sclerosis, amyotrophic lateral sclerosis), centers for cardiac rehabilitation, home health care for bed-bound older people, home care for respirator-dependent infants, and hospice care for the terminally ill are examples of tertiary health care commonly provided in nonhospital settings.

Nursing care is an essential component in each of these settings and for each level of care described. Nursing practice in community settings is similar to nursing practice in acute care facilities because nurses perform assessments, administer procedures, teach clients and their caregivers, counsel, and work to ensure that clients receive needed care and services.

Nursing practice in community settings, however, may differ significantly from nursing practice in the hospital. The community setting is often characterized by less structure, less formality, and more independence. Reliance on technology and a "controlled" environment is greatly reduced and recognition of the importance of knowing and understanding the client's unique situation and individual needs is enhanced. Thus the application of the nursing process (assessment, analysis, planning, intervention, evaluation) must take into account information beyond the immediate physical and psychosocial needs that are addressed in the formal and controlled hospital setting. In community-based practice, environmental threats, availability of resources, financial burdens, family concerns, lifestyle choices, and various management issues for clients and their caregivers are often of primary concern.

COMMUNITY-BASED NURSING AND COMMUNITY HEALTH NURSING

Within the discipline of nursing, confusion regarding what comprises CBN practice and how it differs from CHN is common. **Community-based nursing** practice refers to the application of the nursing process in caring for individuals, families, and groups where they live, work, or go to school or as they move through the health care system. In CBN, all levels of prevention are emphasized (i.e., primary, secondary, and tertiary), but its focus is more on secondary and tertiary levels. Home health nursing and nursing in outpatient or ambulatory settings are examples of CBN.

Community health nursing is a synthesis of nursing practice and public health practice applied to promoting and preserving the health of populations (ANA, 1986). The CHN practice is continuous and comprehensive and considers the impact of the environment on health. In CHN, the dominant responsibility is to the population as a whole, but care is directed to individuals, families, or groups, thus contributing to the health of the total aggregate or population. Public health nursing, school nursing, and occupational health nursing are examples of CHN.

In an excellent discussion, Zotti, Brown, and Stotts (1996) compared CBN and CHN. They explained that the goals of the two are different because CHN emphasizes preservation and protection of health, whereas in CBN, the emphasis is on managing acute or chronic conditions. In CHN, the primary client is the community and in CBN, the primary clients are the individual and the family. Also, services in CBN are largely direct and in CHN, services are both direct and indirect. Thus, although both community-based nurses and community health nurses work in the community, they have different goals, methods, and purposes in delivering nursing care.

EDUCATION FOCUS

As mentioned, nursing educators have recognized the need to enhance community content and clinical experiences for nursing students. Matteson (2000) and Hamner (1999) identified several content areas that should be enhanced in all programs to address the need for CBN education. This content includes knowledge of health-promotion strategies, concepts of risk reduction and disease prevention, illness and disease management, continuum of health services, family health care, self-care, community resources, collaboration, delegation, health care systems, and policy development. Areas for expanded clinical experiences include ambulatory care facilities, college health facilities, correctional facilities, genetic clinics, geriatric clinics, and home health nursing.

DIFFERENTIATED PRACTICE ISSUES

The movement of nursing out of traditional, structured roles found in acute care settings has given new direction to the debate on "differentiated practice," sparking questions on whether associate degree or diploma-prepared nurses are educationally equipped to practice in less structured, community-based settings. Although the ANA's published 1965 and 1984 position statements outlining two entry levels for nursing practice (the "technical" nurse and the "professional" nurse) were widely debated, little action has been taken toward an official distinction in levels of practice. Since the late 1990s, only North Dakota required a baccalaureate degree for a professional nurse's license (Kovner, 1999).

Discussion of the merits of differentiated practice is beyond the scope of this book. When appropriate, however, specific educational requirements and recommendations for nurses using advanced knowledge, working with designated populations, or in specialized settings are included.

EMPLOYMENT OPPORTUNITIES IN COMMUNITY SETTINGS

CURRENT TRENDS IN NURSING EMPLOYMENT

In the case study at the beginning of the chapter, what Martha discovered when she began her job search is not unusual. As a result of cost-containment measures and medical practice modifications, nursing employment has changed over the past several years. The Public Health Service's Division of Nursing has chronicled this change in practice settings through periodic surveys of RNs. The 2000 National Sample Survey of Registered Nurses (U.S. Department

of Health and Human Services/Division of Nursing [USDHHS/DON], 2001) discovered the following:

- The rate for RNs who work outside of hospitals is 40.1% (up from 33.5% in 1992).
- Although the number of RNs working in hospitals increased, the proportion of nurses working in hospitals declined between 1992 and 2000.
- The number of nurses employed in community/public health settings showed a 36% increase between 1992 and 2000, which was largely the result of an increase in nurses working in home health care and managed care organizations (MCOs).

Reforms in health care delivery appear to dictate that these trends will continue well into the twenty-first century. Table 1-2 presents data detailing employment settings for RNs practicing in the United States.

Another finding of the National Nursing Survey (USDHHS/DON, 2001) was that the supply of RNs, like that of other health care providers, has a problem with geographic maldistribution. States in the Southwest and mountain regions have approximately half the number of nurses per 100,000 people as states in New England and the Midwest.

TABLE **1-2** Summary of Employment Settings for All Registered Nurses

SETTING	ESTIMATED PERCENT
Hospitals	59.1
Nursing home/extended care facilities	6.9
Nursing education	2.1
Community/public health settings (includes home health agencies, school health, and occupational health)	18.3
Ambulatory care settings	9.5
Other	3.6

From U.S. Department of Health and Human Services Division of Nursing, Bureau of Health Professions (USDHHS/DON). (2001). *The registered nurse population: National sample survey of registered nurses, March, 2000.* Washington, DC: Government Printing Office.

For example, Montana, Nevada, Utah, Oklahoma, and Texas have 520 to 630 RNs per 100,000 people. In contrast, Massachusetts, Rhode Island, and the Dakotas have 1101 to 1194 RNs per 100,000 people. It is interesting to note that the District of Columbia has the greatest per capita concentration, with 1675 RNs per 100,000 people. Rural areas, in particular, are understaffed with RNs because some 80% of all nurses work in urban areas (USDHHS/DON, 2001).

EMPLOYMENT OPPORTUNITIES

The movement from an illness-oriented "cure" perspective in hospitals, to a focus on health promotion and primary health care in community-based settings—combined with changing

---

BOX 1-2 Community-Based Employment Opportunities for Registered Nurses

AMBULATORY CARE

Physician's (offices solo, partnership, or private group practice)
Managed health care organizations/insurers
HMOs
Utilization review
Case management
Hospital-based ambulatory services
Hospital clinics
Day surgery
Freestanding ambulatory surgery centers
Freestanding emergi-centers
Categorical clinics and services (may be hospital-based or freestanding)
Intravenous therapy and chemotherapy clinics
Dialysis units
Adult day care centers
Day care centers for ill children
Mental health clinics
Family planning clinics
Cardiac rehabilitation programs
Neurological rehabilitation programs (spinal cord injuries, multiple sclerosis, amyotrophic lateral sclerosis)
Geriatric clinics
Migrant health clinics
AIDS clinics
Diabetes management and education services
Pulmonary clinics (asthma, chronic obstructive pulmonary disease, cystic fibrosis)
Genetic screening and counseling services
Bloodmobiles
Freestanding diagnostic centers
Diagnostic imaging centers
Mobile mammography centers

HEALTH DEPARTMENT SERVICES

Maternal/child health clinics
Family planning clinics

Communicable disease control programs
HIV/AIDS (testing, counseling, and treatment)
Tuberculosis (testing, treatment, and surveillance)
Sexually transmitted diseases (testing, counseling, and treatment)
Immunization clinics
Neighborhood clinics serving disenfranchised populations
Mobile clinics serving disenfranchised populations
Substance abuse programs
Jails and prisons
Indian health services

HOME HEALTH CARE SERVICES

Skilled nursing care
Intravenous therapy
High-risk pregnancy/neonate care
Maternal/child newborn care
Private duty (hourly care)
Respite care
Hospice care

LONG-TERM CARE

Skilled nursing facilities
Hospital-based facilities
Freestanding/nursing home-based facilities
Hospice facilities
Nursing homes
Skilled nursing care
Assisted living

OTHER COMMUNITY HEALTH SETTINGS

School health programs
Occupational health programs
Parish nursing programs
Summer camp programs
Childbirth education programs

AIDS, Acquired immunodeficiency syndrome; *HIV,* human immunodeficiency virus.

demographics (i.e., an aging population), cost-consciousness, and changes in medical technology and treatments—have dramatically changed employment opportunities for today's RNs. This shift of emphasis to primary care and outpatient treatment and management of both acute and chronic health conditions will continue. As a result, employment growth in a variety of ambulatory care settings, home health care, nursing homes, occupational health, school health, and parish care programs can be expected. Box 1-2 lists current and future employment options for RNs in nonacute-care settings.

As shown in Box 1-2, nursing opportunities in community settings are extensive and varied. New graduates and experienced nurses should have a number of alternatives to explore to meet individual professional interests. For instance:

- If pediatrics is the nurse's primary area of interest, employment choices include working in a pediatrician's office, a pediatric hospital-based clinic, a school health program, and a well-child clinic.
- If the nurse enjoys working with older people, there are many options, including adult day care, geriatric clinics, home health, and nursing homes.
- If surgery is an interest, the nurse should realize that about half of all surgical procedures are now performed on an outpatient basis (Mezey and Lawrence, 1995).

As a result, employment opportunities in both freestanding and hospital-based day surgery centers have increased and include not only operating room nursing, but also postanesthesia care, intake/admissions, and patient education positions. In addition, postday surgery home care is becoming increasingly popular (see the Research Highlight "Future of Nursing Employment").

CHARACTERISTICS OF COMMUNITY-BASED NURSING

Although opportunities for employment in community-based settings are impressive, a baccalaureate degree may be required for some positions. Many school health programs and most public health departments, for example, will hire only nurses with a Bachelor of Science

---

Research Highlight

Future of Nursing Employment

Buerhaus and Staiger (1997) conducted a large scale, nationwide study of health executives. In this study, the researchers examined how the work environment of nurses is changing, the underlying forces driving change, and how these forces are expected to affect employment of nurses in the future. They reported that the executives perceived a rapidly changing nurse labor market and employer requirements. Indeed, they observed that although hospital restructuring has resulted in a decrease in the number of RNs in hospitals, RNs are finding employment in home health care, nursing homes, and with MCOs.

Future employment opportunities for nurses are "bright," but changing. Because hospitals are discharging patients earlier, follow-up care in the home has become more intensive and "high tech." Many RNs are providing more education to patients and families and are using advanced skills. Among other observations for the future were that information systems and new technology will become increasingly important and nurses will need to assimilate the use of technology into their practice. There is also a need to increase education and experience in the areas of palliative care, pain control, patient education, chronic illness monitoring, case finding, and surveillance.

The researchers concluded that nurse educators need to respond quickly to prepare nurses for rapidly changing employer requirements. Schools of nursing should revamp their curricula to fit the environment in which graduates will practice in the future, particularly in the area of CBN.

Buerhaus, P. I., & Staiger, D. O. (1997). Future of the nurse labor market according to health executives in high managed-care areas of the United States. *Image: Journal of Nursing Scholarship*, 29(4), 313-318.

in nursing (BSN) degree. Furthermore, experience may be necessary for many nursing positions in nonhospital settings. Home health agencies, for example, typically prefer 1 to 2 years of recent, acute care experience for new-hire RNs.

Practicing in community settings has several advantages. Many nurses prefer the emphasis on health promotion and illness prevention that is a major focus of primary health care. The opportunity to get to know clients and their families by seeing them in their own homes, workplaces, schools, or communities and to provide more holistic care has also been cited as an advantage of nursing in the community setting. Another advantage has been the customary Monday-to-Friday daytime work schedule. Although a hospital must be staffed around the clock, 7 days per week, few nonacute-care facilities have required staffing for night shifts, weekends, and holidays. As more services are provided in the community, however, hours may expand.

Wages and salaries have tended to be somewhat lower for RNs in community-based practice. This is, in part, reflective of the lack of evening, night, and weekend differential payment. Also, some nurses report concern over the relative lack of a controlled environment and lack of immediate access to support from other nurses when providing nursing care in some community-based settings. This lack of support, or structure, may be a difficult adjustment for some nurses.

NATIONAL HEALTH GOALS

Healthy People: The Surgeon General's Report on Health Promotion and Disease Prevention was initially published in 1979 as a national prevention initiative of the U.S. Department of Health and Human Services (USDHHS) (2000). The 1979 version included a set of goals: reduce mortality among four different age groups—infants, children, adolescents and young adults, and adults—and increase independence among older adults.

An updated version, *Healthy People 2000*, was published in 1990. *Healthy People 2000* contained three broad goals:
1. Increase the span of healthy life for Americans.
2. Reduce health disparities among Americans.
3. Achieve access to preventive services for all Americans (USDHHS, 1990).

Healthy People 2000 was developed to provide direction for individuals to change personal behaviors and for organizations and communities to use to improve health through health-promotion policies. It was organized under the broad approaches of health promotion, health protection, and preventive services and contained more than 300 objectives organized into 22 priority areas. Although only a portion of the objectives was met, the initiative was extremely successful in raising providers' awareness of health behaviors and health-promotional activities. The objectives were used by states, local health departments, and private sector health workers to determine the relative health of their community and to set goals for the future.

A third edition, **Healthy People 2010**, was introduced in January, 2000. It expands upon the objectives from *Healthy People 2000* through a broadened scientific base and improved surveillance and data systems. There is also a heightened awareness of preventive health services, which is reflective of changes in demographics, science, technology, and disease. *Healthy People 2010* lists two broad goals:

Goal 1: Increase quality and years of healthy life.
Goal 2: Eliminate health disparities.

Goal 1 moves beyond the idea of increasing life expectancy to incorporate the concept of "health-related-quality-of-life" (HRQOL), a concept of health that includes aspects of both physical and mental health and their determinants and measures functional status and well-being. By integrating mental and physical health concepts, it provides a way to expand the definition of health beyond simply being the opposite of the negative concepts of disease and death (USDHHS, 2000).

In *Healthy People 2010*, some 467 objectives are divided into 28 focus areas (see the *Healthy People 2010* box). The objectives may be used as a framework to guide health-promotion activities in schools, clinics, worksites, and so forth, and for community-wide initiatives (USDHHS, 2000). All health care practitioners should review *Healthy People 2010* objectives, focusing on those areas relevant to their practice. Whenever possible, objectives should be incorporated into programs, events, and publications and should be used as a framework to promote healthy individuals, families, groups, and communities.

healthy people **2010**

Priority Areas

1. Access to quality health services
2. Arthritis, osteoporosis, and chronic back conditions
3. Cancer
4. Chronic kidney disease
5. Diabetes
6. Disability and secondary conditions
7. Educational and community-based programs
8. Environmental health
9. Family planning and sexual health
10. Food safety
11. Health communication
12. Heart disease and stroke
13. HIV
14. Immunizations and infectious diseases
15. Injury and violence prevention
16. Maternal, infant, and child health
17. Medical product safety
18. Mental health and mental disorders
19. Nutrition and overweight
20. Occupational safety and health
21. Oral health
22. Physical activity and fitness
23. Public health infrastructure
24. Respiratory diseases
25. Sexually transmitted diseases
26. Substance abuse
27. Tobacco use
28. Vision and hearing

From U.S. Department of Health and Human Services (USDHHS). (2000). *Healthy People 2010: National health promotion and disease prevention objectives.* Washington, DC: Government Printing Office.

Leading health indicators used to measure progress toward the *Healthy People 2010* goals focus on positively impacting physical activity, overweight and obesity, tobacco use, substance abuse, responsible sexual behavior, mental health, injury and violence, environmental quality, immunizations, and access to health care. These indicators are intended to help all Americans understand the importance of health promotion and disease prevention and to encourage participation in improving health in the next decade.

Implementation of activities and interventions to achieve most of the goals for *Healthy People 2010* rests on health care providers in community-based practice. Furthermore, meeting these objectives requires changing the focus of practice from illness and cure to health promotion and illness prevention. Throughout this book, related objectives from *Healthy People 2010* are presented and practical methods to achieve them are discussed (see the Research Highlight "*Healthy People 2010*").

SUMMARY

Health care at all levels is becoming increasingly community based. In response, nurses, such as Martha from the chapter-opening case study, must be educationally and experientially prepared to provide care in very diverse settings.

Research Highlight

Healthy People 2010

Hill (2000) reported on efforts to meet *Healthy People 2010* objectives for breastfeeding. She explained that in the United States, the breastfeeding initiation rate is 64% and the duration rate at 6 months postpartum is 29%. This falls significantly short of the *Healthy People 2010* goals of 75% initiation and 50% at 6 months. Factors identified that influence breastfeeding include sociodemographics, maternal attitudes toward breastfeeding, influence of significant others, and the workplace environment.

Hill, P. D. (2000). Update on breastfeeding: *Healthy People 2010* objectives. *MCN: American Journal of Maternal/Child Nursing, 25*(5), 248-251.

Indeed, like Martha, nurses are learning that in most localities, RNs are desperately needed to fill positions in home health agencies, HMOs, a large variety of outpatient clinics, and in acute care settings.

This chapter introduces the recognition of, and rationale for, enhancing educational opportunities for all nurses in community-based settings. Related information is presented in Chapter 2, which discusses differences and similarities between nursing roles and interventions in acute care settings and community settings.

KEY POINTS

- The health care delivery system is changing; care is becoming more focused on health promotion and illness prevention and moving from acute care and hospital-based delivery to prevention and management in community-based settings.
- Nurses have recognized the need to adapt delivery of care and nursing education to meet the needs of the population and the changing health care system.
- Like primary health care (preventive services and diagnosis and treatment of common acute episodic illnesses), secondary health care (relatively serious or complicated care traditionally provided in hospitals), and tertiary health care (management of chronic, complicated, long-term health problems) are increasingly being delivered in community-based settings.
- Although most nurses still work in hospitals, the proportion is changing with nurses increasingly being employed in community-based settings. This trend is expected to continue.
- Opportunities for nurses to work in community-based settings are numerous and diverse.
- *Healthy People 2010* has two goals: (1) to increase quality and years of healthy life for U.S. residents and (2) to eliminate health disparities. Community-based health care providers are responsible for the implementation of activities and interventions to achieve most of the goals.

Learning Activities & Application to Practice

1. Obtain a copy of *The Registered Nurse Population: National Sample Survey of Registered Nurses* (USDHHS, 2001). Review changes in your geographic region. Compare local statistics with those of other regions of the United States.
2. Obtain a copy of *Healthy People 2010* (USDHHS, 2000). With classmates, discuss the document and the implications for nursing practice.
3. Research employment opportunities for RNs in both hospital and community-based settings in your area. Where are more opportunities? Are there differences in salaries? Hours? Experience requirements? Share your findings with classmates.

REFERENCES

American Nurses' Association (ANA). (1986). *Standards of community health nursing practice.* Washington, DC: American Nurses' Association.

American Nurses' Association (ANA). (1991). *Nursing's agenda for health care reform.* Washington, DC: American Nurses' Association.

Buerhaus, P. I., & Staiger, D. O. (1997). Future of the nurse labor market according to health executives in high managed-care areas of the United States. *Image: Journal of Nursing Scholarship, 29*(4), 313-318.

Hamner, M. B. (1999). Associate and baccalaureate degree preparation for home health care in an era of managed care. In M. E. Tagliareni & B. B. Marckx (Eds.), *Teaching in the community: Preparing nurses for the 21st century* (pp. 95-109). Sudbury, MA: Jones & Bartlett Publishers.

Hill, P. D. (2000). Update on breastfeeding: *Healthy people 2010* objectives. *MCN: American Journal of Maternal/Child Nursing, 25*(5), 248-251.

Kovner, C. (1999). The health care workforce. In A. R. Kovner & S. Jonas (Eds.), *Jonas's and Kovner's health care delivery in the United States* (6th ed., pp. 64-115). New York: Springer Publishing Co.

Matteson, P. (2000). Preparing nurses for the future. In P. S. Matteson (Ed.), *Community-based nursing education* (pp. 1-7). New York: Springer Publishing Co.

Mengel, A., & Donnelly, G. (1999). Associate degree and baccalaureate nursing education. In M. E. Tagliareni & B. B. Marckx (Eds.), *Teaching in the community: Preparing nurses for the 21st century.* Sudbury, MA: Jones & Bartlett Publishers.

Mezey, A. P., & Lawrence, R. S. (1995). Ambulatory care. In A. R. Kovner (Ed.), *Jonas's health care delivery in the United States*. New York: Springer Publishing Co.

National League for Nursing (NLN). (1993). *A vision for nursing education*. New York: National League for Nursing.

National League for Nursing/Council of Associate Degree Programs (NLN/CADP). (1994). *Web of inclusion: Faculty helping faculty—evaluation summary*. National Video Conference, October 14, 1994. New York: National League for Nursing.

Tagliareni, M. E., & Murray, J. P. (1995). Community-focused experiences in the ADN curriculum. *Journal of Nursing Education, 34*(8), 366-371.

Tri-Council (American Association of Colleges of Nursing, American Nurses' Association, American Organization of Nurse Executives, National League for Nursing). (2001). *White paper: Strategies to reverse the new nursing shortage*. Retrieved 7/26/2001 from http://www.ana.org/pressrel/2001/sta0205.htm.

U.S. Department of Health and Human Services, Division of Nursing (USDHHS/DON), Bureau of Health Professions, Public Health Service. (2001). *The registered nurse population: National sample survey of registered nurses*, March 2000. Washington, DC: Government Printing Office.

U.S. Department of Health and Human Services (USDHHS). (1990). *Healthy people 2000: National health promotion and disease prevention objectives*. Washington, DC: Government Printing Office.

U.S. Department of Health and Human Services (USDHHS). (2000). *Healthy people 2010*. Washington, DC: Government Printing Office.

Zotti, M. E., Brown, P., & Stotts, R. C. (1996). Community-based nursing versus community health nursing: What does it all mean? *Nursing Outlook, 44*(5), 211-217.

Roles and Interventions in Community-Based Nursing Practice

Upon completion of this chapter, the reader will be able to:

1. Discuss the various roles used by registered nurses in community-based practice.

2. Compare and contrast the emphasis placed on various roles in community-based practice and practice in acute care settings.

3. Give examples of nursing interventions used in various community-based settings and explain how they are similar to and different from acute care nursing interventions.

Advocate

Collaborator

Counselor

Direct care provider

Educator

Leader

Manager

Nursing Interventions
Classification (NIC)
system

Researcher

Role model

See Glossary for definitions.

Sally Smith is a home health nurse for a hospital-based agency in a small city. Last Tuesday, Sally saw five clients: (1) Mrs. Black, to perform a fasting blood glucose tolerance test and to teach about type 2 diabetes; (2) Mr. Johnson, for twice-a-day dressing changes following an amputation of his left great toe; (3) Mrs. Garcia, to teach about anticoagulant therapy and to draw blood to monitor clotting times; (4) Mrs. Gray, who has a diagnosis of Alzheimer's disease, and her family, who are considering placing her in a nursing home because they can no longer care for her at home; and (5) Mr. Jones, who was recently discharged from the hospital following an episode of congestive heart failure (CHF) and who needs to be evaluated for fluid retention, hypertension, and heart and lung function.

Sally performs several roles and interventions in her practice as a home health care nurse. In preparation, Sally must schedule the day's visits on the basis of several factors. For example, she needs to see Mrs. Black before breakfast to obtain an accurate fasting glucose value and allow her to maintain her normal insulin and breakfast schedule. Mr. Johnson must be seen fairly early too because his dressing changes are scheduled for early to midmorning and early evening. To ensure accuracy, Mrs. Garcia's blood sample must be taken to the laboratory within 30 minutes and the results should be reported to her physician by 3:00 PM. Finally, the visit to Mrs. Gray and her family is to be coordinated with one of the agency's medical social workers. Sally must consider each of these factors, calculate the distance that must be covered between the clients' residences, ensure that all supplies are available (dressing materials, laboratory supplies), and schedule with other providers when planning the day's visits. Therefore management of self, time, client's care needs and schedules, and resources is a key component of Sally's workday.

In addition to her management roles, Sally performs numerous skilled nursing interventions, such as physical assessment, wound care, blood glucose monitoring, and venipuncture. She continually teaches her clients about their health and health care management. She also collaborates closely with clients, their caregivers, the social worker, physicians, other home health care nurses, and various other providers (e.g., aides, therapists, laboratory technicians) and she routinely acts as a counselor, advocate, and role model for her clients, their families, and other caregivers.

Nursing practice in community settings differs considerably from practice in the hospital. Just as nursing practice in acute care institutions varies greatly from one area to another (the operating room differs from the intensive care unit [ICU], which differs from postpartum care, which differs from acute psychiatric care), it can be very different between community settings. Home health nursing is very different from school nursing, which, in turn, is very different from working in a health maintenance organization (HMO) or clinic. But, just as there are similarities in nursing practice in acute care settings (i.e., following physician orders, medication administration, and taking vital signs), there are similarities throughout community settings (i.e., emphasis on health promotion, teaching, counseling, advocacy, and ensuring continuity of care).

NURSING ROLES IN COMMUNITY SETTINGS

Shortened hospital stays, proliferation of day surgery, emphasis on health promotion, recognition of the unique health care needs of older clients and the underserved, and the desire to decrease costs have changed the health care system and nursing practice (see Chapter 1). Although performing traditional nursing skills (e.g., administering injections, taking vital signs,

changing dressings) in the role of "direct care provider" is still an integral part of nursing practice, the importance of other roles is increasing. Although the variety of roles that make up nursing practice is the same no matter what the setting, the emphasis varies greatly. This chapter describes some of the roles common to nursing practice and explains how these roles differ in community-based practice compared with hospital-based practice and how they differ among community settings.

DIRECT CARE PROVIDER

The **direct care provider** role involves the direct delivery of care. Performing tasks or skills for which the nurse has been trained and that are typically associated with nursing practice (e.g., client assessment, taking vital signs, medication administration, changing dressings, and inserting catheters) is the essence of the role of direct care provider.

This role constitutes much of nursing practice in acute care settings, where patients are typically hospitalized after surgery or for treatment of serious or complex medical conditions. For example, most of an ICU nurse's time (about 70% to 80%) is spent in direct care provision. A nurse working on a "general medicine" floor devotes about 50% of the time in direct delivery of care; in contrast, the amount of time spent in direct care delivery for a nurse working in a postpartum unit is 40% to 50% and for the nurse working in an inpatient psychiatric unit, it is 20% to 30%.

Although direct care provision is an important part of community-based nursing practice, this task tends to occupy less time than in acute care settings. In community settings, direct care provision might be most time intensive for the nurse in home health (35% to 40%); it is less significant in occupational health or school health (10% to 15%); and it might be minimal at an HMO practice. As a result, many nursing students and registered nurses (RNs) who are new to community-based practice often discount the nurse's importance in health care delivery in these settings because the nurses are not observed giving direct care (i.e., giving medication, performing hygiene procedures, managing intravenous lines). It is important that nurses recognize the difference in emphasis on roles in the various settings.

EDUCATOR

Regardless of the setting, health education is an essential component of quality nursing care. Education in hospitals typically focuses on patient instructions for posthospital discharge and is often severely restricted because of time limitations as hospital stays have become shortened. The limited amount of time for teaching, coupled with the acuity level of the patient and stress on the family, often means that health teaching is marginally effective. Incorporation of written discharge instructions with verbal explanations and other techniques, including post-discharge telephone calls, has helped improve the assimilation of information by clients and caregivers in acute care settings.

Although health education is an important role for nursing in acute care settings, it is often the most significant role of the nurse working in community settings. Teaching individuals, families, and groups about maintenance of health, threats to health, and relevant lifestyle choices that affect health is integral in all community settings. The information presented should allow clients to make informed decisions on health matters and to direct self-care to follow treatment regimens.

The **educator** role makes up much of community-based nursing practice, as noted by the following:

- School nurses often spend 30% to 40% of their time providing health education in areas such as prevention of sexually transmitted diseases (STDs), basic hygiene, and dental care.
- Occupational health nurses instruct clients on issues such as accident prevention, ergonomics, smoking cessation strategies, and the importance of physical fitness.
- Home health nurses spend much of their time teaching clients and families self-care strategies (e.g., dressing changes, diabetes management, colostomy care).
- Nurses in ambulatory clinic settings teach infant nutrition to new parents, signs and symptoms of infection to clients with acquired immunodeficiency syndrome (AIDS), principles of a low-fat diet to clients with coronary artery disease, and medication management to clients with CHF.

Health education goes beyond simple dissemination of information. Whether the information is instruction concerning the schedule and potential side effects of a prescribed medication, nutritional principles to reduce blood lipids, or breastfeeding, it must be presented appropriately for the individual client. As health educators, nurses should consider such factors as the client's developmental stage, learning readiness, language, educational level, and perceived learning needs. Additionally, the nurse must evaluate the learner's level of understanding accurately and reinforce it accordingly.

All RNs should be familiar with basics of client teaching. Theories, models, and principles of teaching and experience in applying principles needs to be part of every introductory or nursing fundamentals course. Various tools (e.g., written materials, visual aids, models) and techniques (e.g., demonstration, observation, repetition) should be incorporated into the teaching plan. Use of appropriate, familiar terminology (i.e., avoidance of medical jargon), consideration of cultural variables, and encouraging or enabling the client to ask questions are essential. Evaluation of the client's level of understanding is accomplished through questioning, the use of return demonstration, or both.

COUNSELOR

A nurse in the role of a **counselor** listens to clients and their families, encourages them to explore issues and options, and enables them to manage their personal situations. Assistance with identification of problems and possible solutions and guidance through the problem-solving process are functions of nurses in most community-based settings. Indeed, counseling represents a significant component of quality, community-based nursing care. For example, a clinic nurse may discuss contraception options with a young mother; a school nurse might talk with a high school student perceived to be "at risk" for using drugs or alcohol; or a hospice nurse might discuss the importance of respite care and caring for the caregiver with the family of a terminally ill client.

In contrast, nurses in acute care settings typically spend considerably less time counseling clients. Because much of the care in hospitals is directed by hospital procedure or physician orders, there tends to be less emphasis on this role. Exceptions may include nursing care in psychiatric settings, where counseling might constitute the greatest percentage of the nurse's time, and nursing care for families of very seriously ill clients for whom the family must weigh options for treatment and long-term care.

ADVOCATE

A nurse **advocate** is one who acts on behalf of, or intercedes for, the client. Frequently, clients—particularly children, elderly people, and the disadvantaged—are unable to obtain needed care and services within today's health care system.

Advocates ensure that clients receive necessary care and services.

Nurses act as client advocates in all settings. In hospitals, nurses work as advocates through creative interventions, such as:

- Ensuring that patients are as pain free as possible by phoning a physician at 1:00 AM to change a medication.
- Working with administrators to plan visiting hours to accommodate individual and family needs.
- Helping parents to stay in hospital rooms with small children.
- Protecting a client's desires regarding advanced directives.

In community settings, the nurse's role as an advocate is vital. Because they often work with vulnerable populations, nurses in community settings serve as client advocates constantly (Box 2-1). For example, it is often the school nurse who identifies a source of funding to pay for eyeglasses for the child whose parents cannot afford them or who identifies and reports suspected child abuse or neglect. The occupational health nurse's responsibility is to ensure that Occupational Safety and Health Administration (OSHA) guidelines for employee safety are carried out. The home health nurse may be the one who finds a way to provide insulin for an older client who cannot afford to pay for medications and the nurse in the homeless shelter clinic ensures that clients receive blankets and coats in the winter.

MANAGER

The role of the nurse as **manager** in a community-based practice is possibly most similar to the role of the nurse in an acute care setting. Nursing care in both hospital and community settings involves management of the nurse's time, limited resources, other personnel, and program organization and coordination, as well as the management of the client's care. The management role includes planning, organizing, coordinating, marketing, controlling, and evaluating care and care delivery.

BOX 2-1 The Nurse as Advocate

According to Schroeter (2000), advocacy refers to the act of pleading for, supporting, urging by argument, recommending publicly, and active espousal. Advocacy implies taking action to achieve a goal on behalf of another and in nursing it is directly related to client care. As client advocates, nurses should continually strive to ensure the quality and continuity of care and to make certain that client's needs are being met. Nurses must also be advocates for each other, co-workers, family members, and students. The following concepts are keys to advocacy:

- *Understanding advocacy as an ethical concept.* In nursing, advocacy is an ethical practice based on individual values and nursing's code of ethics.
- *Understanding the place of advocacy within nursing practice.* Nurses must recognize that advocacy is an important component of basic practice standards.
- *Analyzing personal communication skills.* Nurses should recognize their own strengths and weaknesses in interpersonal skills and develop them as needed.
- *Identifying situations in which advocacy is necessary.* Nurses should follow their own values and ethical perspectives in identifying advocacy situations, but they should also recognize differing perspectives and adapt accordingly.
- *Taking action.* Advocacy involves taking some type of action (physical, written, verbal) and nurses should be willing to take action when appropriate.

From Schroeter, K. (2000). Advocacy in perioperative nursing practice. *AORN Journal, 71*(6), 1207-10, 1213, 1215-18.

For example, in community settings, school nurses do the following:

- Manage clinics.
- Ensure that student records are complete.
- Perform and document legally mandated services, such as vision and hearing screenings.
- Direct clinic volunteers.

As described in the case study earlier, home health nurses:

- Coordinate scheduled visits based on client needs (i.e., fasting blood glucose or three times daily intravenous administration), estimating distances between client's homes and services to be provided.

- Ensure that other professional services are delivered when necessary and monitor or oversee the practice of a home health aide.
- Use each client's resources to develop a plan of care.

Nurses in clinics or physician offices perform triage so that clients in need of immediate help are treated first, ensure that supplies and equipment are available, and assist in ensuring that clients are seen on a timely basis.

OTHER ROLES IN COMMUNITY-BASED NURSING

Direct care provider, educator, manager, counselor, and advocate are the roles most often performed by nurses. Additional roles that all nurses should perform routinely or occasionally are the following:

- Collaborator
- Role model
- Researcher
- Leader

Each role is described briefly and examples for application of each role to community-based nursing practice are presented.

Collaborator

Changes in health care delivery have included a move from the reliance on an individual physician as the sole director of care who is thereby responsible for all aspects of care, to a more comprehensive, interdisciplinary approach wherein several health care team members are responsible for various facets of care. The nurse in the role of **collaborator** participates in the process of making decisions regarding health care management with individuals from various professions, working with the client and the family or caregivers to jointly determine the course of care. Through interaction, discussion, and coordination, goals are set and a plan of care is formed to meet those goals.

For clients with a complex or chronic health problem, such as coronary artery disease, Alzheimer's disease, or renal failure, the nurse must work with other health providers to

From Collette, C. (1999). A multidisciplinary approach to breast biopsy. *AORN Journal, 69*(4), 810-821.

> ### BOX 2-2 The Nurse as Collaborator
>
> Collette (1999) described a situation in which a multidisciplinary approach was used in an ambulatory surgery unit to develop a program for caring for women undergoing breast biopsy. For development of the program, a committee that included surgeons, radiologists, nurses, and radiology technologists was formed. Guidelines were developed that resulted in a collaborative approach to breast biopsy, which provided clients with the most expedient, accurate, cost-effective diagnoses with the least amount of physical and psychological trauma.

deliver the most comprehensive, effective, cost-conscious care possible. Caring for a stroke victim, for example, may involve collaboration between physicians, nurses, physical therapists, occupational therapists, speech therapists, and possibly others in both community and hospital settings.

Similarly, health-promotion interventions need to be collaborative. For example, a team of professionals in a senior health clinic might work with an elderly client with diabetes to teach principles of nutrition, medication management, and foot care. The nurse in this setting might collaborate with a dietitian, pharmacist, diabetes educator, and others to seek the best management of client care (Box 2-2).

Role Model

A **role model** is a person who demonstrates an action or behavior that is learned by others. Role modeling is both conscious and unconscious and nurses in all settings, whether "on the job" or at home, demonstrate to others both positive and negative actions and attitudes related to health and health care.

In community-based practice, nurses serve as role models to clients, their caregivers, and other health professionals. For example, a student receiving helpful, therapeutic, understanding care from the school nurse might be motivated to become a nurse; the caregiver of an elderly woman watching the professional, matter-of-fact changing of a sterile dressing may be convinced that he or she, too, may be able to learn to perform this task. In another example, a nurse working with immigrant families in a community clinic can demonstrate care, empathy, and appreciation for cultural differences of clients to new employees and nursing students working in the clinic.

Researcher

Nurses, whatever their practice setting or primary population served, must remain informed of developments that are relative to their individual practice. Nurses should be careful, discriminating consumers of research. In the role of **researcher**, they should critically review research findings for merit and applicability to practice and should determine care accordingly. Nurses in obstetric clinics, for example, should be aware of the latest recommendations regarding dietary guidelines during pregnancy and the rationale behind these recommendations. Similarly, nurses working with new families should share findings about sleeping positions for newborns and nurses who work with adults should be aware of new guidelines and rationale for prostate and breast screenings and exercise and diet recommendations. Often, the client is unaware of recent discoveries and innovations related to health and it is the nurse's responsibility to share them when relevant.

Occasionally, a nurse in community-based practice may be a part of a research study. Identifying problems or questions for investigation, participating in approved research studies, and disseminating research findings to clients and other professionals are appropriate actions for all nurses.

Leader

Leadership refers to the ability to influence the behavior of others. In community settings, the nurse may assume the role of a leader with clients and their families, other health care providers, public officials, local leaders, or employers.

As a **leader**, the nurse may work with others to identify and assess threats to health and to intervene to remove or lessen these threats. For example, a nurse employed in a manufacturing setting might direct a group in establishing a health-promotion program, a school nurse might lead a coalition of concerned parents to improve the nutritional value of hot lunches, and a nurse working in a clinic for low-income families might undertake the establishment of evening hours to meet the scheduling needs of the working poor.

COMPARISON OF NURSING ROLES IN HOSPITALS AND COMMUNITY SETTINGS

Although each of the many roles should be part of quality, comprehensive nursing care in any setting, role emphasis varies according to each client's needs and from setting to setting. Figure 2-1 visually depicts estimates of time spent by nurses in various roles in selected community and acute care settings. The time spent in any role varies according to each client's specific needs. Remember, these are estimates and are not meant to be examples of ideal amounts of time spent in each role; furthermore, they are not necessarily accurate for each nurse in each setting. Instead, the purpose of the diagrams is to illustrate the various nursing roles in different settings.

NURSING INTERVENTIONS IN COMMUNITY SETTINGS

Nursing interventions have been defined as "any treatment, based upon clinical judgment and knowledge, that a nurse performs to enhance patient/client outcomes," and they include both direct and indirect care that may be nurse-initiated, physician-initiated, or other provider-initiated treatments (McCloskey and Bulechek, 2000, p. xix). Because nursing roles vary, often dramatically, between acute care and community settings and among different community settings, nursing interventions also vary.

The **Nursing Interventions Classification (NIC) system** (McCloskey and Bulechek, 2000) is the most comprehensively developed taxonomy

of nursing interventions. The NIC system lists 484 nursing interventions that have been defined and developed to include examples of appropriate nursing activities (behaviors or actions that implement the intervention) for each. The identified nursing interventions are divided into seven "domains":

1. Physiological (basic): care that supports physical functioning.
2. Physiological (complex): care that supports homeostatic regulation.
3. Behavioral: care that supports psychosocial functioning and facilitates lifestyle changes.
4. Safety: care that supports protection against harm.
5. Family: care that supports the family unit.
6. Health system: care that supports effective use of the health care delivery system.
7. Community: care that supports the health of the community.

Each domain is further divided into "classes" into which individual interventions are grouped. Some interventions fall into more than one class or domain. The remainder of the chapter describes some of the similarities and differences in nursing interventions in community and in acute care settings.

"UNIVERSAL" NURSING INTERVENTIONS

Certain nursing interventions are required of virtually all nurses in almost all settings (McCloskey and Bulechek, 2000). Examples of universal nursing interventions are as follows:

- Documentation: recording of pertinent patient data in a clinical record.
- Environmental management (safety): monitoring and manipulation of the physical environment to promote safety.
- Anticipatory guidance: preparation of the patient for an anticipated developmental and/or situational crisis.
- Infection control: minimizing the acquisition and transmission of infectious agents.
- Laboratory data interpretation: critical analysis of patient laboratory data to assist with clinical decision making.

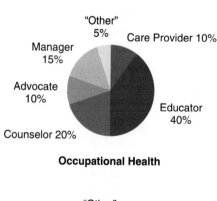

Occupational Health

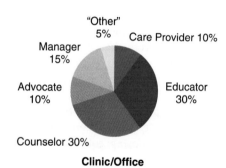

Clinic/Office

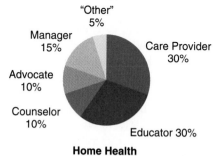

Home Health

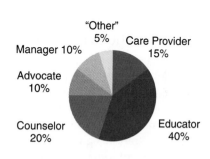

School Nursing

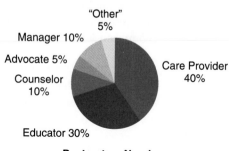

Postpartum Nursing

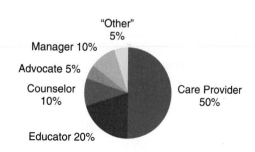

General Medical/Surgical

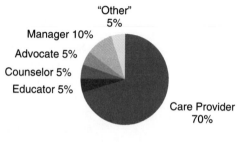

Critical Care

Figure 2-1. Comparison of nursing roles in selected settings.

- Learning facilitation: promoting the ability to process and comprehend information.
- Client rights protection: protection of health care rights of a patient, especially a minor, or an incapacitated or incompetent patient unable to make decisions.
- Physician support: collaborating with physicians to provide quality client care.
- Vital signs monitoring: collection and analysis of cardiovascular, respiratory, and body temperature data to determine and prevent complications.

NURSING INTERVENTIONS IN ACUTE CARE

Some nursing interventions are very specialized and nurses would provide those related activities only when delivering care in certain settings. For example, in critical care settings, nurses frequently perform many of the nursing interventions, termed "physiological complex" (e.g., acid-base management, cerebral edema management, circulatory care, mechanical assist device), but rarely perform many from the "behavioral" domain (e.g., behavior modification, learning readiness enhancement, health education).

Alternatively, many of the interventions in the "family" domain are directed specifically to the practice of perinatal nursing, including the following:

- Cesarean section care
- Electronic fetal monitoring: intrapartum care
- High-risk pregnancy care

Some nursing interventions are performed only rarely outside the acute care setting, as illustrated by the following examples:

- Anesthesia administration
- Autotransfusion
- Artificial airway management
- Cardiac care: acute
- Cerebral edema management
- Circulatory care
- Electronic fetal monitoring
- Endotracheal extubation
- Gastrointestional intubation
- Hemorrhage control
- Intrapartal care: high-risk delivery

- Mechanical ventilation
- Traction and immobilization care
- Tube care: chest

NURSING INTERVENTIONS FREQUENTLY USED IN COMMUNITY PRACTICE

A number of nursing interventions are commonly used throughout all community settings and more often than in acute care settings. For example, abuse protection support (identification of high-risk, dependent relationships and actions to prevent further infliction of physical or emotional harm) is appropriate for home health nurses who see caregivers of seriously ill or infirm clients who need respite care. In the same manner, school nurses and nurses in geriatric or pediatric clinics and similar settings should monitor for signs of neglect or unexplained illness or injury and should seek to identify parents or caregivers who might be at risk of being abusers (i.e., alcoholics or substance abusers or those abused as children) (McCloskey and Bulechek, 2000).

Other nursing interventions identified by McCloskey and Bulechek (2000) commonly found throughout community-based practice are the following:

- Health education: developing and providing instruction and learning experiences to facilitate voluntary adaptation of behavior conductive to health in individuals, families, groups, or communities.
- Health screening: detecting health risks or problems by means of history, examining, and other procedures.
- Health system guidance: facilitating a patient's location and use of appropriate health services.
- Medication administration: preparing, giving, and evaluating the effectiveness of prescription and nonprescription drugs.
- Teaching (prescribed medication): preparing a patient to safely take prescribed medications and monitoring for their effects.
- Nutritional counseling: using an interactive helping process, focusing on the need for diet modification.

- Referral: arranging for services by another care provider or agency.
- Risk identification: analysis of potential risk factors, determination of health risks, and prioritization of risk-reduction strategies for an individual or group.
- Teaching (individual): planning, implementation, and evaluation of a teaching program designed to address a client's particular needs.
- Telephone consultation: eliciting patient's concerns; listening and providing support, information, or teaching in response to patient's stated concerns. (See the Community Application box about telephone consultation.)

Although not all of these interventions are implemented by all nurses working in community settings, they are performed by most nurses.

Table 2-1 compares typical nursing interventions for several settings, both hospital-based settings and community-based settings. As with

the comparison of nursing roles in various settings, these are examples only and the lists are by no means comprehensive or exclusive. Nursing in each area involves many more interventions than are presented here and there may be significant overlap and exceptions in all areas.

SUMMARY

A number of nursing roles and nursing interventions are required to deliver comprehensive, competent, appropriate, and effective client care in any setting. As a home health nurse, Sally, from the opening case study, is an advocate and role model in addition to acting as a direct care provider. In these roles, she performs multiple nursing interventions.

This chapter describes some functions— manager, health educator, counselor—of the most important nursing roles and has shown

---

COMMUNITY APPLICATION
Nursing Intervention: Telephone Consultation

Robinson, Anderson, and Acheson (1996) described the process for implementing a telephone health advice program. They suggested the following steps:

- *Define the scope of the problem.* Conduct a descriptive, prospective study of trends in telephone calls including chief complaints, temporal distribution of calls (are calls heaviest in the morning, evening, weekends, etc.), the profile of the caller (gender, age, client or family member), and type of problem(s).
- *Identify problems to be addressed via telephone.* Prepare a list of the chief symptoms reported by callers and determine whether advice can be provided over the telephone.
- *Develop protocols or guidelines.* Telephone protocols or guidelines should be developed to evaluate, classify, advise, educate, and intervene in advice calls. Nurses may develop their own protocols or use those marketed for telephone consultation. If existing protocols are used, the standards of care for the community should be incorporated. Protocols should be comprehensive, current, authoritative, user friendly, symptom based, and conservative.

- *Develop a file system for protocols.* Protocols should be filed alphabetically according to the symptom(s) addressed. A computer database that can search and find the appropriate protocol on the basis of key words is ideal. A copy of the protocols and reference material should be placed at the telephone station.
- *Determine a method for documentation.* A log of calls and advice given should be maintained to minimize the legal risk. Documentation should include date and time of call, name of caller/client, demographic information about the caller/client, brief statement of illness history and signs and symptoms, statement of advice given/protocol followed, any warning given regarding time frame within which the caller should be seen, and any warnings regarding the severity of the illness.
- *Set quality controls.* Formal orientation should be provided for those providing telephone consultation. Phone logs should be audited periodically to track trends and critique the quality of information given by the RN.

From Robinson, D. L., Anderson, M. M., & Acheson, P. M. (1996). Telephone advice: Lessons learned and considerations for stating programs. *Journal of Emergency Nursing, 22*(5), 409-415.

TABLE 2-1 Commonly Used Nursing Interventions in Selected Settings

PHYSIOLOGIC	BEHAVIORAL	SAFETY	FAMILY	HEALTH SYSTEM	COMMUNITY
Home Health					
Teaching prescribed medications Wound care Cardiac care: rehabilitative Phlebotomy: venous blood sample IV teams IV therapy Medication administration Chemotherapy management	Anxiety reduction Teaching: disease process Teaching: preoperative Teaching: prescribed medication Teaching: prescribed activity/exercise Teaching: prescribed diet	Risk identification Fall prevention Abuse protection support: elder	Caregiver support Home maintenance assistance Normalization promotion Family involvement Respite care	Culture brokerage Discharge planning Health system guidance Insurance authorization Supply management Multidisciplinary care conference Referral Telephone consultation	Case Management Risk Identification
School Nursing					
Oral health promotion Medication administration: oral Heat/cold application Exercise promotion	Substance use prevention Behavior management: overactivity/inattention Teaching: group Teaching: sexuality Distraction	First aid Abuse protection: child Immunization/vaccination administration Risk identification	Developmental enhancement Family involvement Family integrity promotion Parent education: childrearing family Parent education: adolescent	Health policy monitoring Supply management Multidisciplinary care conference Referral	Health screening Health education Program development
Ambulatory Care Nursing (Clinic or Physician's Office)					
Phlebotomy: venous blood sample Exercise program Weight management Weight reduction assistance Medication administration	Self-responsibility facilitation Smoking cessation assistance Substance use prevention Substance use treatment Communication enhancement: hearing deficit	First aid Triage Abuse protector: child Abuse protector: elder Health screening Immunization/vaccination administration Risk identification	Caregiver support Family mobilization Developmental enhancement Family involvement Family integrity promotion Parent education: childrearing family	Referral Telephone consultation Insurance authorization Health system guidance Controlled substance checking Supply management Health care information exchange	Community disaster preparedness Surveillance: community

Occupational Health Nursing					
Coping enhancement					
Decision-making support					
Teaching: disease process					
Teaching: preoperative					
Teaching: prescribed diet					
Teaching: safe sex					
Weight management	Health education	Environmental management: worker safety	Role enhancement	Referral	Community disaster preparedness
Exercise promotion	Self-responsibility facilitation	First aid	Family integrity promotion	Telephone consultation	Environmental risk protection
Weight reduction assistance	Smoking cessation assistance	Emergency care	Parent education: childrearing family	Insurance authorization	Program development
Stress management	Substance use prevention	Health screening	Family support	Health system guidance	
	Coping enhancement	Risk identification		Controlled substance checking	
	Decision-making support	Surveillance: safety		Supply management	
	Teaching: safe sex			Health policy monitoring	

Critical Care Nursing					
Acid-base management	Dying care	Code management	Family involvement	Delegation	Environmental risk protection
Airway suctioning	Emotional support	Area restriction	Family process maintenance	Emergency cart checking	Environmental management: worker safety
Artificial airway management	Presence		Family mobilization	Order transcription	
Bowel management				Shift report	
Cardiac care: acute				Visitation facilitation	
Cerebral edema management				Bedside laboratory testing	
Circulatory care				Technology management	
Electrolyte management					
Phlebotomy: arterial blood sample					
Tube care: chest					
IV therapy					
Embolus precautions					
Pain management					

Data from McCloskey, J. C., & Bulechek, G. M. (2000). *Nursing interventions classification (NIC)* (3rd ed.). St. Louis: Mosby. IV, Intravenous.

continued

TABLE **2-1** Commonly Used Nursing Interventions in Selected Settings—cont'd

PHYSIOLOGIC	BEHAVIORAL	SAFETY	FAMILY	HEALTH SYSTEM	COMMUNITY
General Medical/Surgical Nursing					
Exercise therapy: ambulation Self-care assistance Cough enhancement IV therapy Incision site care Venous access device maintenance Self-care assistance	Anxiety reduction Teaching: disease process Teaching: preoperative Teaching: prescribed medication Teaching: prescribed activity/exercise Teaching: prescribed diet	Code management	Family involvement Family process maintenance Family mobilization Normalization promotion	Admission care Discharge planning Bedside laboratory testing Delegation Emergency cart checking Order transcription Shift report	Case management Environmental management: worker safety
Postpartum Nursing					
Perineal care Constipation management Pelvic floor exercise Self-care assistance Pain management Bleeding reduction: postpartum uterus	Grief work facilitation: perinatal death Support system enhancement Family planning: contraception Parent education: childbearing family Teaching: infant care	Code management Area restriction	Postpartum care Attachment promotion Breastfeeding assistance Environmental management: attachment process Infant care Newborn monitoring Caregiver support Family integrity promotion	Admission care Discharge planning Bedside laboratory testing Delegation Emergency cart checking Order transcription Shift report	Environmental management: worker safety

how they are distinctive in both acute care and community settings. Likewise, nursing interventions are numerous and diverse and their implementation may vary significantly from setting to setting. Similarities and differences are discussed to encourage nurses to recognize and appreciate some of the unique characteristics of nursing care in a wide variety of settings.

KEY POINTS

- Nursing practice in community-based settings differs considerably from practice in the hospital and nursing practice also differs across various community settings.
- Nursing roles in community-based practice that are most frequently used are educator, counselor, manager, advocate, and care provider. The amount of time spent in each role varies from setting to setting, client to client, and day to day.
- Nursing interventions vary, often dramatically, between acute care and community-based settings and among different community settings.

Learning Activities & Application to Practice
In Class

1. With classmates, discuss or debate how the various roles of the nurse differ from setting to setting. What role or roles are seen as most important in each setting? Why?

2. Obtain a copy of *Nursing Interventions Classification*, 3rd edition (McCloskey and Bulechek, 2000). Outline examples of nursing interventions that would be appropriate in several situations in both hospital and community settings. Discuss similarities and differences.

In Clinical

3. Estimate the amount of time you spend during your clinical day in each of the nursing roles described. Keep track of these estimates in a log or diary. Do nursing roles change between settings? How and why? Compare observations with classmates in other settings.

4. List nursing interventions that you have performed in each clinical setting in a log or diary. How are interventions different in each setting? Do you feel some interventions are more important or necessary than others? Why or why not?

REFERENCES

Collette, C. (1999). A multidisciplinary approach to breast biopsy. *AORN Journal, 69*(4), 810-821.

McCloskey, J. C., & Bulechek, G. M. (2000). *Nursing interventions classification (NIC)* (3rd ed.). St. Louis: Mosby.

Robinson, D. L., Anderson, M. M., & Acheson, P. M. (1996). Telephone advice: Lessons learned and considerations for stating programs, *Journal of Emergency Nursing, 22*(5), 409-415.

Schroeter, K. (2000). Advocacy in perioperative nursing practice. *AORN Journal, 71*(6), 1207-10, 1213, 1215-18.

Nursing Care in Ambulatory Settings

objectives

Upon completion of this chapter, the reader will be able to:

1. Discuss specific aspects of nursing care in clinics, offices, schools, worksites, rural areas, parishes, and correctional facilities.

2. Discuss specific aspects of nursing care in ambulatory oncology centers, outpatient surgical centers, and public health departments.

3. Compare and contrast nursing practice in different ambulatory care settings.

4. Explain education and certification issues related to ambulatory nursing practice.

key terms

Ambulatory care
Ambulatory nursing practice
Ambulatory oncology nursing practice
Ambulatory surgery
Correctional nursing

Education for All Handicapped Children Act (PL 94-142)
Occupational health nursing
Occupational Safety and Health Act (PL 91-596)

Parish nursing
Public health nursing
Rural nursing
School nursing
Workers' compensation

See Glossary for definitions.

case study

Bill Barnett is a registered nurse (RN) working in a postanesthesia care (recovery) unit (PACU) in a day surgery center. The day surgery center is a freestanding facility located in a small city. The center houses six operating rooms and 30 to 40 surgical procedures are performed there daily.

The various surgical procedures performed at the center involve virtually all surgical specialties. On a typical day, general surgery procedures (e.g., laparoscopic cholecystectomy, inguinal hernia repair), orthopedic procedures (e.g., arthroscopy), gynecological procedures (e.g., laparoscopy, cervical dilation, curettage), ophthalmic procedures (e.g., cataract extraction, radial keratotomy), plastic surgery (e.g., blepharoplasty, rhinoplasty), otolaryngology procedures (e.g., tonsillectomy, myringotomy/placement of pressure equalization [PE] tubes), and others are performed.

Bill is one of seven PACU RNs employed at the day surgery center and has worked there 5 years. During that time, he has seen the caseload grow dramatically, with many of the procedures becoming increasingly complex. The first surgical cases are scheduled to begin at 07:30 and continue until about 15:00. The RNs work staggered shifts. Bill begins his day at 10:00 and is responsible for recovering patients from the later cases.

On a recent Thursday, Bill cared for Tony Mitchell, a 17-year-old high school football player who tore his left medial meniscus during practice. The surgeon performed arthroscopic surgery on Tony's left knee and shaved the torn part of the meniscus. The surgery was done under general anesthesia and lasted about an hour.

Tony was beginning to awaken from anesthesia when he was brought into the PACU by the anesthesiologist and the circulating nurse. His endotracheal tube had been removed in the operating room, but he still had an oral airway in place and was breathing without difficulty. Bill placed a blood pressure cuff on Tony's right arm and took his vital signs (blood pressure, 110/56; pulse, 88; respirations, 20; temperature, 97°F). His blood oxygen levels were monitored by a pulse oximeter and remained at 98.

When Bill called Tony's name and instructed him to open his eyes, Tony complied. He gagged slightly and reached toward his mouth to remove the oral airway. Bill assisted him and discarded the airway in a nearby container. Tony responded appropriately to questioning and stated that his left leg hurt a little. The left leg had been wrapped in a heavy dressing and Ace bandage in the operating room and then propped on two pillows. Bill assessed the foot and toes for swelling, color, and capillary refill. All were "normal." When asked, Tony moved his left toes without difficulty.

Bill received a report from the anesthesiologist and circulating nurse, both of whom stated that the procedure was uneventful. The anesthesiologist detailed the medications that had been used during the procedure and gave Bill the anesthesia records and operative report and both left to prepare for their next cases.

Bill monitored Tony's vital signs and pulse oximeter every 5 minutes for about 20 minutes and then every 10 to 15 minutes for the next hour. By that time, Tony was alert and requested something to drink. Within 2 hours after admittance to the PACU, Tony was sitting up in a recliner and drinking an iced soft drink; his intravenous line had been removed and his parents were present. Bill used that time to reinforce the postoperative instructions that Tony and his parents had already been given. They repeated the instructions and stated that they would take Tony to the surgeon's office the next day for postoperative evaluation. They had already filled a prescription for pain medication given to them earlier and correctly verbalized the appropriate dosage. Tony was discharged from the day surgery center about an hour later and left on crutches with his parents.

The term **ambulatory care** refers to "personal health care provided to an individual who is not a bed patient in a health care institution" and generally includes all health services provided to noninstitutionalized patients (Mezey and Lawrence, 1995, p. 122). Today, approximately 60% of all surgical procedures are performed on an outpatient basis. Likewise, chemotherapy and other parenteral medications are delivered in homes and outpatient centers; diagnostic tests and procedures are performed in freestanding clinics and centers; and health promotion and health education services are provided in convenient settings such as home, work, church, and school.

Many of the objectives of *Healthy People 2010* (U.S. Department of Health and Human Services [USDHHS], 2000) involve health teaching, symptom monitoring and management, and risk reduction activities that are most effectively delivered during primary care office visits, formal or informal health education classes, individual

healthy people **2010**

Examples of Objectives Appropriate for Community-Based Settings (e.g., Clinics, Schools, Work Sites, Churches)

OBJECTIVE		BASELINE (1998)	TARGET
6.9:	Increase the proportion of children and youth with disabilities who spend at least 80% of their time in regular education programs	45%	60%
7.1:	Increase high school completion	85%	90%
7.4a:	Increase the proportion of the nation's elementary, middle, junior high, and senior high schools that have a nurse-to-student ratio of at least 1:750	28%	50%
7.6:	Increase the proportion of employees who participate in employer-sponsored health-promotion activities	28%	50%
14.23g:	Maintain measles vaccination coverage levels for children in kindergarten through the first grade	96%	95%
15.39:	Reduce weapon carrying by adolescents on school property	8.0%	6.0%
19.16:	Increase the proportion of work sites that offer nutrition for weight-management classes or counseling	55%	85%
24.5:	Reduce the number of school days missed by people with asthma from asthma	NA	NA

Data from U.S. Department of Health and Human Services. (2000). *Healthy people 2010: Conference edition.* Washington, DC: Government Printing Office.

counseling sessions, or other health-promotion situations. The *Healthy People 2010* box lists some of the objectives that relate to ambulatory health care settings.

This chapter explores some of the numerous settings for community-based health care delivery and briefly describes nursing practice in those settings. The settings and descriptions of nursing practice are by no means all inclusive. Settings, clientele, and nursing practice vary greatly by geographical area, population needs, nursing practice guidelines and protocols, and a number of other factors. The purpose of this chapter is to give a general overview of practice opportunities for RNs apart from acute care, long-term care, and home health settings. Included is nursing care in clinics and physicians' offices, schools, work sites, and churches, and specialty practices such as oncology care, surgery, public health, and others.

NURSING PRACTICE IN SELECTED SETTINGS

Community-based nursing practice often involves being a member of a group or practice concerned with the provision of comprehensive, primary care for individuals or families in a geographically or institutionally defined area. In these instances, nursing care is largely focused on health promotion, primary prevention, screening for early identification of disease, and assisting in treatment regimens for both acute and chronic illnesses (e.g., colds, influenza, ear infection, hypertension, diabetes).

Again, it is important to note that nursing roles and interventions may vary significantly in similar settings by organizational or institutional policy, state practice regulations or requirements, and other factors. For example, in one occupational setting, the nurse's practice may primarily be concerned with monitoring Occupational Safety and Health Association guidelines and workers' compensation cases and providing first aid to injured employees, whereas in another company, the occupational health nurse's practice focuses on health promotion and illness-prevention activities, such as conducting screenings and health education classes and providing counseling. This section briefly describes nursing practice in selected settings.

HEALTH CARE PROVIDER OFFICE OR CLINIC

Probably the most familiar role of the nurse in community-based practice is that of the office or clinic nurse. Nurses working in physician-based practices, nurse-based practices, and health maintenance organizations collectively account for the largest group of nurses working outside hospitals. In the United States, approximately 9.5% of all RNs are employed in clinic or office settings (USDHHS/Division of Nursing [DON], 2001). The most common types of practice are the physician-based solo practice, group practice or partnership, and the health maintenance organization.

Nursing Practice in Ambulatory Clinics and Offices

As mentioned previously, the roles and responsibilities of the nurse vary greatly between clinics because the practice, focus, and clients are often very different. Physicians may be general or family practitioners who provide preventative care and diagnose and treat clients of all ages and for all types of health problems. Other general areas of practice include pediatrics, obstetrics and gynecology, and internal medicine. Practitioners in these areas provide "primary care" to more focused groups (i.e., children, women, and adults, respectively), but care is still comprehensive, covering multiple body systems. The many medical and surgical specialists (e.g., surgeons, cardiologists, dermatologists, ophthalmologists, psychiatrists, orthopedists) see clients with more specific health problems.

The roles and interventions that nurses practice in physicians' offices obviously are based on the type of care provided in that office or clinic. For example, a nurse working in a surgeon's office may assist with surgical procedures, provide follow-up through phone calls, remove sutures, and help with preprocedure and postprocedure assessments. A nurse working in a cardiologist's office might assist in monitoring stress tests and perform electrocardiograms and other tests, and a nurse working in a pediatric office may assist in physical and developmental assessment, collect specimens (e.g., finger sticks, strep cultures), teach parents about infant care, and administer immunizations.

The scope of **ambulatory nursing practice** includes such activities as measurement, specimen collection, client follow-up, assessment, health teaching, provision of comfort measures, coordination of services, and preparation of patients for surgical or nonsurgical procedures. Box 3-1 lists some of the roles and responsibilities in practice in ambulatory care clinics.

The American Academy of Ambulatory Care Nursing (AAACN) has published practice standards for ambulatory care nursing administration. The nine standards for practice outlined by the organization relate to structure and organization of ambulatory care nursing, staffing, competency, ambulatory nursing practice, continuity of care, ethics and patient's rights, environment, research, and quality management (AAACN, 2000).

Education, Experience, and Certification Recommendations for Clinic Nurses

There are few requirements for employment in physicians' offices and clinics. Although some physicians prefer that the nurses they employ have at least 1 year of hospital experience, many hire new RNs. A baccalaureate degree is usually not required for nurse's positions in ambulatory settings. Certification for ambulatory care nurses is available through the American Nurses Credentialing Center (ANCC).

BOX 3-1 Examples of Nursing Practice Roles and Interventions in Ambulatory Care

ENABLING OPERATIONS

Maintaining safe work environment
Setting up the room
Ordering supplies
Providing emotional support
Taking vital signs

TECHNICAL PROCEDURES

Preparing the client for procedures
Assisting with procedures
Chaperoning during procedures
Informing the client about treatment
Witnessing signing of consent forms
Administering medications
Collecting specimens

NURSING PROCESS

Developing the nursing care plan
Using nursing diagnosis
Completing the client history
Assessing client learning needs
Evaluating client care outcomes
Charting each client encounter

TELEPHONE COMMUNICATIONS

Performing telephone triage
Calling the pharmacy with prescription
Calling the client with test results

ADVOCACY

Making the clients aware of rights
Acting as a client advocate
Referring the client to an appropriate provider

TEACHING

Instructing the client on medical/nursing regimen
Instructing the client on home and self-care

CARE COORDINATION

Acting as a resource person
Coordinating client care
Assessing needs and initiating referrals
Finding resources in the community
Instructing on health promotion

Adapted from Hackbarth, D. P., Haas, S. A., Kavanagh, J. A., and Vlasses, F. (1995). Dimensions of the staff nurse role in ambulatory care: Part I—Methodology and analysis of data on current staff nurse practice. *Nursing Economics, 13*(2), 89-98. Reprinted from *Nursing Economics,* 1995, vol. 13, no. 2, p. 92. Reprinted with permission of the publisher, Jannetti Publications, Inc., East Holly Avenue, Box 56, Pitman, NJ 08071-0056; Phone (609) 256-2300; Fax (609) 589-7463. (For a sample issue of the journal, contact the publisher.)

SCHOOLS

Documentation of efforts to promote student health through school health services began in New York City in the late 1800s. The distinguished public health nurse, Lillian Wald, is credited with convincing New York City's school board to use a public health nurse to decrease absenteeism. As a result of her support, Lina Rogers was employed as the first school nurse in 1902. Reportedly, Miss Rogers was so successful that 25 additional nurses were hired over the next several years and the use of public health nurses in school-based practice spread rapidly to other cities, including Boston, Chicago, and Philadelphia (Pollitt, 1994). Currently, more than 40,000 school nurses practice in the United States, accounting for about 2.2% of all RNs (Hootman, 1998).

The early emphasis in school health programs was on control of communicable diseases such as tuberculosis, smallpox, diphtheria, whooping cough, pediculosis, scabies, and ringworm. As measures to control communicable diseases proved successful, attention moved toward sanitation, safety issues, and early detection and remediation of physical problems (e.g., vision and hearing deficits) that might impede learning. Throughout the next 40 to 50 years, **school nursing** roles and activities expanded to include assisting the physician with examination of students; counseling of students, parents, and teachers; and developing and implementing health education programs. School nurses also made home visits, provided in-service education for teachers, and served as a resource for school administration.

The roles and practice of school nurses have continued to evolve. Most recently, school health service programs have concentrated on the following components:

- Prevention of illness and disease transmission and early detection of possible disease
- Intervention in identified problems such as alcohol and drug use, sexually transmitted diseases (STDs), pregnancy, family violence, and the adaptation of children with special health needs to the school setting
- Promotion of healthy lifestyles
- Health education, both formal and informal

School health programs and the role of school nurses have strengthened and expanded during the past 2 decades. Currently, school-based teams are used nationwide in numerous ways, including caring for disabled children, investigating suspected child abuse, improving health education, promoting the safety of school children, implementation and management of school-based clinics, and research and evaluation of school health programs.

School Nursing Practice

The school nurse is responsible for maintaining the school health program. The American School Health Association (ASHA) (2001) has identified the following key components of a comprehensive school health program:

- Prevention and control of communicable diseases
- Care of ill or injured students
- Responsibility for administration or oversight of procedures for students with special health needs
- Administration of screening programs
- Providing and monitoring for a safe and healthful environment
- Health promotion
- Health counseling
- Health office management
- School health program evaluation and quality assurance and improvement

Each of these components is discussed briefly in the following sections.

PREVENTION AND CONTROL OF COMMUNICABLE DISEASES. Communicable disease control and prevention in school health programs typically involves monitoring immunization records to ensure student compliance with school district and state requirements, exclusion for communicable disease, and efforts for infection control (e.g., universal precautions for all individuals who contact body fluids, hand washing protocols for cafeteria workers, monitoring incidence of illness and absenteeism).

Although requirements vary, completion of a basic set of childhood immunizations is necessary for school attendance in all states (Lewis and Thomson, 1986). Exceptions to these requirements are occasionally made for religious or health reasons (e.g., having had a documented case of measles).

It is usually the responsibility of the school nurse to monitor the immunization records of each child to ensure compliance. When a deficiency is observed, the nurse follows school district guidelines to ensure remediation of the deficiency. In some districts, this simply involves gaining parental permission and providing the vaccination at the school. In other settings, the nurse sends a letter to the child's parent or guardian that explains which vaccinations are not current. Often, this letter includes consequences (e.g., exclusion from school) if the immunization is not completed in a timely manner and information on where to go for low-cost or free immunizations.

Exclusion from school of students who contract communicable diseases is based on school district policy and state laws. Therefore it is essential that the nurse be aware of these requirements and understand under what conditions a child is to be excluded from school and under what conditions he or she may return. For example, children with chicken pox are generally excluded from attending school until after 7 days from onset of the rash and children with strep infections are excluded until 24 hours has passed following initiation of antibiotic therapy and after fever subsides.

CARE OF ILL OR INJURED STUDENTS. The school nurse is responsible for monitoring the health of students, providing first aid and emergency care when indicated, and administering treatments and medications when prescribed, following school district procedures and standard protocols. The nurse should maintain a file of basic information, health records, and emergency information for each student.

Providing simple first aid for minor injuries is common in school nursing practice. Normally, each school district develops a set of first aid protocols or instructions to follow when caring for simple problems such as scrapes, blisters, sprains, or stings. A first aid kit should be well stocked and readily available for treatment of minor injuries. When more serious emergencies occur, it is often the school nurse's responsibility to provide first aid, inform the parents, and make arrangements to transport the student to the emergency room or physician's office, if necessary. School districts should also have guidelines for the nurse to follow in emergency situations.

For students with acute or chronic illnesses or conditions, administration of medication or treatments at school may be necessary. School districts maintain policies on who is to administer medications and treatment, the process to be followed, and guidelines for record keeping. Sometimes it is the responsibility of the nurse to perform these services, but often the nurse must train others to perform these tasks and monitor their care, per district policy.

RESPONSIBILITY FOR ADMINISTRATION OR OVERSIGHT OF PROCEDURES FOR STUDENTS WITH SPECIAL HEALTH NEEDS. Congress enacted the **Education for All Handicapped Children Act (PL 94-142)** in 1975. Public Law 94-142 "gives all students between the ages of 6 and 18 years the right to a 'free and appropriate public education' in the least restrictive environment possible regardless of physical or mental disabilities" (Kub and Steel, 1995, p. 752). The law was amended in 1986, expanding the eligible population to include preschool students. This amendment was added to reduce developmental delays, minimize institutionalization, and help families meet the special needs of children with disabilities. Handicapping conditions covered by this Act include: auditory impairment, visually handicapped, mentally retarded, orthopedically impaired, seriously emotionally disturbed (e.g., inability to build interpersonal relationships, inappropriate behavior or feelings, depression), and specific learning disability (e.g., dyslexia) (Lewis and Thomson, 1986).

Requirements of Public Law 94-142 that specifically relate to school nursing are: (1) a provision that efforts must be made to screen or identify children in need of special education and related services; (2) completion of an "individualized education plan," which is developed by an interdisciplinary team and includes current educational level, goals, and specific services to be provided; and (3) provision of "designated instruction and services" (DIS), which outlines services required to help the child benefit from education. The DIS includes nursing care.

As part of, or in addition to, the activities cited here, the school nurse may be called on to monitor ventilator-dependent children, perform or supervise intermittent catheterization, and administer gastrostomy feedings. As with medication administration, performance of these procedures must be within the state's Nurse Practice Act, follow district policy, be authorized by parents, and be prescribed by a physician (ASHA, 2001).

ADMINISTRATION OF SCREENING PROGRAMS. Screening for actual and potential health problems and hindrances to education is a very important component of a school health program. State mandates, staff resources, rate of incidence of certain conditions, resources, time, and facilities determine screening programs and procedures.

In most school health programs, screening includes vision, hearing, height and weight, and scoliosis. Additional screening programs may be required or provided by the state (e.g., early, periodic screening, diagnosis, and treatment

[EPSDT] [see Chapter 9] for Medicaid-eligible children).

Comprehensive vision screening programs should be performed annually or minimally in kindergarten, grades 1, 2 or 3, 4 or 5, 7 or 8, and 10 or 11. Additional evaluation can be performed at the request or recommendation of the child's parents or teachers. Vision screening should test for the following:

- Anomalies or conditions of the external eye
- Defects of visual acuity at distance
- Defects of visual acuity at near points
- Refractive error
- Ocular misalignment
- Binocularity defects
- Color discrimination (National Association of School Nurses [NASN], 1992)

After identification of a suspected vision problem, the school nurse should make a referral following district protocol. As with all school referrals, a follow-up should be made within 4 weeks to ensure that the child has had further evaluation and treatment if indicated.

Hearing screening programs, according to the NASN (1993), are conducted to promote a high level of hearing acuity for all students, minimize the number of students with hearing loss, and provide for individual education needs of students with permanent hearing impairment. Hearing screening should be routinely performed in students in kindergarten, grades 1, 2 or 3, 5 and/or 7, 9 or 11; for those with known hearing loss; following academic failure; after a child has failed previous screenings; when speech patterns suggest a hearing problem; or if the child has a history of recurrent middle ear infections or has risk factors for hearing loss (NASN, 1993).

Hearing screening should be performed by nurses or other professionals (e.g., audiologists) trained in hearing screening and should include visual examination through an otoscope (to detect cerumen, foreign bodies, or a perforation of the tympanic membrane), audiometric testing or pure-tone screening (records the softest level at which a tone can be heard), and acoustic emit-

tance testing (used to measure middle ear pressure). As with vision screening, a referral is made following identification of a possible problem.

Optimally, height and weight of each child should be measured and recorded annually to detect potential problems. Recording of growth measurements should be completed and referrals made following district guidelines.

Scoliosis usually develops slowly and may go unrecognized in children. Scoliosis occurs more frequently in girls than in boys and often begins during periods of active growth (e.g., 10 to 16 years). Because of this growth period and the potential for developing scoliosis, the Scoliosis Research Society recommends annual screening of all children 10 to 14 years of age (U.S. Preventative Services Task Force, 1996). As with vision and hearing screening, screening for scoliosis is largely dependent on school district and state mandates and, as with other screening programs, follow-up for suspected scoliosis is essential.

PROVIDING AND MONITORING FOR A SAFE AND HEALTHFUL ENVIRONMENT. For school nurses, provision of a safe and healthful environment includes being aware of fire codes, sanitation measures for the school, and disaster plans for student evacuation and protection. Knowledge of restrictions, laws, and regulations regarding weapons, illegal substances, and other harmful practices (e.g., smoking) is also an essential component of school nursing practice. The school nurse's participation in setting and enforcing rules is also important in maintaining a healthy environment.

HEALTH PROMOTION, EDUCATION, AND COUNSELING. Promoting and encouraging positive health practices through health education is a central component of school nursing. Additionally, the school nurse should be available to perform health counseling for students, parents, staff, and others.

HEALTH OFFICE MANAGEMENT. The school nurse's office should be amply equipped and supplied to allow for comprehensive and appropriate services. Minimally, the health offices should contain a desk and chair, locked filing cabinet for student files, locked cabinet for medications, cots for ill students, hot and cold running water, and private office space for conferences.

SCHOOL HEALTH PROGRAM EVALUATION AND QUALITY ASSURANCE AND IMPROVEMENT. A school health program evaluation should be conducted periodically to assess the achievement of program objectives, identify program strengths and weaknesses, and monitor the quality of practice. School health service evaluations should demonstrate the contribution of nursing service to education programs, compare the existing program to standards, improve procedures and practices, identify community needs for resources, involve community members in the school program, and improve communication between the school and the community.

Education and Experience Recommendations for School Nurses

A baccalaureate degree in nursing is recommended by the American Nurses' Association (ANA) and the NASN as the entry level for practice as a school nurse and many school districts require it. Throughout the United States, however, many diploma- or associate degree-

prepared school nurses are currently practicing (USDHHS/HRSA, 1998). Some school districts require a minimum of 1 year of experience, preferably in pediatrics, before employment.

OCCUPATIONAL HEALTH

Occupational health (industrial) nursing (OHN) in the United States began in the late 1800s. Reportedly, "a group of coal mining companies in Pennsylvania hired a nurse named Betty Moulder...to care for ailing miners and their families" (Rogers, 1994, p. 22). At approximately the same time, Ada Mayo Steward was hired as an "industrial health nurse" by the Vermont Marble Company. By 1912, 38 nurses were employed by businesses and industries, and that number had grown to 11,000 by 1943 (Rogers and Travers, 2001). Currently, between 19,000 and 23,000 occupational health nurses are practicing in the United States (USDHHS/HRSA, 1998). The Research Highlight "Occupational Health" provides details about deaths from injuries suffered in an occupational setting.

Occupational Health Nursing Practice

The American Association of Occupational Health Nurses (AAOHN) has stated that OHN is an

---

Research Highlight

Occupational Health

The CDC (2001a) reported that between 1980 and 1997, almost 104,000 persons died in the United States from occupational injuries (an average of 16 work-related deaths per day). However, there were some positive findings, as it was observed that the rate for occupational injury deaths for all workers decreased 45% during that time. Additional findings included the following:

- Males accounted for 93% of all occupational injury deaths.
- Although 85% of the deaths were among white workers, blacks had a slightly higher fatality rate (5.6 per 100,000 black workers compared with whites at 5.0 per 100,000 workers).

- Workers aged 25 to 34 accounted for the largest number of occupational injury deaths.
- Motor vehicle crashes accounted for 24% of all deaths.
- Homicides were the second leading cause of occupational deaths (14%), followed by machine-related deaths (13%), falls (10%), and electrocutions (7%).
- Industries with the largest number of deaths were construction (19%); transportation, communication, and public utilities (17%); and manufacturing (15%).
- The highest death rates were for mining, agriculture, forestry, fishing, and construction.

From Centers for Disease Control and Prevention (2001a). Fatal occupational injuries—United States, 1980-1997. *MMWR Morbid Mortal Wkly Rep, 50*(16), 317-320.

autonomous specialty in which nurses make independent nursing judgments in providing health care services. Further, OHN is "the specialty practice that focuses on promotion, prevention, and restoration of health within the context of a safe and healthy environment. It includes the prevention of adverse health effects from occupational and environmental hazards. It provides for and delivers occupational and environmental health and safety services to workers, worker populations and community groups." (AAOHN, 1999, p. 2).

Occupational health nursing practice is a synthesis of knowledge from nursing, medicine, public health, occupational health, epidemiology, environmental health, social and behavioral sciences, management, and administration and includes legal and ethical principles (Rogers and Travers, 2001). The OHN practice is directed by a combination of federal and state regulations, company policy and philosophy, the type of work or setting, worker input, nurse interest and expertise, and available resources.

Specific roles and functions of the OHN include the following (Rogers, 1994):

- Assessing the work environment for threats to health and safety.
- Assessing the health status of workers.
- Performing physical examinations, including those for job placement, "return to work," and termination or retirement.
- Conducting appropriate laboratory tests.
- Providing nursing care for occupational and nonoccupational injuries and illnesses.
- Counseling and health education.
- Helping the worker set goals and objectives for his or her care plan.
- Collaborating, communicating, and consulting with other members of the occupational health team and other health care providers in the community.
- Maintaining accurate and complete health records of the workers.
- Developing and implementing programs to correct or reduce identified health and safety hazards.

- Instituting appropriate personal protection programs (e.g., safety glasses, safety shoes, hearing protection).
- Conducting screening programs.
- Developing and implementing health-promotion programs.
- Evaluating various programs.
- Managing workers' compensation claims.
- Training for cardiopulmonary resuscitation (CPR) and first aid.

Legislation Affecting Occupational Health Nursing Practice

As mentioned, much of the practice of the OHN is directed by or in response to federal legislation and state mandates. Several of the most significant laws affecting OHN practice are described here.

WORKERS' COMPENSATION ACTS (DATES VARY BY STATE). **Workers' compensation** is an insurance system operated by the states, with each state having its own law and program. The first workers' compensation law was passed in New York in 1910 and, subsequently, all 50 states and the District of Columbia have enacted workers' compensation laws (Rogers, 1994).

Workers' compensation insurance is "no fault" and benefits are provided through employer-carried insurance plans. Benefits are awarded to individuals who sustain physical or mental injuries from their employment, regardless of who or what was the cause of the injury or illness. Although they vary by state, workers' compensation laws generally allow for ongoing payment of wages and benefits to the injured or disabled worker or dependent survivor for wages lost, medical care and related costs, funeral and burial costs, and some rehabilitation expenses.

OCCUPATIONAL SAFETY AND HEALTH ACT (1970). The **Occupational Safety and Health Act (PL 91-596)** is a comprehensive, multifaceted, and far-reaching piece of legislation. The purpose of the Occupational Safety and Health Act is to "assure so far as possible every working man and woman in the Nation safe and healthful working conditions and to preserve our human resources" (Public Law 01-596, 91st Congress, December 29, 1970; cited in Rogers, 1994, p. 433).

To accomplish the stated purpose, the Occupational Safety and Health Act did the following:

1. Formed the Occupational Safety and Health Administration (OSHA), which sets and enforces standards of occupational safety and health (Department of Labor).
2. Formed the National Institute for Occupational Safety and Health (NIOSH), which researches and recommends occupational safety and health standards to OSHA and funds educational centers for the training of occupational health professionals (USDHHS).
3. Established the National Advisory Council on Occupational Safety and Health, a consumer and professional council that makes occupational safety and health recommendations to OSHA and NIOSH.
4. Established federal occupational safety and health standards.
5. Established the Occupational Safety and Health Review Commission to advise OSHA and NIOSH regarding the legal implications of decisions or actions.
6. Created a mechanism for imposition of fines and other punitive measures for violation of federal occupational safety and health regulations.
7. Requires employers to maintain records of work-related deaths, injuries, and illnesses (Rogers and Travers, 2001).

The party responsible for promulgating legally enforceable standards that employers must meet to be in compliance with the Occupational Safety and Health Act is OSHA. The responsibilities of OSHA are to perform the following:

- Develop and update mandatory occupational safety and health standards.
- Monitor and enforce regulations and standards.
- Require employers to keep accurate records on work-related injuries, illnesses, and hazardous exposures.

- Maintain an occupational safety and health statistics collection and analysis system (in collaboration with NIOSH).
- Supervise employer and worker education and training to identify and prevent unsafe or unhealthy working conditions (in collaboration with NIOSH).
- Provide grants to states to assist in compliance with the Occupational Safety and Health Act (Adams, 2001).

Education, Experience, and Certification Recommendations for Occupational Health Nurses

A baccalaureate degree is recommended for OHN practice. In addition to a baccalaureate degree, the AAOHN recommends a minimum of 2 years of professional nursing experience (preferably in ambulatory, emergency, community health, or critical care) before beginning OHN practice (Clemen-Stone, Eigsti, and McGuire, 1995). Certification in OHN is available through the American Board for Occupational Health Nurses (ABOHN). To be eligible for certification, RNs must have worked at least 4000 hours as an occupational nurse during the past 5 years, have completed 50 contact hours of continuing education in occupational health nursing-related areas during the past 5 years, and successfully pass a certification examination (ABOHN, 2001).

RURAL HEALTH

Like school nursing, early efforts to develop organized nursing practice in rural areas are traced to Lillian Wald. Miss Wald is credited for helping establish the Rural Nursing Service in 1912. A few years later, in 1925, Mary Breckinridge began the Frontier Nursing Service. These efforts focused on improving public health, primary health care, and midwifery services in rural areas (Weinert and Long, 1991). Currently, approximately 2000 nurses are employed in rural health centers (USDHHS/ HRSA, 1998). Many other nurses practice in home health care and county or state public health agencies in rural areas.

The term *rural* is somewhat difficult to define. Typically, rural is defined based on geographic location and population density or in terms of distance or time needed to commute to an urban center. In general, rural areas are communities having less than 20,000 residents or fewer than 99 persons per square mile (Bushy, 2000a).

In 13 states, more than 40% of the population live in federally defined rural areas. The states with the greatest percentage of residents in rural areas (based on the 1990 census) are Vermont, West Virginia, Maine, Mississippi, South Dakota, Montana, North Carolina, and New Hampshire (U.S. Census Bureau, 2001). Although significant regional variations occur, several distinctive characteristics are common to rural populations in general that are important to nurses. Box 3-2 compares characteristics of residents of rural and urban settings.

Issues in Rural Health Care

Distance, isolation, and sparse resources are inherent in rural life and rural residents learn to manage these issues through innovative coping strategies (Bushy, 2000b). As with barriers to health care in other settings and populations, barriers to health care for individuals living in rural settings include availability and accessibility to health care providers and institutions, affordability of health care because many residents are uninsured or underinsured, and acceptability. Lack of transportation, inequitable reimbursement policies for providers, weather conditions, lack of understanding of entitlements and services, and lower education levels also contribute to problems for rural residents in obtaining health care.

One critical issue for rural health care is the shortage of nurses in many areas. Indeed, there is an average of 349 nurses per 100,000 persons in counties with fewer than 10,000 residents, compared with an average of 675 nurses per 100,000 persons in all U.S. counties (Turner and Gunn, 1991). In addition, of the 619 counties designated "nurse shortage counties" in 1990, 92.4% were in nonurban areas (ANA, 1996).

Likewise, the high number of hospital closings and shortage of physicians is of concern in many rural areas. Between 1986 and 1988, more than 50% of the hospitals closed were rural hospitals. Some rural communities have a physician-to-population ratio of 53:100,000 versus 163:100,000 for the nation overall. Counties with less than 10,000 inhabitants have about one third of the physician availability of all U.S. counties (Hartwell, Parker, Korn, and Polich, 1991).

BOX **3-2** Comparisons of Rural and Urban Americans

- A higher proportion of whites live in rural areas (82%) than in urban areas (62%) (however, this varies markedly by region).
- Rural communities have higher percentages of younger and older residents.
- Adults in rural areas have fewer years of formal education.
- Rural families tend to be poorer (more than 25% of rural Americans live in or near poverty and nearly 40% of all rural children are impoverished).
- Rural Americans are more likely to be uninsured or underinsured.
- Rural residents are more likely to have chronic illnesses (e.g., hypertension, arthritis, diabetes, cardiovascular disease, cancer).
- Rural residents have higher infant and maternal morbidity and mortality rates.
- Several health care risks are unique to rural occupations (e.g., machinery accidents, skin cancer from exposure to the sun, pulmonary and other problems related to exposure to chemicals and pesticides).
- Rural adults are less likely to have preventative health care (e.g., Pap smears, breast examinations, prostate specific antigen, cholesterol screenings).

Data from Bushy, A. (2000a). Community health nursing in rural environments. In M. Stanhope & J. Lancaster (Eds.), *Community and public health nursing* (5th ed.). St. Louis: Mosby; Bushy, A. (2000b). Rural health. In C. M. Smith & F. A. Maurer (Eds.), *Community health nursing: Theory and practice* (2nd ed.). Philadelphia: W. B. Saunders.

Rural Nursing Practice

Nurses practicing **rural nursing** most often practice in clinic settings, home health, or a combination. Skills needed by nurses in rural settings include technical and clinical competency; adaptability; flexibility; refined assessment skills; organizational abilities; independence; good decision-making skills; leadership ability; self-confidence; and skill in handling emergencies, teaching, and public relations. Box 3-3 presents characteristics of nursing practice in rural settings.

It is important that rural health nurses be willing to be cross-trained and educated to acquire competencies outside their primary specialty area. Rural nurses must also be able to remain current and competent in practice in an environment characterized by sparse resources. Furthermore, it is recommended that all nurses in rural settings have training in trauma care and advanced life support, which may be required to assist in the stabilization of emergency cases. Finally, rural nurses need case management skills for transfer, referral, and coordination of care in areas characterized by the lack of specialized health care resources (Turner and Gunn, 1991).

Education and Experience for Rural Nursing Practice

Nurses who practice in rural settings should have experience in a variety of areas, including rehabilitation, obstetrics, medical-surgical nursing, geriatrics, pediatrics, and emergency care. A knowledge of available resources and ability to coordinate formal and informal services is very important in rural health nursing (Bushy, 2000b).

There are no specific educational recommendations for rural nursing practice. Educational preparation, however, should include public health principles, the process of community assessment, and content in health promotion and illness prevention, which historically has been a component of baccalaureate nursing education. Recently, nursing authorities have recognized the need to consider changes in nursing education to develop curricula at each education level to address the unique needs of rural nursing. In particular, "schools and colleges of nursing which are situated in rural areas, or whose graduates tend to serve rural residents, have an obligation to structure their programs to include rural content and clinical experiences in rural settings" (ANA, 1996, p. 24).

BOX **3-3** Characteristics of Nursing Practice in Rural Environments

- Variety/diversity in clinical experiences
- Broader/expanding scope of practice
- Generalist skills
- Flexibility/creativity in delivering care
- Sparse resources (e.g., materials, professionals, equipment, fiscal)
- Professional/personal isolation
- Greater independence
- More autonomy
- Role overlap with other disciplines
- Slower pace
- Lack of anonymity
- Increased opportunity for informal interactions with patients and co-workers

- Opportunity for client follow-up on discharge in informal community settings
- Discharge planning allows for integration of formal with informal resources
- Care for clients across the life span
- Exposed to clients with a full range of conditions/diagnoses
- Status in the community: Viewed as an occupation of prestige
- Viewed as a professional "role model"
- Opportunity for community involvement and informal health education

From Bushy, A. (2000a). Community health nursing in rural environments. In M. Stanhope & J. Lancaster (Eds.), *Community and public health nursing* (5th ed., pp. 330-348). St. Louis: Mosby.

PARISH NURSING

Parish nursing is both a new and an old model of health care delivery. Indeed, the history of nursing is full of examples of religious orders or congregations providing care for the sick (Schank, Weis, and Matheus, 1996). The concept of modern-day parish nursing in the United States is attributed to a Lutheran chaplain, Granger Westberg, who reportedly advanced the role beginning in 1983 (Miskelly, 1995).

The philosophy of parish nursing is "to promote the health of a faith community (churches or synagogues) by working with the pastor and staff to integrate the theological, psychological, sociological, and physiological perspectives of health and healing into the work, sacrament and services of the congregation" (Solari-Twadell, Djupe, and McDermott, 1990, p. 51). Parish nursing programs are supported by many different denominations. There are thought to be at least 3000 parish nurses practicing in the United States (Siegrist, 2001).

The growing interest in parish nursing is attributed to several factors, including the following:

- Increasing focus on health promotion, disease prevention, and health and illness management.
- Problems of fragmentation of health care and the reemergence of the "wholeness" concept regarding health care.
- Increased emphasis on self-care and individual responsibility.
- Problems with access and cost.
- Increasing numbers of people with chronic illness.
- Recognition of the need to identify and work with people in the community and in institutions (Schank, Weis, and Matheus, 1996).

Miskelly (1995) describes the following four models of parish nursing:

1. Institutional/paid model: The parish nurse is employed by a hospital, community agency, or long-term care facility that provides salary, benefits, support, and supervision and contracts with one or more churches to deliver care.

2. Institutional/volunteer model: A relationship exists between a church and an institution, whereby the institution provides a stipend to the nurse or congregation and/or education and supervision; the nurse(s) are volunteers.

3. Congregational/paid model: The nurse is employed by the congregation and receives benefits and supervision from the church itself.

4. Congregational/volunteer model: The parish health care program is supported by nurses volunteering their time.

Parish Nursing Practice

The goal of parish nursing is the enhancement of quality of life for all members of the congregation (Schank, Weis, and Matheus, 1996). Parish nurses coordinate and train volunteers. They organize and facilitate support groups, provide referrals to community resources, provide health education and counseling, and serve as a liaison within the health care system. In addition, parish nurses provide health education, advocacy, counseling, and screenings. Invasive nursing procedures and/or home health care are not usually components of parish nursing programs.

Through research, several health education needs appropriate for parish nursing care have been identified. These include stress management, development of a durable power of attorney and living wills, nutrition, grief support, cancer risk factors and prevention, CPR training, parenting skills, alcohol abuse, and infertility (Miskelly, 1995). Interventions include health counseling and screening (e.g., cholesterol, blood pressure, skin cancer, occult blood screening), support group facilitation (e.g., grief, parenting, caregiver), education (e.g., stress management, nutrition, exercise, CPR), and community resource referrals (e.g., weight control groups, infertility support groups, violence resources, alcohol abuse support groups). Provision and facilitation of information on health-related topics through use of a monthly newsletter and maintenance of a health section in the church library can be used to disseminate timely information on safety tips, home health care, health insurance, prevention of heart disease, and many other topics (Miskelly, 1995).

The parish nurse should develop the practice and program in response to the unique needs and priorities of the congregation and its members. Leadership, organizational, clinical, counseling, and teaching skills are essential.

Education and Experience for Parish Nursing Practice

A baccalaureate degree is recommended for parish nurses. Three to five years of experience in nursing practice, spiritual maturity, and ability to practice independently are important attributes for a parish nurse (Siegrist, 2001). It is recommended that all parish nurses complete a formal program of study. These are typically offered in universities, hospitals, or established parish nursing programs, and may be taken for college credit, continuing education, or postgraduate certification (Solari-Twadell and McDermott, 1999). (See the Research Highlight "Educational Requirements for Parish Nurses.")

The curriculum for parish nursing courses should be comprehensive. Among others, topics for inclusion are an overview of the role of the church in health care, the history and philosophy of parish nursing, models of parish nursing, and roles and functions of the parish nurse. Other important issues and interventions for parish nurses are community assessment, health-promotion concepts, philosophy of self-care, legal and ethical issues (i.e., confidentiality, accountability, documentations, and end-of-life issues), how to be a part of a ministerial team, and how to start a parish nursing program (International Parish Nurse Resource Center, 1998).

CORRECTIONAL INSTITUTIONS

According to Droes, "The number of individuals incarcerated in the United States is the highest since data were first available in 1925" (1994, p. 201). In the United States, the judicial system has mandated that correctional facilities have the responsibility to provide health care to all individuals confined to their facilities (Hufft and Fawkes, 1994). In many cases, nurses are the primary health care providers in correctional facilities. Currently, approximately 9000 RNs work in correctional institutions, including jails, prisons, and juvenile detention facilities (USDHHS/Health Resources and Services Administration, Bureau of Health Professions/Division of Nursing [HRSA/BHP/DON], 1998).

Issues in Caring for Persons in Correctional Facilities

In general, members of ethnic and racial minorities and people from lower socioeconomic groups are disproportionally represented in

---

Research Highlight

Educational Requirements for Parish Nurses

McDermott, Solari-Twadell, and Matheus (1998) conducted a longitudinal study that examined education for parish nurses. Findings showed that at least 52 educational courses are offered for parish nurses in the United States. Of these, 12 were university based (primarily in schools of nursing), one was based in a seminary, and 32 were sponsored by health care institutions. Other educational programs were provided through parish nurse networks or congregational sponsors.

From their study, the researchers drafted guidelines for educating parish nurses to help regulate the process. To this end they made a number of recommendations on the course content for programs. Among others, recommended topics for parish nurse preparation programs were budget development, grant writing, marketing, human resource management, orientation, program evaluation, documentation, working with volunteers, and networking.

From McDermott, M. A., Solari-Twadell, P. A., & Matheus, R. (1998). Promoting quality education for the parish nurse and the parish nurse coordinator. *Nursing and Health Care Perspectives, 19*(1), 4-6.

correctional facilities. Additionally, residents of correctional institutions experience a higher rate of diseases and disability than the general population. Infectious diseases (e.g., respiratory infections, influenza, gonorrhea, tuberculosis, hepatitis, and human immunodeficiency virus [HIV]), conditions related to the use and abuse of drugs and alcohol, seizure disorders, and acute mental health problems are particularly common. Trauma and chronic problems such as cirrhosis of the liver, gastritis, pancreatitis, and cardiac pathology are also prevalent (Powell, 2001).

One of the many distinctive characteristics of providing health care in correctional facilities is that clients usually have no choice in the selection of the health care providers and may have no choice in the services provided. Likewise, a great deal of professionalism is needed for **correctional nursing**, in that providers in prison settings must have the ability to separate the action of the crime or offense of the individual inmate from his or her illness or health care needs (Hufft and Fawkes, 1994).

Nursing Practice in Correctional Facilities

Health services in correctional settings vary from health screening to full hospital services. In general, the main component of nursing practice

in correctional facilities is the provision of primary care and emergency services for the inmates. Primary health care in these facilities typically includes screening activities, direct health care services, analysis of individual health behaviors, teaching and counseling, and assisting individuals in assuming responsibility for their own health (ANA, 1995) (see the Community Application box).

Because of the situation and population encountered in this type of nursing practice, client needs and related nursing interventions in correctional facilities are quite unique. The ANA (1985) described the following specific interventions:

- Health education: Promotion of individual and group well-being through health education activities (e.g., health counseling, health teaching, and formal programs in health education).
- Suicide prevention: Ongoing assessment of suicide risk and planning and coordination of interventions that prevent suicidal behaviors.
- Communicable disease control: Promotion of a healthful environment to reduce the incidence of communicable disease within the correctional setting.
- Alcohol and drug rehabilitation: Collaboration with other members of the health care

---

COMMUNITY APPLICATION
Nursing in Correctional Facilities

The CDC (2001b) described changes in health care delivery at a correctional facility following an outbreak of hepatitis B (HBV) among inmates. It was reported that in one of the prison's dormitories, 23 of 97 inmates were discovered to have either chronic HBV infection, acute infection, or resolved infection. Following that discovery, HBV testing was offered to all inmates (a total of 1247). Of those tested, almost 20% had either acute, chronic, or resolved HBV infection. The study also identified risk behaviors among the inmates. These included injecting drugs, having sex with another inmate, using a razor that

had been used by another inmate, and receiving a tattoo in prison.

To control the outbreak, the state's department of corrections offered HBV vaccination to all susceptible inmates. Also, acutely and chronically infected inmates were notified of their infection status and each received a clinical assessment and treatment as appropriate; postexposure prophylaxis was provided to their contacts. Finally, the state's department of health and department of corrections are collaborating to implement routine HBV vaccination for all inmates in the correctional system.

From Centers for Disease Control and Prevention. (2001b). Hepatitis B outbreak in a state correctional facility, 2000. *MMWR Morbid Mortal Wkly Rep, 50*(25), 529-532.

team to treat inmates who have substance abuse problems.

- Medication administration: Supervision of the administration of medications in accordance with state regulations and national standards.
- Psychosocial counseling: Provision of crisis intervention and episodic and ongoing psychosocial counseling.
- Emergency care: Initiation of emergency care as needed, according to community standards of care.
- Environmental health: Ongoing monitoring of the environment for conditions that would have a negative impact on health and safety within the facility and reporting of significant findings to the institution's management.

Nurses who work in correctional facilities must work toward the goal of preserving and promoting the health of the incarcerated individual within the institution's broader goal of security. However, it is important to note that these nurses should provide only health care services—it is inappropriate for nurses to be involved in the security functions or disciplinary decisions of the setting (e.g., conducting body cavity or strip searches) (ANA, 1995). The institution should have a well developed and periodically revised set of policies and procedures developed jointly by nurses, physicians, prisoners, and institution personnel (Stevens, 1993).

Education and Experience Recommendations for Nursing Practice in Correctional Facilities

Experience in mental health nursing is desirable for nurses who wish to practice in correctional facilities. Likewise, experience in emergency services, medical/surgical nursing, and community or public health nursing is also very beneficial. Educationally, the ANA recommends a baccalaureate degree in nursing for the practice of nursing in correctional facilities (ANA, 1985). Finally, because of the unique characteristics described here, Stevens (1993) suggests that "nurses considering this practice setting should first observe a colleague who practices in the setting" (p. 6).

NURSING PRACTICE WITH SELECTED POPULATIONS

In contrast to the provision of care to individuals and families in geographical settings, organizations, clinics, or agencies, community-based nursing care often involves caring for individuals or families undergoing directed care to treat specified illnesses or to prevent certain illnesses or health threats. Practice in these settings is often limited to single encounters to provide treatment or preventative services (e.g., day surgery, immunizations, STD treatment) or multiple visits providing care for a chronic illness (e.g., ambulatory oncology, tuberculosis management, renal dialysis). This section describes nursing practice in specialized, community-based settings.

PUBLIC HEALTH DEPARTMENTS

Public health departments safeguard the health of the public and improve the health status of the community. Local health departments are given the authority by the state to protect the health and welfare of their residents and are funded through local taxes and fees and grants from their state and federal sources.

Approximately 3000 local health departments exist in the United States. Of these, 66% serve populations of less than 50,000, 46% have fewer than 10 full-time employees, and 10% have 100 or more employees. Additionally, 90% of local health departments employ RNs (either directly or through contracted services) (Maurer, 2000). State, county, and local health departments combined employ approximately 44,000 RNs (about 2.5% of all RNs) (USDHHS/HRSA/BHP/DON, 2001).

The scope of services provided by public health departments varies considerably across the country. In general, health departments have traditionally been responsible for environmental sanitation, communicable disease surveillance and prevention, and other services to prevent illness and promote health. Public health efforts include a variety of services and interventions, such as regulation of water and air quality; solid waste disposal; supervision of restaurants, grocery stores, and other food processors and handlers; and control of vectors that might spread disease (e.g., mosquitoes, rats).

To control communicable diseases, health departments are required to monitor them (see Chapter 16) and are usually involved in their prevention as well. This often includes provision of immunizations; easily accessible (affordable) treatment for STDs; and screening, diagnosis, and treatment of certain communicable diseases such as tuberculosis, AIDS, and Hansen's disease. In addition to these programs, again varying greatly by area, many public health departments provide prenatal and family planning services, well-baby care, community mental health services, and home health care.

Public Health Nursing Practice

Nursing practice in public health departments varies greatly, depending on the nurse's assigned area. Much of **public health nursing** practice focusing on control of communicable disease is described in detail in Chapter 16. Home health, family planning, maternal child health, and community mental health are covered in Chapters 4, 11, and 15, respectively. The reader is referred to those chapters to learn more about public health nursing practice.

Education and Experience Recommendations for Public Health Nurses

Because public health theory and practice are included in baccalaureate nursing programs, a baccalaureate degree in nursing is preferred by most health departments. However, most nurses currently working in public health departments were educated in diploma or associate-degree programs.

One or more years of nursing experience is often required for employment in public health departments. Practical experience in maternal and child health, primary health care, mental health care, infection control, and management of clients with HIV and AIDS is particularly helpful in public health nursing.

AMBULATORY ONCOLOGY CARE

According to Lin and Martin (1994), "over 80% of all cancer care is delivered in the outpatient setting" (p. 227). Sites for delivery of care and some services offered for patients with cancer include the following:
- Physicians' offices: Services may include chemotherapy administration, procedures, laboratory and x-ray facilities, counseling, and educational programs.
- Outpatient clinics: Services performed include radiation therapy, chemotherapy, biotherapy, physician and psychosocial services, symptom control, bone marrow transplantation, and rehabilitation.
- Twenty-three-hour and 24-hour clinics and day hospitals: These provide urgent care and may include an emergency room for oncology patients, an outpatient procedure unit, observation, an investigational treatment area, an after-hours telephone triage center, and on-call physician support (Lamkin, 1994).

The following health care services are related to care of oncology patients:
- Prevention, screening, and detection
- Chemotherapy
- Radiation therapy
- Blood component therapy
- Patient and family education
- Discharge planning and referral
- Nutritional support
- Group or individual counseling
- Physical therapy and rehabilitation
- Outpatient surgery
- Prescription supply and procurement
- Survivor services
- Treatment planning
- Symptom management (Lamkin, 1994)

Nursing Practice in Ambulatory Oncology Settings

Nursing interventions in **ambulatory oncology nursing practice** include client counseling (e.g., client advocacy, emotional support during visitations and by telephone), health care maintenance (e.g., general assessment of health, assessment of compliance, measurement of physiological indices), primary care (e.g., triage in person or by telephone, obtaining client history, performing physical examination), client education (e.g., group educational programs, explanation of plan of care, reinforcement of physician instructions), therapeutic care (e.g., administration of treatments such as irrigations, dressing changes, specimen collection; administration of medications), normative care (e.g., preparing client for physician, assisting physician, providing follow-up appointment), nonclient-centered care (e.g., maintaining supplies and equipment, developing educational materials and standards of care for staff, maintaining knowledge of new care practice), communication (e.g., providing information to other health care providers regarding client care issues), and documentation and planning (Cooley, Lin, and Hunter, 1994).

Ambulatory oncology nurses often provide telephone triage, which includes follow-up, symptom management, patient education, scheduling appointments and tests, and contacting physicians to discuss patient care issues. Well-defined assessment skills, incorporating physical, psychosocial, and financial aspects, are the cornerstone of practice (Cooley, Lin, and Hunter, 1994).

Client and family education is essential to accomplish one important goal of outpatient oncology care: to prepare the client for self-care. Client education needs include treatment options, information about specific treatments and diagnostic tests, symptom management, nutrition, pharmacology, accessing social services, technical skills (e.g., caring for catheters, central lines, self-injection), and how and when to access assistance when needed (Lamkin, 1994).

Education, Certification, Experience, and Recommendations for Ambulatory Oncology Nurses

Nurses who practice in ambulatory oncology centers should have at least 1 year of clinical experience in oncology or chronic illness. They must have good clinical skills, be certified in CPR, and be able to handle emergency situations.

Certification in oncology nursing is available at three different levels: (1) oncology certified nurse (ONC), (2) certification in pediatric oncology (CPON), and (3) advanced oncology certified nurse (AOCN) for those with graduate degrees (Oncology Nursing Certification Corporation, 2001). Some agencies require baccalaureate-level preparation (Cooley, Lin, and Hunter, 1994).

AMBULATORY SURGERY

Ambulatory surgery refers to the process in which "patients have surgery, recover, and are discharged home the same day" (Groah, 1996, p. 367). Ambulatory surgery is not a new concept (it reportedly dates back to ancient Egypt), but it has increased dramatically in recent years because of advances in anesthesia and surgical techniques and a desire for convenience and cost containment. Indeed, it is estimated that almost 30 million ambulatory surgical procedures are performed each year in the United States (Fortunato, 2000).

Cost containment is one of the primary reasons for the proliferation in same-day surgical procedures. Indeed, many third-party payers require that certain procedures be done on an outpatient basis unless documentation can be provided that this would be unsafe for the patient (Mezey and Lawrence, 1995). To determine eligibility for having a surgical procedure performed on an ambulatory basis, considerations should include general health status (patients should be evaluated to determine possibility of complications during and after the surgical procedure), results of preoperative tests (e.g., laboratory tests, chest x-ray, electrocardiogram), willingness and acceptance by the patient and family (including provision for competent care at home), anticipated recovery period, and reimbursement sources (Fortunato, 2000).

Several terms can be used to describe ambulatory surgical care facilities. These include outpatient surgery centers, same-day surgical units, one-day surgery centers, or ambulatory surgery centers. Several different organizational structures are available for ambulatory surgery facilities, including the following:

- Hospital-based dedicated unit: Patients are admitted to an autonomous, independent, self-contained unit within or attached to the hospital, but physically separated from the inpatient operating room suite.
- Hospital-based integrated unit: Patients share the same operating room suite and other hospital facilities with inpatients, but have a separate preoperative holding area.
- Hospital-affiliated satellite surgery center: Patients are cared for at an ambulatory surgery center owned and operated by the hospital, but are physically separated from it.
- Freestanding ambulatory surgery center: Patients are cared for at a totally independent facility that is privately owned and operated for the purpose of providing surgical care.
- Office-based center: Patients are seen at a physician's office that is equipped for surgery. Many general surgeons, dermatologists, plastic surgeons, periodontists, podiatrists, and others perform surgical procedures in their offices (Fortunato, 2000).

Freestanding postsurgical recovery centers provide short nonhospital stays for less-intensive recovery and for less-complex surgical cases (Williams, 1999). These centers are designed for individuals who are otherwise well, but may need monitoring or services that cannot be easily, safely, or economically provided in the home. For example, a patient who has undergone extensive plastic surgery may need to be monitored for a day or two and treated for pain and to prevent complications (e.g., infection), but may not require hospitalization. For this person, a short stay in a recovery center would be appropriate. Likewise, if a day surgery patient has no one to provide care at home, an overnight stay in a recovery center might help avoid an otherwise unnecessary hospitalization.

Advantages of ambulatory surgery include decreased cost to the patient and institution, increased bed availability for seriously ill patients, decreased risk of acquiring a nosocomial infec-

tion, and less disruption to the patient's personal life (Fairchild, 1996). Disadvantages include increased anxiety of the patient and caregiver, complications (e.g., allergic responses to drugs and anesthetics, prolonged procedures, secondary diagnosis), and unrealistic patient expectations of physical capabilities postoperatively. Occasionally, patients require hospitalization because of prolonged procedures, secondary diagnosis, surgical accident, or other complications (e.g., excessive pain, nausea and vomiting, bleeding, swelling) (Fortunato, 2000). Contraindications to ambulatory surgery include patients who are physically unstable, morbidly obese, acute substance abusers, or individuals who do not have adequate support at home (Groah, 1996). Box 3-4 lists surgical procedures commonly performed on an outpatient basis.

Nursing Practice in Ambulatory Surgery

Nursing care during ambulatory surgery is typically provided in three phases: (1) preoperative care, (2) intraoperative care, and (3) postanesthesia care.

PREOPERATIVE CARE. In the preoperative phase, the patient is admitted to the facility, given preoperative instructions, and prepared for the procedure. Any tests that have been performed in preparation are reviewed and other tests may be performed at that time. The nurse conducts a preoperative interview to verify information about past medical and surgical history, the pending procedure(s), current medications, drug allergies, and other pertinent information (e.g., whether the patient wears contact lenses or has dental work or any prostheses). The nurse confirms that any instructions regarding eating or drinking before admission have been followed.

The nurse then allows the patient to change into a gown and escorts him or her to the holding area, where baseline vital signs are taken (Figure 3-1). In the holding area, the patient may be given preoperative medications and further prepared for the procedure (e.g., the operative site may be shaved or an intravenous line started). Agency protocol determines how the

BOX **3-4** Commonly Performed Outpatient Procedures

GYNECOLOGY

Conization of cervix
Dilation and curettage
Salpingectomy
Hymenal ring lesion excision
Salpingogram
Therapeutic abortion
Tubal ligation
Hymenotomy
Examination under anesthesia
Culdoscopy
Vaginoplasty
Minilaparotomy
Bartholin cyst excision

ORTHOPEDIC SURGERY

Arthroscopy
Nail removal
Cast change
Ligament repair
Metacarpal wire removal
Plate (bone) removal
Ganglion excision
Ulnar nerve transplant
Median nerve decompression
Release de Quervain's fracture
Release Dupuytren's contracture
Release trigger thumb
Fracture reduction
Bunionectomy
Excision exostosis
Bursa removal
Tendon repair

OPHTHALMOLOGY

Eye cyst excision
Examination under anesthesia
Cataract procedures

Ptosis
Tear duct probe
Enucleation
Eyelid surgery
Eye muscle surgery
Chalazion
Iridectomy

THORACIC SURGERY

Esophageal dilation
Pacemaker battery replacement

NEUROSURGERY

Carpal tunnel release
Median nerve decompression
Ulnar nerve transfer

DENTAL/ORAL SURGERY

Dental extraction
Curettage of maxilla
Intraoral biopsy
Closed reduction jaw fracture

OTOLARYNGOLOGY

Nasopharyngoscopy
Nasal septum repair
Otoplasty
Tonsillectomy and adenoidectomy
Adenoidectomy
Bronchoscopy and laryngoscopy
Nasal fracture reduction
Foreign body removed from ear

PLASTIC SURGERY

Augmental mammoplasty
Nose reduction
Blepharoplasty
Skin grafts

Redundant tissue removal
Basal cell carcinoma excision
Contracture release
Ganglionectomy
Otoplasty
Scar revision
Tendon repair

GENERAL SURGERY

Breast biopsy
Laryngoscopy
Esophagoscopy
Gastroscopy
Endoscopy
Node biopsies
Herniorrhaphy
Lipoma removal
Nevus removal
Lesion excision
Polyp excision
Bronchoscopy
Brachial arteriogram
Pilonidal cyst excision
Debridement
Hemorrhoidectomy
Abscess incision and drainage
Sigmoidoscopy

UROLOGY

Cystogram and pyelogram
Biopsy bladder tumor
Transurethral resection
Circumcision
Vasectomy
Cystoscopy
Orchiectomy
Prostate biopsy
Testicular biopsy

Adapted from Katz, R. (1987). Issues in outpatient surgery. *Seminars in Anesthesiology,* 258. From Fairchild, S. S. (1996). Topics and issues affecting practice. In S. S. Fairchild (Ed.), *Perioperative nursing: Principles and practice* (2nd ed.). Boston: Little, Brown & Co.

consent forms for surgery and other paperwork are completed and who is responsible. The nurse should ensure that all consent forms are complete and accurate.

INTRAOPERATIVE CARE. As with perioperative nursing care in the hospital, the intraoperative team usually consists of a circulating nurse, a scrub nurse, an anesthesiologist or certified registered nurse-anesthetist (CRNA), and the surgeon.

Often the surgeon has an assistant. In most agencies, it is the responsibility of the circulating nurse to ensure that the procedure runs smoothly. The circulating nurse typically retrieves the patient from preoperative holding when the anesthesiologist or CRNA is ready. The circulating nurse assists the scrub nurse and the anesthesiologist or CRNA with their preparatory work while helping reduce the patient's anxiety.

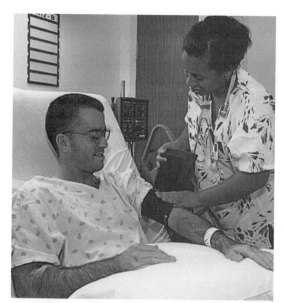

Figure 3-1. Nurse taking the blood pressure of a patient before surgery in an ambulatory surgical facility. (Courtesy Rick Brady, Photographer, Riva, Maryland.)

Both the circulating nurse and the scrub nurse assist the surgeon throughout the procedure. At the end of the procedure, the circulating nurse attends the anesthesiologist or CRNA while the patient awakens if general anesthetic is used. The circulating nurse assists the patient to a stretcher (a wheelchair may be used for procedures done under local or regional anesthesia) and takes the patient to the postanesthesia care area.

POSTANESTHESIA CARE AND DISCHARGE. Following the procedure, the patient is taken to the designated PACU or recovery area for observation; for management of pain, nausea, and vomiting; and to ensure maintenance of fluid and electrolyte balance. In the PACU, the vital signs are taken periodically, and the patient is monitored for complications related to surgery, anesthesia, or the presenting health condition.

Discharge is based on the absence of indications of serious complications (e.g., bleeding, unusual pain), when the patient is alert and able to walk safely, and a responsible person is in attendance. Discharge criteria include the patient being alert and oriented and having

stable vital signs; no respiratory distress; no hoarseness or cough following endotracheal intubation; a gag reflex; ability to swallow and cough; no dizziness, nausea, or vomiting; no bleeding and minimal swelling or drainage on dressings; ability to tolerate fluids and having been able to void; no excessive pain that will not be alleviated with oral medications at home; ability to ambulate (based on developmental age or physical limitations); capable of self-care or accompanied by a responsible adult and appropriate mode of transportation (Fortunato, 2000).

The PACU nurse is usually responsible for reviewing postprocedure instructions with the patient and the caregiver(s). It is essential that they be aware of signs and symptoms of complications and when to call the surgeon or go to the hospital. Instructions should also include pain management, bathing instructions, wound care (if applicable), activity limitations, diet, and the importance of a follow-up appointment with the surgeon. Instructions should be written and explicit to ensure that they are easily understood (Groah, 1996).

Experience, Education, and Certification for Ambulatory Surgery Nursing Practice

There are no specific educational requirements for RNs practicing in ambulatory care surgery. However, many ambulatory surgery centers require a minimum of 1 year of experience in either the operating room or postanesthesia care.

Certification in operating room nursing care is definitely an advantage. The Association of Operating Room Nurses (AORN) grants certification through the Certification Board of Perioperative Nursing to qualifying operating room nurses and RN first assistants.

NURSING CARE IN "OTHER" AMBULATORY SETTINGS

Additional settings in which nurses are employed in community-based practice are nursing in poison control centers, ambulatory diagnostic centers (e.g., outpatient imaging and radiology services for diagnosis and treatment), community hotlines (e.g., suicide, AIDS, drug and alcohol abuse, family violence), summer camps, and migrant health centers. Nurses who desire to practice in nonacute care settings should be alert to the variety of opportunities. For more information, see the Resources box at the end of the chapter that lists organizations for the various ambulatory settings described in this chapter.

SUMMARY

Most health care is provided to clients who are not inpatients in health care facilities. Indeed, the majority of care is provided in ambulatory settings. Increasingly, in addition to services such as health-promotion and illness-prevention interventions, which have traditionally been provided in community settings, many surgical procedures, chemotherapy, and diagnostic procedures are taking place in ambulatory settings. As a result, many nurses, such as Bill, the PACU nurse from the case study, are needed to fill positions in these areas.

The type and practice of nurses in ambulatory settings are incredibly variable. Settings include health care offices or clinics, schools, occupational settings, rural health clinics, parish practices, correctional facilities, public health departments, ambulatory oncology centers, and many others. The practice and focus of the nurses in ambulatory settings is wide and whatever their area of specialization or interest, nurse are encouraged to examine opportunities to work in ambulatory settings.

Resources

Ambulatory Health Care Nursing

Ambulatory Care Nursing
American Academy of Ambulatory Care Nursing

Ambulatory Oncology Nursing
Oncology Nursing Society
Oncology Nursing Certification Corporation
American Cancer Society
National Cancer Institute

Ambulatory Surgery
Association of Operating Room Nurses
American Society of Perianesthesia Nurses

Occupational Health Nursing
American Association of Occupational Health
    Nurses
Occupational Safety and Health Administration
National Safety Council

Parish Nursing
International Parish Nursing Resource Center
Health Ministries Association
Marquette University Parish Nurse Institute

Public Health Nursing
American Public Health Association
Centers for Disease Control and Prevention

School Nursing
American School Health Association
National Association of School Nurses

Rural Nursing
Department of Agriculture/Office of Community
    and Rural Development
Department of Health and Human Services/
    Office of Rural Health Policy
National Rural Health Association

Visit the book's website at
www.wbsaunders.com/SIMON/McEwen
for a direct link to the website for each
organization listed.

KEY POINTS

- Ambulatory care refers to personal health care or health services (e.g., outpatient surgery and chemotherapy, diagnostic tests and procedures) provided to noninstitutionalized patients.
- Ambulatory nursing care is largely focused on health promotion, primary prevention, screening for early identification of disease, and assisting in treatment regimens for both acute and chronic illnesses. Care is usually ongoing and comprehensive.
- About 9.5% of all RNs practice in a health care office or clinic (with a provider such as a physician, nurse practitioner, or physician

assistant). Clinic or office nurses assist with assessments and procedures, provide education, collect specimens, and administer medications. Coordination of services and preparation of patients for procedures are other roles and responsibilities.

- Currently, about 2.2% of all RNs are school nurses. School nurses work to prevent illnesses, intervene in identified problems, promote healthy lifestyles, and provide health education. Caring for students with special health needs (e.g., urinary catheterization, tube feedings, tracheotomy care) is becoming increasingly common.

- Occupational health nurses provide health care services to workers, focusing on health promotion and protection from injury and illness within the context of a safe and healthy work environment. Occupational health nurses provide assessment of the environment for threats to health and safety, assessment of the health status of workers, nursing care for occupational and nonoccupational injuries and illnesses, counseling, and health education. Several laws directly affect the practice of the occupational health nurses. These include Workers' Compensation Acts and the Occupational Safety and Health Act.

- Delivery of nursing and health care to clients in rural areas has a number of distinctive characteristics and challenges. Distance, isolation, and sparse resources, combined with shortage of nurses and other health care providers in rural areas, are particular challenges. Rural nurses must be clinically competent in a very broad number of areas and are typically cross-trained to manage client needs in areas including trauma, routine obstetrical care, care of children and elders, and care of clients with mental health needs.

- Parish nurses seek to promote the health of a community (centered in a church or synagogue) by integration of theological, psychological, sociological, and physiological perspectives of health. Parish nurses work to enhance the quality of life for members of a congregation and often the surrounding neighborhood. Parish nursing interventions include organization of support groups, provision of referrals to community resources, health education, counseling, and acting as a liaison within the larger health care system.

- The U.S. government requires health care services for all inmates in correctional facilities. As a result, approximately 9000 RNs work in jails, prisons, and juvenile detention facilities. The main component of nursing practice in correctional facilities is provision of primary care and emergency services for the inmates.

- Approximately 44,000 nurses practice in local, county, and state public health departments. Depending on mandates of the individual locality, health departments are responsible for diverse areas, including environmental sanitation, communicable disease surveillance and prevention, and maternal and child health.

- Ambulatory oncology care allows cancer patients to receive diagnosis and treatment as outpatients. Nurses may care for oncology clients in physicians' offices, outpatient clinics, and day hospitals. Health care services may include prevention, screening, chemotherapy, radiation therapy, education, discharge planning, nutritional support, counseling, and outpatient surgery.

- More than half of all surgical procedures can be performed on an ambulatory basis; thus, nursing in outpatient surgical centers continues to grow. Nurses who work in outpatient surgical centers may provide preoperative care, intraoperative care, or postanesthesia care. Preoperative care involves giving the patient and family preoperative instructions and preparing them for the procedure. Intraoperative nursing consists of acting as circulating nurse; scrub nurse; or, in some cases, first assistant during the surgical procedure. During postanesthesia care, the nurse observes the patient for complications, manages complications and side effects (e.g., nausea, pain), and prepares him or her for discharge.

Learning Activities & Application to Practice

In Class

1. Interview a nurse who practices in an ambulatory setting. What roles and responsibilities does the nurse have? What are common interventions? Describe positive and negative aspects of practice. What are education and experience requirements? What are employment opportunities, work hours, and salaries? Share findings with the class.

In Clinical

2. Spend one or more days in one or more of the ambulatory settings described. If possible, select an acute or chronic care setting (e.g., ambulatory surgery, oncology) and a primary care setting (e.g., physician office, school, parish nursing). In a log or journal, compare and contrast nursing practice in the two settings.

REFERENCES

Adams, C. (2001). Promoting and protecting the health of adults and the working population. In J. A. Allender & B. W. Spradley (Eds.), *Community health nursing: Concepts and practice* (5th ed., pp. 581-599). Philadelphia: Lippincott.

American Academy of Ambulatory Care Nursing (AAACN). (2000). *Ambulatory care nursing administration and practice standards.* Pitman, NJ: American Academy of Ambulatory Care Nursing.

American Association of Occupational Health Nurses (AAOHN). (1999). *Standards of occupational and environmental health nursing.* Atlanta, GA: American Association of Occupational Health Nurses.

American Board for Occupational Health Nurses (ABOHN). (2001). *Certification eligibility.* Retrieved 07/07/2001 from http://www.abohn.org.

American Nurses' Association. (1985). *Standards of nursing practice in correctional facilities.* Kansas City, MO: American Nurses' Association.

American Nurses' Association. (1995). *Scope and standards of nursing practice in correctional facilities.* Washington, DC: American Nurses' Association.

American Nurses' Association. (1996). *Rural/frontier nursing: The challenge to grow.* Washington, DC: American Nurses' Association.

American School Health Association. (2001). Retrieved 07/10/2001 from http://www.ashaweb.org.

Bushy, A. (2000a). Community health nursing in rural environments. In M. Stanhope & J. Lancaster (Eds.), *Community health nursing: Promoting the health of aggregates, families and individuals* (5th ed., pp. 330-340). St. Louis: Mosby.

Bushy, A. (2000b). Rural health. In C. M. Smith & F. A. Maurer (Eds.), *Community health nursing: Theory and practice* (2nd ed., pp. 870-898). Philadelphia: W. B. Saunders.

Centers for Disease Control and Prevention. (2001a). Fatal occupational injuries—United States, 1980-1997. *MMWR Morbid Mortal Wkly Rep, 50*(16), 317-320.

Centers for Disease Control and Prevention. (2001b). Hepatitis B outbreak in a state correctional facility, 2000. *MMWR Morbid Mortal Wkly Rep, 50*(25), 529-532.

Clemen-Stone, S., Eigsti, D. G., & McGuire, S. L. (1995). *Comprehensive community health nursing* (4th ed.). St. Louis: Mosby.

Cooley, M. E., Lin, E. M., & Hunter, S. W. (1994). The ambulatory oncology nurse's role. *Seminars in Oncology Nursing 10*(4), 245-253.

Droes, N. S. (1994). Correctional nursing practice. *Journal of Community Health Nursing 11*(4), 201-210.

Fairchild, S. S. (1996). Topics and issues affecting practice. In S. S. Fairchild (Ed.), *Perioperative nursing: Principles and practice* (2nd ed., pp. 634-640). Boston: Little, Brown & Co.

Fortunato, N. H. (2000). Ambulatory surgery. In N. H. Fortunato (Ed.), *Berry & Kohn's operating room technique* (9th ed., pp. 161-167). St. Louis: Mosby.

Groah, L. K. (1996). Ambulatory surgery. In L. K. Groah, *Perioperative nursing* (3rd ed., pp. 367-375). Stamford, CT: Appleton & Lange.

Hackbarth, D. P., Haas, S. A., Kavanagh, J. A., & Vlasses, F. (1995). Dimensions of the staff nurse role in ambulatory care: Part I—Methodology and analysis of data on current staff nurse practice. *Nursing Economics, 13*(2), 89-98.

Hartwell, S., Parker, M., Korn, K., & Polich, C. L. (1991). Rural health care delivery and financing: Results of eight case studies. In A. Bushy (Ed.), *Rural nursing* (pp. 128-140). Newbury Park, CA: Sage Publications.

Hootman, J. (1998). Only the best will do for our children! *School Health Newsletter,* Winter/Spring 1998. Retrieved 07/12/2001 from http://www.school-health.org/research.html.

Hufft, A. G., & Fawkes, L. S. (1994). Federal inmates: A unique psychiatric nursing challenge. *Nursing Clinics of North America, 29*(1), 35-41.

International Parish Nurse Resource Center. (1998). *Role of the parish nurse, mission and resources.* Ridge Park, IL: International Parish Nurse Resource Center.

Kub, J., & Steel, S. A. (1995). School health. In C. M. Smith & F. A. Maurer (Eds.), *Community health nursing: Theory and practice* (pp. 747-775). Philadelphia, W. B. Saunders.

Lamkin, L. (1994). Outpatient oncology settings: A variety of services. *Seminars in Oncology Nursing, 10*(4), 229-235.

Lewis, K. D. & Thomson, H. B. (1986). *Manual of school health.* Menlo Park, CA: Addison-Wesley.

Maurer, F. A. (2000). State and local health departments. In C. M. Smith & F. A. Maurer (Eds.), *Community health nursing: Theory and practice* (2nd ed., pp. 91-112). Philadelphia: W. B. Saunders.

McDermott, M. A., Solari-Twadell, P. A., & Matheus, R. (1998). Promoting quality education for the parish nurse and the parish nurse coordinator. *Nursing and Health Care Perspectives, 19*(1), 4-6.

Mezey, A. P., & Lawrence, R. S. (1995). Ambulatory care. In A. R. Kovner (Ed.), *Jonas's health care delivery in the United States* (5th ed., pp. 122-161). New York: Springer Publishing Co.

Miskelly, S. (1995). A parish nursing model: Applying the community health nursing process in a church community. *Journal of Community Health Nursing, 12*(1), 1-14.

National Association of School Nurses. (1992). *Vision screening guidelines for school nurses.* Scarborough, ME: National Association of School Nurses.

National Association of School Nurses. (1993). *Hearing screening guidelines for school nurses.* Scarborough, ME: National Association of School Nurses.

Oncology Nursing Certification Corporation. (2001). Certification requirements for oncology nurses. Retrieved 01/21/2002 from http://www.oncc.org.

Pollitt, P. (1994). Lina Rogers Struthers: The first school nurse. *Journal of School Nursing, 10*(1), 34-36.

Powell, J. (2001). Correctional health. In M. A. Nies & M. McEwen (Eds.), *Community health nursing: Promoting the health of populations* (pp. 761-771). Philadelphia: W. B. Saunders.

Rogers, B. (1994). *Occupational health nursing: Concepts and practice.* Philadelphia: W. B. Saunders.

Rogers, B., & Travers, P. H. (2001). Occupational health. In M. A. Nies & M. McEwen (Eds.), *Community health nursing: Promoting the health of populations* (pp. 730-760). Philadelphia: W. B. Saunders.

Schank, M. J., Weis, D., & Matheus, R. (1996). Parish nursing: Ministry of healing. *Geriatric Nursing, 17*(1), 11-13.

Siegrist, B. C. (2001). Parish health. In M. A. Nies & M. McEwen (Eds.), *Community health nursing: Promoting the health of populations* (3rd ed.). Philadelphia: W. B. Saunders.

Solari-Twadell, P. A., & McDermott, M. A. (1999). *Parish nursing: Promoting whole person health within faith communities.* Thousand Oaks, CA: Sage.

Solari-Twadell, P., Djupe, A., & McDermott, M. (Eds.), (1990). *Parish nursing: The developing practice.* Park Ridge, IL: National Parish Nurse Resource Center.

Stevens, R. (1993). When your clients are in jail. *Nursing Forum, 28*(4), 5-8.

Turner, T. A., & Gunn, I. P. (1991). Issues in rural health nursing. In A. Bushy (Ed.), *Rural nursing* (pp. 107-127). Newbury Park, CA: Sage Publications.

U.S. Census Bureau (2001). Urban criteria for census 2000. Retrieved 07/09/2001 from www.census.gov/geo/www/ua/ua_2k.html.

U.S. Department of Health and Human Services. (2000). *Healthy people 2010: National health promotion and disease prevention objectives.* Washington, DC: Government Printing Office.

U.S. Department of Health and Human Services/Health Resources and Services Administration, Bureau of Health Professions/Division of Nursing. (2001). *The registered nurse population, March 2000.* Rockville, MD: Government Printing Office.

U.S. Department of Health and Human Services/Health Resources and Services Administration, Bureau of Health Professions/Division of Nursing. (1998). *The registered nurse population: Findings from the sample survey of registered nurses, March, 1996.* Rockville, MD: Government Printing Office.

U.S. Preventative Services Task Force. (1996). *Guide to clinical preventive services* (2nd ed.). Washington, DC: U.S. Department of Health and Human Services.

Weinert, C., & Long, K. A. (1991). The theory and research base for rural nursing practice. In A. Bushy (Ed.), *Rural nursing* (pp. 21-38). Newbury Park, CA: Sage Publications.

Williams, S. J. (1999). Ambulatory health care services. In S. J. Williams & P. R. Torrens (Eds.), *Introduction to health services* (5th ed., pp. 227-256). Albany, NY: Delmar Publishers.

Home Health Care Nursing

objectives

Upon
completion of
this chapter,
the reader will
be able to:

1. Discuss home health care nursing and explain its connection to other types of nursing practice.

2. Explain the impact of Medicare regulations on home health nursing.

3. Describe the importance of documentation in home health nursing.

4. Discuss skills and knowledge necessary for the home health nurse including discharge planning, case management, coordination of community resources, and interdisciplinary collaboration.

5. Explain the three stages of a home visit.

6. Discuss different types of specialized home health nursing including infusion therapy, chronic wound care, perinatal home care, psychiatric home care, and hospice care.

key terms

Case management
Conditions of participation
Coordination of community
  resources
Discharge planning
Enterostomal care

Home health care
Home health nursing
Hospice care
Infusion therapy
Interdisciplinary
  collaboration

Perinatal home care
Psychiatric home health
  care
Qualifications for home care
Skilled nursing services

See Glossary for definitions.

case study

Penny Mitchell has been a home health nurse for 2 years and is employed by a hospital-based agency in a small city. Before taking this position, she worked for 5 years as a staff nurse—primarily in a coronary care unit.

Each day Penny sees four to six clients, mostly elderly, with a variety of health problems. One recent Thursday, she saw four clients: Mr. Carter, who has congestive heart failure, to monitor his blood pressure and weight and perform medication teaching; Mrs. Kirk, who is homebound because of osteoporosis and receives monthly calcitonin injections; Mrs. Thomas, to change her Foley catheter, which her caregiver reported to be leaking; and Mr. Wilson, for admission to home care services following discharge from the hospital the day before and to initiate PRN dressing changes for a granulating abdominal wound.

Penny prepares for each day by calling her scheduled clients the night before to set up times, outline the services she will be providing, determine if she needs to bring any special supplies, and learn if there are any specific instructions regarding the client's care of which she is not aware. Because Mr. Wilson is a new client and Penny has never been to his home, she is careful to obtain specific directions from his wife. She confirms with Mrs. Kirk that her medication is at her home and that it is not necessary to stop at the pharmacy. She inventories her car stock of dressings, gloves, solutions, and other supplies to identify anything she might need that is not readily available. Finally, she determines what forms will be needed for documentation of each client's care and gathers educational materials that will be beneficial in client teaching.

Each visit consists of a general assessment followed by implementation of the prescribed skilled nursing services. The clients and their family members or caregivers are given instruction on their illness, treatment regimen, and self-care. Referrals for additional services are made as appropriate and physicians and/or others involved in the care of each client are called to report findings, clarify orders, and request assistance. Also, the process of admitting new clients, like Mr. Wilson, into agency service necessitates additional assessments (e.g., complete physical assessment; health history; and medication, functional, social needs) and explanation and completion of several documents related to home health services and Medicare reimbursement.

After she has seen each client and made necessary notifications and referrals, Penny carefully completes documentation of all findings and services. Her orientation to the agency, 2 years of experience, and several related training sessions have taught her the importance of precise and thorough documentation. Therefore she painstakingly completes and reviews all documentation and organizes each case folder to return to the agency. Finally, she contacts the agency to give a brief report on each client and receive her assignment for the following day.

With recent reforms in health care financing and delivery, hospital occupancy rates have declined dramatically, outpatient surgery has increased markedly, and clients are being discharged "sicker and quicker." This in turn has resulted in a huge increase in home health care. Indeed, home care is the fastest growing specialty of nursing. According to the Public Health Service's Division of Nursing, between 1988 and 1996, the number of nurses working in home health care increased by 50% (U.S. Department of Health and Human Services [USDHHS], 1998). The growth in home health care is also demonstrated by the rapidly increasing number of Medicare-certified agencies, clients, and visits over the past decade. The growth in home care peaked in 1997, but because of changes in Medicare reimbursement, it has declined somewhat over the past few years. Table 4-1 illustrates the dramatic growth in home health care since 1967.

HISTORY OF HOME HEALTH CARE DELIVERY AND FINANCING

Until the early 1900s, care for the ill and injured was provided almost exclusively in the home by family members, friends, or trained health care providers. In the United States, organized home health nursing services began when the first visiting nurse associations (VNAs) were established in Buffalo, Boston, and Philadelphia during the mid-1880s. The early VNAs were established to care for the poor and disenfranchised suffering from illness or injury. The renowned public health nurse, Lillian Wald, is credited with starting a visiting nursing service for New York City

TABLE **4-1** Growth in Medicare-Certified Home Health Care

YEAR	NUMBER OF HOME HEALTH AGENCIES	MEDICARE EXPENDITURES (MILLIONS)	NUMBER OF CLIENTS (THOUSANDS)	NUMBER OF VISITS (THOUSANDS)
1967	1753	$46	N/A	N/A
1980	2924	$662	957	22,428
1992	6004	$7878	2565	135,012
1998	8080	$10,446	3062	154,992

Data from National Association for Home Care. (2000). *Basic statistics about home care.* Washington, DC: National Association for Home Care.

TABLE **4-2** Medicare-Certified Home Health Agencies by Sponsor: 1967, 1990, and 1999

	1967		1990		1999	
SPONSOR	NUMBER	PERCENTAGE	NUMBER	PERCENTAGE	NUMBER	PERCENTAGE
Visiting Nurse Association (VNA)	642	36.6	521	9.1	487	6.3
Public	939	53.6	985	17.3	918	11.8
Proprietary	0	0	1884	33.1	3192	41.2
Private (nonprofit)	0	0	710	12.5	621	8.0
Hospital-based	133	7.6	1486	26.1	2300	29.7
Other	39	2.2	109	2.0	229	3.0
Totals	1753	100	5695	100	7747	100

Data from National Association for Home Care. (2000). *Basic statistics about home care.* Washington, DC: National Association for Home Care.

in 1893 and persuading the Metropolitan Life Insurance Company to furnish home nursing services for policyholders in 1908 (Rice, 2001a). Provision of home health nursing services for insured clients became increasingly common during the following decades. Public health departments, the Red Cross, and philanthropic efforts funded many of the earliest home health agencies.

Initially, home health nursing services and interventions were determined by the nurse. Teaching on hygiene and infant care; instituting measures to control communicable disease; assistance with self-care; performance of activities of daily living for persons with serious or chronic illnesses; and caring for elderly, ill, and dying patients were among the services provided.

Passage of Medicare in 1965 dramatically changed home health care. In the early years, home health care was directed and delivered vir-

tually exclusively by nurses; physician guidance and oversight were not required. With Medicare, the payment source, client eligibility, purpose of home care, and provision of home care changed. Medicare developed very stringent requirements for eligibility, services, and physician oversight. Physician-prescribed and physician-directed care became a necessity and guidelines for services were defined and requirements for eligibility predetermined. The independent practice of nurses providing care to individuals and families in their homes was greatly altered and home health care services were determined by physician directives.

Until recently, home health care in the United States was largely provided by "official" (governmental or public) or voluntary (private, nonprofit agencies such as VNAs funded by fees-for-service, united community funds, grants, and other sources) agencies. As Table 4-2 shows, however, the majority of home health agencies now are proprietary or hospital based. This trend also reflects the changes in the health care system. As care moved from acute care institutions, largely because of the advent of diagnoses-related group reimbursement policies, both proprietary and nonprofit hospitals and providers have recognized the need for home care services and the potential for revenue generation.

DEFINITIONS RELATED TO HOME HEALTH CARE

Home health care has been defined as the following:

that component of a continuum of comprehensive health care whereby health services are provided to individuals and families in their places of residence for the purpose of promoting, maintaining or restoring health, or maximizing the level of independence, while minimizing the effects of disability and illness, including terminal illness. Services appropriate to the needs of the individual client and family are planned, coordinated, and made available by providers organized for the delivery of home care through the use of employed staff, contractual arrangements or a combination of the two patterns (Warhola, 1980, p. 9).

Emphasis is placed on the premise that "health care" (not medical care) should be "comprehensive" and designed to "promote, maintain or restore health" with the objective being to "maximize independence."

Home health nursing combines aspects of community health nursing with selected technical skills from other specialty nursing practices and delivers care for individuals in collaboration with the family and/or designated caregivers. Home health nursing refers to "the practice of nursing applied to a client with a health condition in the client's place of residence" and a "specialized area of nursing practice with its roots firmly placed in community health nursing" (American Nurses' Association [ANA], 1999, p. 3). A conceptual model for home health nursing is presented in Figure 4-1. This model visually depicts the integration of medical/surgical, community health, parent-child, gerontological, and psychiatric-mental health nursing into home health care nursing practice.

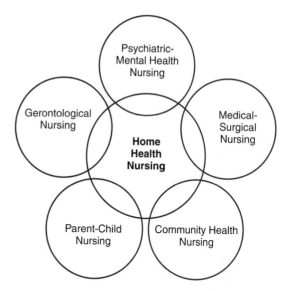

Figure 4-1. Conceptual model of home health nursing. (From American Nurses' Association. [1992]. *A statement on the scope of home health nursing practice.* Washington, DC: American Nurses' Association.)

The home health nurse's role is to be care manager in coordinating and directing all involved disciplines and caregivers to optimize client outcomes. This is accomplished through sharing information of community health resources with the client and caregivers (ANA, 1999). Additionally, a comprehensive knowledge base incorporating aspects of the specialty areas within nursing is required to deliver holistic care in the home.

Unlike other types of nursing practice, home health care nursing is not limited to a particular age group or diagnosis. Depending on the specific client's needs, care may be episodic or continuous and may be primary, secondary, and/or tertiary in nature. Home health nursing should be holistic and focused on the individual client, integrating family/caregiver, environmental, and community resources to promote optimal well-being for the client (American Nurses Credentialing Center [ANCC], 2000).

STANDARDS AND CREDENTIALING FOR HOME HEALTH NURSING

Similar to other nursing practice standards, the Home Health Nursing standards endorsed by the ANA follow the steps of the nursing process, addressing assessment, diagnosis, outcome identification, planning, implementation, and evaluation. Additionally, standards of professional performance relate to quality of care, performance appraisal, education (i.e., knowledge and competency), collegiality, ethics, collaboration, research, and resource utilization (ANA, 1999). Certification in home health nursing is offered by the ANCC (a subsidiary of the ANA) to enhance professional development and recognize professional achievement. Eligibility requirements for certification as a generalist in home health nursing are the following:

1. An active registered nurse (RN) license in the United States
2. A baccalaureate or higher degree in nursing
3. A minimum of 2 years of practice as an RN
4. A minimum of 1500 hours of practice as an RN in home health nursing during the past 3 years
5. Thirty contact hours of continuing education during the last 3 years; following validation that these criteria have been met, the candidate is eligible to sit for the ANCC Board examination (ANCC, 2000)

HOME HEALTH CARE REIMBURSEMENT AND DOCUMENTATION

Public sources (Medicare and Medicaid) finance more than 54% of home health services (Health Care Financing Administration [HCFA], 1999); therefore the discussion related to financing and documentation is directed toward meeting Medicare requirements. To be reimbursed by Medicare for services rendered to clients, home health agencies must be "Medicare certified." Medicare certification is awarded only to those agencies that have successfully demonstrated that they meet Medicare's **conditions of participation** for home health agencies. These conditions are regulations that consist of explicit rules, standards, and requirements established at the federal level of the government and are therefore constant within all states. These regulations outline requirements for virtually all aspects of home health care and detail such areas as personnel qualifications, notifying clients of their rights, acceptance of clients, plan of care, medical supervision, types of services that are offered by the agency, and the duties of each service provider (e.g., skilled nursing, various therapies, home health aide) (HCFA, 2001).

If a home health care agency meets the conditions of participation, it may choose to seek accreditation. The accreditation process is very rigorous and includes a thorough self-study and a site visit by a team of professionals from the accrediting agency. If the home health agency is accredited, it is awarded "deemed status" and is eligible to receive Medicare reimbursement (Milone-Nuzzo, 2000).

To process Medicare claims, the Centers for Medicare & Medicaid Services (CMS), formerly the HCFA, contracts with regional insurance companies, or fiscal intermediaries. The home health agency sends the fiscal intermediary a bill for services each month accompanied by the required documentation. These materials are reviewed by the intermediary and, if all documentation is included and appropriately meets the coverage criteria for home care, the bill is paid. Often there are questions regarding client eligibility or appropriateness of services. In these cases, more information may be requested by the intermediary (Clark, 1999).

For eligibility for coverage under Medicare guidelines, the following **qualifications for home care** must be met (HCFA, 2001):

- The person to whom the services are provided must be eligible for Medicare.
- Services must be "reasonable and necessary" in relation to the client's health status and medical needs, as reflected in the medical records and home health plan of care.

- The client's care must require intermittent skilled nursing care, physical therapy, or speech therapy.
- The client must be homebound.
- The client must be under the care of a physician who develops and monitors a home health plan.
- The home health agency must be certified to participate in Medicare.

Each home health professional service (e.g., nursing, physical therapy, speech therapy) has guidelines on what Medicare defines as covered services. To be covered by Medicare, the RN makes the initial evaluation visit, regularly reevaluates the client's nursing needs, initiates the plan of care, plans necessary revisions, provides services requiring specialized nursing skills, initiates appropriate preventive and rehabilitative nursing procedures, prepares clinical and progress notes, coordinates services, informs the physician and other personnel of changes in the client's condition, counsels the client and family, and supervises and teaches other nursing personnel. Examples of **skilled nursing services** that are reimbursable (HCFA, 2001) under defined circumstances are listed in Box 4-1.

HOME HEALTH CARE DOCUMENTATION

When asked what they like most about home health care, nurses often cite the autonomy, being able to spend more time caring for clients, or the hours. When asked what they like least about home health care, nurses almost always mention the paperwork. Completion of all required documentation has several purposes:

- Recording services rendered
- Describing the client's condition and response to care
- Promoting continuity of care
- Validating reimbursement claims
- Forestalling legal actions

For reimbursement by Medicare, documentation of all services and care given must be meticulously completed. To standardize and coordinate reimbursement, in 1985 HCFA (now CMS) instituted the requirement of completion of several forms to document home health care. These forms documenting each skilled nursing visit must be completed and submitted to the fiscal intermediary.

The CMS Form 485 is entitled "Home Health Certification and Plan of Treatment." It contains the signed physician's orders and certifies that the client meets the eligibility requirements for home health care reimbursement. Orders for specific skilled services and goals are listed. Form 486 updates medical and client care information and is completed at the time of certification or billing for services or for recertification. Specific instructions on completion of each of these forms are included in orientation to the agency.

To develop the requisite plan of care (CMS Form 485) and provide the information needed to ensure client eligibility certification for home care (CMS Form 486), each home health care agency has additional forms to be completed for each client. Individual agencies design forms for

---

BOX **4-1** Medicare-Reimbursable Skilled Nursing Services

- Observation and assessment of a client's condition
- Management and evaluation of a client care plan
- Teaching and training activities for the client and the client's family or caregivers
- Tube feedings
- Tracheotomy aspiration
- Insertion and irrigation and replacement of catheters in selected clients

- Wound care
- Ostomy care
- Heat treatments
- Administration of medical gasses
- Rehabilitation care
- Venipuncture
- Psychiatric evaluation, therapy, and teaching (by a psychiatrically trained nurse)

documentation that best meet the needs of their particular clientele and nurses' preferences. Documentation of a thorough nursing assessment, including physical, psychosocial, functional, nutritional, and safety components, and gathering information on all medications, is necessary. Other materials specified by Medicare include written documentation of notification of client rights, notification of client liability for payment and charges, and advisement of a state-established home health hotline for complaints or questions.

Orientation of nurses new to home health care practice or to a new agency demands in-depth instruction on documentation requirements, including specifics on how to complete all forms thoroughly and accurately. Table 4-3 presents information to guide home health nurses in documentation of home health care services.

ELEMENTS OF HOME CARE NURSING PRACTICE

Home health care nursing practice requires unique skills and knowledge. Home health care nursing responsibilities are varied and numerous. A few basic and essential activities that comprise home health care nursing are described in the following sections.

DISCHARGE PLANNING

Discharge planning is the process of determining and planning to meet client needs following release from a health care facility. The discharge planning process allows client and family needs to be identified and evaluated, with responsibility for meeting those needs being transferred to the client, the client's caregiver or significant others, or other health care providers. The purposes of discharge planning include promoting continuity of care to improve client health status and coordinating the client's needs with available resources (Clark, 1995). Reduction in average length of service, lower cost, efficient use of resources, fewer requests for additional services, improved communication, and better informa-

tion on client needs are benefits attributable to discharge planning.

Ideally, the discharge planning process should begin before the client is hospitalized, with anticipation of the client's needs during recovery. When the course of recovery is predicted to be difficult for any of several reasons and follow-up care through a home health agency is anticipated or requested, comprehensive discharge planning is beneficial. Discharge planning as a service is performed by different health professionals, including nurses, social workers, physicians, and chaplains (Clark, 1995). Many institutions employ professionals—usually nurses or social workers—for this position. These individuals are responsible for identifying clients in need of ongoing care following discharge, consulting with caregivers (both in the institution and when the client is discharged), educating staff regarding discharge plans, and coordinating activities. Many health care institutions utilize assessment instruments to identify clients who need more.

CASE MANAGEMENT

Case management has been defined as "a process of identifying needs for and arranging, coordinating, monitoring, and evaluating quality, cost-effective, primary, secondary, and tertiary prevention services to achieve designated health outcomes" (Clark, 1999, p. 216). According to Horn and Horn (1993), in case management, "one professional is responsible for assessing needs, targeting services to meet the needs, and monitoring and evaluating client status to ensure that needs are met adequately" (p. 48). The goals of case management are to provide quality health care, decrease fragmentation, enhance client's quality of life, and contain costs.

The case manager's role is comprehensive and includes assessment of the client's needs and resources, outlining a plan of care to meet the identified needs, arranging for the most cost-effective complement of services and providers to meet the identified needs, and coordinating the activities of various health care providers (Clark, 1999). In home health care nursing, case

TABLE **4-3** Guidelines for Medicare Documentation to Validate the Need for Home Care Services

AVOID THE FOLLOWING WORDS	USE INSTEAD
Monitor, supervise. Denotes a stable client.	**Assess, evaluate**. "Monitor" may be used when managed care is ordered and the skilled nurse is supervising paraprofessionals to ensure safe delivery of the therapeutic regimen.
Healing well. Suggests that visits are unnecessary and supports client discharge from home health services.	Objectively describe the wound in terms of size, depth, drainage, color, and odor.
Discussed. Does not require the skills of a professional; anyone can discuss.	Teach, educate, instruct; demonstrate.
Prevent/prevention. Not covered. Must be done incidental to a skilled service such as assessment teaching and treatment.	Focus on **restorative**, **rehabilitative**, and/or **palliative** (hospice) interventions.
Stable, independent. Negates medical necessity and supports client discharge from home health services.	Document response to treatment.
Feeling better. Subjective and supports client discharge from health services.	Focus on the client's physical assessment, functional ability, and problems/needs.
Noncompliant/uncooperative.	Document specific problems with coping or refusal to follow the plan of care as a source of referral to a psychiatric home health nurse or social worker. Document refusal to follow the plan of care as a justification for a learning contract or, per home health agency policy, client discharge.
Went to the market/going to church, etc. Negates homebound status.	Document equipment, manual assistance, and number of people required for client to leave home. Verify homebound status each visit. If the client leaves the home, explain why trips were taken as related to lifestyle or medical necessity.
Client not at home.	**Not available for visit or no answer to locked door.** Document on next visit why client was not available for visit.
Continue care plan.	Describe what your next visit plans are based on (e.g., assess cardiopulmonary status of client with congestive heart failure).
Maintenance. Never use this word because it negates the necessity of visits and supports client discharge from home health services.	Document response to the plan of care of case-management needs.
Confused.	Describe disorientation to person, place, or time. Describe ability to follow commands and short- and long-term recall.
Chronic condition. Is indicative of a stable condition.	Describe exacerbation of the chronic condition that requires the services of a skilled nurse.
Reinforce, reinstruct. Repetitive instruction will not be covered unless learning difficulties are documented.	Document comprehension difficulties, attention deficit, or other problems that hamper ability to learn and necessitate repeating instructions. Use words such as **demonstrate**, **teach**, **instruct**, or **educate**.
Observed. Anyone can observe.	Use **assess** or **evaluate**. Skilled observation may be used as a component of client education to document client/caregiver return demonstration.

From Rice, R. (2000). *Manual of home health nursing procedures* (2nd ed.). St. Louis: Mosby.

management generally refers to the comprehensive supervision of the care given to each client. The case manager, usually the RN, functions as the team leader who provides or arranges primary care, supervises paraprofessionals, and collaborates with other health professionals (e.g., a physical or occupational therapist or medical social worker). The case manager is responsible for maintaining communication between the disciplines and with the client and monitoring and evaluating client goals.

COORDINATION OF COMMUNITY RESOURCES

Coordination of community resources requires the nurse to be knowledgeable about services offered by his or her own agency and any resources available in the community that would benefit clients. In addition to being aware of resources, the home health nurse must understand the referral process.

During the referral process, a client is directed to appropriate agencies or organizations for information or assistance with care. To make effective and appropriate referrals, the nurse must do the following:

- Be aware of community services available for needs related to home health nursing practice.
- Determine if the client is eligible for the services offered by the agency or organization.
- Have an understanding of how to refer a client for a particular service and who may refer a client (e.g., some services or service providers require a referral from a physician only).
- Know the costs of services and payment mechanism.
- Be aware of the location, telephone number, hours of operation, and contact person.

Often, the nurse provides the client or their caregiver with the necessary information for the referral and allows him or her to make initial contact. At other times, it may be appropriate for the nurse to call the individual, agency, or organization directly.

To identify sources for community referrals, the home health nurse may use a directory of community services, which is available in many cities and towns. In addition, home health agencies often provide nurses with a list of available community resources. Experienced home health nurses usually develop a personal listing of service providers that have been helpful for clients in the past. Names of agencies, contact persons, and their telephone numbers are essential. Examples of commonly utilized community resources are various government programs (e.g., Medicaid; Veteran's Affairs; Women, Infants, and Children [WIC] program); Meals on Wheels; adult day care providers; area hospices, if not provided by the nurse's agency; organizations that assist with financial obligations; and transportation providers for the handicapped or elderly.

INTERDISCIPLINARY COLLABORATION

Home health nursing practice requires the nurse to initiate and maintain a collegial and collaborative relationship with all health care providers working with the client. In health care, collaboration implies joint decision making regarding the plan of care with all professionals involved with the client's care. **Interdisciplinary collaboration** is integrated within the roles and functions of the home health nurse discussed here and is vitally important in the process of discharge planning and case management. To comply with Medicare requirements and to best direct client care, the nurse must work with the physician to receive orders and outline the plan of care. As the case manager, the nurse must share the plan of care with all involved in the client's care and make recommendations and modifications based on their input. Case conferences should be held regularly, particularly for clients with complicated or prolonged care, to share information among the providers and discuss the client's response to the treatment plan. In addition, the nurse may oversee, evaluate, or supervise the care of others. Professionals involved in home health care planning and delivery are described in Box 4-2. See a discussion of the Home Care Bill of Rights in the Community Application box.

BOX 4-2 Professionals Involved in Home Health Care Planning and Delivery

Nurses: Registered nurses have been the traditional providers of health care in the home. As described, nurses provide skilled nursing services, coordinate care as case managers and referral agents, and act as client advocates.

Physicians: Most clients are referred for home care services by physicians, and, as stated, physician oversight of the plan of care is required for Medicare reimbursement and for payment from other insurers.

Physical therapists: Most home care agencies employ physical therapists to assess client's needs for assistive devices that will support rehabilitation and safety, evaluate neuromuscular and functional ability, prescribe and administer therapy procedures to meet client needs, and teach the client or caregivers to perform these therapies and related activities.

Occupational therapists: Whereas physical therapists usually concentrate on gross motor skills and rehabilitation, occupational therapists assist the client in restoration of small motor coordination and improving physical tasks related to activities of daily living and reaching the highest level of functioning possible.

Speech therapists/speech pathologists: Speech therapists work with clients with communication problems related to speech, language, hearing, and swallowing difficulties to treat, manage, or alleviate these problems.

Social workers: Social workers assist clients with social, emotional, and financial needs. In addition, social workers often serve as advocates and refer clients to available community resources.

Registered dietitians/nutritionists: Dietitians provide direct counseling and teaching for clients with special dietary needs and problems. In addition, they may act as consultants or resource persons for nurses and other health care providers.

Home health aides: Home health aides are paraprofessionals who assist in the home with the client's personal care, basic nursing (e.g., vital signs, assistance with self-administered medication), light housekeeping, and related tasks (e.g., shopping, meal preparation). For Medicare reimbursement, home health aides must be supervised by an RN.

Other providers: Other professionals and paraprofessionals that occasionally provide care to clients in the home or might assist home health nurses include pharmacists, phlebotomists, laboratory technicians, respiratory therapists, enterostomal therapists, chaplains, and massage therapists.

COMMUNITY APPLICATION
Home Care Bill of Rights

One of the Medicare funding provisions mandated by the HCFA requires that the Home Health Agency provide the client with a written notice of the client's rights in advance of furnishing care to the client or during the initial evaluation visit before the initiation of treatment. Before treatment, each home health client must be informed of his or her "right" for health care treatment and this must be documented on the client's permanent record. To comply with this requirement, the National Association of Home Care (NAHC) has established a "bill of rights" for clients and their families to inform them of the ethical conduct they can expect from home care agencies. Copies of the Home Care Bill of Rights can be obtained from NAHC's website, which can be accessed directly from the book's website. See the Resources box at the end of the chapter for this information.

THE PROCESS OF HOME HEALTH NURSING

Home health nursing may be specialized or generalized and is always detail intensive. Orientation, education, and training of nurses in home health nursing practice should be comprehensive and specific and include significant time spent with preceptors. This section focuses on the process of the home health nursing visit and gives specific instructions on how to conduct a home visit and what may be expected and required of the provider.

The process of the home health nursing visit is typically divided into three levels or stages: (1) the previsit/planning stage; (2) the visit, or implementation, stage; and (3) the postvisit stage. Each of these stages and the home health nurse's activities are described in the following sections.

PLANNING FOR THE HOME HEALTH NURSING VISIT

To be efficient, safe, and productive, home health care nursing requires a significant amount of previsit planning. Previsit planning involves determining which clients are to be seen during the day and prioritization of the scheduled visits based on a number of factors. For example, one client needs a blood sugar drawn before breakfast, another client needs dressing changes twice a day, and the caregiver of a third client will only be present in the morning to let the nurse into the residence. Other factors to be considered in scheduling include distance between visits, the need to take specimens to the laboratory, the need to coordinate care with other health professionals, and the need to work with physicians. In addition to scheduling, the nurse must be aware of supplies, equipment, medications, teaching materials, and anything else that might be needed and make arrangements for obtaining materials that are not immediately at hand.

The previsit/planning phase consists of those activities that prepare the nurse to accomplish the required tasks of the home visits scheduled. This phase requires several considerations as the nurse plans care for all clients to be seen each day. These considerations and activities are outlined.

Caseload Scheduling

Assignments and scheduling guidelines for home health clients differ among agencies. The plan of care developed by the admitting nurse and/or "case manager," in collaboration with the physician, determines how often the client will be seen and what services are to be provided during each visit. Often, agencies assign home health nurses a caseload of clients and each nurse determines which clients to see on which days. In other agencies, all assignments are made from the central office, based on individual client needs and available personnel. Typically, the agency assigns nurses based on geographical or distance considerations (e.g., one nurse sees clients in a given area) or based on specialized needs of the client or abilities of the nurse (e.g., infusion therapy or wound care).

Home health nurses usually see four to six clients each day, although this may vary somewhat based on client acuity and prescribed services (e.g., an intravenous infusion may take 2 hours or more) or distances that must be traveled (e.g., in rural areas, the nurse may drive 100 miles or more to see one client). When planning the day's schedule, the nurse begins with a list of all clients that will be seen that day. This list should include the following:
- A synopsis of the client's diagnosis(es)
- What services need to be provided during the day's visit
- Any supplies, equipment, or medications needed in the home that are not at hand
- General directions regarding location of each residence (e.g., map coordinates)

From this list, the nurse can begin the process of scheduling client visits. This is typically accomplished during the afternoon or evening before the day's visit.

Telephone Contact

After the day's preliminary schedule is determined, each client is contacted to inform him or her of the anticipated time for the nursing visit and to briefly explain the purpose of the visit. In addition, the nurse should get specific directions to the residence if this is the first visit and determine if any special additional instructions, requests, or information regarding each client may be needed; for example, scheduling around the presence of a caregiver or the need to bring additional supplies.

Occasionally, it is impossible to contact the client to schedule the visit. For example, the client may not have a telephone or may not be able to answer it, or he or she may not speak English. In these cases, contacting a relative, neighbor, or other caregiver to establish the time and purpose of the visit should be attempted. Each agency has guidelines on what to do if telephone scheduling is not possible. If no problems (e.g., the client has a physician's appointment or requests an earlier or later time to avoid a conflict) are encountered with the preliminary schedule, the nurse uses this schedule when seeing the day's caseload.

Review of the Client's Chart

Following scheduling, the home health nurse should familiarize himself or herself with the client's plan of care. Chart or case review is a very important step in the care of the home health client. However, this may not be a simple process. Many providers from the home health agency may see the same client. Depending on agency protocols, the client's comprehensive chart may be at the agency or in the possession of the case manager. In many instances, other providers see the client without seeing the master chart and need as much information as possible regarding that client, his or her condition, and the plan of care. Each agency uses different methods to deliver this information. Voice mail or other recorded reports, faxed information, and charts and data left in the home are methods used to manage information about each client and deliver it to health care team members.

The nurse scheduling the visit should review all available information before seeing the client. If anything is unclear or if the nurse has any questions regarding the care plan, the case manager (if someone other than the scheduled nurse), the physician, the nurse's supervisor, or other appropriate individual should be contacted to answer questions or clarify information, plans, or procedures before the nurse sees the client. This enables the nurse to be prepared for and to better expedite each visit and ensures that all concerns and questions regarding the client's care are addressed.

Assessment of Personal Supplies and Equipment

Another important step in previsit planning involves daily inventory of the nurse's bag and routine periodic inventory of the car stock of supplies. The accompanying Community Application boxes detail what should be included in each one. Based on agency guidelines and variations in the nurse's practice (e.g., if he or she is a member of the intravenous team or is a wound specialist),

---

COMMUNITY APPLICATION
Suggested Contents of a Home Health Nurse's Bag

Large shoulder bag with multiple compartments and zippered closure

Medical Equipment/Supplies

Antimicrobial soap (preferably liquid) and paper towels; alcohol foam
Stethoscope
Sphygmomanometer
Thermometer (oral and rectal or tympanic) and appropriate covers
Penlight or flashlight
Tape measure and/or small ruler
Alcohol wipes
Nonsterile gloves (dozen pairs)
Nonsterile disposable gown or apron
Nonsterile waterproof pads (chux)
Disposable masks
Goggles
Sterile gloves (three or four pairs)
Dressing supplies (4-inch gauze squares [4 × 4s], 2-inch gauze squares [2 × 2s]), 3-inch and 4-inch dressing gauze, sterile applicators, silk and paper tape, sterile saline, adhesive bandages)

Venipuncture supplies (e.g., assortment of vacutainer needles, tubes, syringes, tourniquet)
Glucometer and strips
Sterile specimen cup, culture tubes
Bandage scissors
Forceps
Biohazard containers and bags

Other Materials

Map
Agency and Medicare required forms and charting materials and information
Laboratory forms and plastic pouches for transporting laboratory specimens
Teaching materials
Pocket medication reference book
Pocket nursing interventions reference book
Plastic trash bags
Bathroom scale

COMMUNITY APPLICATION
Suggested Contents of a Home Health Nurse's Car Stock

Dressing Supplies

Two or three dozen packages of sterile 2 × 2s and
4 × 4s
3-inch and 4-inch gauze dressings (6 to 12 packages
of each)
Sterile abdominal dressing (ABD) pads (box)
Hypertonic dressing gauze
Nonstick dressing gauze (e.g., telfa, adaptic)
Hydrocolloid dressings (several boxes in a variety
of sizes)
Adhesive bandages (one box of assorted sizes;
"spots" for venipunctures)
Alcohol wipes (one box)
Sterile gloves (one or two boxes)
Nonsterile gloves (one or two boxes)
Assortment of tapes
Sterile scissors (two or three pairs)
Sterile forceps (two or three pairs)
Staple remover (one or two)
Suture removal kit(s)
Steri strips (several sizes)
Sterile saline (several containers)
Hydrogen peroxide (two or three bottles)
Other dressings, ointments, solutions, and supplies
based on factors such as client needs and
physician preferences

**Catheters and Related Equipment
and Supplies**

Adult briefs (variety of sizes)
Catheter insertion kits (two)
Indwelling catheters (variety of sizes)

Red rubber catheters (variety of sizes)
Catheter drainage bags (two)
Catheter irrigation kit (two)
Sterile water for irrigation (three or four bottles)
Catheter leg bag (two)
Underpads (waterproof pads—chux) (two
packages)
Urine specimen containers (sterile; three or four)

**Miscellaneous Equipment and Supplies
for Routine Visits**

Variety of needles and syringes
Lancets and chemstrips for glucometer (if used)
Restraints
Lubricating jelly
Levine tube (two)
Trash bags (one box)
Pill boxes (two)
Disposable masks and aprons or gowns (several
of each)

**Miscellaneous Equipment and Supplies
for Specialized Home Care (When Applicable)**

Enterostomal therapy supplies (e.g., colostomy,
ileostomy bags, stomahesive)
Infusion therapy supplies (e.g., variety of
administration sets, syringes, injectable solutions)
Respiratory therapy or tracheotomy supplies (e.g.,
suction tubes, suction tips and catheters,
tracheotomy care trays)
Gastrointestinal feeding supplies (e.g., variety of
bags, tubings)

these supplies may vary. The car stock should be checked periodically for expired supplies and to ensure that no supplies are damaged and should be replenished as necessary. The bag should be inventoried and replenished daily.

Safety Concerns and Previsit Planning

It is important to note that several safety concerns apply to home health care nurses. Typically, home health nurses work alone; they may go into questionably safe neighborhoods; they may drive many miles in adverse weather conditions; and some may encounter threatening situations. To enhance communication between the nurse and the agency and to promote safety, most agencies supply nurses with cellular telephones and pagers. To assist in minimizing threats, the Community Application box "Safety Tips for Home Health Nurses" provides general information on safety in home health.

The final aspect of previsit planning should include notification of the agency of the nurse's anticipated schedule. This allows the agency to trace or monitor the movement of the nurse and, with the use of the beeper or cellular telephone, to contact him or her if necessary.

COMMUNITY APPLICATION
Safety Tips for Home Health Nurses

- Maintain car; keep gas tank at least half full
- Lock all car doors at all times; keep windows rolled up
- Park as close to the entrance to the client's residence as possible
- Use a map; know where clients live; get directions
- Keep purse in the car trunk; carry change and identification in a pocket
- Dress appropriately, conservatively, professionally (according to agency guidelines); wear comfortable shoes, minimal jewelry, and name tag
- Pay attention to uncomfortable, intuitive "feelings"; if the setting or situation seems unsafe, leave at once

- Avoid walking by groups of individuals loitering near building entrances and/or isolated places
- Never walk into a home uninvited; always knock and wait at the door to be let in either physically or verbally
- If pets are annoying or threatening, request that they be removed to another room before entering the home
- Know the agency's policy regarding safety; some agencies will provide a security guard, assistant, or escort to accompany providers in questionably safe areas
- Visit only during scheduled hours; if exceptions must be made, notify supervisor

THE HOME VISIT ACTIVITIES

Smith (1995) divides the home health visit into three phases: (1) initiation, (2) implementation, and (3) termination. Specific activities for each are described in the following sections.

Initiation Phase

The initiation phase begins as the nurse knocks on the door and gains entrance into the residence. The nurse should identify herself or himself and the agency and briefly review the purpose of the visit. For example, the nurse might say "Good morning, Mrs. Johnson, I'm Mary Smith from the Visiting Nurses' Association and I am here to change Mr. Johnson's dressing." The nurse should greet all in attendance and determine who is the primary caregiver for the client, if appropriate. (Often, the client lives alone.)

There may a brief social phase that can be used to begin assessments and establish rapport. A standard greeting, such as "How are you doing this morning," allows the nurse to begin collecting data on the client's physical, psychological, and social well-being (Figure 4-2). A brief discussion about the weather, holidays, or news events allows the nurse to assess cognitive status. Talking for a few minutes with the caregiver(s) can convey caring, assist with assess-

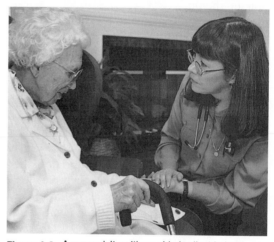

Figure 4-2. A nurse visits with an elderly client in her home. (Courtesy Rick Brady, Photographer, Riva, Maryland.)

ment of the family situation, and assist with the concerns, abilities, and understanding level of the caregiver. At this point and throughout the visit, the nurse should continually assess the surroundings to determine potential threats to the client's condition or safety.

During this brief social phase, the nurse should review the chart or records left in the home. He or she should make sure that permissions are signed or should obtain them if this is the initial visit. At this time, the nurse may open his or her bag and begin removing needed equipment, such as a blood pressure cuff and stethoscope. The nurse should also remove the soap and paper towels from the bag and excuse himself or herself briefly to the bathroom or kitchen to wash hands. The nurse is now ready to begin the physical assessment and implement the plan of care.

Implementation Phase

The implementation phase is the working component of home health care provision. During this phase, assessments are conducted, skilled nursing care is provided, and teaching is accomplished.

ASSESSMENT. Assessment in home health nursing involves several different areas. In addition to thorough physical assessment, assessment of psychosocial needs, functional abilities, medication, nutrition, safety issues, and the client's environment is essential. Home health agencies typically develop their own assessment tools and provide the requisite forms for documentation of assessment in each of these areas.

Typically, a thorough database is completed during the initial admission visit. From this database, the plan of care is developed to address identified needs and appropriate skilled nursing interventions and other therapies (e.g., physical therapy, occupational therapy) and ancillary assistance (e.g., home health aide assistance with activities of daily living) that will be administered as appropriate. During subsequent visits, less comprehensive, more directed assessments are conducted. During each visit, the nurse takes vital signs and performs a routine head-to-toe assessment, including assessment of the respiratory system (e.g., listening to breath sounds, quality of respirations, assessing presence or absence of cough), cardiovascular system (e.g., rate, rhythm, heart sounds, presence or absence of chest pain, peripheral pulses, capillary refill, edema), neurological system (e.g., whether the client is alert and oriented, reactivity of pupils, ability to move extremities, and equal strength of same), gastro-

intestinal system (e.g., abdomen; bowel sounds; any distention, masses, or tenderness; nausea, vomiting, or diarrhea; last bowel movement; and appetite), urinary system (e.g., frequency of urination, any burning, unusual odor), and skin integrity (e.g., turgor, temperature, color, any redness, open areas or wounds). Particular attention is given to those areas related to identified problems or potential problems. For example, if the client has diabetes, the nurse should very carefully assess the feet for adequate circulation and evidence of skin breakdown, or if the client has been diagnosed with congestive heart failure, careful attention to cardiovascular and respiratory function, including monitoring of weight and signs of peripheral edema, is essential.

After the home health nurse has washed his or her hands, the assessment is begun. An individual routine is usually established, wherein the nurse develops a pattern to ensure that all systems and areas are covered during the assessment. Most nurses usually begin by taking and charting vital signs. Comparison with previous readings and notation of significant changes may dictate unplanned actions or interventions (e.g., if the client has developed a temperature since yesterday or if the blood pressure is unusually high, the physician may need to be called immediately). While taking the vital signs and throughout the physical assessment, the nurse can take the opportunity to question the client to obtain additional information (e.g., "When did you last have a bowel movement?" "What did you eat for breakfast?" "Have you noticed any dizziness or pain?"). Follow-up questions to the client's responses of change or identification of possible problems allows the nurse to obtain more information (e.g., "When did you first notice burning when you urinate?" "I see your ankles are a little swollen—have you been up quite a lot?" "Your blood pressure is a little higher than it has been—did you take your medication this morning?"). Any problems should be noted in the visit record and discussed with the physician or case manager as appropriate.

Following the initial visit, much less documentation is required. A revisit summary outlining the routine assessment and all findings should be included. This should be followed by narrative description of the purpose of the visit and details of the skilled nursing care given.

PROVISION OF SKILLED NURSING CARE. As described earlier, skilled observation and assessment are essential services for Medicare reimbursement. Other covered services include wound care, venipuncture, administration of medications, tracheotomy and catheter care, and teaching clients and caregivers various skills and services. During each visit, the nurse performs the identified and assigned tasks and documents them according to agency guidelines.

Often, the nursing care performed requires the nurse to use materials carried in his or her bag (e.g., drawing blood, removing sutures or staples) or supplies left in the home (e.g., changing dressings, performing tracheotomy care, administering intravenous medications). As in the acute care setting, the nurse must treat the bag and stock of supplies as clean and carefully avoid contamination and cross-contamination. It is important to remember to remove the supplies and equipment from the bag or stock before beginning the procedures and not to return to the bag without washing hands or removing contaminated gloves. In addition, the nurse should be careful to place the bag on a clean surface (not the floor) and to ensure that children or pets cannot reach it. When leaving equipment and supplies in the home, the same guidelines and procedures should apply, and manufacturer's recommendations regarding storage should be carefully maintained. Dressing supplies, for example, should be placed in a clean cupboard or on a shelf away from the reach of pets and children and away from moisture or extreme heat. Likewise, medications, formulas, and solutions should be stored according to guidelines. If the nurse is unsure of the ability of the client to store supplies properly, he or she should make other arrangements. For example, occasionally a family may not have reliable electricity or a working refrigerator and cannot properly store solutions for total parenteral nutrition (TPN). In such a case, the nurse may need to arrange to pick up the prescribed solutions at a pharmacy and bring them with him or her or to store them at a neighbor's residence.

When performing sterile procedures (e.g., dressing changes, insertion of catheters, hanging solutions), it is as important that meticulous technique be followed in the home as in the hospital. In addition, the nurse should ensure that all contaminated materials and waste be disposed of properly. The client and the caregivers should be taught proper management of infectious wastes and the rationale behind such management. Containers for handling sharps should be provided, and methods for appropriate disposal should be taught to the client and the caregiver.

TEACHING. In home health care, teaching is one of the most important functions of the nurse. The nurse teaches the client and the caregivers general information about their illness or condition, care or treatment regimen, medications, and identification and reporting of symptoms or complications. In addition, clients and their caregivers may be given specific instructions on a variety of health-related topics, such as self-administration of insulin or other injectable medications, management of an American Diabetic Association diet, self-catheterization, administration of gastrostomy tube feedings, tracheotomy care, bowel training, wound care, or colostomy or ileostomy care.

As discussed in Chapter 2, it is very important to realize that health teaching goes beyond information dissemination. In home health care, the nurse must assess the readiness and ability of the client or caregiver to perform the necessary tasks; present the information in a manner that is understandable to the learner; possibly use several methods, tools, and materials in the instruction process; and carefully, accurately, and thoroughly evaluate the level of understanding and response to the teaching. Observation of the client as he or she performs a sterile dressing change, use of return demonstration in drawing up insulin, and verbalization of principles of infection control are evaluation techniques that the nurse may use to determine how well the client understands the instructions.

Many agencies provide and encourage the use of written materials to assist their nurses in teaching clients and caregivers in home settings. Written instructions are particularly helpful for clients who will be required to perform procedures without the presence of the nurse. Step-by-step guides can be reviewed and discussed with the client and often prove to be very helpful tools. Providing written instruction on areas such as the steps in monitoring blood sugar and self-administration of insulin, the signs and symptoms of complications of anticoagulant therapy and when to notify the physician, the signs and symptoms of urinary tract infection for the client with an indwelling catheter, and the management of congestive heart failure can assist in enhancing the client's understanding of his or her health problems; in treating or alleviating symptoms; and in preventing, identifying, or recognizing changes or complications to the condition.

Termination Phase

Following completion of the skilled nursing interventions and teaching, the home health nurse evaluates the client's response to care and briefly summarizes the continuing plan of care with the client and caregiver. If care is to be ongoing, the nurse can set up a time for the next home visit. During this phase, the nurse should be careful to gather all equipment and supplies that he or she will take. If any specimens have been collected, these should be placed in appropriate containers and requisite paperwork should be completed.

At this point, the nurse should also review potential health emergencies and appropriate actions to take. For example, the nurse might say, "Mrs. Cooper, if you experience any chest pain or shortness of breath or if you gain more than 2 pounds when you weigh yourself in the morning, call your doctor immediately."

Before departure, the nurse should ask the client and caregiver if they have any questions and clarify once more when he or she will return and the purpose of the next visit (e.g., "Good-bye for now, Mrs. Charles. Another nurse will see you this evening, but I will be back about the same time tomorrow to change your dressing" or "Mrs. McClure, I will call your doctor today to report on your laboratory findings. If there are no changes in your Coumadin schedule, I will be back in 2 or 3 weeks to check your clotting times again. I will call you and let you know").

POSTVISIT ACTIVITIES

After each visit, several activities must be completed to fulfill the responsibilities of the home health care nurse. These activities include communication of findings to other health care providers (reporting and referral) and documentation (completion of all forms and charting).

Communication

Reporting of important assessment and evaluation findings to all appropriate personnel or referral to other providers for follow-up of identified concerns is a very important component of home health care practice. If the nurse seeing the client is the case manager, typically, he or she reports findings or significant changes in the client's condition to the physician. Other providers may also be contacted to refer or initiate services (e.g., occupational therapy, speech therapy). Also, current care providers may be contacted to discuss their assessment of the client (e.g., the nurse might call Mrs. Thornton's physical therapist to discuss whether additional visits might be appropriate to do more in-depth teaching of range-of-motion exercises).

The home health care nurse should keep the physician informed of the client's condition. Any changes in health status and any significant findings should be reported immediately. If the home health nurse seeing the client is not the case manager, he or she should also report to that nurse, usually following agency guidelines.

Referrals to nonagency providers (e.g., Meals on Wheels, adult day care centers) should be made as appropriate and following agency guidelines. As nurses gain experience in home health care practice, they maintain a list or booklet of community resources to share with their clients.

Documentation

The importance of complete, concise, and accurate documentation in home health nursing cannot be overstated. All forms and documents must be completed according to Medicare or other third-party payer guidelines and the home health care agency's requirements. An experienced home health nurse may be able to complete most of the paperwork while in the client's home. However, the nurse should comprehensively review each client's chart at the end of the day.

Documentation should include date and time of reporting to the physician and/or case manager described previously and any actions based on that reporting. For example, "Mrs. Cooper's B/P—160/94; Dr. Black notified @ 13:00; he stated that no changes be made in medication at present, requests that pt's B/P be reevaluated in 2 days. Plan—SNV on Thursday to reevaluate" or "Dr. Brown contacted @ 9:30 and informed that wound edges were reddened, drainage malodorous, and pt reports increased pain. M.D. requested wound C & S be performed and client seen again tomorrow. C & S to lab at 10:30; results available in 24 hrs. Plan—contact lab tomorrow a.m. and schedule p.m. SNV." Often, home health agencies periodically review home care nurses' documentation to ensure comprehensiveness.

SPECIALIZED HOME HEALTH CARE

Related to changes in the health care system, specialized home health services have been added and expanded over the past decade. For example, infusion therapy, which includes TPN, chemotherapy, and administration of other pharmacotherapeutics, has become increasingly common. Other areas of specialized care now being provided in the home include care of ventilator-dependent clients, high-risk prenatal clients, routine postpartum clients, clients with chronic mental health problems, and clients with chronic wounds. Hospice, or care of the terminally ill, is also becoming more commonplace. Basic components of each of these areas are described in this section.

INFUSION THERAPY

Home **infusion therapy** is a very significant component of home health care. With shortened hospital stays, many patients are discharged needing additional or prolonged parenteral medication. Home health care agencies have responded by adding home infusion nurses or teams or incorporating home infusion therapy into specialized orientation or training for their regular home care nurses. In addition, many home health agencies have developed that specialize in infusion therapy.

The growth in home infusion or intravenous therapy programs has been phenomenal since the 1980s. Reasons cited for the growth include the following:

- Increased complexity of cases
- More aggressive treatments available in the home
- Improved technology (e.g., portable infusion pumps, flexible silicone catheters)
- Efforts to reduce costs through decreasing inpatient hospitalization
- Consumer awareness, whereby clients and their families are more willing to participate in the recovery process (Watkins and Rice, 1996)

Types of Home Infusion Therapy

Several types of infusion therapy are routinely delivered in homes. Antibiotics, pain medication, TPN, hydration, and chemotherapy are the most routinely administered home intravenous therapies. Therapies less commonly provided in the home include administration of human growth hormones, cardiac drugs, blood and blood components, and aminophylline (Humphrey and

Milone-Nuzzo, 1991). The largest percentage of home infusion involves antibiotics and other antiinfectives (68%); antineoplastics and pain medications account for another 15%, with the remainder being hydration, TPN, and other therapies (Balinsky, 1995). Table 4-4 lists common diagnoses for routine intravenous therapy.

Home Infusion Therapy Management

Home infusion therapy is nursing intensive and can be very complex. Orientation of new nurses to home infusion services should be comprehensive and cover specific procedures for each type of care (e.g., TPN, chemotherapy, antibiotic therapy). Resources for assistance, supervision, and consultation should be available at all times and procedures for complications must be reviewed routinely and followed painstakingly.

In addition to delivering the prescribed medications, the nurse must evaluate the client for complications (e.g., medication reactions or infection) related to the illness or the treatment regimen. Management of the plan of care requires consideration of the drug therapy schedule, presence or absence of other caregivers who may be needed to assist, additional or preliminary medications or therapies, availability or source of the medication; preparation of the medication, use of an infusion pump if prescribed, and assessment and maintenance of the administration port.

Pain Management

In home health care, pain medications including narcotics are used to manage severe pain usually caused by cancer, acquired immunodeficiency syndrome (AIDS), or neurological or orthopedic conditions. Narcotics may be administered intravenously, intramuscularly, subcutaneously, intrathecally, or epidurally when oral or rectal drug administration is no longer adequate. In home care, use of client-controlled analgesia pumps is becoming more common. Pain management is discussed in more detail later in this chapter in the section on hospice care.

TABLE **4-4** Home Infusion Therapy

TYPE OF INFUSION THERAPY	EXAMPLES OF MEDICAL DIAGNOSES
Antibiotic therapy	AIDS-related infections Bacterial endocarditis Cystic fibrosis Osteomyelitis Pneumonia
Parenteral nutrition	AIDS-related enteropathy Colitis Crohn's disease Pancreatitis Various cancers (e.g., colon, liver, stomach)
Chemotherapy	Leukemias Lymphomas Sarcomas Various carcinomas (e.g., breast, lung, pancreas)
Pain management	Chronic intractable pain (secondary to cancer) Various AIDS-related diagnoses
Hydration therapy	Gastroenteritis Hyperemesis gravidarum Intractable diarrhea

From Humphrey, C. J., & Milone-Nuzzo, P. (1991). *Home care nursing: An orientation to practice.* New York: Appleton & Lange.

Total Parenteral Nutrition

Use of TPN may be indicated when oral nutrition is not sufficient. The TPN requires a physician's order specifying the type of solution, frequency of administration, frequency of vital sign assessment, and periodic serum chemistry assessment. The TPN solutions are prepared in a pharmacy and must be refrigerated. An infusion pump is always used to ensure constant flow rates.

Enteral Nutrition Therapy

Enteral nutrition therapy is indicated for those clients who cannot receive sufficient oral nutrition. Enteral nutrition is the treatment of choice for clients with functioning lower gastrointestinal tract, but for whom food intake is not possible, is not adequate, or is too difficult. Home-based enteral nutrition is most commonly seen when providing care to clients with conditions such as pharyngeal or esophageal strictures or neurological disorders resulting in dysphagia, anorexia, and coma.

The client's diagnosis, condition, long-term needs, and prognosis determine the type of feeding tube and placement. In acute care facilities, nasogastric or orogastric tubes are often used to insert nutrients directly into the stomach. Surgically implanted feeding tubes (gastrostomy or jejunostomy tubes) are used for clients with long-term nutrition assistance and/or conditions that necessitate bypassing portions of the gastrointestinal system. In home care, as in institutional settings, the feeding regimen is determined and prescribed by the physician or an interdisciplinary team including a nutritionist, physician, and possibly a pharmacist. Choice of feeding solutions or formulas requires consideration of the metabolic needs of the client, financial limitations, learning ability of the client or caregivers, and other necessary therapies. Instruction for enteral therapy should include the specific supplements, amount, time, route, and procedure. Feedings may be prescribed as continuous, intermittent, or bolus. As in other areas of home health care, much of the nurse's responsibility lies in teaching the

client or caregiver procedures for home nutrition therapy and supporting and monitoring the care.

WOUND MANAGEMENT

Wound care is one of the most common services provided by home health nurses. In the home, nurses typically work with wounds that are difficult to heal, usually because of underlying disease processes (e.g., diabetes, peripheral vascular disease), anemia, poor nutrition, wound contamination, chemical irritants, neglect, medications, age, and other factors (Rice, 2001b). When wounds do not respond to care or when providing care to a client with an ostomy, nurses with special training or experience may be used.

Chronic Wound Care

Basic wound care, including frequency of dressing change, type of dressing used, cleaning solutions, and topical medications, is generally determined by the physician. Nurses who specialize in wound care, however, often have latitude to make decisions based on their expertise. Goals for wound treatment and management include the following:

1. Prevention of further tissue destruction by reducing or controlling predisposing causes of tissue destruction
2. Prevention of infection
3. Planning treatments as appropriate for (a) type of wound (pressure, venous, or surgical) and (b) condition and size of the wound (stage, amount of drainage, and related factors) (Rice and Wiersema, 1996, p. 222)

In addition to changing dressings, nursing interventions in wound care include assessment of the wound and evaluation of the efficacy of treatment, cleansing and debridement, obtaining cultures when indicated, teaching the client and/or caregiver how to change the dressing using sterile technique, and teaching caregivers signs and symptoms of infection and how to prevent further tissue breakdown.

A number of wound care products are available and used by home care nurses to treat and prevent wounds. These include transparent dressings, hydrocolloid dressings, nonadherent dressings, and hypertonic saline gauze. The nurse may assist in securing specialized equipment or supplies to prevent pressure sores. Gel pads, foam mattresses, and air support mattresses, for example, may be helpful.

Enterostomal Care

Many home care agencies employ enterostomal nurses or enterostomal therapists to assist clients with a colostomy, an ileostomy, or a urostomy. Client and caregiver education and support and monitoring for complications or side effects are primary functions of **enterostomal care**.

In addition to providing client education for ostomy care, enterostomal nurses are often specialists in wound care and management. Typically, ET nurses case manage clients with ostomies and act as a resource for other home health nurses. Often, the ET nurse is consulted to assist in preventing skin breakdown for high-risk clients (e.g., those who are bed bound, very frail, paraplegic, or quadriplegic) or if a wound is not healing as anticipated.

CARE OF VENTILATOR-DEPENDENT CLIENTS

As with areas of specialized care, home health care for ventilator-dependent clients is growing. Individuals with conditions such as severe chronic obstructive pulmonary disease or other chronic lung problems (e.g., cystic fibrosis or complex pneumonia) or spinal cord injuries or defects who are ventilator dependent or need ventilator assistance are sometimes discharged from acute care or long-term institutions into the home. Home health nurses who work with ventilator-dependent clients must have intensive training and consistent agency support. When providing care to ventilator-dependent clients, the home health nurse must work closely with the physician, respiratory therapist, and family members. The nurse's role in the care of ventilator-dependent clients is largely supportive and includes the following:

- Assessing the home situation for the availability of 24-hour caregivers who are properly

trained, competent, and able to perform cardiopulmonary resuscitation.
- Working with the physician and respiratory therapist to outline guidelines for concern (e.g., complications such as infection or respiratory difficulty) and appropriate interventions to teach the caregivers.
- Implementing and periodically reviewing emergency plans with the care providers.
- Coordinating referrals with social workers, physical or occupational therapists, respite caregivers, support groups, or others as appropriate.
- Teaching and monitoring tracheotomy care and suctioning.
- Providing skilled nursing care for other needs of the client.
- Assisting in monitoring blood gas levels and acid-base balance as ordered or needed.

Ventilator-dependent clients are at risk for problems and complications such as infection, fluid volume overload, impaired skin integrity, and injury (e.g., tracheostomal trauma from suctioning, overinflation of the tracheostomy tube cuff, tissue adhesions and stricture) (Rice, 2001c). Agency policy and physician orders dictate care for these clients. In general, the stoma should be cleaned daily, with the skin being assessed for signs of infection. Needed suctioning using disposable or properly cleaned catheters should be performed using aseptic technique and tracheotomy tubes should be changed at least monthly. Knowledge of commonly used equipment and supplies is essential for nurses who work with ventilator-dependent clients.

PERINATAL HOME CARE

Home care for pregnant and postpartum clients has increased dramatically during the past few years. Technologically advanced care for high-risk pregnancies and for neonates with identified breathing difficulties is now delivered in the home under certain conditions. In addition, postpartum care for clients, particularly following shortened hospital stays, is becoming increasingly common and even mandated in some locations. High-tech perinatal home care, apnea monitoring for high-risk infants, and postpartum home care are discussed briefly.

Home Care of High-Risk Perinatal Clients

One of the newest areas for home health nursing involves the care of high-risk perinatal clients. Until very recently, high-risk maternity clients were hospitalized for extended periods for monitoring or treatment. In many cases, they are now being cared for in the home. **Perinatal home care** services include the following components:

- Uterine monitoring: A portable monitor may be used to assess contractions. The monitor may then be taken back to the provider, agency, or institution for evaluation or the information may be transmitted to a receiving center via telephone lines.
- Fetal monitoring: A portable fetal monitor may be used to perform a nonstress test to assess fetal development and condition. Like the uterine monitor, the fetal monitor produces a printed strip that can be transmitted or carried to the institution or agency for interpretation.
- Ultrasound: A portable ultrasound machine is used to perform a biophysical profile to evaluate fetal movement, fetal heart rate, muscle tone, and fluid volume.
- Infusion pump treatment: Subcutaneous infusion therapy utilizes a microinfusion pump to deliver continuous or intermittent low doses of a prescribed medication. For example, a medication such as terbutaline can be administered to control uterine contractions associated with preterm labor; an insulin pump may be used to administer insulin subcutaneously for an uncontrolled, brittle diabetic; or heparin may be administered via pump for a pregnant woman prone to developing blood clots.
- Infusion therapy: Antibiotics may be needed for severe infection; hydration therapy and TPN may be administered for hyperemesis.
- Hypertension monitoring: The nurse can teach the client or family to monitor blood pressure and report findings. As with uterine or fetal monitors, remote blood pressure

monitors enable the client to transmit findings to a center or provider for interpretation (Dahlberg, Blazek, Wikoff, Tuckwell, and Koloroutis, 1995).

Postpartum Home Care

Increasingly, shortened postpartum hospital stays, attributable to health care reform and cost containment, have led to steady growth in postpartum home care. Evans (1995) reported that during the past decade, hospital stays for women experiencing vaginal delivery have declined from 3 to 4 days to 24 hours or less and hospital stays for women who have undergone cesarean delivery decreased from 5 to 7 days to 72 hours. Benefits attributable to early discharge are quicker reestablishment of family routines, decreased separation from the family, decreased costs, decreased risk of nosocomial infection, emotional and psychological benefits from familiar surroundings, and increased confidence in learning to care for the neonate in the normal setting. Disadvantages include decreased educational opportunities; need for increased help at home to provide meals and other home maintenance services; lack of rest for the mother; lack of nursing guidance for breastfeeding and neonatal care; and potential for undiagnosed complications, such as neonatal hyperbilirubinemia, low neonatal temperature, maternal hemorrhage, and excessive maternal pain.

Postpartum nursing care, whether in the hospital or home, includes monitoring the physical and emotional well-being of family members; identification of potential or developing complications; and bridging the gap between discharge and ambulatory follow-up for mothers and infants (Lynch, Kordish, and Williams, 2001). To meet the educational, physiological, and supportive needs of the childbearing family, several different models of postpartum home health care have been developed. In general, postpartum home care services include health promotion and health education activities that have been within the traditional scope and functions of postpartum care. Postpartum home care services described by

Evans (1995) include follow-up telephone calls 1 to 3 days after discharge, home visits 1 to 3 days after discharge, new parent information telephone lines staffed by a nurse and available 24 hours a day, lactation consultation to assist with problems encountered with breastfeeding, and organized support groups and outpatient clinics that encourage the first visit 3 to 4 days postdischarge to assess both mother and infant and provide relevant teaching and interventions.

Many providers and agencies have programs that offer a combination of these services. For example, Williams and Cooper (1993) described a program for maternity clients that includes an RN case manager who coordinates care with physicians, discharge planning nurses, and community agencies; home visits 1 to 3 days postdischarge for assessment of the mother, infant, and family and provision of interventions as warranted; use of a risk management documentation tool; postvisit telephone call(s); and a 24-hour help line.

During postpartum home visitation, the most common concerns of the mother are pain associated with episiotomy or cesarean incision, breast engorgement, backache, and uterine cramping. In addition, teaching regarding nutritional needs and avoidance of infection and constipation is also warranted. Infant concerns and questions are typically related to nutrition—particularly ineffective breastfeeding and bottle-feeding problems—and hyperbilirubinemia (Williams and Cooper, 1993).

Apnea Monitoring

Apnea monitoring is most often indicated for premature infants with apnea, infants who have experienced or are at risk for experiencing a life-threatening event, and infants at risk for sudden infant death syndrome (Humphrey and Milone-Nuzzo, 1991). In home care, the primary role of the nurse is in educating the parents or caregivers about normal infant breathing patterns, recognition of and response to apnea episodes, infant cardiopulmonary resuscitation, and use and maintenance of the apnea monitor. Additionally,

the home care nurse should review the infant's cardiopulmonary status, review teaching, evaluate the parents' level of understanding, and assess the parents' stress. Referral for social services or respite care may be appropriate.

PSYCHIATRIC HOME CARE

Although **psychiatric home health care** was first recognized as a reimbursable treatment alternative by the HCFA (now known as the Centers for Medicare & Medicaid) and thereby eligible for Medicare reimbursement in 1979, it has only very recently become widely available for clients (Carson, 1996). Psychiatric home care is appropriate for individuals with diagnosed or suspected mental illness who need psychiatric services, but cannot use traditional outpatient mental health services. For example, psychiatric home care can prevent or shorten psychiatric hospitalization, particularly for acutely depressed individuals and those diagnosed as schizophrenic (Hauk, 1996). The goals of psychiatric home health care are the following:

- Reduce the need for hospitalization or rehospitalization of clients in psychological crisis.
- Promote the client's adjustment to the community and home.
- Monitor medication compliance, effectiveness, and side effects.
- Provide assistance with problem solving to families.
- Reinforce predischarge therapy and treatment.
- Provide education to clients and their families regarding issues such as disease process, medication, diet, and community resources.
- Provide in-home respite services to the client's family (Gilkison and Neathery, 1995).

The elderly, many of whom have been previously hospitalized or institutionalized, make up the largest population served by psychiatric home care (Dittbrenner, 1994). Much of psychiatric home care, like much of home health care in general, is reimbursed by Medicare.

To be eligible for Medicare reimbursement for psychiatric home care services, several criteria must be met regarding the client and the care provider. For example, the client must be home-bound and have a diagnosed psychiatric condition. In addition, the plan of care must be directed by a psychiatrist and the care must be delivered by a "specially trained" or "experienced" nurse. Special training or experience includes a Master's degree in psychiatric nursing or community health nursing, or a bachelor's degree in nursing with 1 year of adult or geriatric psychiatric experience, or a diploma or associate degree in nursing and 2 years of adult or geriatric psychiatric experience, or ANA certification in psychiatric or community health nursing (Carson, 1996; Hauk, 1996).

Client conditions or diagnoses in which home care might be beneficial, or even preferable to traditional outpatient or inpatient care, include confusion or disorientation, severe depression, altered perception or cognition, risk for self-harm, vulnerability in the community, requirement of 24-hour supervision, excessive fear or anxiety, agoraphobia, need for assistive devices for mobility, or inability to leave home independently (Carson, 1996). (See the Community Application box "Nursing Interventions and Services in Psychiatric Home Health Care.")

HOSPICE CARE: HOME CARE OF THE TERMINALLY ILL

The hospice movement in the United States is relatively recent, beginning in the 1970s (Clemen-Stone, Eigsti, and McGuire, 1995). **Hospice care** is a philosophy intended to provide palliative care to the terminally ill. Most hospice patients have a diagnosis of cancer, but other diagnoses commonly seen in hospice care include AIDS, severe chronic obstructive pulmonary disease, terminal heart conditions, and neurological conditions such as amyotrophic lateral sclerosis or multiple sclerosis.

Hospice programs may be located either at a client's place of residence or in an inpatient facility. Models for hospice care include hospice-based programs within a hospital or within an

---

COMMUNITY APPLICATION
Nursing Interventions and Services in Psychiatric Home Health Care

- Individual psychotherapy, as appropriate, to improve self-concept, decrease fear or anxiety, decrease hopelessness, increase motivation, increase spiritual well-being, improve eating patterns, improve sleep patterns, increase social interaction, and promote diversional activities
- Ongoing assessment and monitoring of psychiatric and emotional status
- Medication administration and management (including injection of medications such as haloperidol or fluphenazine decanoate) and assessment for medication effectiveness, compliance, and side effects
- Teaching about medication regimens, disease process, communication skills, and signs and symptoms of exacerbation of illness

- Crisis and symptom management
- Laboratory services (e.g., medication blood levels, white blood counts for clozapine)
- Case management to link clients and caregivers to community resources
- Assessment of family and community support systems and their effectiveness
- 24-hour on-call nursing support
- Development, implementation, and evaluation of a nursing care plan
- Coordination with other home care services, such as pharmacy, support, therapy, social service, and home care aide services

Data from Carson, V. B. (1996). The journey through home mental health care. In V. B. Carson & E. N. Arnold (Eds.), *Mental health nursing: The nurse-patient journey.* Philadelphia: W. B. Saunders; Dittbrenner, H. (1994). Psychiatric home care: An overview. *Caring,* June, 26-30; Hauk, D. O. (1996). The mental health patient. In R. Rice (Ed.), *Home health nursing: Concepts and application* (2nd ed.). St. Louis: Mosby; Lima, B. (1995). In-home psychiatric nursing: The at-home mental health program. *Caring,* July, 14-20.

extended care facility, a free-standing hospice, or home care hospice programs.

Although hospice care is frequently delivered to clients and their families in the home, there are distinctive differences between hospice care and traditional home health care. For example, in hospice nursing the primary focus is on quality of life and palliation, whereas in conventional home health the primary focus is on rehabilitation and restoration. In hospice, the nurse sees the client intermittently, with visits intensifying in frequency until death. In conventional home health, the nurse sees the client intermittently, with the number of visits decreasing in frequency until the client is medically stable. Finally, hospice care requires expertise in managing terminal symptoms with active efforts to try alternative comforting approaches in contrast to treating acute or chronic illnesses.

Hospice care focuses on the client and the family. According to the ANA (1987), hospice care emphasizes the following:

1. Assistance in dealing with emotional, spiritual, and medical problems
2. Support of the family
3. Keeping the client in his or her home for as long as is feasible while making his or her life as comfortable and as meaningful as possible
4. Coordinated home care; inpatient, acute, and respite care; and bereavement services
5. Coordinated professional services and volunteer services appropriate to the individual client
6. Palliative care focusing on pain management

Eligibility for Hospice Care

Medicare Part A reimburses providers for hospice care. To be eligible for hospice benefits, clients must have life expectancy of 6 months or less, according to a physician's estimate, and they must not be undergoing or contemplating active treatment for their disease. In addition, they must have decided to forgo resuscitative measures at the time of death (Nichols and Rice, 2001).

Caregiver Support

Caregiver support involves teaching about the course and progression of the disease and pain and symptom management. In addition, reassurance and provision of respite care or relief for the caregivers is very important. The hospice nurse can assist by referring the caregiver to providers of respite care or by instructing other family members or intermediate caregivers how to care for the client. Reassurance that the care is appropriate and that they are "doing the right thing" is emotionally beneficial. Common reactions seen in caregivers of the dying include grief, loneliness, isolation, feelings of uselessness or helplessness, anxiety, anger, depression, and fatigue. The hospice nurse can anticipate these and be prepared to intervene (Kemp, 1999).

Symptom Management

Control of symptoms is one of the primary goals in caring for hospice clients. Symptoms encountered can be the result of treatment and palliative measures taken (e.g., constipation from pain medications or nausea from radiation therapy) or the disease process and progression. Among the most frequently encountered problems are anorexia, weakness, fatigue, constipation, edema, urinary problems, dyspnea, skin problems, insomnia, dry mouth, dysphasia, coughing and confusion (Nichols and Rice, 2001). The nurse should anticipate these problems and take preventative measures whenever possible. Teaching the caregivers symptom prevention and/or management is essential.

Pain Management

According to Kemp (1999), pain is the most problematic and feared symptom in terminal care. Effective pain management includes accurate assessment of the pain and establishment of an effective, individualized pain management plan. Thorough assessment of a client's pain should include information regarding each of the following elements:

• Location of the pain
• Extension or radiation

- Onset and pattern
- Duration
- Character or quality
- Precipitating, aggravating, or alleviating factors
- Intensity
- Associated symptoms
- Effect on activities of daily living
- Methods of pain relief (Matassarin-Jacobs, 1993)

Often, pain treatment is inadequate and inconsistent because of failure to routinely assess pain and pain relief; lack of knowledge among nurses and physicians of pain management; social or cultural fears; persistent myths (e.g., that pain is inevitable or use of opioids will result in loss of control or addiction); fear of respiratory depression; social or legal impediments to using opioids; communication problems among clients, caregivers, and professional staff; disease characteristics; and client characteristics (Kemp, 1999). To assist in developing a pain management plan, Box 4-3 contains basic principles for pain management.

Nurses who care for hospice clients should be very knowledgeable about pain management in general and about pharmacological management in particular. Utilization of appropriate drugs, dosages, and combinations requires experience and may require experimentation (e.g., some drugs or combinations of drugs or routes

of administration work better for different clients or for different diagnoses). Hospice nurses must be well informed of the different types of pain medications and adjuvant medications and appropriate dosages and combinations. It is important to note that dosages and schedules may vary dramatically for terminally ill clients and opioid doses may seem very high to nurses who do not routinely work with clients with severe pain. To assist in understanding the uses of different pain medications, Figure 4-3 presents the World Health Organization's three-step program to manage cancer pain.

Psychological and Spiritual Support of the Dying Client

Addressing the psychological and spiritual needs of the dying client can be extremely difficult for the nurse and the caregiver. Review of Kubler-Ross' (1969) stages of death and dying (denial, anger, bargaining, depression, and acceptance) can be helpful. Recognition of these stages in the client and the family can assist in determining appropriate interventions. When observing a dying client, the nurse can expect feelings of loss and grief, loneliness, uselessness, anger, anxiety, fear, and depression.

Spiritual care involves understanding the client's spiritual beliefs and recognizing spiritual needs. Interventions can include listening to fears and concerns, helping the client understand the

---

BOX 4-3 Principles of Effective Pain Management

- Use medications or techniques appropriate to the severity and specific type of pain.
- Give medications in amounts sufficient to control the pain and at intervals appropriate to the medication's duration of action.
- Use oral medications when possible.
- Give medications around the clock at regular intervals (prophylactically) to achieve a constant titer.
- Use adjuvant medications (e.g., nonsteroidal anti-inflammatory drugs, corticosteroids, anticonvulsants, antidepressants, phenothiazines).

- Assess and treat side effects or complications.
- Anticipate side effects (e.g., constipation from narcotics, nausea).
- Assess for tolerance.
- Assess for and intervene in psychosocial and spiritual issues related to pain.
- Approach each patient as an individual and assess unique beliefs, strengths, and weaknesses.
- Teach the client and family principles of pain management.

From Kemp, C. E. (1999). *Terminal illness: A guide to nursing care* (2nd ed.). Philadelphia: J. B. Lippincott.

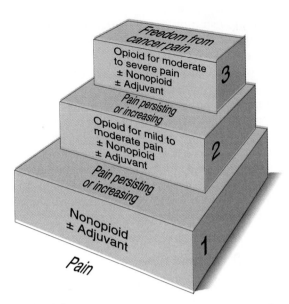

Figure 4-3. World Health Organization three-step analgesic ladder. *Step 1:* Nonopioid ± adjuvant. When pain persists or increases, proceed to Step 2. *Step 2:* Opioid for mild-to-moderate pain ± nonopioid ± adjuvant. When pain persists or increases, proceed to Step 3. *Step 3:* Opioid for moderate to severe pain ± nonopioid ± adjuvant. (Reproduced with permission from the World Health Organization [WHO]. [1996]. *Cancer pain relief* [2nd ed.]. Geneva: World Health Organization.)

meaning of death, praying with the client, reading to him or her from the Bible or literature from another religion, expressing hope, and affirming the importance of spiritual concerns at the end of life. Referral to a minister, priest, rabbi, or other spiritual care provider should be offered.

Kemp (1999) describes personal qualities the nurse can demonstrate that are helpful in providing spiritual care at the end of life: realism (e.g., death is the end of a life on earth), hopefulness (i.e., includes hope of a better life in the present and in the future), truthfulness, faith, resourcefulness (i.e., ability to use the available resources), advocacy, sensitivity (e.g., acceptance of the client's uniqueness), and openness to the client's needs. Presence, or simply being near the client, can also be very comforting.

Interventions at Death

Infection, organ failure, lung or heart infarction, electrolyte imbalance, and hemorrhage are the most common causes of death in cancer clients (Kemp, 1999). Teaching the family what to expect as death nears and what to do following death are very important functions of the hospice nurse. Common signs of impending death include progressive anorexia, refusal of fluids, dreams and visions of persons who have died previously, withdrawal, changes in symptoms (e.g., increase or decrease in pain), respiratory symptoms (e.g., increasingly shallow and/or labored respirations, with periods of apnea, dyspnea, increased secretions), increased pulse rate, and changes in consciousness (e.g., drowsiness, unresponsiveness, confusion, agitation) (Kemp, 1999). The client's skin may become progressively cyanotic, cool, and mottled. The nurse should reassure the family that these signs are expected and manage them appropriately with comfort measures.

As death nears, families are instructed to call the primary hospice nurse or agency and not to call any emergency services. Depending on community or state requirements and agency policy, the nurse usually calls the physician, religious leader, funeral home, or others who have been identified in advance. Following the client's death, the nurse may bathe the client, remove all tubes and equipment, cover the body, and stay with the family until all arrangements have been made. It is appropriate for the nurse to cry or express grief with the family if he or she needs to do so. Frequently, hospice nurses attend the client's wake, mass, funeral, or memorial service.

SUMMARY

Home health care is a dynamic, growing field for nursing practice that can be fun, autonomous, flexible, and very rewarding. Like Penny, the nurse in the opening case study, RNs who desire to work in home health care should be experienced and must be well trained and supported by agency management. A comprehensive orientation and ongoing assistance and supervisory support enhance the transition into home health practice and promote high quality nursing care.

As health care delivery continues to evolve and become increasingly community based, more and different types of care will be provided in the home. Emerging technology will allow for greater use of telecommunications, which, in turn, may dramatically change the types of care delivered in homes. Other factors, such as the aging of the population and the increasing numbers of clients with chronic diseases, will dictate an increased need for more home health agencies and providers. In particular, those that offer specialized care as described here will be in demand.

Because the knowledge base and information necessary for the practice of home health care nursing is vast, only a small portion has been discussed here; many issues and topics are beyond the scope of this book. The Resources box that follows presents a list of organizations that are excellent sources for more information on home health care nursing practice.

Resources

Home Health Care Nursing

National Association for Home Care
Centers for Medicare & Medicaid (formerly HCFA)
Medicare
Visiting Nurses' Association of America
National Hospice and Palliative Care
   Organization
Children's Hospice International

Visit the book's website at **www.wbsaunders.com/SIMON/McEwen**
for a direct link to the website for each organization listed.

KEY POINTS

- Home health nursing integrates medical/surgical, community health, parent-child, gerontological, and psychiatric-mental health nursing into home health care practice. It refers to comprehensive nursing care provided to individuals and families in their place of residence, focusing on the environmental, psychosocial, economic, cultural, and personal health factors affecting health status.

- With the passage of Medicare in 1965, the practice of home health care nursing changed dramatically. Until recently, home health care was largely provided by official (governmental or public) or voluntary (private, nonprofit) agencies. This has changed in the past decade and the majority of home health agencies are now proprietary or hospital based.

- Public sources (Medicare and Medicaid) finance more than 50% of home health services. To be reimbursed by Medicare, home health agencies must be Medicare certified, follow Medicare's conditions of participation (explicit rules, standards, and requirements), and be certified by an accreditation organization.

- To qualify for coverage under Medicare, services must be "reasonable and necessary"; the client's care must require intermittent skilled nursing care, physical therapy, or speech therapy; the client must be homebound and under the care of a physician who develops a home health plan; and the agency must be certified to participate in Medicare.

- Thorough and accurate documentation is essential in home health nursing to record services, describe the client's condition and response to care, promote continuity of care, validate reimbursement claims, and forestall legal action. Completion of the required Medicare forms is necessary for payment.

- Home health care nursing requires unique skills and knowledge. Basic and essential activities include discharge planning (the process of determining the planning to meet client needs following release from a health care facility), case management (the process of ensuring that the services provided are appropriate for the client's needs), coordination of community resources, and interdisciplinary collaboration.

- Previsit planning involves determining which clients are to be seen and prioritization of the scheduled visits. Planning includes caseload scheduling, making contact by telephone or another method if necessary, review of the client's chart, assessment of supplies and equipment needed and what is on hand, and consideration of safety concerns.

- During the implementation stage, the scheduled plan of care is completed, which includes a comprehensive assessment, provision of skilled nursing care, health teaching as necessary, and other interventions. Following completion of the skilled nursing interventions and teaching, the nurse evaluates the response of the client to care, summarizes the continuing plan of care with the client and caregiver, and may set up a time for the next visit.
- Postvisit activities include communication of findings to other health care providers and completing requisite documentation.
- Home infusion therapy is a very significant component of home health care and includes delivery of antibiotics, pain medication, TPN, hydration, and chemotherapy.
- Home-based care of clients with chronic wounds is an important component of home health care. Nursing interventions in wound care typically include assessment of the wound and evaluation of the efficacy of treatment, cleaning and debridement, obtaining cultures, and teaching the client and/or caregiver how to change the dressing using sterile techniques.
- Enterostomal nurses are specialists in wound care and management and they provide specialized care for clients with a colostomy, an ileostomy, or a urostomy.
- Home care of ventilator-dependent clients may be necessary for persons with severe chronic obstructive pulmonary disease or other chronic lung problems, spinal cord injuries, or other defects, who have been discharged from acute care or long-term institutions into the home.
- Home care for pregnant and postpartum clients has increased dramatically during the past few years. Technologically advanced care for high-risk pregnancies (e.g., uterine monitoring, fetal monitoring, ultrasound, infusion pump treatment, and infusion therapy and hypertension monitoring) and care for neonates with compli-

cations (e.g., apnea monitoring) are becoming fairly routine. Postpartum care for uncomplicated clients following shortened hospital stays is also growing.

- Psychiatric home care is appropriate for individuals with diagnoses of suspected mental illnesses who need psychiatric services, but cannot use traditional outpatient mental health services. Psychiatric home care can prevent hospitalization for clients with diagnoses such as severe depression, schizophrenia, and Alzheimer's disease.
- Hospice care provides palliative care to the terminally ill and is frequently provided in the home. Hospice care focuses on the family and the client and provides assistance in dealing with emotional, spiritual, and medical problems; coordinates professional and volunteer services; and makes the client as comfortable as possible through pain and symptom management.

Learning Activities & Application to Practice

In Class

1. With classmates, practice conducting a home visit. One student can act as the client, one or two can act as caregivers, and one or two can act as the nurses. Practice each stage of the home visit and critique each other.

2. Talk with a nurse who routinely works in one of the specialized home health care areas examined in the chapter. Encourage the nurse to describe the types of clients seen, sources of reimbursement, changes in home health care in recent years, and anticipated changes. What professional experience is necessary for this type of practice? What strategies must be used to assist in teaching caregivers to provide the necessary care?

3. Box 4-4 lists a sample daily caseload for a home health nurse. Study the caseload and set a tentative schedule for ordering the visits. You will need to anticipate the amount of time needed for each visit and allow time for travel. Discuss the schedule with classmates.

> ## **4-4** Sample Home Health Nursing Daily Caseload

Mrs. E. Cooper: Map coordinates, 37G; admit visit; dx—CHF, HTN
Assess: V.S., C/P status, weight, edema—lower extremities, nutrition status, medication compliance
Teaching: HTN, low-Na diet, medication regimen
Special considerations: Daughter to be in the home 09:00-12:00—requests SNV when she is present

Mr. C. McClure: Map coordinates, 38D; return visit; dx—postCVA (anticoagulant therapy)
Assess: V.S., C/P status, neuro status, weight, nutrition status, medication compliance
Teaching: Anticoagulant therapy (s/sx of complications, medication regimen, safety)
Special considerations: Lab draw—protime—specimen to lab within 30 minutes; call M.D. with results before 14:00.

Mr. T. Johnson: Map coordinates, 23A; return visit; dx—diabetes
Assess: V.S., C/P status, weight, nutrition/diet, blood sugar (fasting), medication compliance
Teaching: IDDM (review materials left in home), observe DFS and self-administration of insulin, ADA diet
Special considerations: Requests SNV around 7:30 to allow breakfast by 8:30

Mrs. M. Charles: Map coordinates, 38M; return visit; dx—wound right foot—BID dressing changes (early A.M. and late afternoon)
Assess: V.S., C/P status, neuro status, nutrition status, medication compliance, wound—right foot
Wound care: Location—right foot; wet-to-dry dressing—cleanse with NS, pack with 2 4 × 4s and secure with 4" gauze
Teaching: s/sx of infection, safety
Special considerations: Pt had 99.8 temp yesterday—M.D. notified—requests to be called following visit regardless of findings; needs 1 week supply of gauze, NS, sterile gloves, and 4 x 4s

Mrs. G. Grace: Map coordinates, 36A; return visit; dx—urinary incontinence—indwelling catheter
Assess: V.S., C/P status, elimination status, neuro status, nutrition status, skin integrity
Teaching: s/sx of infection, monitoring fluid intake, catheter care
Special considerations: c/g reports catheter leaking—requests change

ADA, American Diabetes Association; *BID,* twice a day; *c/g,* caregiver; *CHF,* congestive heart failure; *C/P,* cardiopulmonary; *CVA,* cerebrovascular accident; *DFS,* diabetic finger stick; *dx,* diagnosis; *HTN,* hypertension; *IDDM,* insulin-dependent diabetes mellitus; *lab,* laboratory; *M.D.,* physician; *Na,* sodium; *neuro,* neurological; *NS,* normal saline; *pt,* patient; *s/sx,* signs and symptoms; *SNV,* skilled nursing visit; *V.S.,* vital signs.

In Clinical

4. Work with a practicing home health care nurse for a minimum of 6 days. Keep a log or a diary recording the types of clients seen. What skilled nursing interventions were performed? What practical experiences and skills are helpful for nurses considering home health practice? Describe the process of documentation.

5. In a log or diary, list the activities that were accomplished for one home visit within the three stages of a home visit described. Outline what preparations were made during the planning stage, what skilled nursing interventions and teaching were provided during the implementation stage, and describe postvisit activities. If possible, include the rationale chosen for scheduling of the case-load (i.e., what factors were considered in ordering the schedule?).

6. Work with a home health nurse who provides "specialty" care as described in this chapter.

REFERENCES

American Nurses' Association. (1987). *Standards for hospice nursing practice.* Kansas City, MO: American Nurses' Association.

American Nurses' Association. (1992). *A statement on the scope of home health nursing practice.* Washington, DC: American Nurses' Association.

American Nurses' Association. (1999). *The scope and standards of home health nursing practice.* Washington, DC: American Nurses' Association.

American Nurses Credentialing Center. (2000). *ANCC certification catalog.* Washington, DC: American Nurses' Association.

Balinsky, W. (1995). High-tech homecare. *Caring*, May, 7-9.

Carson, V. B. (1996). The journey through home mental health care. In V. B. Carson & E. N. Arnold (Eds.), *Mental health nursing: The nurse-patient journey* (pp. 1151-1170). Philadelphia: W. B. Saunders.

Clark, M. J. (1995). *Nursing in the community* (2nd ed.). Norwalk, CT: Appleton & Lange.

Clark, M. J. (1999). *Nursing in the community* (3rd ed.). Norwalk, CT: Appleton & Lange.

Clemen-Stone, S., Eigsti, D. G., & McGuire, S. L. (1995). *Comprehensive community health nursing* (4th ed.). St. Louis: Mosby.

Dahlberg, N. L. F., Blazek, D., Wikoff, B., Tuckwell, B. L., & Koloroutis, M. (1995). High-tech, high-touch perinatal home care. *Caring*, May, 36-39.

Dittbrenner, H. (1994). Psychiatric home care: An overview. *Caring*, June, 26-30.

Evans, C. J. (1995). Postpartum home care in the United States. *Journal of Obstetric, Gynecologic, and Neonatal Nursing*, 24(2), 180-186.

Gilkison, J. R., & Neathery, M. B. (1995). Mental health in the home and community. In D. Antia-Otong (Ed.), *Psychiatric nursing: Biological and behavioral concepts* (pp. 521-541). Philadelphia: W. B. Saunders.

Hauk, D. O. (1996). The mental health patient. In R. Rice (Ed.), *Home health nursing: Concepts and application* (2nd ed., pp. 399-420). St. Louis: Mosby.

Humphrey, C. J., & Milone-Nuzzo, P. (1991). *Home care nursing: An orientation to practice.* Norwalk, CT: Appleton & Lange.

Health Care Financing Administration (HCFA). (1999). *A profile of Medicare home health: Chartbook.* (Publication # FCFA 10138). Washington, DC: DHHS/HCFA.

Health Care Financing Administration (HCFA). (2001). Home Health Agency Manual (Publication #11). Washington, DC: HCFA. Retrieved 07/06/2001 from http://www.hcfa.gov/pubforms/11_hha/hh00.htm.

Horn, B. J., & Horn, B. M. (1993). The health care system. In J. M. Swanson & M. Albrecht (Eds.), *Community health nursing: Promoting the health of aggregates.* Philadelphia: W. B. Saunders.

Humphrey, C. J., & Milone-Nuzzo, P. (1991). *Home care nursing: An orientation to practice.* Norwalk, CT: Appleton & Lange.

Kemp, C. E. (1999). *Terminal illness: A guide to nursing care* (2nd ed.). Philadelphia: J. B. Lippincott.

Kubler-Ross, E. (1969). *On death and dying.* New York: Macmillan.

Lima, B. (1995). In-home psychiatric nursing: The at-home mental health program. *Caring*, July, 14-20

Lynch, A. M., Kordish, R. A., & Williams, L. R. (2001). Maternal-child nursing: Postpartum home care. In R. Rice (Ed.), *Home health nursing: Concepts and application* (3rd ed., pp. 379-398). St. Louis: Mosby.

Matassarin-Jacobs, E. (1993). Pain assessment and intervention. In J. M. Black & E. Matassarin-Jacobs (Eds.), *Luckmann and Sorensen's medical-surgical nursing: A psychophysiologic approach* (4th ed., pp. 311-358). Philadelphia: W. B. Saunders.

Milone-Nuzzo, P. (2000). Home health care. In C. M. Smith & F. A. Maurer (Eds.), *Community health nursing: Theory and practice* (2nd ed.). Philadelphia: W. B. Saunders.

National Association for Home Care. (2000). *Basic statistics about home care.* Washington, DC: National Association for Home Care.

Nichols, G., & Rice, R. (2001). The hospice patient. In R. Rice (Ed.), *Home health nursing: Concepts and application* (3rd ed., pp. 430-456). St. Louis: Mosby.

Rice, R. (2000). *Manual of home health nursing practice* (2nd ed.). St. Louis: Mosby.

Rice, R. (2001a). Home care nursing practice: Historical perspectives and philosophy of care. In R. Rice (Ed.), *Home health nursing practice: Concepts & application* (3rd ed., pp. 3-14.) St. Louis: Mosby.

Rice, R. (2001b). The patient with chronic wounds. In R. Rice (Ed.), *Home health nursing practice: Concepts & application* (3rd ed., pp. 239-264). St. Louis: Mosby.

Rice, R. (2001c). The ventilator-dependent patient. In R. Rice (Ed.), *Home health nursing practice: Concepts & application* (3rd ed., pp. 215-238). St. Louis: Mosby.

Rice, R., & Wiersema, L. A. (1996). The patient with chronic wounds. In R. Rice (Ed.), *Home health nursing practice: Concepts & application* (2nd ed., pp. 211-234). St. Louis: Mosby.

Smith, C. M. (1995). The home visit: Opening the doors. In C. M. Smith & F. A. Maurer (Eds.), *Community health nursing: Theory and practice* (pp. 179-204). Philadelphia: W. B. Saunders.

U.S. Department of Health and Human Services, Division of Nursing, Bureau of Health Professions, Public Health Service. (1998). *The registered nurse population: Findings for the national sample survey of registered nurses,* March, 1996. Washington, DC: Government Printing Office.

Warhola, C. (1980). *Planning for home health services: A resource handbook.* (DHHS Publication No. [HRA] 80-14017). Washington, DC: U.S. Department of Health and Human Services.

Watkins, L. B., & Rice, R. (1996). The patient receiving home infusion therapy. In R. Rice (Ed.), *Home health nursing practice: Concepts & application* (2nd ed., pp. 283-298). St. Louis: Mosby.

Williams, L. R., & Cooper, M. K. (1993). Nurse-managed postpartum home care. *Journal of Obstetric, Gynecologic, and Neonatal Nursing*, 22(1), 25-31.

World Health Organization (WHO). (1996). *Cancer pain relief* (2nd ed.). Geneva: World Health Organization.

Factors That Influence Health and Health Care

Overview of the Health Care Delivery System

objectives

Upon completion of this chapter, the reader will be able to:

1. Describe the public sector and private sector components of the health care delivery system.

2. Explain the different organizations (e.g., hospitals, ambulatory health centers, nursing homes, home health) and providers (e.g., nurses, physicians, therapists, pharmacists) that comprise the health care system.

3. Describe financing of health care delivery, including third party payers, managed care options (i.e., health maintenance organizations, preferred provider organizations), Medicare, and Medicaid.

4. Compare and contrast Medicare and Medicaid.

5. Discuss factors that have contributed to the high costs of health care.

key terms

Capitation	Health maintenance organization (HMO)	Preferred provider organization (PPO)
Coinsurance		Third party reimbursement
Copayment	Independent practice association (IPA)	Utilization review
Deductible	Managed care	
Diagnosis-related group (DRG)	Medicaid	*See Glossary for definitions.*
Gatekeeper	Medicare	

case study

Carol Clark is employed as a head nurse for the evening shift in the emergency department of a large, nonprofit hospital in an urban area. Carol has been a nurse for 20 years and during that time she has witnessed dramatic changes in health care provision and in the health care delivery system. Carol knows that reimbursement issues are extremely important to the hospital, but she finds it confusing and even unfair that a client's care is often affected by his or her health care insurance coverage or lack of coverage. It concerns her that one of the first questions she must ask clients as they come into the emergency department is "Do you have health insurance?"

One recent Monday, Carol saw Melissa Mills, a 34-year-old woman, for lower abdominal pain; George Green, a 76-year-old man with chest pain; Beth Bell, a 12-year-old girl who had sprained her ankle; Nancy Nelson, a 19-year-old prima gravida in active labor; and Andy Adams, a 46-year-old man experiencing an acute asthma attack. During the evening, Carol wondered whether the care given each of these clients was influenced by insurance coverage and insurer requirements. Following the shift, Carol reviewed the disposition of each case from a financial standpoint and this is what she learned:

Ms. Mills is insured through a large health maintenance organization (HMO). It was determined that her pain was caused by ovulation and she was sent home with pain medication. Because she was not referred to the emergency department by her primary care provider, it is unlikely that the HMO will pay for the visit.

Mr. Green is insured by Medicare parts A and B. He was admitted into the coronary care unit for observation. Hospital coverage is fairly comprehensive and based on the prospective payment system. Medical coverage is at 80% following a deductible.

Beth Bell's health care is financed by traditional insurance through her father's employer. Hospital and medical coverage will be 80% to 100% after a predetermined deductible.

Ms. Nelson has no health insurance. Because it was determined that delivery was not imminent, she was sent to the local public hospital, which provides care for indigent clients. She is eligible for Medicaid, but has not applied.

Mr. Adams has no health insurance. Because his asthma attack was severe and he was in danger of respiratory arrest, Mr. Adams was kept for treatment and observation. Although Mr. Adams has no insurance, he is responsible for the costs of his health care and will be billed. Because he is only sporadically employed, Mr. Adams will be unable to pay most of the bill, which totals several thousand dollars, and the hospital will incur the cost of his care as bad debt. (Bad debt is covered by increasing charges to paying clients.)

Carol, like many other health care providers, is struggling to understand the health care delivery system and to be informed about financing of health care and differing health plans and reimbursement methods. She, along with other providers, must learn to practice within the context of constant change and to work with multiple insurance plans and providers.

To better understand the context in which they practice, it is essential that all nurses—particularly nurses working in primary care or community-based settings (including emergency departments as in the case study)—acquire a working knowledge of the health care delivery system (HCDS). This chapter presents basic concepts, information, illustrations, and tables to reinforce the nurse's understanding of the HCDS, including its structure, health care settings and organizations, provider roles, and health care financing. Understanding these concepts will assist the nurse to deliver the highest quality, most cost-effective care possible.

Like the Holy Roman Empire, which was neither Holy nor Roman nor an Empire, the Health Care System refers not to health, nor to care, nor is it a system. Ninety-five percent of the medical effort in the United States goes to disease, not health, provides medical treatment, not care; and is in no way a system. Rather it is a vast haphazard conglomeration of medical entrepreneurs, be they doctors, pharmacies, pharmaceutical manufacturers, hospitals or insurance companies.—Earl Ubell, 1974

STRUCTURE OF THE HEALTH CARE DELIVERY SYSTEM

Organizationally, the HCDS can be divided into public sector and private sector components. The public sector of the HCDS can be subdivided into federal, state, and local level divisions and is typically concerned with the health of populations and the provision of a healthy environment. The private sector includes nonprofit and proprietary organizations (e.g., hospitals, clinics, home health agencies, voluntary groups) and providers (e.g., physicians, dentists, therapists) whose primary focus is health care for individuals and families.

PUBLIC SECTOR

The U.S. Department of Health and Human Services (USDHHS) is the federal cabinet department that directly or indirectly oversees most components of the HCDS. Most USDHHS agencies have regional, state, or local offices that may be contacted for specific needs or questions. For example, regional or local offices of the Social Security Administration, the Administration on Aging, and Aid to Families with Dependent Children (AFDC) should be accessed to obtain information on services, eligibility, and other issues.

Agencies within the USDHHS include the Centers for Disease Control and Prevention (CDC), the Food and Drug Administration (FDA), and the National Institutes of Health (NIH). Each of these agencies and organizations is responsible for oversight or regulation of differing issues related to health and health care delivery. The NIH, for example, finances a significant amount of research related to health; the FDA is responsible for monitoring and regulating the safety of pharmaceuticals, food additives, other consumer goods, and health care products and equipment; and the CDC monitors infectious diseases and directs programs to control and prevent diseases. The impact of these agencies and other components of the USDHHS on health and the health care system cannot be overstated and all nurses should be familiar with the various components of the USDHHS. Therefore listings and functions of most of the offices and agencies within the USDHHS are presented in Table 5-1.

Each state maintains a state health department, usually located in the state capitol. Most state health departments are headed by a health officer or commissioner and are funded through state taxes and federal monies (e.g., grants, matching funds). Local health departments may reside within a city, county, municipality, or district. State legislatures generally define the responsibilities and roles of the local health agency. Funding for local activities comes from a combination of local and state taxes and federal grants. Although roles, functions, and services vary, state and local health departments are typically responsible for the activities listed in Box 5-1.

PRIVATE SECTOR

The private sector of the HCDS is composed of various providers (e.g., physicians, nurses, dentists, pharmacists), organizations (e.g., American Red Cross, American Heart Association, American Cancer Society), institutions (e.g., hospitals, clinics), industries and corporations (e.g., pharmaceutical companies, hospital equipment manufacturers), and insurers (e.g., Blue Cross/ Blue Shield, Cigna). Although most components of the private sector of the HCDS are income producing or for profit, others are designated nonprofit and thus tax exempt. Nonprofit, private sector organizations include voluntary agencies, such as the Red Cross and the American Cancer Society, and direct care providers, including the visiting nurses' associations and many hospitals and community clinics.

The individuals and organizations that compose the private sector of the HCDS work more or less independently to produce goods and services to promote the health of U.S. residents and to treat and manage health threats, diseases, and related conditions. However, the public component of the HCDS maintains a degree of control over the private sector through a variety of means, as described previously. Licensure of most direct providers (e.g., physicians, nurses, dentists) is required by all states; federal approval is needed for all new medications and devices used in medical treatment before marketing; and recommendations and federal and state requirements

TABLE **5-1** U.S. Department of Health and Human Services—Selected Agencies and Units

AGENCY OR ORGANIZATION	FUNCTION
Department of Health and Human Services	Oversees, manages, and finances most of the products, organizations, and interests related to health.
Centers for Disease Control and Prevention	Monitors and supports programs to prevent and control infectious diseases and promote health.
Food and Drug Administration	Provides surveillance for the safety of pharmaceuticals and other consumer goods.
Health Resources and Services Administration	Provides health care for medically underserved populations and maintains the National Health Service Corps.
National Institutes of Health	Conducts and funds health-related research.
Substance Abuse and Mental Health Services Administration	Supports research and programs related to substance abuse and mental health.
Agency for Health Care Research and Quality	Provides evidence-based information on health care outcomes, quality, cost, use, and access.
Office of Disease Prevention and Health Promotion	Carries out the goals of *Healthy People 2010* and provides other information services.
Centers for Medicare and Medicaid (formerly known as the HCFA)	Administers Medicare, Medicaid, and Child Health Insurance Program.
Administration for Children and Families	Coordinates efforts for children and families, including Head Start, Job Opportunities and Basic Skills Training (JOBS), and Aid to Families with Dependent Children (AFDC).
Indian Health Services	Supports hospitals and health centers that provide services to 1.5 million Native Americans.
Administration on Aging	Represents the concerns of older U.S. residents.

Direct links to the website for each agency can be accessed by visiting the book's website at

www.wbsaunders.com/SIMON/McEwen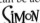

BOX **5-1** Functions and Services of State and Local Health Departments

STATE HEALTH DEPARTMENTS
Administer Medicaid
Operate state mental hospitals
Provide licensure and regulation of health practitioners and health facilities
Regulate insurance companies
Control and monitor communicable diseases
Enforce and oversee environmental programs
Direct health planning and development
Maintain vital records for the state

LOCAL HEALTH DEPARTMENTS
Provide direct health services (i.e., family planning and Women, Infants, and Children [WIC])
Record local vital statistical data and report them to the state
Control and prevent communicable diseases
Direct environmental services (i.e., monitor water quality, inspect food services, and vector control)

for communicable disease prevention, management, and reporting are examples of how the public sector of the HCDS directly affects the private sector in health care delivery. The following sections provide more examples and details about various organizations and providers.

HEALTH CARE PROVIDER ORGANIZATIONS

The U.S. HCDS is composed of a multitude of providers and organizations serving the population at many levels and for a vast array of needs. Chapter 1 included a discussion of primary, secondary, and tertiary heath care. Recall that *primary health care* refers to basic care for preventive services or treatment of common acute illnesses and conditions (e.g., sore throat, otitis media, pregnancy) or routine chronic conditions (e.g., diabetes, hypertension, arthritis) in ambulatory settings. *Secondary health care* refers to more intensive or complicated care, usually provided in acute care settings (typically a hospital [e.g., open-heart surgery, treatment of complications of diabetes]). Finally, *tertiary health care* is long-term care for complex, chronic, and complicated health problems (e.g., burn units, skilled nursing facilities, nursing homes). Facilities, organizations, and providers for each of these levels are described here.

AMBULATORY HEALTH CARE

Primary health care is provided to ambulatory clients in community-based settings. Ambulatory care is commonly thought of as health care provided to an individual who is not a bed patient in a health care institution.

The numbers and types of ambulatory care settings and providers are rapidly growing. There are two basic types of ambulatory care: (1) care provided by private physicians in solo, partnership, or group practice on a fee-for-service basis or preferred provider organization (PPO)-type arrangement; and (2) care provided in organized settings that "have an identity independent from that of the individual physicians practicing in it"

(Mezey, 1999, p. 187). These include some types of HMOs, hospital-based ambulatory services, hospital-sponsored group practices, surgicenters, urgicenters or emergicenters, neighborhood health centers, organized home care, and school and workplace health services.

Providers of care in ambulatory settings include physicians, dentists, nurses, nurse practitioners, physician assistants (PAs), social workers, therapists, pharmacists, optometrists, and chiropractors. Specific information regarding some of the many health care providers is presented later in this chapter.

According to a survey performed in 1996, U.S. residents averaged six physician contacts each year and 78% of U.S. residents reported that they had seen a physician in the previous year (USDHHS, 1997). The number of yearly physician contacts varied greatly based on age (approximately 7 contacts per year for infants and small children; 3.5 contacts per year for young and middle-aged adults; and 10 to 12 contacts per year for those older than 65 years), gender (males had 5 contacts per year; females, 7 contacts per year), and income (surprisingly, those with annual incomes under $14,000 averaged almost 8 contacts per year and those with incomes greater than $50,000 per year averaged 6 contacts per year). Other factors, such as race and geographical region, however, had very little influence on the number of physician contacts. Williams (1999) reported that the 10 most common principal diagnoses for office visits in 1997 were the following:

1. Essential hypertension
2. Acute upper respiratory infection
3. Health supervision of infant or child
4. Normal pregnancy
5. Malignant neoplasms
6. General medical examination
7. Otitis media
8. Arthritis and related disorders
9. Diabetes mellitus
10. Allergic rhinitis

Residents of the United States average about two visits each year for dental care. In contrast to physician care, dental visits are fewest for small children (less than one visit per year) and greatest between the ages of 5 and 14 and 45 and 64 (average, 2.3 visits per year). Although the number of yearly dental visits varies little between men and women, there is marked difference between races (whites, 2.1 visits per year; blacks, 1.3 visits per year) and with family income (those with annual incomes less than $10,000, 1.3 visits per year; those with annual incomes greater than $35,000, 2.7 per year) (Aday, 1993). Most dental visits are for preventive care (e.g., cleaning and fluoride treatment) and to obtain fillings.

Innovations in anesthesiology and surgical techniques have led to rapid growth in the number of outpatient surgery and day surgery procedures. Begun in the early 1970s as a cost-cutting measure, ambulatory surgery is now very common. Indeed, it is estimated that more than half of all surgical procedures are performed on an outpatient basis.

Likewise, the growth of freestanding emergicenters is attributed to attempts to lower costs by decreasing the use of expensive hospital emergency rooms for nonurgent primary care. Emergicenters offer convenient locations, flexible hours, and short waiting periods at significantly lower costs for services. As emergicenters have increased in number and in acceptance by clients, they have evolved to offer a combination of walk-in and appointment services. They provide a wide range of primary care, including preventive care (e.g., physical examinations) and diagnosis and treatment of acute, episodic illnesses (e.g., bronchitis, influenza) and injuries (e.g., minor lacerations, sprains, and strains).

HOSPITALS

Acute care hospitals are the principal settings for provision of secondary health care. "Hospitals differ from one another with respect to size, mission, ownership, complexity, competitive environment, population served, endowment and financial situation, physical facilities, costs per day for care, or cost by patient diagnostic cat-

egory" (Kovner, 1999, p. 162). Hospitals may range in size from less than 30 beds to more than 500 beds, serve special populations (e.g., children, elders, disabled), care for clients with specific diagnoses (e.g., acquired immunodeficiency syndrome [AIDS], tuberculosis, cancer), and/or support a defined mission of service (e.g., hospice, rehabilitation). Hospitals in which the average stay is less than 30 days are called short-term hospitals.

Collectively, hospitals are among the largest industries in the United States in terms of the number of employees and revenue. About half of health care personnel work in hospitals and about 40% of health care expenditures are to hospitals (Dowling, 1999).

Hospitals may be publicly or privately funded. Those that are privately funded may be nonprofit or proprietary. Examples of each are found in Table 5-2. The distinction between public and privately funded institutions is not absolute because virtually all public facilities accept private-pay clients and many private hospitals will take uninsured clients and/or may be reimbursed by public monies.

It is important to note that the total number of hospitals decreased rather significantly during the past two decades. Cost containment strategies, the increasing use of outpatient care, and many other factors have resulted in hospital closures throughout the nation. These same factors have prompted a reduction in hospital beds in many other hospitals. Table 5-3 illustrates the trend in reduction in the number of hospitals over the past decade.

LONG-TERM CARE FACILITIES

Tertiary, or long-term, care includes institutional health services, mental health services, and residential services provided to temporarily or chronically disabled persons over an extended period. The goal of long-term care is to provide services that enhance the functional ability of these individuals.

Functional ability refers to a person's capacity to perform basic self-care activities such as

TABLE **5-2** Types of Hospitals

PUBLIC			PRIVATE	
FEDERAL	STATE	LOCAL	NONPROFIT	PROPRIETARY
Veterans Administration hospitals	State mental facilities	City/county general or charity hospitals	Religious based (e.g., Catholic, Christian, or Jewish)	Corporately owned (e.g., Humana, Columbia/HCA, National Medical Enterprises)
Federal prison hospitals	Tuberculosis hospitals		Foundation, charity, or voluntary (e.g., many children's hospitals, Masonic hospitals)	Group owned (typically physician groups)
Military hospitals	Teaching hospitals associated with state universities (also local)			
Special hospitals (e.g., Native Americans, Hansen's disease)				

TABLE **5-3** Hospital Facts: 1981, 1991, 1999

TYPE OF HOSPITALS	HOSPITALS 1981 (*N*)	HOSPITALS 1991 (*N*)	HOSPITALS 1999 (*N*)
Public			
Federal	348	334	264
State psychiatrics	549	800	649
State respiratory	11	4	NA
Long-term general	146	124	NA
State and local government	1744	1429	1197
Private			
Nonprofit	3340	3175	3012
Proprietary	729	738	747

Data from American Hospital Association. (2001). *Hospital statistics.* Chicago: American Hospital Association.

eating, dressing, and personal care (e.g., bathing, showering, oral care, and maintenance of bowel and bladder control). These activities are generally termed activities of daily living (ADL). Long-term care may also assist the client in performance of instrumental activities of daily living (IADL) (e.g., shopping, housekeeping, meal preparation, managing of monetary affairs) (Evashwick, 1999).

The need for long-term care may be temporary (e.g., an older person's recovery from joint replacement surgery or rehabilitative care for a client with a spinal cord injury) or permanent (e.g., institutional care for an individual who is profoundly mentally retarded or for a bedbound, frail older person). Functional disability, particularly in the elderly, often results from chronic conditions such as arthritis, hearing impairment, vision impairment, diabetes, and respiratory or cardiac disease. The need for more and higher quality long-term care facilities and providers is evident with the increase in the number of elderly and chronically ill. Examples of long-term care facilities and some of the services they provide are listed in Box 5-2.

In general, long-term care is financed through governmental programs (Medicaid, Medicare, and state funding for care of the mentally ill) and out-of-pocket payment. Nursing home care of the elderly, for example, is largely financed through a combination of Medicaid and out-of-pocket payment. It is important to note that approximately 47% of Medicaid expenditures are for nursing home care, largely for older people (Evashwick, 1999). Detailed information on financing of health care services is discussed later in this chapter.

BOX 5-2 Examples of Long-Term Care Facilities and Services

NURSING HOMES

Generic term that includes a wide spectrum of facilities such as retirement centers, convalescent homes, and skilled nursing facilities. Nursing homes are utilized by individuals who are not able to remain at home because of physical health problems, mental health problems, or functional disabilities.

SKILLED NURSING FACILITIES

Long-term care establishments that are designed to provide a higher level of care than custodial care facilities, but at a level less intensive than care provided in short-term, acute care hospitals. Skilled nursing facilities must have a licensed nurse available at all times and are eligible for Medicare reimbursement.

HOME HEALTH CARE

Consists of a variety of nursing, therapy, and social support services provided to individuals and their families at their place of residence. Home health care can include skilled nursing care, nurse's aide services, physical therapy, occupational therapy, and speech therapy. Home health care must include a plan of care prescribed by a physician for Medicare reimbursement.

ADULT DAY CARE

Refers to a variety of health and social services for the elderly during the day and out of the home. Adult day care provides respite care to delay or prevent institutionalization, particularly for elders in families in which the caregivers work or when the elder lives alone.

RESPITE CARE

Provides a temporary respite, or break, for the caregivers of frail elderly or disabled chronically ill. Respite care may be provided in or out of the client's home and may include homemaker services and/or assistance with ADL. Medicaid and Medicare will pay for respite care in some circumstances.

HOSPICE

Refers to the provision of care for the terminally ill. Hospice care may be delivered at home or in an institutional setting and is directed toward symptom management; pain control; and psychological, social, and spiritual care for the client and the family.

ASSISTED LIVING ARRANGEMENTS

Refers to a group or residential setting (licensed or unlicensed) that provides personal care and meets unscheduled needs for older, disabled persons. Assisted living facilities vary greatly with regard to size, funding sources, target populations, services, and staffing. There are several models, including:

Congregate living arrangements—provide group-living and supportive service facilities, typically multi-unit apartment complexes, where residents can live and eat independently.

Board-and-care homes—provide rooms, meals, assistance with ADL, and some protective oversight and may be licensed or unlicensed.

Continuing care communities—comprehensive service settings providing three levels of living: (1) independent, (2) assisted, and (3) nursing home care; a resident can join a continuing care community as an independent resident and progress through the services if physical or mental disabilities dictate.

Data from Evashwick, C. J. (1999). The continuum of long-term care. In S. J. Williams & P. R. Torrens (Eds.), *Introduction to health services* (5th ed., pp. 295-348). Albany, NY: Delmar Publishers; Richardson, H., Raphael, C., & Barton, L. (1999). Long-term care. In A. R. Kovner & S. Jonas (Eds.), *Jonas' & Kovner's health care delivery in the United States* (6th ed., pp. 206-242). New York: Springer Publishing.

HEALTH CARE PROFESSIONALS

When people consider health care professionals, they most often think of nurses and doctors; however, in reality, health care in the United States is provided by more than 200 different occupational groups. Consumers have a general understanding of the roles and functions of providers, but there remains much room for misunderstanding. For example, what are the educational requirements for a nurse? What is the difference between a psychologist, a psychiatrist, and a psychotherapist or between an MD and a doctor of osteopathy (DO)? Does a specific client need to see an audiologist or a speech therapist?

Because of the importance of collaboration and coordination in their practice, nurses working in community settings need to understand the practice parameters, roles, education, and credentialing requirements of the many health care providers. Knowledge of the different disciplines can assist the nurse in the planning and implementation of health care. Information on education, practice, and licensure for many health care providers is described here. The *Healthy People 2010* box presents information about objectives related to increasing the number of health professionals from racial and ethnic minority groups, which hopefully will contribute to better health care access for those groups.

PHYSICIANS, PHYSICIAN ASSISTANTS, AND DENTISTS

Doctor of Medicine

Allopathic doctors of medicine (MDs) prevent, diagnose, and treat disease and injury. They prescribe medications, perform surgery, and direct many other health services (e.g., laboratory services, hospital use) and providers. Education requirements are 3 to 4 years of college (most have a bachelor's degree) and 4 years of medical school, followed by a 1-year internship. The MDs who stop training at this point are nonspecialists, or general practitioners. However, most MDs (80% to 90%) specialize. Specialization requires 3 to 4 years of additional, residency training. Medical specialties include internal medicine, general surgery, obstetrics, pediatrics, and radiology. Subspecialties include hematology, oncology, cardiology, orthopedic surgery, and thoracic surgery.

All states require physicians to be licensed. Requirements for licensure include graduation from an accredited professional school, passage of a licensing examination administered by the National Board of Medical Examiners, and successful completion of an accredited graduate

---

healthy people **2010**

Health Professions and *Healthy People 2010*

The USDHHS has recognized that certain racial and ethnic groups and low-income communities lag behind the overall U.S. population on virtually all health status indicators. Among other factors, this can be tied to a lack of a specific source of care. One way to help achieve the goal of eliminating health disparities is proposed in Objective 1-8 of *Healthy People 2010*—to increase the proportion of all health professions' degrees awarded to members of racial and ethnic minority groups. Although members of racial and ethnic minority groups make up about 25% of the U.S. population, only about 10% of health professionals are from these groups. Many believe that increasing the number of health professionals from racial and ethnic minority groups will help improve access to care.

Several suggestions have been proposed to help accomplish this. First, enhanced efforts are needed to provide financial assistance for students from underrepresented racial and ethnic groups to pursue health care degrees. Secondly, health care practitioners, particularly those from minority groups should encourage mentor relationships with health profession students. Third, efforts should be made to promote early recruiting of students from certain racial and ethnic groups. Finally, the number of minority faculty members in schools that train health care professionals needs to be increased.

medical education program (internship or residency).

Doctor of Osteopathy

Like MDs, DOs prevent, diagnose, and treat diseases. Osteopathy, however, emphasizes that the body can make its own remedies given normal structural relationship, environmental conditions, and nutrition. Education requirements and specialties are similar to those for an MD and include instruction in body mechanics and manipulative methods in diagnosis and treatment and medicinal and surgical treatments.

Physician Assistant

The role of the PA developed in the 1960s in response to a shortage of primary care physicians in certain areas. The PA's practice includes physical examination, ordering and interpretation of laboratory tests, and making tentative diagnoses and prescribing treatments under protocol and direct and/or indirect supervision of physicians. Education requirements are 3 to 4 years of college (a bachelor's degree is usually required) and 2 years of PA school. The PA programs are located in medical schools, universities, or schools of allied health. Most offer a bachelor's degree as the basic degree, although some offer a master's degree. A few PA programs award a certificate.

Almost all states require licensure to practice as a PA. Graduation from an accredited professional school is necessary for licensure. Specialization is possible and specialty areas include surgery, emergency medicine, and orthopedics.

Doctor of Dental Surgery and Doctor of Dental Medicine

Dentists may obtain one of two degrees: doctor of dental surgery (DDS) and doctor of dental medicine (DDM). Dentists prevent, diagnose, and treat problems of the teeth and tissues of the mouth. Education requirements are similar to those for an MD, with an additional 4 academic years in dental school. Most dentists (85%) are generalists. Specialization requires 2 years or more of additional training and includes endo-

dontics (treatment of the roots of teeth), orthodontics (straightening of teeth), periodontics (treatment of the gums and bone supporting the teeth), and pedodontics (children's dentistry).

All states require dentists to be licensed. Licensure requires graduation from an accredited dental school and successful completion of a licensing examination, including written and practical components.

NURSES

Nurses use the nursing process in the promotion and maintenance of health; management of illness, injury, or infirmity; restoration of optimum function; or achievement of a dignified death. Nursing practice varies depending on education, licensure, and credentialing.

Licensed Practical Nurse or Licensed Vocational Nurse

Education programs for licensed practical nurses (LPNs) or licensed vocational nurses (LVNs) are 12 to 18 months and are available in trade, technical, and vocational schools and community colleges. All states require LPNs/LVNs to be licensed and requirements include graduation from a state-approved program in practical nursing or vocational nursing and successful completion of a licensing examination.

Registered Nurses

Education for a registered nurse (RN) may be in associate degree (2 years of community college), diploma (2- to 3-year hospital-based training), or baccalaureate programs (4 to 5 years in colleges or universities). All states require RNs to be licensed. Requirements include graduation from a state-approved nursing program and successful completion of the National Council Licensure Examination (NCLEX), a written examination administered by each state.

Advanced Practice Nurses

Advanced practice nurses (APNs) may be nurse practitioners, clinical nurse specialists, certified nurse-midwives, or certified RN-anesthetists.

They conduct assessments and diagnose and treat clients, usually following a predefined protocol. Most APNs are in specialty practices such as anesthesia, pediatrics, geriatrics, gynecology, and obstetrics. Education requirements generally include a basic undergraduate degree in nursing, with additional graduate education. Most APN programs award master's degrees. Licensure requirements vary between states, but typically include graduation from an accredited APN program, completion of a certification examination conducted by a nationally recognized organization, and completion of a requisite number of hours in advanced practice. Scope of practice parameters for APNs in such areas as prescriptive authority and third party reimbursement also vary between states and are detailed in each state's Nurse Practice Act.

THERAPISTS

A number of different types of therapists practice in the U.S. HCDS. Some of those more commonly encountered in community-based practice are described.

Physical Therapists

Physical therapists (PTs) plan, organize, and administer treatments to restore functional mobility, relieve pain, and prevent or limit permanent disability. In addition, some PTs perform diagnostic testing to determine joint measurement, functional activity, and voluntary muscle power. Although education requirements vary somewhat, the minimum educational requirement for practice is a bachelor's degree. Some programs confer a certificate (for those who hold a degree in another field) and others confer a master's degree. All states require PTs to be licensed and requirements include graduation from an accredited professional school and successful completion of a licensing examination. Specialization requires additional educational preparation, 2 years or more of practice experience, and successful completion of a certification examination. Specialization areas include pediatrics, sports therapy, geriatrics, and orthope-

dics. Physical therapy technicians usually have a 2-year associate degree education.

Occupational Therapists

Occupational therapists (OTs) employ a number of techniques to help clients who are mentally, physically, developmentally, or emotionally disabled maintain daily living skills and cope with physical and emotional effects of disability. The OTs assist clients in learning or relearning ADL and help them establish as independent, productive, and satisfying a lifestyle as possible. Educational preparation requires a bachelor's degree. Some programs confer a master's degree if the student is postbaccalaureate. Most states regulate OTs through licensure. Requirements include degree or certificate from an accredited program and successful completion of the OT National Certification Examination.

Speech Therapists and Audiologists

Speech therapists (STs), or language pathologists, diagnose and treat persons experiencing speech or language problems resulting from conditions such as hearing loss, brain injury (cerebrovascular accident), cleft palate, and voice pathology. Audiologists assess, diagnose, treat, and work to prevent hearing problems. Educational preparation for STs and audiologists is generally at the graduate level. Specialty areas include pediatrics, geriatrics, and linguistics. Most states mandate licensure for STs and audiologists and requirements include graduation from an accredited master's degree program, completion of a licensing examination, and supervised clinical experience.

OTHER HEALTH CARE PROVIDERS

Nurses in community-based practice may work with several other health care providers. These include optometrists, pharmacists, psychologists, dietitians, and social workers.

Optometrists

Optometrists are primary eye care providers who diagnose and treat common vision problems and prescribe eye glasses, contact lenses, and vision therapy. Most optometrist programs require 2 to 3 years of undergraduate study (most optometrists have a bachelor's degree) followed by completion of a 4-year program to obtain a doctor of optometry degree. All states require optometrists to be licensed.

Psychologists

Psychologists study the behavior of individuals to understand and identify fundamental processes of behavior; develop, administer, and score a variety of psychological tests; provide counseling and therapy to persons suffering emotional or adjustment problems; conduct research to improve diagnosis and treatment of mental and emotional disorders; and study human and animal behavior. A psychologist's education is 7 years or more. Typically, a psychologist has an undergraduate degree in psychology and 3 to 5 years of graduate study. A master's degree (master of arts, master of science, or master of education) allows for provision of supervised psychological services, whereas a doctoral degree (doctor of philosophy [PhD], doctor of psychiatry, or doctor of education) is the standard entry-level degree required for independent practice. A psychiatrist is a physician who has completed a 3-year residency in psychiatry and can diagnose and treat mental illness using a variety of therapies, including pharmacotherapeutics. All states require licensure or certification of psychologists, although requirements vary.

Pharmacists

Pharmacists dispense medicines prescribed by physicians, podiatrists, and dentists, and in some states, PAs and NPs, and advise health professionals on medication selection and use. A bachelor's degree is the standard entry-level requirement for the practice of pharmacy. Graduate preparation confers a master's degree, doctor of pharmacy (PharmD), or a PhD and is necessary for educators, researchers, and specialists. All states require pharmacists to be licensed. Requirements include graduation from an accredited program, successful completion of a

licensing examination, supervised clinical experience or internship, and that the pharmacist be over 21 years of age. Pharmacology technicians generally have an associate degree and work under the supervision of a pharmacist.

Dietitians

Dietitians teach individuals and health professionals about the science of food and nutrition. The entry level for practice as a dietitian is the bachelor's degree. A 6- to 12-month supervised internship is required if the graduate desires licensure.

Social Workers

Social workers work with individuals and families to address a wide variety of social problems and issues. Medical social workers refer clients to community resources, assist clients in attaining needed social and health care services, and help plan for institutional community placement (e.g., nursing home or extended-care facility). Identification of community resources, financial assistance, and referral for additional services are part of the practice of many social workers. The bachelor's degree is the minimum entry level for practice as a social worker. Master's and advanced master's degrees (e.g., doctoral level training) are necessary for licensure in some states and for the provision of some interventions such as counseling. Licensure for practicing social workers is required by all states and most states recognize more than one category of social worker based on education and work experience.

HEALTH CARE FINANCING

Financing of health care is becoming increasingly complex and confusing. Over the past 50 years, the HCDS has evolved from being a simple, fee-for-service enterprise to a very complex entity in which various individuals, groups, corporations, and/or insurers contract with providers and organizations to deliver care to individuals, families, and groups. Because of their important role in coordination and management of care, all nurses should be aware of the payment structure for health care. Understanding of eligibility requirements, copayments, deductibles, and the variety of third party reimbursement strategies can assist nurses in planning and implementing appropriate, cost-effective, and reimbursable care.

THE HIGH COST OF HEALTH CARE

Thorpe and Knickman (1999) report that health care expenditures in 1995 represented an estimated 13.6% of the U.S. gross national product (up from 12.2% in 1990, 9.4% in 1980, and 7.3% in 1970), or about $3600 per capita. Although still very high, the percentage has dropped considerably from 15.6% reported in the early 1990s. This per capita expenditure is by far the highest in the world. By comparison, Switzerland, France, Germany, and Canada spent 8.6% to 9.8% of their gross national products on health care during 1990 and Japan and Great Britain spent about 6.9% to 7.3% (Koch, 1999).

Reasons for the expenditures and the phenomenal growth of the cost of health care are numerous and interrelated. The growth in private insurance and **third party reimbursement** for services and general economic inflation are two of the most often cited reasons for increasing health care costs. In addition, the rapid increase in the income of health care providers, most notably physicians, has profoundly affected the health care expenditures. During the 1980s and 1990s, for example, physician income grew faster than that of any other profession and according to a report by the American Medical Association in 1994, mean physician net income ranges from $110,000 (general/family practice) to $220,000 (surgery) (Kovner and Salsberg, 1999). This represents an almost 100% increase in income since 1982 using constant dollars. During the same time period, the average income of year-round, full-time workers increased from about $25,000 to $30,000 (or about 20%).

Another factor that affects the costs of health care is the changes in population demography. As Americans age, more expensive and intensive health care is required. Lifestyle choices, includ-

ing smoking, alcohol consumption, high-fat diets, obesity, lack of exercise, use of legal (e.g., alcohol) and illegal (e.g., cocaine) substances, and indiscriminate sexual practices have contributed to an increase in chronic diseases such as lung cancer, heart disease, diabetes, and AIDS. Growth in the numbers of uninsured individuals has contributed indirectly to the increase in health care costs, as health care providers raise charges and fees for those able to pay to offset bad debt.

The American public has been warned that medical care may soon have to be rationed...The truth is that medical care is already rationed and it always has been. One of the disgraces of national policy is that the poor and unemployed who cannot afford to pay for medical care or have no medical insurance must often accept inferior treatment, if they can get it at all (John P. Bunker, Stanford University, from Lee and Estes, 1994, p. 273).

Dependence on technology by health care providers and insistence on high-tech care by consumers contributes to misuse and abuse of technology. Overuse of expensive care and procedures (e.g., cesarean section, hysterectomy, cataract surgery, prostatectomy), medications (e.g., use of a very expensive antibiotic when penicillin would produce the same result), and failure to encourage preventative interventions such as immunizations and health-promotion activities (e.g., stopping smoking, lowering cholesterol, exercising regularly) have also contributed to inefficiency, waste, and overuse of care. The increase in costs of health care include the costs incurred in research and development; manufacture and marketing; and profits made on new medications, equipment, and techniques. Finally, malpractice insurance premiums and alterations in practice to address potential litigation and forestall malpractice claims (defensive medicine) have been cited as contributing factors to the rapid increase in health care costs.

The current system of health care financing is composed of a combination of fee-for-service, public sector payment, and third party (e.g., health insurance) reimbursement. Financing sources and distribution of health care expenditures are presented in Figure 5-1. As indicated in

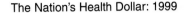

The Nation's Health Dollar: 1999

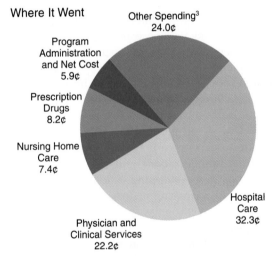

Where It
Came From

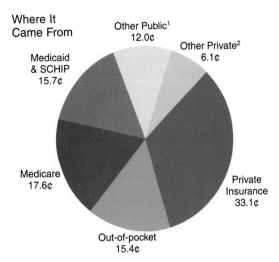

Where It Went

1. "Other Public" includes programs such as workers' compensation, public health activity, Department of Defense, Department of Veterans Affairs, Indian health services, and State and local hospital and school health.
2. "Other Private" includes industrial in-plant, privately funded construction, and nonpatient revenues, including philanthropy.
3. "Other Spending" includes dentist services, other professional services, home health, durable medical products, over-the-counter medicines and sundries, public health, research, and construction.
NOTE: Numbers shown may not add to 100.0 because of rounding.

Figure 5-1. Health care funding sources and expenditures. (From Centers for Medicare & Medicaid, Office of the Actuary, National Health Statistics Group. [2000]. Retrieved 07/11/2001 from http://www.hcfa.gov/stats/nhe-oact/tables/chart.htm.)

this illustration, payment for health care services comes from a combination of governmental sources (e.g., Medicare, Medicaid, Veteran's Administration, military service) and private sources (e.g., private health insurance, direct payment). Additionally, the greatest percentage of payment went to hospital care (32.3%), followed by "other spending" (e.g., dental care, other professional services, home health, durable medical products, over-the-counter medicines, research and construction) and physicians' services.

PUBLIC FINANCING

As discussed, local, state, and federal governments combine to finance about 45% of health care. Because Medicare and Medicaid are very important sources of health care financing, it is imperative that nurses be aware of specific components of these programs, including eligibility parameters, reimbursement requirements, and which services are or are not covered.

Medicare

Medicare is a federal health insurance program for people 65 and older, people with end-stage renal disease, and certain disabled people (USDHHS/Health Care Financing Administration [HCFA], 2001), which was established by Title XVIII of the Social Security Act in 1965. Medicare is financed through tax wages, administered by the Social Security Administration (which is responsible for application and determining eligibility), and funded through the Centers for Medicare and Medicaid Services (CMS) (formerly known as the HCFA).

Medicare is divided into Part A and Part B. Medicare Part A insures qualified individuals for hospital and skilled nursing facility care and for home health, hospice care, and blood. Part A has **deductibles** and **coinsurance**, but most people do not have to pay premiums for coverage. Medicare Part B insures qualified individuals for physician services, outpatient hospital services, home health care, durable medical equipment, and other medical services and supplies not covered by Part A. Part B requires monthly premiums for all subscribers ($50 per month in 2001) and deductibles ($100/year in 2001) and coinsurance (20% of the Medicare-approved amount) for which the individual is responsible (USDHHS/HCFA, 2001).

Medicare Part B also helps pay for ambulance services; artificial limbs and eyes; arm, leg, back and neck braces; limited chiropractic services; emergency care; medical supplies; and transplants. Services that Medicare does *not* cover include dental care and dentures, cosmetic surgery, custodial care at home, health care received while traveling outside of the United States, hearing aids, routine eye care, routine or yearly physical examinations, and some screening tests. One of the most significant costs not covered by Medicare, however, is the cost of prescription drugs (USDHHS/HCFA, 2001).

Most U.S. residents (about 98%) are eligible for premium-free Medicare Part A benefits when they reach age 65, based on their own or their spouse's employment. Medicare Part A benefits are also available for individuals who rely on dialysis for permanent kidney failure or who have had a kidney transplant and for those who are disabled and eligible for Social Security benefits.

Before 1983, Medicare paid physicians and other providers on a fee-for-service basis and hospitals on a cost-based retrospective basis (Koch, 1999). In an attempt to better manage costs and to stop the rapid increase in expenditures, Congress enacted the Social Security Amendment of 1983 (Public Law 98-21). This act ended the cost-plus, fee-for-service system and introduced the prospective payment system for hospital coverage. The prospective payment system uses 468 **diagnosis-related groups (DRGs)** to classify cases for payment and reimbursement is based on a fixed price per case, a fee known as **capitation**. The prospective payment system requires that all providers bill Medicare directly for reimbursement for services. Medicare claims are paid indirectly by the HCFA through the use of fiscal intermediaries. These intermediaries are typically insurance companies who contract with Medicare to review, process, and pay all claims (see the Community Application box "Medigap Insurance").

Medicaid

The Medicaid program was initiated in 1965 by Title XIX of the Social Security Act. **Medicaid** is a public assistance welfare program that provides financial assistance to pay for health care for the poor, blind, disabled, and families with dependent children. Medicaid is funded jointly by the federal government and each state. Eligibility, coverage, and payment for services vary greatly from state to state.

Although covered services vary, federal requirements dictate that Medicaid cover certain services in all states. These include inpatient and outpatient hospital care; skilled nursing care; physician services; family planning services; home health care; and early and periodic screening, diagnosis, and treatment (EPSDT) services for eligible children. Additional services that may be covered in some states include dental care, eye care, and medications. Box 5-3 provides detailed information on Medicaid beneficiaries and services. A comparison of Medicare and Medicaid appears in Table 5-4.

It is important to note that both the legislative and executive branches of the federal government are exploring ways to decrease health care costs. Several states, including Arizona, Massachusetts, Hawaii, and Oregon, are experimenting with plans to reduce costs through a variety of changes (Stanhope, 1996). Reduction of coverage for certain services, prioritizing care based on specified criteria such as effectiveness and benefit, refusal to pay for certain procedures or services, encouraging participants to use managed care, and other efforts have been proposed and are being tested. All health providers and consumers are advised to closely monitor the ongoing debates and support legislative efforts that control costs and maintain quality.

COMMUNITY APPLICATION
Medigap Insurance

A Medigap plan is a health insurance plan that helps fill the gaps in Medicare plan coverage. Medigap may help a beneficiary lower their out-of-pocket costs and get more health insurance coverage. When purchasing a Medigap policy, the individual will pay a premium to the insurance company, but must still pay their monthly Medicare Part B premium. Medigap plans are not sold or serviced by the state or federal government; they are sold by private insurance companies. Medigap plans must meet requirements of the state and each state has a different required set of benefits in their Medigap plans.

Services and items typically covered by Medigap policies include a portion of coinsurance for hospital and skilled nursing stays, the Medicare Part B yearly deductible, and routine yearly checkups. Medigap plans do not generally cover long-term care, vision or dental care, hearing aids, private duty nursing care, and unlimited prescription drugs.

Other helpful information about Medigap plans includes the following:
- Medigap plans are designed to not duplicate coverage provided by Medicare.
- The front of the Medigap policy must identify it as "Medicare Supplement Insurance."
- There may be preexisting condition exclusions in Medigap plans.
- It is illegal for an insurance company to sell a second Medigap plan.
- It is illegal to sell a Medigap plan to someone in a Medicare managed care plan.
- It is illegal for an insurance company or agent to use high pressure tactics to force or frighten someone into buying a Medigap plan
- It is illegal to make false or misleading comparisons to promote switching from one company or plan to another.

Data from Centers for Medicare & Medicaid, Washington, DC, 2001. For more information visit the Medicare website, which is directly accessible through the book's website at **www.wbsaunders/SIMON/McEwen** $SIMON$

BOX 5-3 Medicaid Beneficiaries and Services

FEDERALLY DICTATED RECIPIENTS

All persons in federal aide programs, including Supplemental Security Income (SSI) and AFDC
Pregnant women and children up to 6 years of age with a family income below 133% of the poverty level
Children 18 years of age and younger, born after September 30, 1983, with a family income below the poverty level
Medicare beneficiaries with income below the poverty level (but only for payment of Medicare premiums and cost sharing)

OPTIONAL RECIPIENTS

Pregnant women and infants to age 1 whose family income is below 185% of the poverty level (percentage set by the state)
Optional targeted low-income children
Certain aged, blind, or disabled adults who have incomes above those requiring mandatory coverage, but below the federal poverty level
Low-income, uninsured women diagnosed through a CDC early detection program determined to be in need of treatment for breast or cervical cancer
Medically needy older persons not qualified for income assistance (welfare)

STATE-DETERMINED OPTIONAL SERVICES

Prescription drugs
Dental care
Optometry and eyeglasses
Residential intermediate care facilities for the mentally retarded
Nursing facility services for people under 21 years of age
Prescription drugs
Prosthetic devices

FEDERALLY REQUIRED SERVICES

Inpatient and outpatient hospital care
Physician services
Medical and surgical dental services
Skilled nursing home care
Home health care for persons eligible for nursing facility services
Family planning services and supplies
Rural health clinic services
Laboratory and X-ray services
Pediatric and family nurse practitioner services
Ambulatory services offered by a federally qualified health center
Nurse-midwife services (as authorized under state law)
The EPSDT service for individual under age 21.
Prenatal care and delivery services for pregnant women

From Centers for Medicare & Medicaid Services. (2001). *Medicaid services and Medicaid eligibility.* Retrieved 07/11/2001 from http://www.hcfa.gov/medicaid/meligib.htm.

TABLE **5-4** Comparison of Medicare and Medicaid

MEDICARE	MEDICAID
• A federal health insurance program for persons 65 years and older, disabled persons, and persons with end-stage renal disease	• A welfare-assistance program for the poor; those eligible for Medicaid include families receiving AFDC, individuals receiving benefits for the SSI Program because of age or disability, and the medically needy whose incomes fall below a certain percentage of the poverty level; each state determines eligibility requirements, payment for services, and type of services provided (with some federal restrictions)
• Financed through Social Security taxes and monthly premiums	• Jointly funded by the states and the federal government
• Administered by the CMS (formerly known as the HCFA) within the USDHHS • The CMS contracts with insurance companies to process and pay claims submitted by beneficiaries	• Administered by a designated state agency and CMS
• Medicare Part A covers inpatient hospital care, home health care, hospice care, and skilled nursing care • Medicare Part B covers physicians' services; covered services provided by other health professions, including RNs, nurse practitioners, chiropractors, psychologists, and social workers; outpatient hospital services, ambulance services, ambulatory surgery; outpatient physical, occupational, and speech therapy; radiation therapy; durable medical equipment; surgical dressing; screening examinations are also covered	• Medicaid benefits include inpatient and outpatient hospital services; prenatal care; outpatient diagnostic and laboratory services; home health care; physicians' services; screening, diagnosis, and treatment of children; family planning services; states may add additional benefits, including prescription medications, dental services, ambulance services, psychiatric care, medical supplies, optometrists' services, and eyeglasses
• Medicare enrollees in Part B pay a monthly premium of $50 per month for coverage	• There is no cost to those eligible for Medicaid
• Payment may be fee-for-service or option of enrolling in an HMO or comprehensive medical plan	• Payment to providers is a combination of fee-for-service based on "reasonable charges" and a state-defined "Medicaid fee schedule"
• Payment to hospitals is based on diagnosis-related groups (DRGs) or audited costs	• Payment to hospitals is based on DRGs, with some exceptions

From National Heritage Insurance Company. (1995). *Medicaid provider procedures manual: Texas department of human services.* Austin, TX: National Heritage Insurance Company; U.S. Department of Health and Human Services/Health Care Financing Administration. (2001). *Medicare & you, 2001.* Washington, DC: Government Printing Office.

PRIVATE FINANCING

The greatest percentage of health care is financed by private health insurance (see Figure 5-1). At present, the structure of the private sector health insurance system is very complex. In the United States, health care insurance is frequently provided by employers and has become an expected benefit of employment. Typically, employer-provided health insurance covers both the employee and his or her family and both the employer and the employee contribute to the cost of premiums.

As insurance premium costs have increased dramatically over the past two decades, alterations in the structure and coverage parameters of this system have been and continue to be altered. The result has been an increase in **managed care** plans; changes in premiums, coinsurance, and deductibles; limits to coverage; and refusal to pay for preexisting conditions. Health care insurance programs and options include various financial arrangements, such as traditional, indemnity health insurance coverage; PPOs; and HMOs. Each is described briefly.

Traditional Health Insurance

In the United States, health insurance began when teachers in Dallas, Texas devised a way to finance and share the costs of health care. In 1929, Dallas public school teachers contracted with Baylor Hospital to provide specified health care services for a predetermined cost. By 1939, this insurance plan had grown to include many other groups and became Blue Cross-Blue Shield (Koch, 1999). The idea of health insurance grew very rapidly and currently about 73% of U.S. residents are covered by private health insurance.

Health insurance organizations may be nonprofit (e.g., Blue Cross-Blue Shield) or commercial, for profit (e.g., Aetna, Prudential). Under traditional contracts, the insurance company finances care for enrollees. Premiums, deductibles, and copayments or coinsurance are required by indemnity policies. Premiums have increased dramatically since the 1980s, prompting cost-containment strategies by most employers. These strategies include encouraging the use of managed care, reducing reliance on traditional insurers through increasing self-funding of health benefits, and increasing the share of health care expenses paid by the employees. Many insurers now provide options for enrollees whereby they may choose traditional coverage or care through an HMO or PPO.

Preferred Provider Organizations

Preferred provider organizations (PPOs) are business arrangements, or contracts, between a group of health care providers (e.g., hospitals or physicians) and a purchaser of health care services (e.g., employers or insurance companies). The PPOs began during the mid-1980s to decrease the costs of health care insurance. In these arrangements, the providers agree to supply services to a defined group of patients (e.g., employees of company "X") at a discounted fee-for-service basis. According to Koch (1999), PPOs have five elements:

1. A limited number of physicians and hospitals
2. Negotiated fee schedules
3. **Utilization review** or utilization management

4. Consumer choice of providers with incentives to use participating providers
5. Expedient settlement of claims

As of 1996, about 25% of private insurance was through PPOs (Thorpe and Knickman, 1999) and the percentage is growing.

Health Maintenance Organizations

A **health maintenance organization (HMO)** is an organized health care system that provides health services to enrolled individuals for a fixed, prepaid fee. HMOs typically possess an organized system to provide health care in a particular geographical area, an agreed upon set of services for health maintenance and treatment, voluntarily enrolled membership, and rates similar to those of providers in the community (Clark, 1999). The HMOs provide fairly comprehensive coverage in return for the prepaid fee, usually without deductibles and with minimal **copayments** ($10 to $20 per visit is common). The HMOs are intended to reduce hospitalizations and health care costs by encouraging illness prevention and health maintenance and reducing inappropriate care. There is evidence of success in these goals, as Thorpe and Knickman (1999) report that HMOs have resulted in a 40% reduction in hospital use for enrollees.

In the United States, the concept of the HMO began in 1929 at a private health clinic in Los Angeles, which expanded in 1930 as the Kaiser company provided coverage for workers building the Grand Coulee Dam (Koch, 1999). The number of prepaid insurance plans, however, grew very slowly until the 1970s. The cost of health care had already become a concern, and, in response, the HMO Act of 1973 (Public Law 93-222) was passed. Subsequent amendments have encouraged rapid growth through the 1980s through use of incentives to employers and providers. Estimates indicate that members enrolled in HMO plans have climbed dramatically, growing from 9.1 million (1980), to 18.9 million (1985), to 36.5 million (1990), to 63.3 million (1996), or about 33%

of enrollment in group health plans (Thorpe and Knickman, 1999).

Some basic HMO models are the staff model, the group model, and the **independent practice association (IPA)**, with some variations in each. In the traditional, or staff model, the HMO is an organization that employs physicians and other providers to deliver services to the HMO's enrollees. In the group model, a group or association of physicians contracts with the fiscal agent to provide services to enrollees. Finally, in the IPA model, the fiscal agent contracts with a range of physicians who are not associated with each other and work in independent practices to provide services on a capitated basis.

Because of capitated payments, physicians working in HMOs usually have incentives to use resources efficiently. Reportedly, some HMOs offer bonuses to physicians if services, such as specialists and expensive procedures, are not significantly utilized and HMOs might reprimand providers for overuse of services and specialists.

The HMOs usually require that enrollees designate one primary care provider as a **gatekeeper**. The gatekeeper may be a family practitioner, internist, pediatrician, or, in some cases, an obstetrician/gynecologist. This primary care physician determines when referral to a specialist is needed and provides oversight for all of the client's health care needs. Other cost-containment strategies employed by HMOs, and other health care insurers, include second surgical opinions, preauthorization for most hospital admissions, case management, and utilization review (Torrens and Williams, 1999). The preauthorization requirement and second surgical opinions were developed to correct the practice of unnecessary surgeries and unneeded hospitalizations.

Table 5-5 presents a simplified comparison of HMOs, PPOs, and traditional health insurance. An understanding of the requirements of each increases the nurse's awareness of the similarities and differences in the programs to encourage care planning that is sensitive to the financial needs and resources of the client.

CARING FOR THE UNINSURED

In the United States, an estimated 44 million individuals have no health insurance on any given day (USDHHS, 2000). Furthermore, at any given time in the United States, as many as 25% of Americans have no or inadequate health care coverage. The typical uninsured individual is a member of a family in which the adults are unemployed or underemployed and thereby ineligible for employee-paid health insurance coverage. Children, young adults, and members of minorities are disproportionately represented among uninsured persons.

The lack of insurance affects health and well-being in many ways. Lack of access to timely and affordable health care discourages the use of preventive services and early treatment for acute, episodic illnesses. Failure to seek preventive care (e.g., prenatal care) contributes to an increase in complications of pregnancy, such as low-birth-weight infants. Likewise, failure to adequately immunize infants and small children puts them at risk for a variety of illnesses. People who have no health care coverage often wait to seek care until the illness has progressed to a stage requiring more extensive, and therefore more costly, treatment. Emergency departments are more accessible to the uninsured and are often their only source of health care.

The lack of accessible health care services for those who are uninsured or underinsured has, by default, created health care rationing, in which only those who can afford treatment receive it. Uncompensated care continues to drain many regional and public hospitals and also affects private health providers and society at large. Public hospitals must incur a very large share of uncompensated care, which results in increased taxes and higher insurance costs for everyone. Recognition of these problems has resulted in efforts to reform the HCDS and many proposals have been made to address these issues and institute some form of universal coverage. Nurses are encouraged to stay informed

TABLE **5-5** Comparison of Private Insurance Plans

TRADITIONAL INDEMNITY	PREFERRED PROVIDER ORGANIZATION	HEALTH MAINTENANCE ORGANIZATION: STAFF MODEL	HEALTH MAINTENANCE ORGANIZATION: INDIVIDUAL PRACTICE ASSOCIATION AND GROUP MODELS
Free choice of providers without any restrictions	Free choice of providers; lower costs if providers are within network of preferred providers	Choice of providers limited to physicians and other providers employed by the HMO	Choice of providers limited to physicians under contract with the HMO
No referral necessary for specialty care	No referral necessary for specialty care; use of specialists within PPO encouraged through financial incentives	Designated primary care provider (gatekeeper) must approve treatment and determines when referrals are made to specialists; specialists within the HMO are used whenever possible	Designated primary care provider (gatekeeper) must approve treatment and determines when referrals are made to specialists; Individual Practice Association specialists are used whenever possible
Providers use their own office; referrals for specialized care may not be conveniently located	Providers use their own offices	Centralized facility allows for convenience and coordination of care	Providers use their own offices
Costs of premiums highest of all insurance plans; deductibles required; copayments 20% to 30% of total medical care	Premiums and deductible are lower than traditional insurance; copayment or coinsurance is usually required; costs to the insured if providers are outside of the PPO	Premiums and copayments are lower than traditional indemnity and PPOs	Premiums and copayments are lower than traditional indemnity and PPOs
No coordination of care; each provider works independently	Limited coordination of care	Care coordinated through primary care provider; case management may be utilized	Care coordinated through primary care provider; case management may be utilized
Provider or insured must file claim forms for reimbursement; processing time may be lengthy	May require additional paperwork or approval for some services	No paperwork required for basic services	No paperwork required for basic services
Preventive care may or may not be covered	Preventive care may or may not be covered	Preventive care encouraged	Preventive care encouraged

of legislative efforts at all levels and to support efforts to provide care to all.

SUMMARY

Like Carol, the nurse in the chapter case study, nurses across the country have recognized that it is essential for all health care providers to have a basic understanding of the HCDS. Although it does not seem to fit with predetermined perceptions of nursing practice, nurses must learn to work within the context of change and to understand the different health care reimbursement mechanisms.

Indeed, it has been widely recognized that financial and reimbursement considerations, current and anticipated need for health care, practice parameters for providers, and various other factors influence how health care is delivered in the United States. Each of these issues bears further reflection and study as nurses learn to work within the system to deliver the best possible care.

KEY POINTS

* The HCDS is divided into public sector and private sector components.
* The public sector is subdivided into federal, state, and local levels and is typically concerned with the health of populations and maintaining a healthy environment. At the federal level, the USDHHS oversees many of the issues related to health. Each state maintains a state health department and defines what services will be offered at the state level and at the local level.
* The private sector system is composed of a variety of providers, institutions, industries, corporations, and insurers. It can be further divided into nonprofit or proprietary components.
* The HCDS contains a multitude of organizations that serve the population at many levels and for many needs. These include ambulatory health care settings, hospitals, and long-

term care facilities (e.g., nursing homes, skilled nursing units, hospice care).
* Numerous different health care professionals provide care to members of the population. These include physicians, PAs, dentists, nurses, nurse practitioners, therapists, optometrists, psychologists and counselors, pharmacists, social workers, and many others.
* In the United States, health care is very expensive, representing about 13.6% of the gross national product. Reasons for the high cost of health care include growth in insurance and third party payment for services, general economic inflation, increases in the income of health care providers, changes in population demography (e.g., aging of U.S. residents), lifestyle choices that are detrimental to health (e.g., smoking, drug abuse, poor diet, indiscriminate sexual practices), and dependence on technology.
* Financing of health care is very complex and consists of a combination of fee-for-service, public sector payment, and third party reimbursement. Payment for health care comes from a combination of governmental sources (e.g., Medicare, Medicaid, Veteran's Administration) and private sources (e.g., private health insurance, direct payment).
* Medicare is the federal health insurance program for people 65 years of age and older and persons with certain disabilities. It is divided into parts A and B. Medicare Part A insures individuals for hospital and skilled nursing facility care, home health, and hospice care. Part A has deductibles and coinsurance, but most people do not pay premiums for coverage. Medicare Part B insures individuals for physician services, outpatient hospital services, medical equipment, and other medical services and supplies not covered by Part A. A monthly premium is required.
* Medicaid is a public assistance welfare program that pays for health care for the poor, blind, and disabled and families with dependent children. Medicaid is funded

jointly by the federal government and each state. Eligibility, coverage, and payment for services are set by each state and vary greatly. Medicaid covers inpatient and outpatient hospital care; skilled nursing care; physician services; family planning services; home health care; and early periodic screening, diagnosis, and treatment services for eligible children. Other services that may be covered in some states include dental care, eye care, and medications.

- The greatest percentage of health care is financed by private health insurance. The health insurance system is very complex and is typically provided by an individual's employer and both the employer and the employee contribute to the cost of premiums. Health care insurance programs include a variety of financial arrangements, including indemnity health insurance, PPOs, and HMOs.

- Approximately 25% of U.S. residents have no or inadequate health care coverage. Children, young adults, and members of minorities are disproportionately represented among the uninsured and underinsured.

Learning Activities & Application to Practice

In Class

1. Obtain a copy of the current Medicare Handbook (USDHHS/HCFA, 2001). With classmates, discuss Medicare coverage and related fees. Discuss the importance of Medicare requirements, guidelines, and reimbursement parameters in directing health care payment for services (e.g., DRGs).

2. With classmates, create a list of local health care organizations (e.g., ambulatory care agencies, hospitals, voluntary organizations) according to source of payment (public or private) and whether they are nonprofit or for profit. Identify actual or perceived differences in mission and services provided.

3. Discuss personal sources of health care insurance with other students. Compare coverage, costs, deductibles, and copayments. Share personal experiences with the costs of health care (e.g., recent pregnancy, chronic illness, having a checkup, medications). What are some experiences with managed care?

In Clinical

4. In each setting, gather information on the sources of, and procedure for, reimbursement. What is covered by insurance, Medicare, or Medicaid and what is not? How can services be provided efficiently and cost effectively?

5. Interview a health care professional from another discipline (e.g., PT, medical technologist, pharmacist) encountered during clinical. Question the professional on issues such as education and licensure or certification requirements, practice, salary range, and related information. If possible, spend a few hours observing this individual in practice and share observations with the other students.

REFERENCES

Aday, L. A. (1993). Indicators and predictors of health services utilization. In S. J. Williams & P. R. Torrens (Eds.), *Introduction to health services* (4th ed., pp. 46-70). Albany, NY: Delmar Publishers.

American Hospital Association. (2001). *Hospital statistics*. Chicago: American Hospital Association.

Centers for Medicare & Medicaid Services. (2001). *Medicaid services and Medicaid eligibility.* Retrieved 07/11/2001 from http://www.hcfa.gov/medicaid/meligib.htm.

Clark, M. J. (1999). *Nursing in the community* (3rd ed.). Norwalk, CT: Appleton & Lange.

Evashwick, C. J. (1999). The continuum of long-term care. In S. J. Williams & P. R. Torrens (Eds.), *Introduction to health services* (5th ed., pp. 295-348). Albany, NY: Delmar Publishers.

Dowling, W. L. (1999). Hospitals and health systems. In S. J. Williams & P. R. Torrens (Eds.), *Introduction to health services* (5th ed., pp. 257-294). Albany, NY: Delmar Publishers.

Koch, A. L. (1999). Financing health services. In S. J. Williams & P. R. Torrens (Eds.), *Introduction to health services* (5th ed., pp. 113-150). Albany, NY: Delmar Publishers.

Kovner, A. R. (1999). Hospitals. In A. R. Kovner & S. Jonas (Eds.), *Jonas's & Kovner's health care delivery in the United States* (6th ed., pp. 157-182). New York: Springer Publishing.

Kovner, C., & Salsberg, E. S. (1999). The health care workforce. In A. R. Kovner & S. Jonas (Eds.), *Jonas's & Kovner's health care delivery in the United States* (6th ed., pp. 64-115). New York: Springer Publishing.

Lee, P. R., & Estes, C. L. (Eds.). (1994). *The nation's health* (4th ed.). Boston: Jones and Bartlett.

Mezey, A. P. (1999). Ambulatory care. In A. R. Kovner & S. Jonas (Eds.), *Jonas's & Kovner's health care delivery in the United States* (6th ed., pp. 183-205). New York: Springer Publishing.

National Heritage Insurance Company. (1995). *Medicaid provider procedures manual: Texas Department of Human Services.* Austin, TX: National Heritage Insurance Company.

Richardson, H., Raphael, C., & Barton, L. (1999). Long-term care: Health social and housing services for those with chronic illness. In A. R. Kovner & S. Jonas (Eds.), *Jonas's & Kovner's health care delivery in the United States* (6th ed., pp. 206-242). New York: Springer Publishing.

Stanhope, M. (1996). Economics of health care delivery. In M. Stanhope & J. Lancaster (Eds.), *Community health nursing: Promoting health of aggregates, families and individuals* (4th ed., pp. 65-92). St. Louis: Mosby.

Thorpe, K. E., & Knickman, J. R. (1999). Financing for health care. In A. R. Kovner & S. Jonas (Eds.), *Jonas's & Kovner's health care delivery in the United States* (6th ed., pp. 32-63). New York: Springer Publishing.

Torrens, P. R., & Williams, S. J. (1999). Managed care: Restructuring the system. In S. J. Williams & P. R. Torrens (Eds.), *Introduction to health services* (5th ed., pp. 151-171). Albany, NY: Delmar Publishers.

U.S. Department of Health and Human Services. (1997). *Health United States, 1997.* Washington, DC: Government Printing Office.

U.S. Department of Health and Human Services. (2000). *Healthy people 2010: National health promotion and disease prevention objectives.* Washington, DC: Government Printing Office.

U.S. Department of Health and Human Services/ Health Care Financing Administration. (2001). *Medicare & you, 2001.* Washington, DC: Government Printing Office.

Williams, S. J. (1999). Ambulatory health care services. In S. J. Williams & P. R. Torrens (Eds.), *Introduction to health services* (5th ed., pp. 227-256). Albany, NY: Delmar Publishers.

Epidemiology

Upon completion of this chapter, the reader will be able to:

1. Explain ways in which concepts of epidemiology can be used in community-based nursing practice.

2. Apply models of disease causation in examination of diseases and health problems.

3. Develop primary, secondary, and tertiary prevention strategies for selected health threats.

4. Discuss commonly used rates such as mortality rates, incidence rates, and prevalence rates and give examples of when they are used.

5. Identify sources of information that may be accessed by nurses in community settings.

6. Describe the difference between descriptive epidemiology and analytic epidemiology and give examples of each.

key terms

Agent	Incidence rate	Outbreak
Distribution	Morbidity rate	Prevalence rate
Epidemiology	Mortality rate	
Host	Natural history of disease	*See Glossary for definitions.*

case study

Meg Henderson is a school nurse who cares for children of elementary school age in a small city. One of her primary responsibilities is prevention of communicable diseases. In addition to monitoring each child's immunization status, this includes identifying children with communicable diseases, excluding them from school, and then reinstating them, according to school district policy.

One recent Monday, Meg saw Elizabeth Ellis, a third grader, whose teacher sent her to the clinic because she was seen scratching her head repeatedly. Using applicators, Meg carefully examined Elizabeth's hair and saw evidence of head lice. When questioned, Elizabeth replied that her head had been itching "about 2 or 3 days." Meg learned that Elizabeth lives with her parents and older brother and younger sister, who are also students at the school. Following district guidelines, Meg examined both of Elizabeth's siblings and determined that they were also infected. She called Mrs. Ellis and informed her that she must come to school to get her children and treat the entire family for lice.

When Mrs. Ellis arrived to pick up her children, she was obviously embarrassed. Meg explained that lice are a very contagious parasite, easily passed between children through sharing of brushes, combs, hats, or other items and not an indicator of poor hygiene. She also stated that head lice are easily treatable and gave Mrs. Ellis an information packet that she keeps in the clinic describing the transmission, identification, and treatment of head lice. She reviewed the information with Mrs. Ellis, informed her that the children could return to school after they had all been treated, and pointed out that they should be treated again in 2 weeks.

After the Ellis family left, Meg examined all of the students from each of the Ellis children's classes for head lice. From the three classes, she identified five more children with lice and then called their parents. These children had siblings in three more classes and the children in each of these classes were also examined. At the end of the day, a total of 15 children had been excluded from school.

The following week, Meg reexamined all of the children in each class with an infected student. Two weeks after the incident, she examined all of the excluded children and determined that they had been successfully treated. No more cases of lice were identified that semester.

Much of nursing practice, particularly in community settings, involves prevention, early identification and prompt treatment of health problems, and monitoring for emerging threats and unidentified patterns that might signify health problems. For example, a nurse working in an inner-city women's clinic might note that the diagnosis of cervical dysplasia among teenagers and women in their early 20s has increased over a period, associated with increases in human papillomavirus infection. In addition to assisting with treatment of the clients involved, she would inform officials from the county health department's sexually transmitted disease (STD) program or a regional medical school for further investigation.

Another example would be a nurse working in a manufacturing plant who notes an unusual increase in complaints of back strain. After assisting the workers with reducing their back pain, the nurse should collect data on cases of back strain during the past 6 months and look for trends. Further, the nurse should inform the plant management and work with them to take appropriate steps to identify the cause of the problems and develop plant policy to minimize risks. Recording problems, keeping track of patterns, and working to identify causes are all part of the science and practice of epidemiology.

Epidemiology is the basic science of public health and refers to "the study of the distribution and determinants of health-related states or events in a specified population, and the application of this study to the control of health problems" (Centers for Disease Control and Prevention [CDC], 1992, p. 430). The science of epidemiology is based on the idea that disease, illness, and ill health are not randomly distributed in a population, but rather that "each of us has certain characteristics that predispose us to, or protect us against, a variety of different diseases" (Gordis, 1999, p. 3). Identifying these characteristics and removing or minimizing them if they are harmful, or enhancing them or transferring them if helpful, are basic goals in epidemiology.

Nurses who work with clients in community settings are frequently in a position to assist in identification, management, treatment, and prevention of health problems and, as a result, need a general understanding of the basic principles, theories, and concepts of epidemiology. In addition, a nurse needs to be able to read and interpret data about trends in diseases to carry out responsibilities in client teaching. Valanis (1999)

BOX **Box 6-1** Uses of Epidemiology

- Investigation of disease etiology
- Identification of risks
- Identification of syndromes and classification of disease
- Differential diagnoses and planning clinical treatment
- Surveillance of population health status
- Community diagnosis and planning of health services
- Evaluation of health services and public health interventions

Data from Valanis, B. (1999). *Epidemiology in nursing and health care* (3rd ed.). Norwalk, CT: Appleton & Lange.

outlines seven uses of epidemiology, which are depicted in Box 6-1.

Healthy People 2010 (U.S. Department of Health and Human Services, 2000), introduced in Chapter 1, was written based on epidemiological principles. This document presents health statistics and data; describes health threats; discusses interventions and plans; and sets goals and objectives directed toward prevention, man-

agement, minimization, or elimination of the identified health threats. The *Healthy People 2010* box presents examples of *Healthy People 2010's* objectives demonstrating epidemiological concepts (e.g., primary prevention, rates) described in this chapter.

This chapter presents basic concepts of epidemiology and describes how understanding the course or progression of a disease or health condition is important for nurses who practice in community settings. The use of epidemiological concepts and principles to identify risks and to assist in the prevention and management of disease also is discussed. Box 6-2 defines some common terms used in epidemiology.

MODELS OF DISEASE CAUSATION

Several theories and models describe disease causation and the properties that relate to disease processes and prevention. Four of the most frequently encountered models are briefly discussed in the following sections.

healthy people **2010**

Objectives Related to Epidemiology

OBJECTIVE	BASELINE (1998)	TARGET
3.1: Reduce the overall cancer death rate	201.4 per 100,000	158.7 per 100,000
9.7: Reduce pregnancies among adolescent females	72 pregnancies per 1000	46 pregnancies per 1000
10.1b: Reduce infections caused by *E. coli* 0157:H7	2.1 per 100,000	1.0 per 100,000
12.13: Reduce the mean total blood cholesterol levels among adults	206 mg/dL	199 mg/dL
13.1: Reduce AIDS among adolescents and adult (incidence)	19.5 new cases per 100,000	1.0 new cases per 100,000
14.3a: Reduce hepatitis B among adults 19-24 years (incidence)	24.0 new cases per 100,000	2.4 new cases per 100,000
16.1b: Reduce fetal and infant deaths during perinatal period	7.5 per 1000 live births	4.5 per 1000 live births
19.2 Reduce the proportion of adults who are obese (prevalence)	23%	15%
27.1a: Reduce cigarette smoking by adults (prevalence)	24%	12%

Data from U.S. Department of Health and Human Services. (2000). *Healthy people 2010: conference edition.* Washington, DC: Government Printing Office.

BOX 6-2 Epidemiological Terms and Concepts

Epidemiology is derived from three Greek words: *epi* (upon), *demos* (the people), and *logos* (science). *Epidemiology* is defined as "The study of the distribution and determinants of health-related states or events in a specified population, and the application of this study to the control of health problems" (CDC, 1992, p. 430). The following terms are related to epidemiology, but are not discussed in this chapter:

- *Carrier*: A person or animal without apparent disease who harbors a specific infectious agent and is capable of transmitting the agent to others.
- *Cohort*: A well-defined group of people who have had a common experience or exposure, who are then followed up for the incidence of new diseases or events, as in a cohort or prospective study.
- *Common source outbreak (point source)*: An outbreak that results from a group of persons being exposed to a common noxious influence, such as an infectious agent or toxin. If the group is exposed over a relatively brief time, so that all cases occur within one incubation period, then the common source outbreak is further classified as a point source outbreak.
- *Crude mortality rate*: The mortality rate from all causes of death for a population.
- *Direct transmission*: The immediate transfer of an agent from a reservoir to a susceptible host by direct contact of droplet spread.
- *Endemic disease*: The constant presence of a disease or infectious agent within a given geographical area or population group; it may also refer to the usual prevalence of a given disease within such an area or a group.
- *Epidemic*: The occurrence of more cases of disease than expected in a given area or among a specific group of people over a particular period.
- *Herd immunity*: The resistance of a group to invasion and spread of an infectious agent, based on the resistance to infection of a high proportion of individual members of the group.

- *Indirect transmission*: The transmission of an agent carried from a reservoir to a susceptible host by suspended air particles or by animate (vector) or inanimate (vehicle) intermediaries.
- *Pandemic*: An epidemic occurring over a very wide area (several countries or continents) and usually affecting a large proportion of the population.
- *Propagated outbreak*: An outbreak that does not have a common source, but instead spreads from person to person.
- *Risk*: The probability that an event will occur (e.g., that an individual will become ill or die within a stated period or age).
- *Risk factor*: An aspect of personal behavior or lifestyle, an environmental exposure, or an inborn or inherited characteristic that is associated with an increased occurrence of disease or other health-related event or condition.
- *Universal precautions*: Recommendations issued by the CDC to minimize the risk of transmission of bloodborne pathogens, particularly HIV and hepatitis B virus, by health care and public safety workers. Barrier precautions are to be used to prevent exposure to blood and certain body fluids of all clients.
- *Vector*: An animate intermediary in the indirect transmission of an agent that carries the agent from a reservoir to a susceptible host.
- *Vehicle*: An inanimate intermediary in the indirect transmission of an agent that carries the agent from a reservoir to a susceptible host.
- *Years of potential life lost*: A measure of the impact of premature mortality on a population, calculated as the sum of the differences between some predetermined minimum or desired life span and the age of death for individuals who died earlier than that predetermined age.
- *Zoonoses*: An infectious disease that is transmissible under normal conditions from animals to humans.

From Centers for Disease Control and Prevention (CDC). (1992). *Principles of epidemiology* (2nd ed.). Atlanta: Centers for Disease Control and Prevention.

THE EPIDEMIOLOGICAL TRIANGLE

The classic epidemiological model, particularly useful in the depiction of communicable disease, is the epidemiological triangle (Figure 6-1). This model is often used to illustrate the interrelationships among the essential components of **host**, **agent**, and environment with regard to disease causation. A change in any of the three components can result in the disease process. For example, exposure (environment) of a child who has not been immunized (host) to the measles virus (agent) will probably result in a case of

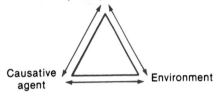

Figure 6-1. The epidemiological triangle.

measles. Another example would be respiratory difficulties resulting after an adult with chronic bronchitis (host) drives to work during rush hour (environment) on a day with excessive atmospheric ozone (agent).

Within the epidemiological triangle, prevention of the disease lies in preventing exposure to the agent, enhancing the physical attributes of the host to resist the disease, and minimizing any environmental factors that might contribute to disease development. Box 6-3 outlines host, agent, and environmental factors that affect health and could influence progression of the disease process.

THE WEB OF CAUSATION

The causes of most diseases are more complex than simply an interaction between a host, agent, and environment. To explain disease and disability caused by multiple factors, MacMahon and Pugh (1970) developed the concept of "chain of causation," later termed the "web of causation." Chronic diseases such as coronary artery disease and most types of cancer are not attributable to one or two factors alone. Rather, the interaction of multiple factors is necessary to produce the disease. An example of the application of the web of causation to the development of coronary heart disease is presented in Figure 6-2.

The web of causation can also be applied to many health-related threats and conditions. The problem of teenage pregnancy, for example, is attributable to a complex interaction between a number of causative and contributing factors, including lack of knowledge about sexuality and pregnancy prevention, lack of easily accessible contraception, peer pressure to engage in sex, low self-esteem, social patterns that encourage early motherhood, and use of alcohol or other drugs. Patterns of family violence, cocaine use, and gang

---

BOX **6-3** Some Host, Agent, and Environmental Factors That Affect Health

HOST FACTORS

Demographic data: Age, gender, ethnic background, race, marital status, religion, education, economic status

Level of health: Genetic risk factors, physiological states, anatomical factors, response to stress, previous disease, nutrition, fitness

Body defenses: Autoimmune system, lymphatic system

State of immunity: Susceptibility versus active or passive immunity

Human behavior: Diet, exercise, hygiene, substance abuse, occupation, personal and sexual contact, use of health resources, food handling

AGENT FACTORS (PRESENCE OR ABSENCE)

Biological: Viruses, bacteria, fungi, and their mode of transmission, life cycle, virulence

Physical: Radiation, temperature, noise

Chemical: Gas, liquids, poisons, allergens

ENVIRONMENTAL FACTORS

Physical properties: Water, air, climate, season, weather, geology, geography, pollution

Biological entities: Animals, plants, insects, food, drugs, food source

Social and economic consideration: Family, community, political organization, public policy, institutions, occupation, economic status, technology, mobility, housing, population density, attitudes, customs, culture, health practices, health services

From Neal, M. T., & Tarzian, A. J. (2000). Epidemiology: Unraveling the mysteries of disease and health. In C. M. Smith & F. A. Maurer (Eds.), *Community health nursing: Theory and practice* (2nd ed., pp. 311-339). Philadelphia: W. B. Saunders.

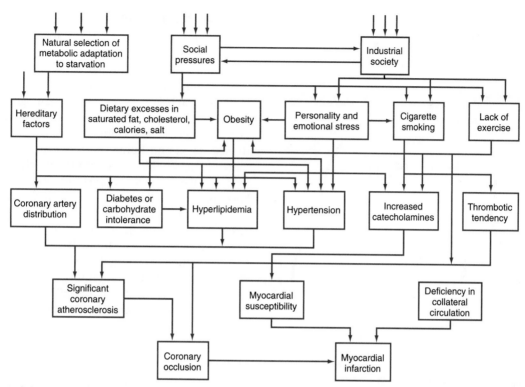

Figure 6-2. The web of causation for myocardial infarction. (From Frideman, G. D. [1987]. *Primer of epidemiology.* New York: McGraw-Hill.)

membership are examples of other threats to health and well-being that can be more accurately explained through a multiple-causation model.

Recognition that many health problems have multiple causes leads to the recognition that simple solutions to these health problems rarely exist. When trying to manage teenage pregnancy, for example, the solution is not as simple as addressing a "knowledge deficit about sexuality and contraception." Many (if not most) teens are well informed about contraception and the mechanics of how one gets pregnant and still fail to take preventative measures.

To prevent heart disease in an individual at risk, interventions include health education addressing a number of areas, including smoking cessation, reduction of blood pressure, weight loss, cholesterol reduction, and exercise.

Interventions might also need to address life-style, stress management, social support, and personality traits, among others. Likewise, to prevent teenage pregnancy, interventions should include health teaching on improving self-esteem; role-playing exercises on how to say "no"; encouraging an orientation to the future; enhancing parental supervision; and providing recreational alternatives (sports and other after-school activities) in addition to giving information on sexuality, the mechanics of reproduction, and methods of contraception.

THE ICEBERG MODEL

The "iceberg model" or "iceberg principle" (Figure 6-3) describes the phenomenon that at any given time there are a small number of known cases of a disease or condition at the early

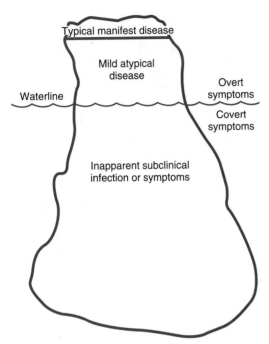

Figure 6-3. The iceberg model. (From Clemen-Stone, S., Eigsti, D. G., & McGuire, S. L. [1995]. *Comprehensive community health nursing* [4th ed.]. St. Louis: Mosby-Year Book.)

and advanced stages. These known cases are those that are visible. However, like the iceberg, the greatest threat comes from the greater amount of unknown cases (i.e., those that are not identified).

Infection with human immunodeficiency virus (HIV) is an excellent illustration of this principle. The clinically diagnosed cases of acquired immunodeficiency syndrome (AIDS) (manifest disease) represent only a small fraction of all cases of those infected. Those known to have HIV infection (mild, atypical disease) make up a more significant part of the whole, but the greatest concern, and possibly the greatest threat, comes from those individuals who have not been diagnosed and may be transmitting HIV unknowingly.

NATURAL HISTORY OF DISEASE

The **natural history of disease** refers to the progress of a disease process in an individual over time. In what is now a classic model, Leavell and Clark (1965) described two periods in the natural history of disease, prepathogenesis and pathogenesis. In this model, the prepathogenesis stage occurs before interaction of the disease agent and human host, when the individual is susceptible. For example, an adult man may smoke, a teenage girl might consider becoming sexually active, or a preschooler attends a party also attended by a sick child. After exposure or interaction, the period of pathogenesis proceeds to early pathogenesis (e.g., alterations in lung tissue, pregnancy, or chicken pox) and on through the disease course to resolution—either death, disability, or recovery (e.g., lung cancer, teenage motherhood, immunity to chicken pox).

LEVELS OF PREVENTION

In addition to the description of the natural history of disease progression, Leavell and Clark (1965) also outlined three levels of prevention that correlate with the stages of disease progression: (1) primary prevention, (2) secondary prevention, and (3) tertiary prevention. These levels are described as follows:

- *Primary prevention* consists of activities directed at preventing a problem before it occurs. Altering susceptibility or reducing exposure for susceptible individuals in the period of prepathogenesis is primary prevention. Primary prevention consists of two categories: (1) general health promotion (e.g., good nutrition, adequate shelter, rest, exercise) and (2) specific protection (e.g., immunization, water purification).
- *Secondary prevention* refers to early detection and prompt intervention in a disease or health threat during the period of early pathogenesis. Screening for disease and prompt referral and treatment are secondary prevention. Mammography, blood pressure screening,

scoliosis screening, and Papanicolaou smears are examples of secondary prevention.

- *Tertiary prevention* consists of limitation of disability and rehabilitation during the period of advanced disease and convalescence, in which the disease has occurred and resulted in a degree of damage. Teaching how to perform insulin injections and teaching disease management to a diabetic, referral for occupational therapy and physical therapy for a head injury victim, and leading a support group for grieving parents are examples of tertiary prevention.

Much of nursing practice in community settings is intended to prevent the progression of disease at the earliest period or phase using the appropriate level or levels of prevention. Thus, when applying "levels of prevention" to AIDS, a nurse would do the following:

- Educate clients on the practice of sexual abstinence or "safer sex" (primary prevention in the period of prepathogenesis).
- Encourage testing and counseling for clients with known exposure or who are in high-risk groups; provide referrals for follow-up for clients who test positive for HIV (secondary prevention in the period of early pathogenesis for early diagnosis and prompt treatment).
- Provide education on management of HIV infection, advocacy, case management, and other interventions (tertiary prevention to limit disability through the periods of advanced disease).

Figure 6-4 illustrates the relationship between the levels of prevention and the natural history of disease, as described by Leavell and Clark (1965).

EPIDEMIOLOGICAL TOOLS

RATES—DESCRIPTION, CALCULATION, AND INTERPRETATION

In epidemiology, rates are used to make comparisons among groups or populations or to compare a subgroup of the population with the total population. Rates are essential tools in identifying actual and potential problems in a given community or population. Rates from a given aggregate or community can be compared with international, national, state, local, or regional rates; age-specific rates; gender-specific rates; or race-specific rates. Just as a nurse working in a hospital compares a complete blood count with a given norm or standard, nurses who work in community settings use rates to compare information on morbidity and mortality in their practice setting or aggregate with "norms," "standards," or "goals."

The use of rates allows the nurse working in any setting to recognize when a health threat or disease encountered is normal or typical, or if a problem or concern that warrants further investigation or intervention exists. For example, an elementary school nurse found that five children in her school of 500 have chicken pox (a rate of 10 children per 1000). Should school be closed to prevent further infection? The nurse called the local health department and discovered that the current state incidence rate was 25 per 1000 children and the county incidence rate was 20 per 1000. Thus, she determined that the rate of chicken pox in her school was actually much lower than rates in comparison groups, so there was no reason to be concerned.

In calculating a rate, the numerator is the number of events and the denominator is the total population at risk. The rate is usually converted to a standard base denominator (1000; 10,000; or 100,000) to permit comparisons between various groups.

Measures of Morbidity

Measurement of morbidity and mortality is an integral part of public health. Different types of **morbidity rates** are used to measure and monitor illnesses. The **incidence rate** refers to the number of new cases of an illness or injury that occur within a specified time. The **prevalence rate** refers to all of the existing cases of an illness at a given point of time. Incidence rates are most helpful in detecting and describing fluctuations in acute diseases and prevalence rates are important in measuring chronic illness.

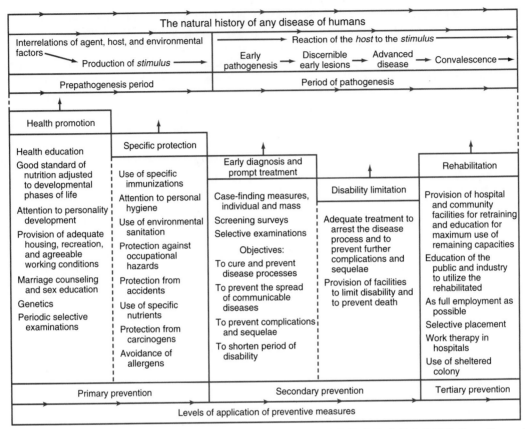

Figure 6-4. Levels of prevention in the natural history of disease. (From Leavell, H. R., & Clark, E. G. [1965]. *Preventive medicine for the doctor in his community: An epidemiologic approach.* New York: McGraw-Hill.)

Table 6-1 provides an example of disease prevalence in describing arthritis in persons 18 years of age and older. As Table 6-1 indicates, approximately 29% of Americans report having arthritis. In addition, arthritis is strongly associated with age and there is a weaker association with gender (i.e., women have a higher prevalence than do men).

Figure 6-5 presents an example of disease incidence by visually depicting the number of reported pediatric AIDS cases for 1999. In reviewing this map, it is somewhat surprising to note that the states with the highest percentage of cases are Florida (39 cases), New York (38 cases), Pennsylvania (23 cases), and New Jersey (22 cases); the states with the largest populations

(California and Texas) had relatively many fewer cases. Figure 6-5 helps show where problems with pediatric AIDS persist, which allows for better targeting with prevention programs.

Measures of Mortality

Just as different types of morbidity rates are used to measure and monitor illnesses, a number of different rates are used to measure attributes regarding death (**mortality rates**). Measures of mortality frequently used in public health are listed in Table 6-2. Of particular interest to nurses working in community settings are the infant mortality rate, crude death rate, and the cause-specific death rate (e.g., how many individuals have died from AIDS or automobile

TABLE **6-1** Example of Disease Prevalence: Prevalence of Arthritis Among Persons Aged 18 Years by Sex and Age

CHARACTERISTIC	PREVALENCE	(95% CI)	ODDS RATIO
SEX			
Women	33%	(32%-34%)	1.4
Men	25%	(24%-26%)	1.0
AGE GROUP (YR)			
18-44	16%	(15%-17%)	1.0
45-64	39%	(37%-40%)	3.4
≥65	53%	(52%-55%)	5.5
Total	29%	(28%-30%)	—

From Centers for Disease Control and Prevention (CDC). (2000a). Health-related quality of life among adults with arthritis—behavioral risk factor surveillance system, 11 states, 1996-1998. *MMWR Morbidity and Mortality Weekly Report, 49*(17), 366-369.
CI, confidence interval.

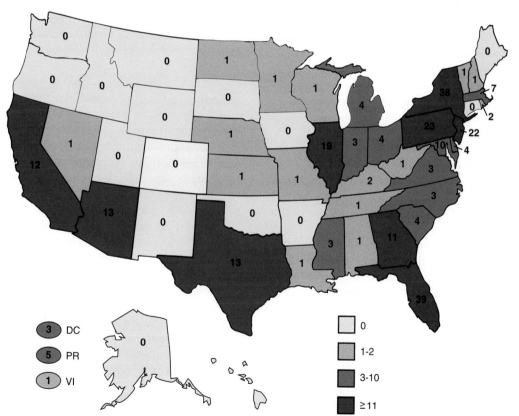

Figure 6-5. Example of disease incidence: acquired immunodeficiency syndrome (AIDS)—reported pediatric cases (children and adolescents aged less than 13 years), United States, Puerto Rico and U.S. Virgin Islands,1999. (From Centers for Disease Control and Prevention [CDC]. [2001]. Summary of notifiable diseases, United States, 1999. *MMWR Morbidity and Mortality Weekly Report, 48*[53], 1-104.)

TABLE **6-2** Frequently Used Measures of Mortality

MEASURE	NUMERATOR (X)	DENOMINATOR (Y)	EXPRESSED PER NUMBER AT RISK (10^N)
Crude death rate	Total number of deaths reported during a given time interval	Estimated midinterval population	1000 or 100,000
Cause-specific death rate	Number of deaths assigned to a specific cause during a given time interval	Estimated midinterval population	100,000
Neonatal mortality rate	Number of deaths under 28 days of age during a given time interval	Number of live births during the same time interval	1000
Postneonatal mortality rate	Number of deaths from 28 days to, but not including, 1 year of age, during a given time interval	Number of live births during the same time interval	1000
Infant mortality rate	Number of deaths under 1 year of age during a given time interval	Number of live births reported during the same time interval	1000
Maternal mortality rate	Number of deaths assigned to pregnancy-related causes during a given time interval	Number of live births during the same time interval	100,000

From Centers for Disease Control and Prevention (CDC). (1992). *Principles of epidemiology* (2nd ed.). Atlanta: Centers for Disease Control and Prevention.

accidents). Table 6-3 presents an example of mortality data.

COLLECTION OF DATA: THE CENSUS, VITAL STATISTICS, AND HEALTH STATISTICS

Sources of population-focused data for nurses in community-based practice include the census and local, state, and national vital statistics and health statistics. Each of these is discussed briefly. Much of the relevant information for nurses is available at local or state health departments and the local library. Sources of data on health issues from federal sources are listed in the Resources box at the end of the chapter.

The Census

The Bureau of the Census is responsible for collection of data on the U.S. population. A census of the population to assess its characteristics has been conducted every 10 years since 1790 as mandated by the Constitution of the United States. Among other reasons, the census is undertaken to establish each state's representation in the House of Representatives.

The methodology of census taking has evolved over the decades. To make the task more manageable and the data more meaningful, census tracts were developed. Census tracts are relatively small, usually homogenous geographic areas that allow for analysis of small units within communities. Maps outlining boundaries for census tracts can be obtained from a local public library.

Census tract information can be extremely valuable for nurses and others involved in health program planning. Information elicited from the census questionnaire includes:

- Name, sex, race, age, ethnicity, and marital status of everyone living in the household (including housemates, foster children, boarders, and live-in employees)
- Housing characteristics, including the type of dwelling (e.g., mobile home, single-family detached, duplex, apartment); age of the dwelling; number of rooms; number of bedrooms; presence of plumbing facilities; kitchen facilities; source of fuel; source of water; sewage system; yearly costs for electricity, gas, and water

TABLE **6-3** Mortality Rate Example: Deaths, Death Rates, and Percent of Total Deaths for the 15 Leading Causes of Death: United States, 1999

RANK	CAUSE OF DEATH (ICD-10)	NUMBER	DEATH RATE	TOTAL DEATHS (%)
—	All causes	2,391,630	877.0	100.0
1	Diseases of heart	724,915	265.8	30.3
2	Malignant neoplasms	549,787	201.6	23.0
3	Cerebrovascular diseases	167,340	61.4	7.0
4	Chronic lower respiratory diseases	124,153	45.5	5.2
5	Accidents (unintentional injuries)	97,298	35.7	4.1
—	Motor vehicle accidents	42,437	15.6	1.8
—	All other accidents	54,862	20.1	2.3
6	Diabetes	68,379	25.1	2.9
7	Pneumonia and influenza	63,686	23.4	2.7
8	Alzheimer's disease	44,507	16.3	1.9
9	Nephritis, nephrotic syndrome, and nephrosis	35,524	13.0	1.5
10	Septicemia	30,670	11.2	1.3
11	Intentional self-harm (suicide)	29,041	10.6	1.2
12	Chronic liver disease and cirrhosis	26,225	9.6	1.1
13	Essential hypertension and hypertensive renal disease	16,964	6.2	0.7
14	Assault (homicide)	16,831	6.2	0.7
15	Aortic aneurysm and dissection	15,806	5.8	0.7
—	All other causes	380,503	139.5	15.9

From National Center for Health Statistics (NCHS). (2001). Deaths: Preliminary Data for 1999. *National Vital Statistics Report, 49*(3), 1-49.
ICD-10, international classification of diseases.
Data are based on a continuous file of records received from the states. Rates per 100,000 population based on the year 2000 standard.

- Information on the ownership of the home (e.g., owned by the resident, rented, mortgaged), estimated value, monthly rent, length of time in residence, property taxes
- Education attainment of all in the household
- Language spoken in the home
- Information related to occupation and work, including location of work, transportation to work (e.g., car, bus, subway, ferry, motorcycle), estimated time to get to work and home, employment information, type of work (e.g., manufacturing, wholesale trade, retail trade, agriculture, construction, service, government), retirement benefits, and income

This information is gathered during April of each new decade (i.e., 1980, 1990, 2000) for all individuals residing in the United States. Information on numerous divisions (e.g., U.S. geographical areas) and subdivisions (e.g.,

states, metropolitan areas, census tract) of the census can be obtained at a regional public library and from the Bureau of the Census. See the Resources box for information on how to directly access the Bureau's website.

Vital Statistics

The term *vital statistics* refers to data collected about the significant events that occur within a population over a period. These data are systematically gathered by agencies at local, state, national, and international levels. Vital statistics data include the data collected from ongoing recording, or registration, of all vital events—births and adoptions; deaths and fetal deaths; and marriages, divorces, legal separations, and annulments (Valanis, 1999). Data on vital events are collected locally and reported to area and state offices through channels dictated by each state. Local vital statistics data can typically be obtained from the county or district records office and are often available at public libraries. State vital statistic information can be gathered from state records departments and national information from the National Center for Health Statistics (NCHS) (see the Resources box).

Health Statistics

The CDC, the National Institutes of Health (NIH), and the NCHS (see the Resources box) are the primary sources for morbidity and mortality data in the United States. Each of these organizations is a component of the Department of Health and Human Services, as discussed in Chapter 5.

The CDC has primary responsibility for monitoring communicable diseases and other actual and potential health threats. The CDC publishes information for health providers in the *Morbidity and Mortality Weekly Report (MMWR)*. Included in this periodical are weekly updates on selected reportable diseases, brief articles on a variety of topics, periodic recommendations for prevention, detection, and treatment of diseases, and field reports detailing current and completed investigations into disease **outbreaks**. The *MMWR* can be found in most medical libraries, in public libraries with significant public document collections, at local health departments, or online through the CDC's website (see the Resources box).

The NIH is essentially concerned with research into numerous areas related to health. Information from the NIH primarily covers federally funded research projects. Information generated from the various studies is typically published in various professional journals. In addition, selected major studies, reports, guidelines, and recommendations are published and available from the Government Printing Office. In addition to maintaining information on vital statistics (e.g., births, deaths) as discussed, the NCHS also monitors and publishes causes of morbidity and mortality.

DESCRIPTIVE AND ANALYTICAL EPIDEMIOLOGY

There are two basic types of epidemiology. *Descriptive epidemiology* examines the amount and **distribution** of a disease in terms of person, place, and time to distinguish characteristics of individuals who have a specific disease from those who do not. Analytical epidemiology investigates the etiology of disease. In *analytical epidemiology*, observational and experimental studies are used to establish a causal relationship between identified threats and development of disease or disability.

DESCRIPTIVE EPIDEMIOLOGY

Descriptive epidemiology considers the amount and distribution of disease within a population by person, place, and time. As implied by the name, it is predominantly used to describe patterns of disease rather than considering or speculating on causality. Table 6-4 details characteristics or descriptors commonly used in the study of the amount and distribution of disease.

In many health reports and records, health problems are often presented with accompanying information on characteristics of those who have the health problem (i.e., data on person, place, and time). Table 6-5, for example, describes characteristics of young smokers by grade (high school, middle school), sex, and race/ethnicity. As Table 6-5 illustrates, epidemiological data are often presented in a manner that allows for interpretation and application to other populations and provides information that can be regathered and compared to analyze trends over time.

ANALYTICAL EPIDEMIOLOGY

Analytical epidemiology focuses on the determinants of disease in a given population. The search for causes and effects, or to quantify the association between exposures and outcomes and to test hypotheses about causal relationships, is the purpose of analytical epidemiology (CDC, 1992). The process of identification of the etiology of a disease occurs following comparison of

TABLE **6-4** Characteristics Assessed in Descriptive Epidemiology: Person, Place, and Time

PERSON	PLACE	TIME
Age	Natural boundaries	Secular trends
Sex	Political subdivisions	Cyclic changes
Ethnic group and race	Environmental factors	Clusters in time and place
Social class	Urban-rural differences	
Occupation	International comparisons	
Marital status		
Family variables (e.g., family size, birth order, maternal age, parental deprivation)		
Personal variables (e.g., blood type, environmental exposure, personality traits)		

Data from Mausner, J. S., & Kramer, S. (1985). *Epidemiology—an introductory text.* Philadelphia: W. B. Saunders.

TABLE **6-5** Percentage of Middle School and High School Students Who Are Current Users of Cigarettes and Smokeless Tobacco, 1999

STUDENT CHARACTERISTIC	ANY TOBACCO	CIGARETTES	SMOKELESS TOBACCO
Middle School			
SEX			
Male	14.2	9.6	4.2
Female	11.3	8.9	1.3
RACE/ETHNICITY			
White	11.6	8.8	3.0
Black	14.4	9.0	1.9
Hispanic	15.2	11.0	2.2
Total, Middle School	12.8	9.2	2.7
High School			
SEX			
Male	38.1	28.7	11.7
Female	31.4	28.2	1.5
RACE/ETHNICITY			
White	39.4	32.9	8.7
Black	24.0	15.9	2.4
Hispanic	30.7	25.8	3.7
Total, High School	34.8	28.5	6.6

From Centers for Disease Control and Prevention (CDC). (2000b). Youth tobacco surveillance—United States, 1998-1999. *MMWR Morbidity and Mortality Weekly Report, 49*(SS-10), 1-93.

COMMUNITY APPLICATION
Preventing Emerging Infectious Diseases

The CDC (1998) has recognized that infectious diseases are a continuing threat to all persons, regardless of age, sex, lifestyle, ethnic background, and socioeconomic status. In recognition of the potential problem of emerging infections, the CDC has identified these emerging threats:

- New variant Creutzfeldt-Jakob disease, which is possibly transmitted by ingestion of beef from animals afflicted with bovine spongiform encephalopathy (mad cow disease)
- A new and virulent strain of influenza in Hong Kong
- Several multistate foodborne outbreaks including hepatitis A on frozen strawberries and *Escherichia coli* 0157:H7 in apple cider, lettuce, alfalfa sprouts, and ground beef
- *Staphylococcus aureus* with reduced susceptibility to vancomycin
- A new strain of multidrug-resistant tuberculosis (strain W); appears more frequently in persons with HIV infection and has become endemic in New York

A set of goals was established to address these emerging infections. These goals include strategies for surveillance and response, applied research, infrastructure and training, and prevention and control. It is hoped that achieving these goals will promote understanding of infectious diseases and enhance their detection, control, and prevention.

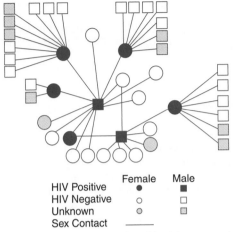

Figure 6-6. Example of analytic epidemiology: sex network of seven persons with HIV infection—Mississippi, 1999. (From Centers for Disease Control and Prevention [CDC]. [2000d]. Cluster of HIV-infected adolescents and young adults—Mississippi, 1999. *MMWR Morbidity and Mortality Weekly Report, 49* [38], 861-864.)

groups through epidemiological studies (see the Community Application box "Preventing Emerging Infectious Diseases"). Epidemiological studies are typically experimental or observational and may involve significant amounts of time.

One example of analytic epidemiology was a CDC (2000c) study that examined the relationship between alcohol use and the incidence of gonorrhea. In this study, multiple statistical analyses suggested that the incidence of gonorrhea decreased in states when the minimum drinking age was raised. In addition, states with higher beer taxes also had lower gonorrhea rates among 15- to 24-year-olds. The study concluded that a beer tax increase of $0.20 per six pack could reduce overall gonorrhea rates by 8.9%.

Another example of analytic epidemiology is a study of a cluster of HIV infection among adolescents and young adults (CDC, 2000d). Contact investigations of sex partners and social contacts of two HIV-positive persons identified by the health department identified five additional HIV-positive young people in a small town in rural Mississippi (Figure 6-6). Of the seven infected, five were young women (median age, 21 years). The wide-scale study examined several factors including age; gender; history of other STDs; coinfection with other STDs; drug and alcohol use; and exchange of sex for alcohol, drugs, or money. Common characteristics of infected women included low socioeconomic status, absentee fathers, truancy, school failure, and having sex partners who were greater than 10 years older than themselves. It was concluded that among adolescents, disadvantaged black women have some of the highest HIV infection rates in the United States and this cohort must be a high priority for prevention activities.

COMMUNITY APPLICATION
Cancer Clusters

A disease cluster is the occurrence of a greater than expected number of cases of a particular disease within a group of people, a geographical area, or time. Cancer clusters may be suspected when people report that several family members, friends, neighbors, or co-workers have been diagnosed with cancer.

Various statistical methods are used to determine whether the reported number of cancer cases is really a larger number than would normally be expected to occur. Central cancer registry data are used to compare cancer rates to determine whether an actual excess of cases has occurred. Reported disease clusters may be investigated by epidemiologists.

The first level of response to inquiries about suspected cancer clusters involves state health departments and other relevant state agencies. Various federal agencies, centers, and institutes may provide assistance in responding to special inquiries about suspected cancer clusters. These include National Institute for Occupational Safety and Health, the National Institute of Environmental Health Sciences, the National Cancer Institute, and the Environmental Protection Agency.

From Centers for Disease Control and Prevention (CDC). (1997). *Cancer clusters.* Retrieved 7/20/01 from http://www.cdc.gov/cancer/npcr/clusters.htm

For an example of another type of disease cluster, see the Community Application box, "Cancer Clusters."

SUMMARY

This chapter presents some of the basic elements of epidemiology. Recognition of the causes and course of a disease or health problem and identification of methods to prevent progression of the disease are very important components of nursing practice in any setting and they are essential when practicing in the community. Indeed, this principle was illustrated by the case study in which Meg, a school nurse, was called upon to deal with an outbreak of head lice.

Many of the concepts included here are carried throughout the remainder of this book. Each of the chapters on health promotion (Chapters 9 to 12), for example, includes several primary, secondary, and tertiary prevention interventions. Additionally, Chapter 16 takes a closer look at disease transmission and epidemiology when discussing communicable disease.

Resources
Population Data

Centers for Disease Control and Prevention
National Center for Health Statistics
U.S. Census Bureau
National Institutes of Health

Visit the book's website at
www.wbsaunders.com/SIMON/McEwen
for a direct link to the website for each organization listed.

KEY POINTS

- Epidemiology is defined as the study of the distribution and determinants of disease in humans and application of this information to control health problems. Identification of characteristics or risk factors that predispose persons to, or protect them against, disease and removing or minimizing them if harmful or enhancing them if helpful, are basic goals in epidemiology. The use of epidemiological concepts and principles to identify risks and assist in the prevention and management of disease is important for nurses working in community-based practice.

- A basic understanding of disease causation is important to assist in identification of risk factors and development of prevention strategies. Models of disease causation include the epidemiological triangle (host, agent, and environment triad), the web of causation (explains diseases of multiple causation), and the natural history of disease (demonstrates how a disease progresses through stages of prepathogenesis and pathogenesis).

- Much of nursing practice in community settings is intended to prevent the progression of disease at the earliest period or phase using the appropriate level of prevention. Nursing interventions can be delivered at three different levels of prevention: (1) primary prevention (activities that prevent a problem before it occurs), (2) secondary prevention (early detection and prompt intervention during the period of early pathogenesis), and (3) tertiary prevention (efforts to limit disability and promote rehabilitation during the period of advanced disease and convalescence).

- Rates are statistical tools used to make comparisons between groups or populations or compare a subgroup of a population with the total population. Rates that measure the amount of morbidity associated with a particular illness include incidence and prevalence rates. Commonly used measures of mortality include the infant mortality rate, crude death rate, and cause-specific death rates.

- Sources of data on health-related issues include the census (population characteristics such as sex, race or ethnicity, age, housing characteristics, education levels, occupation information), vital statistics (e.g., registration of births, deaths), and health statistics (maintained by state health departments and the CDC).

- Descriptive epidemiology refers to the amount and distribution of a disease in terms of person, place, and time. Analytical epidemiology investigates the etiology of disease through observational and experimental studies to identify causal relationships between identified threats and development of subsequent disease or disability.

Learning Activities & Application to Practice
In Class

1. Select one or two timely illnesses or syndromes (e.g., bovine spongiform encephalopathy [BSE], autism, AIDS, skin cancer). Examine the illness using the models of disease causation described. Which model best fits each illness? Are the models useful for determining appropriate interventions?

2. For the illnesses or health conditions discussed in the previous exercise or other similar conditions, discuss primary-, secondary-, and tertiary-level interventions that nurses might be expected to deliver in community-based settings. With classmates, come up with examples of each level of prevention.

3. Complete the calculation exercises in Box 6-4.

In Clinical

4. With a small group of classmates, obtain selected census and vital statistics data on a local community or group. Determine what data are pertinent to the health of members of the community or to management of health care resources (e.g., presence or absence of running water, number of persons in the household, number of small children, number of elders, number of deaths, number of live births). Share findings with other groups and compare.

5. Observe for clusters of health problems that might indicate the need for comparison with other groups. For example, if working in a school, observe how many children seem to be having breathing difficulties or are being diagnosed with asthma. A comparison should be done with another school to see if one has higher rates of asthma than does the other.

6-4 Exercises for Calculation of Rates

During 2001, 215 *new* cases of AIDS were reported in Grand River, a city of 500,000. This brought the total of active cases of AIDS to 2280. During that time, 105 deaths were attributable to the disease.

1. What is the incidence rate per 100,000 for AIDS during 2001?
2. What was the prevalence rate of AIDS per 100,000?
3. What is the cause-specific death rate for AIDS per 100,000?

Sun City is a small city with a mid2001 population of 120,000. During 2001, 342 live births and 515 deaths occurred in Sun City. Sun City has a large elderly population, with approximately 24,000 of the population being older than 65 years. Of the 515 deaths during 2001, 425 were in individuals older than 65.

4. What is the crude birth rate for Sun City for 2001 per 1000?
5. What is the crude death rate for Sun City for 2001 per 1000?
6. What is the age-specific death rate for individuals older than 65 for Sun City for 2001 per 1000?

Answers are at the end of the chapter, after the References.

REFERENCES

Centers for Disease Control and Prevention (CDC). (1992). *Principles of epidemiology* (2nd ed.). Atlanta: Centers for Disease Control and Prevention.

Centers for Disease Control and Prevention (CDC). (1997). *Cancer clusters*. Retrieved 7/20/01 from http://www.cdc.gov/cancer/npcr/clusters.htm.

Centers for Disease Control and Prevention (CDC). (1998). Preventing emerging infectious diseases: A strategy for the 21st century overview of the updated CDC plan. *MMWR Morbidity and Mortality Weekly Report, 47*(RR15), 1-14.

Centers for Disease Control and Prevention (CDC). (2000a). Health-related quality of life among adults with arthritis—behavioral risk factor surveillance system, 11 states, 1996-1998. *MMWR Morbidity and Mortality Weekly Report, 49*(17), 366-369.

Centers for Disease Control and Prevention (CDC). (2000b). Youth tobacco surveillance—United States,

1998-1999. *MMWR Morbidity and Mortality Weekly Report, 49*(SS-10), 1-93.

Centers for Disease Control and Prevention (CDC). (2000c). Alcohol policy and sexually transmitted disease rates—United States, 1981-1995. *MMWR Morbidity and Mortality Weekly Report, 49*(16), 346-349.

Centers for Disease Control and Prevention (CDC). (2000d). Cluster of HIV-infected adolescents and young adults—Mississippi, 1999. *MMWR Morbidity and Mortality Weekly Report, 49*(38), 861-864.

Centers for Disease Control and Prevention (CDC). (2001). *Summary of notifiable diseases, United States, 1999. MMWR Morbidity and Mortality Weekly Report, 48*(53), 1-104.

Clemen-Stone, S., Eigsti, D. G., & McGuire, S. L. (1995). *Comprehensive community health nursing* (4th ed.). St. Louis: Mosby.

Frideman, G. D. (1987). *Primer of epidemiology*. New York: McGraw-Hill.

Gordis, L. (1999). *Epidemiology* (2nd ed.). Philadelphia: W. B. Saunders.

Leavell, H. R., & Clark, E. G. (1965). *Preventive medicine for the doctor in his community: An epidemiologic approach* (2nd ed.). New York: McGraw-Hill.

MacMahon, B., & Pugh, T. F. (1970). *Epidemiologic principles and methods*. Boston: Little, Brown & Co.

Mausner, J. S., & Kramer, S. (1985). *Epidemiology: An introductory text*. Philadelphia: W. B. Saunders.

National Center for Health Statistics (NCHS). (2001). Deaths: Preliminary Data for 1999. *National Vital Statistics Report, 49*(3), 1-49.

Neal, M.T., & Tarzian, A. J. (2000). Epidemiology: Unraveling the mysteries of disease and health. In C. M. Smith & F. A. Maurer (Eds.), *Community health nursing: Theory and practice* (2nd ed., pp. 311-339). Philadelphia: W. B. Saunders.

U.S. Department of Health and Human Services. (2000). *Healthy people 2010, conference edition*. Washington, DC: Government Printing Office.

Valanis, B. (1999). *Epidemiology in nursing and health care* (3rd ed.). Norwalk, CT: Appleton & Lange.

ANSWERS TO CALCULATIONS FOR BOX 6-4

1. $215/500,000 \times 100,000 = 43$ cases per 100,000
2. $2280/500,000 \times 100,000 = 456$ cases per 100,000
3. $105/500,000 \times 100,000 = 21$ deaths per 100,000
4. $342/120,00 \times 1000 = 2.85$ births per 1000
5. $515/120,000 \times 1000 = 4.29$ deaths per 1000
6. $425/24,000 \times 1000 = 17.71$ deaths over age 65 per 1000

Environmental Health Issues

objectives

Upon completion of this chapter, the reader will be able to:

1. Discuss potential environmental health threats related to housing and living patterns.

2. Discuss potential environmental health threats related to air pollution.

3. Discuss potential environmental health threats related to water pollution.

4. Discuss potential environmental health threats related to food quality.

5. Discuss potential environmental health threats related to radiation.

6. Discuss environmental problems related to solid waste.

7. Describe primary, secondary, and tertiary prevention strategies for individuals, families, and communities for each of the areas presented above.

key terms

Atmospheric quality	Indoor biological	Ozone depletion
Carbon monoxide (CO)	contaminants	Radon
Chlorofluorocarbons	Intentional food additives	Secondhand smoke
(CFCs)	Lead poisoning	Ultraviolet radiation
Foodborne pathogens	Occupational health risks	Unintentional food additives
Hazardous waste	Ozone	

See Glossary for definitions.

case study

Susan Baldwin is a registered nurse working in a pediatric, primary care clinic in an inner city. On Tuesday of this week, Susan assisted the pediatric nurse practitioner with a routine well-child examination on Billy Benson, a 2-year-old boy who lives with his mother and three siblings in an area housing project. The health care professionals at the clinic follow the American Academy of Pediatrics recommendations for preventative care. In addition to overall physical assessment, the health professionals in the clinic perform various screenings, such as height and weight and vision and hearing testing, on the children, based on these recommendations.

One of the screening examinations recommended by the American Academy of Pediatrics is to test the level of lead in each child's blood. These recommendations have been established because an estimated 10% of inner-city children have serum lead levels above those recommended and lead has been cited as the most common cause of mental impairment and mental retardation in children.

Susan understands the importance of lead screening and explained the problem of lead exposure and the rationale for testing to Billy's mother. She provided Mrs. Benson with pamphlets kept at the clinic explaining the basics of lead poisoning and prevention measures. While discussing the written materials with Mrs. Benson, Susan reviewed some of the main sources of lead contamination. These include paint in homes built before 1960, lead smelters, battery recycling plants, and hobbies that expose individuals to lead (e.g., ceramics, furniture refinishing, and stained glass work). Susan questioned Mrs. Benson and discovered that their residence was built in the late 1970s, which is not a problem, but learned that Billy regularly visits his grandmother, whose home was built in the 1940s. Mrs. Benson stated that she does not participate in any of the mentioned hobbies and knows of no area lead smelters or battery recycling plants.

Following guidelines set by the state health department, Susan drew a small tube of blood from a prick in Billy's finger, carefully labeled it, and completed the required forms. The specimen and accompanying paperwork were sent to the state laboratory for analysis. Susan explained to Mrs. Benson that the state health department has outlined a course of action for children with elevated lead levels based on Centers for Disease Control and Prevention (CDC) recommendations and, if Billy's serum lead levels are elevated, further testing may be necessary.

Environmental factors play an important role in the processes of human development, health, and disease. Historically, public health efforts have addressed measures to improve or ensure adequate and safe supplies of food and water, manage waste disposal and sewage, and control or eliminate vectorborne illnesses (U.S. Department of Health and Human Services [USDHHS], 2000). Nationally, these efforts have been phenomenally successful and are largely responsible for the increase in life expectancy witnessed during the twentieth century (McKeown, 1995).

According to the environmental health report in *Healthy People 2010*, "human exposures to hazardous agents in the air, water, soil, and food and to physical hazards in the environment are major contributors to illness, disability and death worldwide...[and] poor environmental quality is estimated to be directly responsible for approximately 25% of all preventable ill health in the world" (USDHHS, 2000, p. 8.5). Population growth, urbanization, technology, industrialization, and modern agricultural

methods have demonstrated unprecedented progress in many areas, but have concurrently created a number of hazards to human health. Risks from synthetic chemicals, naturally occurring radiation, and biological contamination of food and water supplies remain potential threats to the health of U.S. citizens. In response to these potential threats to health, one priority area of *Healthy People 2010* is environmental health; consequently, a series of related objectives have been published. The *Healthy People 2010* box presents selected goals related to issues of environmental health.

Environmental threats to the health of individuals may come from various sources. Stevens and Hall (2001) categorize environmental health issues and concerns into nine areas, which are listed and defined in Table 7-1. Assessment and intervention strategies, along with general information for health education for each of these areas, with the exception of violence risks, are discussed briefly. Violence risks and related nursing interventions are discussed in Chapters 9 and 11.

healthy people 2010

Selected Objectives for Environmental Health, Food Safety, and Occupational Health and Safety

OBJECTIVE	BASELINE (1997)	TARGET
8.1a: Reduce the proportion of persons exposed to air that does not meet the EPA's health-based standards for harmful air pollutants (ozone).	43%	0%
8.6: Reduce waterborne disease outbreaks arising from water intended for drinking among persons served by community water systems.	6 outbreaks per year	2 outbreaks per year
8.11: Eliminate elevated blood lead levels in children.	4.4% of children aged 1-5	0%
8.15: Increase recycling of municipal solid waste.	27%	38%
8.18: Increase the proportion of persons who live in homes tested for radon concentrations.	17%	20%
10.2b: Reduce outbreaks of infections caused by key foodborne bacteria (Salmonella).	44 outbreaks per year	22 outbreaks per year
10.5: Increase the proportion of consumers who follow key food safety practices.	72%	79%
15.7: Reduce nonfatal poisonings.	348.4 per 100,000	292 per 100,000
16.15: Reduce the occurrence of spina bifida and other neural tube defects.	6 per 10,000 live births	3 per 10,000 live births
20.1c: Reduce deaths from work-related injuries (construction).	14.6 per 100,000 workers	10.2 per 100,000 workers
20.10: Reduce occupational needle stick injuries among health care workers.	600,000	420,000

Data from U.S. Department of Health and Human Services. (2000). *Healthy people 2010: Conference edition.* Washington, DC: Government Printing Office.

TABLE **7-1** Areas of Environmental Health

AREA	DEFINITION
Living patterns	The relationships among persons, communities, and their surrounding environments that depend on habits, interpersonal ties, cultural values, and customs
Work risks	The quality of the employment environment and the potential for injury or illness posed by working conditions
Atmospheric quality	The protectiveness of the atmospheric layers, the risks of severe weather, and the purity of the air available for breathing purposes
Water quality	The availability and volume of the water supply and the mineral content levels, pollution by toxic chemicals, and the presence of pathogenic microorganisms; consists of the balance between water contaminants and existing capabilities to purify water for human use and plant and wildlife sustenance
Housing	As an environmental health concern, refers to the availability, safety, structural, strength, cleanliness, and location of shelter, including public facilities and individual or family dwellings
Food quality	The availability and relative costs of foods, their variety and safety, and the health of animal and plant food sources
Waste control	The management of waste materials resulting from industrial and municipal processes and human consumption and efforts to minimize waste production
Radiation risks	Health dangers posed by the various forms of ionizing radiation relative to barriers preventing exposure of humans and other life forms
Violence risks	The potential for victimization through the violence of particular individuals and the general level of aggression in psychosocial climates

From Stevens, P. E., & Hall, J. M. (2001). Environmental health. In M. Nies & M. McEwen (Eds.), *Community health nursing: Promoting the health of populations* (3rd ed.). Philadelphia: W. B. Saunders.

HOUSING AND LIVING PATTERNS

Numerous actual and potential threats to health related to housing and living patterns exist. Some common concerns include overcrowding, household chemical exposure, potential for poisoning, presence of firearms,

and violence. Table 7-2 describes sources of home pollution. Several related issues (e.g., radon gas, exposure to various chemicals) are listed elsewhere in this chapter. This section discusses potential problems in housing and living conditions related to indoor air quality and lead exposure.

TABLE **7-2** Sources of Home Pollution

POLLUTANT	DESCRIPTION AND SUGGESTIONS	SOURCE AND EXAMPLES OF SUBSTANCE IN HOME
Radon	Colorless, odorless, radioactive gas from the natural breakdown (radioactive decay) of uranium; it is estimated that radon causes up to 20,000 lung cancer deaths per year	Soil or rock under the home; well water; building materials
Asbestos	Mineral fiber used extensively in building materials for insulation and as a fire retardant; asbestos should be removed by a professional if it has deteriorated; exposure to asbestos fibers can cause irreversible and often fatal lung diseases, including cancer	Sprayed-on acoustical ceilings or textured paint; pipe and furnace insulation materials; floor tiles; automobile brakes and clutches
Biological contaminants	Include bacteria, mold and mildew, viruses, animal dander and saliva, dust mites, and pollen; these contaminants can provide infectious diseases or allergic reactions; moisture and dust levels in the home should be kept as low as possible	Mold and mildew; standing water or water-damaged materials; humidifiers; house plants; household pets; ventilation systems; household dust
Indoor combustion	Produces harmful gases (i.e., CO, nitrogen dioxide), particles, and organic compounds (e.g., benzene); health effects range from irritation to the eyes, nose, and throat, to lung cancer; ventilation of gas appliances to the outdoors will minimize risks	Tobacco smoke; unvented kerosene or gas space heaters; unvented kitchen gas stoves; wood stoves or fireplaces; leaking exhaust flues from gas furnaces and clothes dryers; car exhaust from an attached garage
Household products	Can contain potentially harmful organic compounds; health effects vary greatly; the elimination of household chemicals through the use of nontoxic alternatives or by using only in well-ventilated rooms or outside minimizes risks	Cleaning products; paint supplies; stored fuels; hobby products; personal care products; mothballs; air fresheners; dry-cleaned clothes
Formaldehyde	Widely used chemical that is released to the air as a colorless gas; it can cause eye, nose, throat, and respiratory system irritation; headaches, nausea, and fatigue; may be a central nervous system depressant and has been shown to cause cancer in laboratory animals; remove sources of formaldehyde from the home if health effects occur	Particleboard, plywood, and fiberboard in cabinets, furniture, subflooring, and paneling; carpeting, durable-press drapes, other textiles; urea-formaldehyde insulation; glues and adhesives

From Primomo, J., & Salazar, M. K. (2000). Environmental illness: At home, at work and in the community. In C. M. Smith & F. A. Maurer (Eds.), *Community health nursing: Theory and practice* (2nd ed.). Philadelphia: W. B. Saunders.

continued

TABLE **7-2** Sources of Home Pollution—cont'd

POLLUTANT	DESCRIPTION AND SUGGESTIONS	SOURCE AND EXAMPLES OF SUBSTANCE IN HOME
Pesticides	Including insecticides, termiticides, rodenticides, and fungicides—all contain organic compounds; exposure to high levels of pesticides may cause damage to the liver and the central nervous system and increase cancer risks; when possible, nonchemical methods of pest control should be used; if the use of pesticides is unavoidable, they should be used strictly according to the manufacturer's directions	Contaminated soil or dust that is tracked in from outside; stored pesticide containers
Lead	A long-recognized harmful environmental pollutant; fetuses, infants, and children are more vulnerable to toxic effects; if the community health nurse suspects that a home has lead paint, it should be tested	Lead-based paint that is peeling, sanded, or burned; automobile exhaust; lead in drinking water; food contaminated by lead from lead-based ceramic cookware or pottery; lead-related hobbies or occupations

INDOOR AIR QUALITY

Indoor air quality in the home may significantly affect health. Concerns center on combustion pollutants (e.g., carbon monoxide [CO], secondhand smoke) particles (e.g., asbestos, animal dander, pollen), and living organisms (e.g., dust mites, molds, bacteria). Several of these concerns—secondhand smoke, carbon monoxide poisoning, and biological contamination—are addressed in detail.

Secondhand smoke refers to the combination of smoke given off by the burning of a cigarette, pipe, or cigar and the smoke exhaled from the lungs of smokers. Secondhand smoke has been classified by the Environmental Protection Agency (EPA) as a known carcinogen and is estimated to cause approximately 3000 lung cancer deaths in nonsmokers each year (EPA, 1993a). Health threats to infants and children caused by secondhand smoke include increased risk of respiratory tract infection (e.g., pneumonia and bronchitis), decreased lung function, and symptoms of chronic respiratory irritation, middle ear infections, and development and exacerbation of

asthma. In adults, secondhand smoke causes eye, nose, and throat irritation and lung irritation and may affect the cardiovascular system. The Health Teaching box "Reducing the Health Risks of Secondhand Smoking" presents the EPA's recommendations to reduce the health risks of passive smoking.

Pollution from indoor combustion comes from appliances such as space heaters, gas ranges and ovens, furnaces, gas water heaters, and wood- or coal-burning stoves and fireplaces. Potential problems from indoor combustion typically relate to ineffective or improper venting of the appliances, cracked heat exchangers, burning green or treated wood, or using the wrong fuel.

Carbon monoxide (CO) exposure is particularly important because more than 200 deaths each year are caused by accidental CO poisoning (EPA, 1996). Symptoms of CO poisoning include severe headaches, dizziness, confusion, and nausea. If CO poisoning is suspected, the EPA suggests getting all affected into fresh air immediately. Doors and windows should be opened, all combustion appliances should be turned off, and

Reducing the Health Risks of Secondhand Smoking

- Do not smoke in the home and do not permit others to do so.
- If a family member insists on smoking indoors, increase ventilation in the area.
- Do not smoke if children, particularly infants and toddlers, are present.
- Do not smoke in an automobile with the windows closed if passengers are present.
- Find out about the smoking policies of day care centers, schools, and other caregivers of children and take measures to ensure that children are not exposed.
- Teach others about the risks associated with secondhand smoke.

- Encourage and support policies that enact and maintain smoke-free workplaces.
- Prohibit smoking indoors or limit smoking to rooms that have been specially designed to prevent smoke from escaping to other areas of the work site.
- Encourage employer-supported smoking cessation programs.
- Locate designated outdoor smoking areas away from building entrances or building ventilation system air intakes.
- Know the local and state laws regarding smoking in public buildings.
- Support stringent smoking control ordinances in the community.

From the Environmental Protection Agency. (EPA). (1993a). *Secondhand smoke.* (EPA Publication No. 402-F-93-004). Washington, DC: Government Printing Office.

everyone should *leave the house.* A trip to the emergency room may be needed and the physician should be told that CO poisoning is a possibility.

To reduce exposure to combustion pollutants, it is essential that combustion appliances undergo proper selection, installation, inspection, and maintenance. Suggestions to reduce or eliminate exposure to CO and other combustion gases are discussed in the Health Teaching box "Reducing Exposure to Carbon Monoxide and Other Indoor Combustion Pollutants."

Indoor biological contaminants that may be detrimental to health include bacteria, molds, mildew, viruses, animal dander, dust mites, cockroaches, and pollen. Contaminated central air and heating units can become breeding grounds for mold, mildew, and other sources of biological contaminants and can then distribute the contaminants throughout the home. Biological contaminates can trigger allergic reactions including asthma and spread infections and illnesses (i.e. colds, influenza, and chicken pox). Symptoms of health problems caused by biological pollutants include sneezing, watery eyes, coughing, shortness of breath, dizziness, lethargy, fever, and

digestive problems. Children, elderly people, and people with respiratory problems and allergies are particularly susceptible to biological agents in the indoor air.

To reduce exposure to biological contaminants, a number of activities are recommended by the EPA (2000). These are listed in the Health Teaching box "Reducing Exposure to Biological Contaminants."

LEAD EXPOSURE

According to *Healthy People 2010* (USDHHS, 2000), there has been significant success over the past decade in reducing childhood **lead poisoning** in the United States because of measures to decrease lead in gasoline, air, food, and industrial sources. Indeed the fairly dramatic reduction is attributed to identification of those at risk, wide-spread screenings, and effective community efforts to clean up problem areas. More still remains to be done, however, and the risk is disproportionately high in persons having low income and persons from racial and ethnic minorities. Therefore reduction of blood lead levels remains a national priority.

Despite these successes, it is estimated that nearly 1 million children younger than 6 years, particularly minority and poor children from inner cities, have blood lead levels high enough to adversely affect their intelligence, behavior, and development (CDC, 2000a). As a result, the CDC has implemented a multilevel program to screen young children for elevated lead levels; identify possible sources of exposure; monitor the medical management of children with elevated blood

---

health teaching

Reducing Exposure to Carbon Monoxide and Other Indoor Combustion Pollutants

- Choose vented appliances when possible.
- Buy combustion appliances that have been tested and certified to meet safety standards.
- Consider buying gas appliances that have electronic ignitions rather than pilot lights.
- Buy appliances that are the correct size for the area to be heated.
- Have appliances professionally installed.
- If using an unvented gas space heater or kerosene heater, crack open a window and keep doors open to the rest of the house.
- Use a hood fan if using a gas range.
- Make sure vented appliances have the vent connected and nothing is blocking it.
- Do not vent gas clothes dryers or water heaters into the house for heating.

- Read and follow instructions for all appliances.
- Always use the correct fuel for the appliance.
- Never use a range, oven, or dryer to heat the home.
- Never use an unvented combustion heater overnight or in a bedroom while sleeping.
- Never ignore a safety device when it shuts off an appliance.
- Never ignore the smell of fuel.
- Have combustion appliances regularly inspected and maintained.
- Have chimneys and vents inspected when installing or changing vented heating appliances.
- Consider purchasing a CO detector (available at hardware stores).

From U.S. Consumer Product Safety Commission/Environmental Protection Agency and American Lung Association. (1999). *What you should know about combustion appliances and indoor air pollution.* United States: U.S. Consumer Product Safety Commission/Environmental Protection Agency and American Lung Association, Washington, DC. Retrieved 7/13/01 from www.epa.gov.iaq/pubs/combust.html.

---

health teaching

Reducing Exposure to Biological Contaminants

- Maintain a relative humidity of 30% to 50% in the home.
- Remove standing water, water-damaged materials, or wet surfaces.
- Install vented exhaust fans in kitchens and bathrooms.
- Vent clothes dryers outdoors.
- Vent the attic and crawl spaces to prevent moisture build up.
- Keep the house clean (dust mites, pollens, animal dander, and other allergy-causing

agents can be reduced through regular cleaning).
- Use allergen-proof mattresses for those susceptible to allergies.
- Wash bedding in hot water.
- Avoid room furnishings that accumulate dust.
- Use vacuums with high-efficiency filters.
- Clean and disinfect basements regularly.
- Operate a dehumidifier in the basement if needed.

From Environmental Protection Agency. (EPA). (2000). *Biological pollutants in your home.* Retrieved 7/13/01 from http://www.epa.gov/iaq/pubs/bio_1.html.

lead levels; provide health professionals, policy makers, and the public with educational information on preventing lead poisoning; and support community programs to eliminate childhood lead poisoning. (See the Community Application box "Preventing Childhood Environmental Lead Exposure.")

Lead-based paint in homes and buildings built before 1960 has been identified as the major source of lead poisoning. Chipping or peeling

---

COMMUNITY APPLICATION
Preventing Childhood Environmental Lead Exposure

Primary Prevention
Individual/Family Interventions

- Encourage parents to keep children away from peeling or chipping paint.
- Encourage families to remove lead-based paint from older homes.
- Wet mop and wet wipe hard surfaces with a high-phosphate solution.
- Do not vacuum hard surfaces because this might scatter dust.
- Wash children's hands and faces before they eat.
- Wash toys and pacifiers frequently.
- If soil around the home is likely to be lead contaminated (if the house was built before 1960 or is near a major highway), plant bushes next to the house and plant grass or other groundcover to reduce dust
- During remodeling of older homes, be certain children and pregnant women are not in the home until the process is completed; thoroughly clean the house before inhabitants return.
- Do not use pottery or ceramic ware that was inadequately fired or is meant for decorative use for food storage or service.
- Do not store drinks or food in lead crystal.
- Make sure children eat regular meals; lead is more readily absorbed on an empty stomach.

Community Interventions

- Provide education programs and opportunities to learn about lead poisoning and prevention.
- Encourage communities to remove lead-based paint from older homes, particularly in low-income housing.
- Support policymakers who encourage funding for programs to reduce lead exposure.

Secondary Prevention
Individual/Family Interventions

- Recommend screening of high-risk children at age 6 months and at least every year.

- Recommend screening of all children at 12 months and yearly thereafter.
- Identify the source of lead exposure for children with serum lead levels above 10 µg/dl.
- Refer for treatment if needed: If blood lead levels are greater than 20 µg/dl, the child should receive environmental evaluation and remediation and a medical evaluation; drug therapy may also be indicated. If blood lead levels are greater than 45 µg/dl, medical and environmental intervention and chelation therapy are necessary.
- Refer families with identified lead poisoning to local or state-sponsored programs if assistance is needed to remove the source of exposure.

Community Interventions

- Encourage community-sponsored testing for lead-based paint for all homes built before 1950.
- Promote accessibility of screening services.
- Monitor incidence of heavy metal poisoning.
- Educate the public on signs and symptoms of lead poisoning.
- Support government-sponsored financing of lead paint abatement when individual homeowners cannot afford it.

Tertiary Prevention
Individual/Family Interventions

- Monitor progress and effects of treatment.
- Provide assistance in dealing with long-term effects of lead poisoning (i.e., referral for special education programs).
- Advocate lead abatement programs in older residential areas.
- Educate the public on the hazards of lead.
- Promote access to social services needed to manage the effects of lead poisoning.

Data from Centers for Disease Control. (1991). *Preventing lead poisoning in young children.* Atlanta: Centers for Disease Control; Clemen-Stone, S., Eigsti, D. G., & McGuire, S. L. (1995). *Comprehensive community health nursing* (4th ed.). St. Louis: Mosby; U.S. Department of Health and Human Services. (2000). *Healthy people 2010. National health promotion and disease prevention objectives.* Washington, DC: Government Printing Office.

lead-based paint is of concern because it can easily be ingested by children or inhaled through lead-contaminated dust. Anemia, central nervous system disorders, and renal involvement may result from lead exposure. Of particular concern is chronic central nervous system dysfunction, including irreversible deficits in intelligence, behavior, and school performance. The CDC (1997) identifies those at greatest risk for lead poisoning as being children who:

- Live in a house or regularly visit a day care center, preschool, babysitter's home, or other house built before 1960
- Live in or regularly visit a house built before 1960 with recent, ongoing, or planned renovation
- Have a brother, sister, or playmate being treated for lead poisoning
- Live with an adult whose job, hobby, or use of ethnic remedies involves lead
- Live near an active lead smelter, battery recycling plant, or other industry likely to release lead

Maximum permissible blood levels of lead have been revised downward from 30 µg/dl in 1975. Currently, levels greater than 10 µg/dl are denoted as "action" or "intervention levels" (CDC, 1997). Federal, state, and local efforts to decrease lead exposure should be supported by all health professionals.

WORK RISKS

An estimated 5.7 million job-related injuries and illnesses occur each year, with about 2.7 million being severe enough to result in time lost from work (U.S. Department of Labor, 2000). Workers face a variety of job hazards. Use of heavy equipment; exposure to chemicals, biohazards, sunlight, heat, cold, and noise; and potential for assault or violence pose risks to workers. Heavy lifting, working at elevations, and performing repetitive tasks, for example, can lead to serious injuries, such as sprains, fractures, and carpal tunnel syndrome. According to the Department of Labor (1995), sprains and strains are by far the

leading injury and illness category in every major industry, with back sprains being the most common injury. Interestingly, nurses' aides and orderlies had the highest rates of back sprains and lost days from work attributed to overexertion. Other occupations with relatively higher rates of injury include mining, logging, agriculture, construction, manufacturing, trucking, and warehousing.

The extent of illness and injuries directly attributable to occupational risk can be difficult to define because many illnesses may result from prolonged exposure to a noxious substance over decades or a combination of factors. Occupational lung disease, occupational cancers, and noise-induced hearing loss, for example, may take many years to develop. Psychological disorders and cardiovascular changes associated with job stress may be suspected, but are difficult to verify.

To improve occupational health and safety, a combination of federal and state regulations have been implemented during the twentieth century. Probably the most far-reaching piece of legislation was the Occupational Health and Safety Act (1970). The Occupational Health and Safety Act was responsible for the development of the Occupational Safety and Health Administration (OSHA) and National Institute for Occupational Safety and Health (NIOSH). These agencies have been instrumental in setting and enforcing standards to improve worker safety and health and in providing research to address various health issues. Over the last three decades, "OSHA has issued hundreds of occupational health and safety standards covering a wide range of hazards, such as toxic chemicals, hazardous equipment, and working conditions. These standards require employers to use appropriate practices, means, methods, operations or processes to protect employees from hazards on the job" (Rogers, 1994, p. 437).

Prevention of **occupational health risk** hazards includes engineering controls, improving work practices, using personal protective equipment, implementing health-promotion strategies (e.g., programs for smoking cessation or stress reduc-

COMMUNITY APPLICATION
Preventing Work-Related Illness and Injury

Primary Prevention—Health Promotion

Health education—individual and group programs on a variety of topics
Promoting healthful nutrition
Encouraging exercise and fitness
Assisting with stress reduction and coping mechanisms
Providing prenatal monitoring for pregnant workers
Teaching parenting skills

Primary Prevention—Illness Prevention

Health risk appraisal
Assisting with modification of identified risk factors
Promoting smoking cessation
Encouraging weight control
Providing appropriate immunization (e.g., hepatitis B for health workers)

Primary Prevention—Injury Prevention

Accident investigation
Promoting use of safety devices
Removal of safety hazards
Teaching good body mechanics
Safety education
Providing instruction on and monitoring safe handling of hazardous substances

Secondary Prevention—Screening

Preplacement and termination of physical examinations

Environmental and ergonomic screening
Periodic screening for workers at risk

Secondary Prevention—Management of Episodic Conditions

Assisting client in seeking professional health care when needed
Serving as an advocate to correct a health problem
Monitoring recovery from minor illness or injury
Acting as a resource for information on illness, prevention, and treatment

Secondary Prevention—Emergency Response

First aid for minor injuries
Establishing and maintaining a triage system for injuries
Injury diagnosis and treatment
Mobilizing the emergency medical system when appropriate

Tertiary Prevention

Monitoring chronic illness
Preventing or minimizing complications of chronic conditions
Serving as case manager for clients with chronic conditions
Assisting the worker in seeking reimbursement of health costs from health insurers
Providing on-site therapy where possible

---

tion), and monitoring the workplace for emerging hazards. Nurses in community-based practice should be aware of occupational risks and measures that may be taken to prevent or minimize these risks (see the Community Application box "Preventing Work-Related Illness and Injury"). Violence can also be a concern in the workplace, as indicated by the Research Highlight.

ATMOSPHERIC QUALITY

Air pollution threatens the health of humans and animals. It can harm crops and other vegetation; contributes to the erosion, decay, and economic devaluation of buildings and structures; may possibly diminish the protective ozone layer; and contributes to major climatic changes through the greenhouse effect (EPA, 1992). Exposure to air pollutants is associated with increases in morbidity and mortality. Air pollution can cause serious problems to humans including lung damage, inflammatory responses, impairment of defenses, and acute changes in lung function. Major air pollutants affecting **atmospheric quality** are listed in Table 7-3.

In the United States, efforts to detect, monitor, reduce, eliminate, and control air pollution have been in effect since the Clean Air Act was passed

Research Highlight

Violence in the Workplace

Violence in the workplace has received considerable attention in the popular press. Unfortunately, sensational acts of coworker violence are often emphasized by the media to the exclusion of the more common threats involving murder of taxicab drivers, convenience store clerks and other retail workers, security guards, and police officers. These deaths often go virtually unnoticed, yet their numbers are staggering: 1071 workplace homicides occurred in 1994. These included 179 proprietors in retail sales, 105 cashiers, 86 taxicab drivers, 49 managers in restaurants or hotels, 70 police officers or detectives, and 76 security guards. An additional 1 million workers are assaulted each year. These figures indicate that an average of 20 workers are murdered and 18,000 are assaulted each week while at work or on duty.

From U.S. Department of Health and Human Services/Centers for Disease Control/National Institute for Occupational Health and Safety (1996). *Violence in the Workplace.* Retrieved 7/17/01 from http://www/cdc/gov/niosh/violintr.html.

TABLE **7-3** Major Air Pollutants

POLLUTANT	SOURCES	EFFECTS
OZONE A colorless gas that is the major constituent of photochemical smog at the Earth's surface. In the upper atmosphere (stratosphere), however, ozone is beneficial, protecting us from the sun's harmful rays.	Ozone is formed in the lower atmosphere as a result of chemical reactions between oxygen, volatile organic compounds, and nitrogen oxides in the presence of sunlight, especially during hot weather. Sources of such harmful pollutants include vehicles, factories, landfills, industrial solvents, and numerous small sources such as gas stations and farm and lawn equipment.	Ozone causes significant health and environmental problems at the earth's surface, where we live. It can irritate the respiratory tract, produce impaired lung function such as inability to take a deep breath, and cause throat irritation, chest pain, cough, lung inflammation, and possible susceptibility to lung infection. Smog components may aggravate existing respiratory conditions like asthma. Ozone can also reduce yield of agricultural crops and injure forests and other vegetation. Ozone is the most injurious pollutant to plant life.
CARBON MONOXIDE Odorless and colorless gas emitted in the exhaust of motor vehicles and other kinds of engines where incomplete fossil fuel combustion occurs.	Automobiles, buses, trucks, small engines, and some industrial processes. High concentrations can be found in confined spaces like parking garages, poorly ventilated tunnels, or along roadsides during periods of heavy traffic.	Reduces the ability of blood to deliver oxygen to vital tissues, affecting primarily the cardiovascular and nervous systems. Lower concentrations have been shown to adversely affect individuals with heart disease (e.g., angina) and to decrease maximal exercise performance in young, healthy men. Higher concentrations can cause symptoms such as dizziness, headaches, and fatigue.

From Environmental Protection Agency. (EPA). (1992). *What you can do to reduce air pollution.* (EPA Publication No. 450-K-92-002). Washington, DC: Government Printing Office.

TABLE **7-3** Major Air Pollutants—cont'd

POLLUTANT	SOURCES	EFFECTS
NITROGEN DIOXIDE		
Light brown gas at lower concentrations; in higher concentrations, it becomes an important component of unpleasant-looking brown urban haze.	Result of burning fuels in utilities, industrial boilers, cars, and trucks.	One of the major pollutants that causes smog and acid rain. Can harm humans and vegetation when concentrations are sufficiently high. In children, may cause increased respiratory illness such as chest colds and coughing with phlegm. For asthmatics, can cause increased breathing difficulty.
PARTICULATE MATTER		
Solid matter or liquid droplets from smoke, dust, fly ash, and condensing vapors that can be suspended in the air for long periods.	Industrial processes, smelters, automobiles, burning industrial fuels, wood smoke, dust from paved and unpaved roads, construction, and agricultural ground breaking.	These microscopic particles can affect breathing and respiratory symptoms, causing increased respiratory disease and lung damage and possibly premature death. Children, the elderly, and people suffering from heart or lung disease (like asthma) are especially at risk. Also damages paint, soils clothing, and reduces visibility.
SULFUR DIOXIDE		
Colorless gas, odorless at low concentrations, but pungent at very high concentrations.	Emitted largely from industrial, institutional, utility, and apartment-house furnaces and boilers, and petroleum refineries, smelters, paper mills, and chemical plants.	One of the major pollutants that causes smog. Can also, at high concentrations, affect human health, especially among asthmatics (who are particularly sensitive to respiratory tract problems and breathing difficulties that sulfur dioxide can induce). Can also harm vegetation and metals. The pollutants it produces can impair visibility and acidify lakes and streams.
LEAD		
Lead and lead compounds can adversely affect human health through either ingestion of lead-contaminated substances, such as soil, dust, paint, or direct inhalation. This is particularly a risk for young children, whose normal hand-to-mouth activities can result in greater ingestion of lead-contaminated soils and dusts.	Transportation sources using lead in their fuels, coal combustion, smelters, car battery plants, and combustion of garbage containing lead products.	Elevated lead levels can adversely affect mental development and performance, kidney function, and blood chemistry. Young children are particularly at risk because of their greater chance of ingesting lead and the increased sensitivity of young tissues and organs to lead.

continued

TABLE **7-3** Major Air Pollutants—cont'd

POLLUTANT	SOURCES	EFFECTS
TOXIC AIR POLLUTANTS		
Includes pollutants such as arsenic, asbestos, and benzene.	Chemical plants, industrial processes, motor vehicle emissions and fuels, and building materials.	Known or suspected to cause cancer, respiratory effects, birth defects, and reproductive and other serious health effects. Some can cause death or serious injury if accidentally released in large amounts.
STRATOSPHERIC OZONE DEPLETERS		
Chemicals such as chlorofluorocarbons (CFCs), halons, carbon tetrachloride, and methyl chloroform that are used in refrigerants and other industrial processes. These chemicals last a long time in the air, rising to the upper atmosphere where they destroy the protective ozone layer that screens out harmful ultraviolet radiation before it reaches the earth's surface.	Industrial household refrigeration, cooling and cleaning processes, car and home air conditioners, some fire extinguishers, and plastic foam products.	Increased exposure to ultraviolet radiation could potentially cause an increase in skin cancer, increased cataract cases, suppression of the human immune response system, and environmental damage.
GREENHOUSE GASES		
Gases that build up in the atmosphere that may induce global climate change, or the greenhouse effect. They include carbon dioxide, methane, and nitrous oxide.	The main human-made source of carbon dioxide emissions is fossil fuel combustion for energy use and transportation. Methane comes from landfills, cud-chewing livestock, coal mines, and rice paddies. Nitrous oxide results from industrial processes, such as nylon fabrication.	The extent of the effect of climate change on human health and the environment is still uncertain, but could include increased global temperature, increased severity and frequency of storms and other weather extremes, melting of the polar ice cap, and sea-level rise.

in 1963. This legislation set standards for "ambient air quality" (which applies to the air quality in a city or town) and industrial emissions standards. The Clean Air Act was amended most recently in November of 1990. Goals of the 1990 amendments (EPA, 1992) are the following:

- Cut acid rain in half through implementation of systems to reduce sulfur dioxide emissions from power plants.

- Reduce smog and other pollutants through upgrading inspection and maintenance programs for motor vehicles, adoption of clean fuel programs, and limiting use of wood stoves and fireplaces.
- Reduce air toxins (emissions from chemical plants, steel mills, and other businesses) through employment of stringent regulations to reduce industrial emissions.

- Protect the ozone layer through the reduction or elimination of **chlorofluorocarbons (CFCs)** in automobile air conditioners and residential, commercial, and industrial cooling and refrigeration systems.

OZONE DEPLETION

Ozone occurs in two layers in the atmosphere. In the stratosphere, ozone acts to shield the earth from harmful effects of ultraviolet radiation given off by the sun. But, at ground level, high concentrations of ozone are a major health concern because ozone is one of the primary problem gases in air pollution (EPA, 1997a).

The EPA (1997a) explained that there is evidence the Earth's stratospheric ozone layer is being destroyed by CFCs and other ozone-depleting gases found in refrigerants, aerosols, and some solvent cleaning agents. Theoretically, radiation from the sun elicits a chemical reaction between the CFCs and ozone resulting in thinning of the ozone layer. In the early 1980s, a significant depletion of ozone about the size of North America was first observed in the southern hemisphere. At that time, it was estimated that between 50% and 90% depletion in the ozone layer had occurred, creating a hole over Antarctica. A similar thinning of the ozone layer has also been detected over the North Pole.

To reduce the threat posed by the **ozone depletion**, part of the Clean Air Act Amendment of 1990 initiated the phase-out of CFCs (EPA, 1997a). The major concern from a drop in stratospheric ozone levels is the increase in ultraviolet-B light. Increased incidence of skin cancer and cataracts and alterations in the immune system are linked to ozone depletion. Skin cancer is of particular concern. An increase in melanoma and in basal and squamous cell carcinoma is expected. In addition to the harmful effects on humans, there is concern over the effects of increased ultraviolet-B light on animals, plants, and marine ecosystems (EPA, 1994a).

Ground-level ozone is also a serious problem. Ground-level ozone is formed when nitrogen oxides and other volatile organic compounds are emitted from motor vehicles, power plants, and other sources of combustion, in the presence of heat and sunlight. This exchange most readily occurs during hot weather (EPA, 1997b).

When inhaled, ozone can cause acute respiratory problems, aggravate asthma, and cause inflammation of lung tissue. It also impairs the body's immune system, making people more susceptible to respiratory illnesses. Those most at risk from exposure to ozone include children and asthmatics. Excessive ground-level ozone can also be harmful to the environment by making plants susceptible to disease, pests, and environmental stresses (EPA, 1997b).

To combat air pollution, the EPA (1992) has made several suggestions, included in Box 7-1.

WATER QUALITY

The availability of clean, safe water is vitally important in maintaining a healthy environment. According to the USDHHS (2000), only 73% of the community water systems meet safe drinking water standards established by the EPA. Sewage (containing human waste, detergents), industrial processes and wastes (producing heavy metals, detergents, salts, heat, petrochemicals), and agricultural chemicals (e.g., fertilizer, pesticides) are the main sources of water pollution. To ensure and promote water quality, federal legislation was passed in 1948 and has been amended several times (1972, 1974, 1977, 1986, 1987). The Clean Water Act(s) serves to safeguard the quality of the nation's water supply through setting water standards and maximum allowable water contaminant levels.

MICROBIAL CONTAMINATION

Although surface and groundwater treatment through disinfection and filtration has dramatically reduced the incidence of waterborne diseases in the United States during the twentieth century, each year thousands of Americans become ill through drinking contaminated water (CDC, 2000b). For example, a widely publicized outbreak of cryptosporidiosis in Milwaukee

BOX 7-1 What Individuals and Communities Can Do to Reduce Air Pollution

DRIVING TIPS

- Plan ahead: Organize trips to drive fewer miles, combine errands into one trip, avoid driving during peak traffic, and walk or bicycle for short errands.
- Ride share: Participate in carpools or use public transportation.
- Use energy-conserving motor oil and "clean" fuels when possible.
- Drive at minimum and steady speed; do not idle the engine unnecessarily.
- Follow recommendations from the vehicle owner's manual regarding the correct grade of gasoline, shifting gears, and other ways to keep the engine running at maximum efficiency.

CAR MAINTENANCE

- Do not remove or tamper with pollution controls.
- Do not overfill or top off the car's gas tank.
- Get regular engine tune ups and car maintenance checks.

- Keep car filters and catalytic converters clean.
- Consider buying fuel-efficient cars.

REDUCING AIR POLLUTION AT HOME AND WORK

- Conserve electricity: Turn off lights and appliances when not in use, raise the temperature level on air conditioners, turn down heaters in the winter, and purchase energy-efficient appliances.
- Participate in local utilities' conservation programs.
- Use wood stoves and fireplaces wisely and sparingly.
- Properly dispose of household paints, solvents, pesticides, and refrigeration and air conditioning equipment.

GET INVOLVED IN EFFORTS TO REDUCE AIR POLLUTION

- Learn about local efforts and issues.
- Work with community action groups to improve air quality.
- Report air pollution problems to the appropriate local or state agency or the EPA.

From Environmental Protection Agency. (EPA). (1992). *What you can do to reduce air pollution.* (EPA publication: 450-K-92-002). Washington, DC: Government Printing Office.

affected an estimated 400,000 individuals and prompted measures to determine and address the public health concerns and direct new research on ways to detect and control this organism in community water supplies (CDC, 1995).

Waterborne diseases are those diseases that result from ingestion of contaminated water, inhalation of water vapors, body contact through bathing or swimming, and accidental ingestion of water during recreational activities (e.g., swimming, water skiing). Because symptoms are usually mild and short lived, it is assumed that only a small fraction of waterborne illnesses are recognized, reported, and investigated. Bacteria, viruses, and protozoa are the microorganisms of primary concern in waterborne disease. Table 7-4 lists the most common waterborne diseases found in the United States.

Water treatment processes include filtration, disinfection, and treatment of organic and inorganic contaminants. Removal of solids and microorganisms (e.g., Giardia and Cryptosporidium species) is accomplished by filtration

systems (e.g., sand, diatomaceous earth, membrane, or cartridge filtration). Disinfection techniques include use of chlorine, ozone, and chloramines. Granular or powdered activated carbon column aeration, diffused aeration, oxidation, reverse osmosis, and aeration are also used to remove organic contaminants from water supplies (EPA, 1991).

CHEMICAL AND METAL CONTAMINANTS

Chemical contaminants of surface and ground water include pesticides (e.g., insecticides, fungicides, herbicides), petrochemicals and other organic compounds (e.g., improperly disposed of motor oil, paint, antifreeze), and a variety of industrial wastes (e.g., suspended solids, radionuclides, asbestos). Metal contaminants include lead, mercury, copper, arsenic, and iron.

Lead contamination is of particular concern because a significant number of public water systems in the United States provide drinking water that contains lead levels exceeding the action level standard established by the EPA.

TABLE **7-4** Waterborne Diseases of Concern in the United States

DISEASE	MICROBIAL AGENT	GENERAL SYMPTOMS
Amebiasis	Protozoan (*Entamoeba histolytica*)	Abdominal discomfort, fatigue, diarrhea, flatulence, weight loss
Campylobacteriosis	Bacterium (*Campylobacter jejuni*)	Fever, abdominal pain, diarrhea
Cholera	Bacterium (*Vibrio cholerae*)	Watery diarrhea, vomiting, occasional muscle cramps
Cryptosporidiosis	Protozoan (*Cryptosporidium parvum*)	Diarrhea, abdominal discomfort
Giardiasis	Protozoan (*Giardia lamblia*)	Diarrhea, abdominal discomfort
Hepatitis	Virus (hepatitis A)	Fever, chills, abdominal discomfort, jaundice, dark urine
Shigellosis	Bacterium (Shigella species)	Fever, diarrhea, bloody stool
Typhoid fever	Bacterium (*Salmonella typhi*)	Fever, headache, constipation, appetite loss, nausea, diarrhea, vomiting, appearance of an abdominal rash
Viral gastroenteritis	Viruses (Norwalk, rotavirus, and other types)	Fever, headache, gastrointestinal discomfort, vomiting, diarrhea

From Environmental Protection Agency. (EPA). (1993b). *Preventing waterborne disease.* (EPA Publication No. 640-K-93-001). Washington, DC: Government Printing Office.

Also, lead is particularly harmful to infants, young children, and developing fetuses. Lead contamination is largely caused by widespread use of lead in pipes, brass faucets or fittings, and lead solder and is of most concern in homes that are very old or very new. Plumbing installed before 1930 is likely to contain lead. In newer plumbing system construction, lead solder and brass faucets and fittings are often used and can leach lead during the first 5 years of use. Thus, "water in buildings less than five years old... may have high levels of lead contamination" (EPA, 1993c, p. 2).

Recommendations from the EPA (EPA, 1993c) to reduce lead in drinking water include the following:
- Flush pipes before drinking. Run cold water through pipes for 5 to 30 seconds, particularly if the water has been in contact with plumbing for more than 6 hours (e.g., overnight or during a workday).
- Use only cold water for consumption. Use only water from the cold water tap for drinking, cooking, and especially for making baby formula because hot water is more likely to contain higher levels of lead.

- Have water tested. Have the amount of lead in household water tested. This is particularly important for apartment dwellers.
- Consider the use of filtering devices. Filters may help in reducing lead levels if properly used (e.g., filters must be changed as specified by the manufacturer).
- Consider bottled water for consumption. Bottled water is regulated by the Food and Drug Administration (FDA) if sold in interstate commerce and is under state regulation if sold within a state.
- Use only lead-free materials in plumbing repairs and installation. Obtain assurance from a qualified plumber—in writing—that only lead-free materials will be used.

COMMUNITY AND NURSING INTERVENTIONS

Research into improving water treatment and detecting, analyzing, and eliminating contamination is ongoing. Efforts to monitor and improve water quality should be supported by all health care providers and by concerned citizens. Improved public and professional appreciation of the risks of contaminated drinking water and increased willingness of the public to pay for improved drinking water quality are essential (USDHHS, 2000). Suggestions for improving water quality and ensuring safe water include the following:

- Be aware of the community's water source and supplier. How is the water supply treated and tested for contamination? Does the supplier adhere to guidelines and standards set by the EPA?
- Learn about potential contamination sources of ground water and surface water.
- Urge the community water supplier and state and local regulatory and health officials to ensure that the water supply complies with all standards.
- Support efforts to educate the public and elected officials about the need to protect and improve the quality of drinking water.
- Express willingness to pay higher water rates, if necessary, to finance improvements in water quality.
- Support local and state efforts to develop programs and strategies to protect surface and ground water and to develop programs to control contaminating sources and activities.
- Support ongoing research and training efforts to improve water quality.

FOOD QUALITY

The FDA and the Department of Agriculture are responsible for setting standards for food safety, inspection of many foods, regulation of restaurants and food sales, approval of food additives, and for oversight of other aspects of food safety. Although safety of food consumed by U.S. residents is taken for granted, outbreaks of food-related illnesses and threats to health occur occasionally. Food quality and safety concerns include potentially harmful intentional and unintentional additives and biological and chemical contaminants. A variety of other issues related to food, such as genetically engineered foods and misrepresentations of nutrient qualities and substandard inspection, should also be of concern to all nurses.

MICROBIOLOGICAL CONTAMINATION

The USDHHS (2000) estimates that each year some 76 million illnesses, 325,000 hospitalizations, and 5000 deaths are associated with microorganisms in food. Problems cited include emerging pathogens; improper food preparation, storage, and distribution practices; an increasingly global food supply; and an increase in the number of people at risk because of aging and compromised capacity to fight these diseases.

Several **foodborne pathogens** have been cited as being of primary concern with regard to foodborne illnesses. These include *Salmonella, Campylobacter, Escherichia coli* 0157:H7, and *Listeria monocytogenes* (Table 7-5). Campylobacteriosis and salmonellosis are the most frequently reported foodborne illnesses in the United States, but *E. coli* 0157:H7 and *L. monocytogenes* are more severe. The very young, elders, and immunocompromised persons experience the most serious foodborne illnesses. Other high-risk populations include residents in nursing homes; hospitalized cancer and organ transplant patients; and individuals with AIDS, cirrhosis, or reduced stomach acid. Campaigns have been launched to reach all consumers on food safety. The "Seven Commandments of Food Safety" developed by the FDA will help prevent foodborne illnesses (see the Community Application box).

INTENTIONAL FOOD ADDITIVES

Intentional food additives are those substances added to food during processing to enhance the nutritional content of foods (e.g., vitamins and minerals), improve flavor (e.g., monosodium glutamate, salt, sugars, "natural flavors"), enhance color (e.g., dyes), improve texture or consistency (e.g., leavening agents, gums, thickening agents), and/or increase the shelf life (e.g., various preservatives).

The FDA has regulated food additives, to some degree, since the passage of the Food, Drug, and Cosmetic Act in 1938. This law requires food manufacturers to list product ingredients on the food label. Subsequent amendments and

TABLE **7-5** Selected Foodborne Microorganisms

MICROORGANISM	ONSET, DURATION, AND FREQUENCY	ACUTE SYMPTOMS	ASSOCIATED FOODS	PREVENTION
Salmonella species	*Onset of symptoms:* 6-48 hours after ingestion. *Duration of symptoms*: 1-2 days. *Frequency:* 77 reported outbreaks in 1989 involving 2400 individuals. Most cases, however, go unreported, and the FDA estimates 2-4 million annual cases of salmonellosis in the United States.	Nausea, vomiting, abdominal cramps, diarrhea, fever, and headache.	Meats, poultry, eggs, milk and dairy products, fish, shrimp, frog legs, yeast, salad dressings and sauces, cream-filled desserts and toppings, peanut butter, cocoa, and chocolate.	Raw eggs and foods containing raw eggs (e.g., homemade ice cream, Caesar salad, mayonnaise) may cause *Salmonella* infections. Eggs and all meats, particularly poultry, should be thoroughly cooked. Buy refrigerated eggs and keep refrigerated at temperatures less than 40°F. Wash hands, utensils, equipment, and work areas with hot soapy water before and after they come in contact with eggs and poultry. Buy only pasteurized milk and keep refrigerated.
Campylobacter jejuni	*Onset of symptoms:* 2-5 days after ingestion of contaminated food or water. *Duration of symptoms:* 7-10 days, with relapses in about 25% of cases. *Frequency: C. jejuni* is the leading cause of bacterial diarrhea in the United States. Estimates exceed 2-4 million cases per year.	Diarrhea—often bloody and may contain fecal leukocytes— fever, abdominal pain, nausea, headache, and muscle pain.	Raw chicken, raw milk, contaminated water, and raw clams.	Wash and thoroughly cook chicken. Wash hands and cooking utensils that come in contact with raw chicken with hot soapy water. Complete pasteurization of milk and chlorination of drinking water will kill *C. jejuni.*
Escherichia coli 0157:H7 (E. coli 0157:H7)	*Onset of symptoms:* 6-48 hours after ingestion. *Duration of symptoms:* approximately 8 days. *Frequency*: appears to be uncommon; however, probably only the most severe cases are reported.	Severe cramping, abdominal pain, and diarrhea that initially is watery, but becomes grossly bloody. Occasionally vomiting occurs. Fever is low grade or absent.	Raw and undercooked hamburger meat (ground beef) is the primary source. Has also been traced to processed salami. Raw milk and other meats may contain *E. coli* 0157:H7.	Thoroughly cook all beef, particularly ground beef. Maintain cooked beef at appropriately hot or cold temperatures. Do not drink unpasteurized milk.

Adapted from Food and Drug Administration. (1992). *Foodborne pathogenic microorganisms and natural toxins.* Washington, DC: Government Printing Office.

Continued

TABLE **7-5** Selected Foodborne Microorganisms—cont'd

MICROORGANISM	ONSET, DURATION, AND FREQUENCY	ACUTE SYMPTOMS	ASSOCIATED FOODS	PREVENTION
Listeria monocytogenes	*Onset of symptoms:* in general, 7-30 days after exposure, although may be 2-3 days after consumption of heavily contaminated foods. Symptoms in infants may appear hours or days after birth. *Frequency:* appears to be relatively rare—about 1600 cases per year.	Fever, headache, nausea, and vomiting; of particular concern to pregnant women and their unborn children because infection may lead to fetal death, premature labor, or infections in newborns. Major concern—mortality rate is almost 25%.	Dairy products, particularly soft cheeses; also found in some imported seafood (e.g., frozen crab meat, cooked shrimp, and cooked surimi).	Consume only pasteurized milk and dairy products made from pasteurized milk.

COMMUNITY APPLICATION
Seven Commandments of Food Safety

1. Wash hands before handling food.
2. Keep it safe—refrigerate.
3. Do not thaw food on the kitchen counter.
4. Wash hands, utensils, and surfaces after contact with raw meat and poultry.
5. Never leave perishable food out over 2 hours.
6. Thoroughly cook raw meat, poultry, and fish.
7. Freeze or refrigerate leftovers promptly.

Data from U.S. Department of Health and Human Services. (2000). *Healthy people 2010: National health promotion and disease prevention objectives.* Washington, DC: Government Printing Office.

---

legislation have resulted in allowing the FDA to establish and enforce standards for the processing of food, including food additives. The "Delaney clause," added in 1960, forbids the use of any additive shown to cause cancer in humans or animals (Blumenthal, 1990). The Nutrition Labeling and Education Act was passed in 1990 to require listing of color additives by name and the listing of ingredients in standardized foods (Segal, 1993). The Dietary Supplement Act of 1992 set more stringent guidelines for health claims

and nutrition content of foods to ensure that "claims made about the health and nutritional benefits are truthful" (Farley, 1993, p. 2).

Instruction on food additives should be a component of thorough nutrition counseling. Client education should include encouragement to read food labels and to choose foods appropriate for individual nutritional needs.

UNINTENTIONAL (INCIDENTAL) FOOD ADDITIVES

Unintentional food additives refer to those substances that "enter and remain in food as a result of their use as pesticides or herbicides, after being added to animal food, from packaging material, or through chemical changes brought about by processing methods" (Lancaster, 1992, p. 297). Glass chips, insect fragments, mercury and other heavy metals in fish, and residual antibiotics in beef and milk products are examples of food contaminants that have been the source of recent concern (Foulke, 1994; Stevens and Hall, 2001; Wagner, 1992).

To preserve food quality, the FDA has established "food defect action levels," sets and enforces food safety and quality standards, and routinely monitors foods for evidence of "food defects" (Wagner, 1992). Additionally, the EPA and FDA conduct and support research to ensure food safety.

Foulke (1993) summarized FDA findings regarding residual pesticides in food and made recommendations related to these findings. According to this report, an analysis of numerous research studies has shown that residues of pesticide (e.g., herbicides, fungicides, insecticides) were 83% to 99% eliminated from fruits and vegetables through natural means that cause dilution or degradation (e.g., wind, rain, sunlight) and commercial food processing (e.g., washing, blanching, peeling). To further reduce and virtually eliminate ingestion of pesticide residues, the FDA provides the following recommendations (Foulke, 1993):

- Wash fruits and vegetables with large amounts of cold or warm water and scrub with a brush when appropriate (do not use soap).
- Throw away the outer leaves of leafy vegetables such as lettuce and cabbage.
- Peel and cook when appropriate, although some nutrients and fiber are lost when produce is peeled.
- Trim fat from meat and fat and skin from poultry and fish. Residues of some pesticides concentrate in animal fat.

OTHER ISSUES IN FOOD QUALITY

Other concerns and issues in food quality include genetically engineered foods; irradiation of foods; and ongoing development of substances, additives, and chemicals to change food. Recent scientific developments have advanced the production of foods with decreased caloric content, increased nutritive value, and improved shelf life. The Department of Agriculture and the FDA set policy for foods produced from new plant varieties and plant breeding and the FDA must approve new food additives before marketing. Additionally, "all foods are subject to FDA's post-market authority under the 'adulteration' provisions of the act [Food, Drug and Cosmetic Act], and producers have a legal duty

to ensure that the foods they place on the market meet the safety standards of these provisions" (Suddeth, 1993, p. 3). As a result of these efforts, clients should be reassured that efforts are being made to ensure food safety. However, clients should also be encouraged to stay informed on current developments regarding food quality.

WASTE CONTROL

There are two major concerns in the issue of waste control: (1) volume of solid wastes produced in the United States and (2) concerns over the disposal of toxic and hazardous wastes. Each is discussed briefly.

SOLID WASTE MANAGEMENT

The United States is the world's biggest producer of solid wastes. Burying wastes in landfills, incineration, and recycling are the current available options for management of solid wastes. It is estimated that United States residents throw away about 4.4 pounds of garbage per person per day (EPA, 1997c). Figure 7-1 depicts components of America's trash. Besides involving esthetic and practical concerns, effective solid waste management is essential in decreasing pathogen transmission through insect and rodent control and in eliminating potential exposure to toxic and infectious materials.

In response to this growing problem, the EPA has endorsed an "integrated waste management" strategy of source reduction, recycling, waste combustion and landfilling, and community response and activities to produce less waste. Box 7-2 outlines practical ways all citizens can work to manage solid waste more effectively.

TOXIC AND HAZARDOUS WASTE CONTROL

Hazardous materials make up approximately 10% of industrial wastes and include poisons, inflammable materials, infectious contaminants, explosives, and radionuclides. The EPA regulates **hazardous waste** under the Resource Conservation and Recovery Act and, together with the Agency for Toxic Substances and Disease

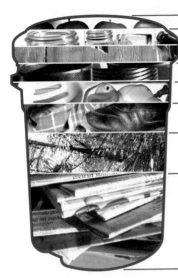

Food scraps, 6.7% = 14.0 million tons

Glass, 6.2% = 12.8 million tons

Wood, 7.1% = 14.9 million tons

Metals, 7.6% = 15.8 million tons

Plastics, 9.1% = 19.0 millions tons

Other, 11.6% = 20.8 million tons
(e.g., rubber, leather, textiles, miscellaneous inorganic wastes)

Yard trimmings, 14.3% = 29.8 million tons

Paper, 39.2% = 81.5 million tons

Total weight = 179.6 million tons
(1988 figures)

Figure 7-1. Total waste generation in the United States. (From Environmental Protection Agency (EPA). (1997c). *Municipal solid waste factbook.* Retrieved 7/17/01 from http://www.epa.gov/epaoswer/non-hw/muncpl/factbook/internet/mswf/gen.htm.

BOX 7-2 Tips for Reducing Solid Waste

REDUCE

Reduce the amount of unnecessary packaging.

REUSE

Consider reusable products.
Reuse bags, containers, and other items.
Borrow, rent, or share items used infrequently.
Sell or donate goods instead of throwing them out.

RECYCLE

Choose recyclable products and containers and recycle them.
Select products made from recycled materials.
Compost yard trimmings and some food scraps.

RESPOND

Educate others on source reduction and recycling practices.
Make preferences known to manufacturers, merchants, and community leaders.
Be creative—find new ways to reduce waste quantity and toxicity.

Registry, is responsible for oversight of hazardous waste disposal and monitoring potential and actual threats posed to health and safety. The EPA has identified 1450 sites as being on the "National Priorities List" designated for cleanup under the Comprehensive Environmental Response, Compensation, and Liability Act of 1980 (the Superfund law). This law requires industry to pay for cleaning up the worst hazardous wastes sites, funded by taxes on industries that produce hazardous wastes (EPA, 2001b).

Some of the most common contaminants include lead (e.g., from paint and glass manufacturing and smelting), mercury (e.g., from batteries, paints, pesticides), polychlorinated biphenyls [PCBs] (e.g., from electrical insulation); chromium (e.g., from copy machines, stainless steel manufacturing, chrome plating), trichlororethane or trichloroethylene (e.g., from dry-cleaning agents), and benzene (e.g., from chemical manufacturing) (EPA, 1994b). To regulate these and other hazardous wastes, the EPA has instituted a tracking system that monitors identified hazardous substances from the time the substance is produced until it reaches an approved site for disposal.

Medical waste is defined by the EPA as cultures and stocks of infectious agents, items contaminated with human blood and blood products, human pathological wastes, contaminated animal carcasses, wastes from clients isolated with highly communicable diseases, and all used sharps. Disposal of medical waste is largely regulated at the state level. Currently, incineration is the method of disposal of choice for medical waste; approximately 90% of hospital waste is currently incinerated on site. The remainder is sterilized in autoclaves or transported off site for treatment (EPA, 2001c).

Hazardous waste management consists of a combination of treatment to reduce toxicity (e.g., incineration, detoxification), storage, and/or disposal following prescribed methods. Additionally, the EPA strongly encourages waste minimization to reduce the volume of hazardous wastes.

LANDFILLS

A landfill is a place where garbage is dumped and covered daily with a layer of soil. The soil cuts down on odor, flies, insects, and animals. Newer landfills, called sanitary landfills, are lined with clay and strong plastic sheets, which are designed to keep the landfill from leaking into the environment—particularly from contaminating ground water. Although some 70% of the garbage in a landfill is biodegradable, most garbage, including food and paper, remains intact for decades because of a lack of light, oxygen, and water that prevents composting.

To minimize potential exposure to contaminants from landfills, nurses and all citizens should be aware of the following safeguards:

- Maintenance of a buffer zone to separate the landfill from surrounding areas
- Surrounding the landfill with a fence
- Installation of gas vents to prevent methane gas build up
- Installation and maintenance of a system to collect and treat leachate (chemicals that leach

out of waste in landfills and may contaminate nearby soil and ground water)
- Establishment and ongoing evaluation of a system to monitor the landfill to ensure adherence to state and federal environmental standards and regulations
- Establishment of an emergency action plan that includes readily available equipment to put out fires and manage other crises (Environmental and Occupational Health Sciences Institute [EOHSI], 1989).

INCINERATION

Incineration as a method of solid and hazardous waste management is controversial. Incineration reduces the volume of waste by up to 90% and is effective in destroying most biological contaminants. However, increasing air pollution, particularly with toxic chemicals, and subsequent disposal processes for residual heavy metals are the primary concerns. Commercial waste incinerators are designed to control emissions into the air. A variety of methods and devices, including filters, "scrubbers," and electrostatic precipitators, are employed to collect particulates and neutralize exhausts. Following incineration, residual ash is tested for toxicity and disposed of accordingly. If no toxins are found, the residue is typically dumped into a regular landfill. If toxins are found, the residue is shipped to hazardous waste landfills. A positive by product of waste incineration that is gaining in acceptance is energy production. Capturing the energy (i.e., heat) that is produced and recycling it is commonplace in newer, state-of-the-art incineration plants.

RADIATION RISKS

Threats to health from ionizing radiation come from several sources. Figure 7-2 illustrates potential sources of exposure to radiation. Unless exposure is occupational in nature (e.g., for radiology technicians, dentists, nuclear plant employees), the most common, and most potentially hazardous, radiation risks come from two sources: (1) radon gas and (2) the sun.

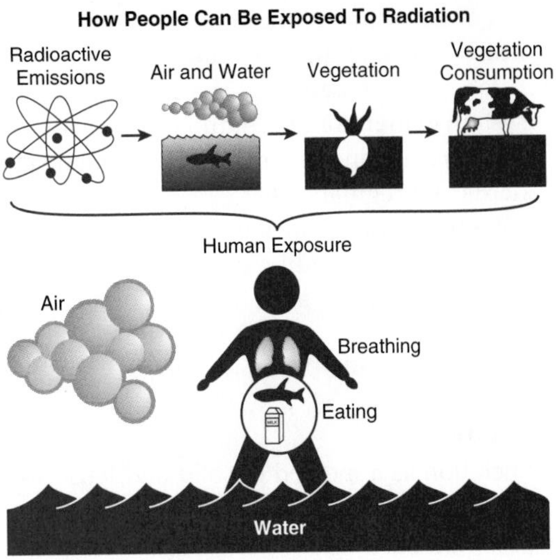

How People Can Be Exposed To Radiation

Figure 7-2. How people can be exposed to radiation. (From Centers for Disease Control and Prevention/National Center for Environmental Health. [1993]. *Radiation studies.* Atlanta: U.S. Department of Health and Human Services, Centers for Disease Control and Prevention.)

RADON GAS

Radon, an odorless, invisible gas, is a by product of the decay of uranium and occurs nearly everywhere in very small amounts. Radon enters buildings through cracks in solid floors, construction joints, cracks in walls, gaps in suspended floors, gaps around service pipes, cavities inside walls, and the water supply (EPA, 2001d). The amount of radon present varies greatly and dangerously high levels can be found in many homes. Millions of homes have elevated radon levels and most homes, particularly in high incidence areas, should be tested for radon. When elevated levels are confirmed, the problems should be corrected (EPA, 1994c).

Indoor radon gas is a national health problem contributing to between 7000 and 30,000 deaths each year. Indeed, about 10% of all lung cancer deaths are linked to radon, making radon the second leading cause of lung cancer in the United States (EPA, 2001e).

Radon is measured in units called picocuries per liter (pCi/L). The average radon level in most houses in the United States is approximately 1 pCi/L. The EPA has established a level of 4 pCi/ L or less as desirable (EPA, 2001e).

To measure radon levels, test kits can be purchased through the mail or from hardware stores and other retail outlets. Test kits should stipulate that they "meet EPA requirements" and should be designated "short term" (to remain in the home for 2 to 90 days) or "long term" (to remain in the home for 90 days or more). Because radon levels tend to vary from day to day, a short-term test is less likely to accurately detect radon. If one short-term test records a level of 4 pCi/L or greater, a second test should be conducted. The EPA recommendations following radon testing are discussed in Box 7-3.

The EPA recommends employing only trained contractors to perform repairs needed to lower home radon levels. Repair costs range from $500 to $2500, depending on the house and choice of radon reduction methods.

BOX 7-3 Environmental Protection Agency Recommendations for Radon Testing

Step 1. Take a short-term test. If the result is 4 pCi/L or higher, take a follow-up test to be sure.

Step 2. Follow up with either a long-term test or a second short-term test:

For a better understanding of the year-round average radon level, take a long-term test.

If test results are needed quickly, take a second short-term test. (If the short-term test results are 10 pCi/L or higher, a second short-term test should be conducted immediately.)

Step 3. If the second test was a long-term test: Home repairs are needed if long-term results are 4 pCi/L or greater.

If the second test was a short-term test: Home repairs are needed if the average of both tests is 4 pCi/L or greater.

Adapted from Environmental Protection Agency/U.S. Department of Health and Human Services. (1994). *A citizen's guide to radon* (2nd ed.). (EPA Publication No. 402-K92-001). Washington, DC: Government Printing Office.

ULTRAVIOLET RADIATION AND SKIN CANCER

Skin cancer is the most common form of cancer in the United States, with approximately 1.3 million new cases diagnosed each year, resulting in approximately 9000 deaths (American Cancer Society [ACS], 2001). Exposure to the sun is associated with three major types of skin cancer: (1) basal cell carcinoma (75% of all cases of skin cancer), (2) squamous cell carcinoma (20% of all cases of skin cancer), and (3) malignant melanoma (4.5% of all cases of skin cancer) (ACS, 2001). Exposure to **ultraviolet radiation** from the sun is believed to cause more than 90% of basal and squamous cell carcinomas (EOHSI, 1991). The correlation between melanoma and sun exposure is less certain.

Rates of skin cancer appear to be rising and an estimated one in six people will develop skin cancer during his or her lifetime. At highest risk are those individuals with a fair complexion, who sunburn easily, and have blond or red hair and blue eyes. As stated, exposure to ultraviolet radiation, particularly during the early years of life, contributes to skin changes that eventually result in development of skin cancer. Indeed, it is estimated that approximately 50% of the ultraviolet radiation damage to the skin occurs by the age of 20 years (EPA, 1998).

SIGNS, SYMPTOMS, AND DETECTION OF SKIN CANCER

Basal and squamous cell carcinomas occur most frequently in older individuals and although basal cell carcinoma rarely metastasizes, squamous cell carcinoma produces regional metastasis in approximately 5% of cases. Skin changes that may indicate basal or squamous cell carcinomas most often occur on the face, head, neck, and hands. The National Cancer Institute recommends observation for any of the following conditions on the skin (EOHSI, 1991, p. 2) and examination of any lesions that last longer than 2 weeks by a primary health care provider:
1. A small, smooth, pale, shiny or waxy lump
2. A firm red lump

3. A lump that bleeds or produces a crust
4. A flat, red spot that is rough, dry, or scaly
Malignant melanoma is the most serious and potentially deadly form of skin cancer, developing in about 51,400 individuals and causing approximately 7800 deaths in the United States annually (ACS, 2001). Melanoma most often occurs in white adults, typically before 50 years of age. Melanoma develops from pigment-forming cells in the skin, most commonly from preexisting or newly developed nevi. Although melanoma can develop virtually anywhere on the body, intermittently sun-exposed areas, such as the back or calf, are the most common sites in whites. In people with very dark skin (e.g., blacks), the palms, soles, and under the nails are the most common sites (ACS, 2001).

The EPA (1998) recommends a simple "ABCD" rule to observe for signs of melanoma in preexisting or new moles, which are listed in Box 7-4.

With early detection and prompt treatment, most skin cancers, including melanoma, can be treated. Treatment options include excisional surgery, cryosurgery, electrodesiccation, and curettage (Clark, 1994). Recommendations for early detection include skin examination by a primary care provider every 1 to 3 years (depending on the client's age) and teaching and encouraging clients to perform monthly skin self-examination. Guidelines endorsed by the ACS (1985) for skin self-examination are the following:
1. Using a full-length mirror, check any moles, blemishes, or birthmarks from head to toes

---

BOX 7-4 ABCD Rule for Signs of Melanoma

A. Asymmetry: One half does not match the other half.

B. Border Irregularity: The edges are ragged, notched, or blurred.

C. Color: The pigmentation is not uniform. Shades of tan, brown, and black are present. Dashes of red, white, and blue may also appear.

D. Diameter: A mole that is greater than 6 mm (about the size of a pencil eraser) is cause for concern.

health teaching

Guidelines for Preventing Skin Cancer

- Limit the time spent in the sun. Ultraviolet radiation is most intense between 10:00 AM and 3:00 PM and in the months of June to September. Limit outdoor activities during these times when possible.
- Use protective clothing. Long sleeves, long pants, and brimmed hats can protect against ultraviolet radiation.
- Use sunscreen. Sunscreen should be applied at least 30 minutes before exposure and should be reapplied every 2 to 3 hours. Waterproof products with an SPF (sun protection factor) rating of 15 or higher provide the best protection.
- Protect children from overexposure. Studies indicate that about 50% of a person's total

lifetime exposure to ultraviolet radiation occurs by age 18.
- Protect skin on hazy days and on sunny days. Clouds normally do not screen out ultraviolet rays.
- Be aware that certain foods, medications, and chemicals can worsen the effects of ultraviolet radiation on the skin. Medications, such as some antihypertensive drugs, antibiotics, and antiinflammatory agents, may produce photosensitivity. Some cosmetics, shampoos, and deodorants may also enhance photosensitivity.
- Avoid indoor tanning. Ultraviolet-A radiation is emitted by sun lamps and can increase the risk of skin cancer, eye injury, and skin aging.

for anything new—changes in size, shape, or color or a sore that does not heal.

2. Examining the body (front and back) in the mirror, then the right and left sides, with the arms raised. A hand mirror should be used to check the back and buttocks.
3. Bending the elbows and looking carefully at the forearms and upper underarms and palms.
4. Looking at the backs of the legs and feet, including the spaces between the toes and the soles.
5. Examining the back of the neck and the scalp with the help of a hand mirror, parting the hair or using a blow dryer to lift the hair and give a closer look.

See the Health Teaching box "Guidelines for Preventing Skin Cancer."

ENVIRONMENTAL HEALTH AND NURSING PRACTICE

Nurses, particularly those who work in community settings, must be knowledgeable about actual and potential threats to health from the environment and should adapt their assessment and diagnostic skills to include community en-

vironmental health issues. Neufer (1994) states that "in the nursing field, environmental health has traditionally been limited to the immediate environment of the individual (e.g., hospitalized patient) or to the family home (e.g., home safety).... Addressing environmental health today requires a systematic assessment of air, soil, surface water, and groundwater quality and the related public health implications of toxic chemicals in the environment..." (p. 156). See the Community Application box "Prevention Interventions for Environmental Safety and Health."

In taking a proactive role in health teaching, counseling, and advocacy regarding actual and potential environmental threats, nurses are indeed able to promote health and prevent illness and disability. To further assist in this, a number of resources relevant to each of the issues discussed in this chapter are presented in the Resources box at the end of the chapter.

SUMMARY

A significant number of potential environmental health problems have been described in this

COMMUNITY APPLICATION
Prevention Interventions for Environmental Safety and Health

Primary Prevention

- Advocate safer environmental design of products, automobiles, equipment, and buildings.
- Teach home safety related to falls and fire prevention, especially to families with children and elderly members.
- Counsel women of childbearing age regarding exposure to environmental hazards.
- Advocate vehicle protection systems, such as seat belts.
- Advocate use of protective devices, such as earplugs for noise.
- Immunize occupationally exposed workers for hepatitis B.
- Develop work site health and safety programs.
- Develop programs to prevent back injuries at work.
- Support the development of exposure standards for toxins.
- Support disclosure of radon and lead concentrations in homes at time of sale.
- Advocate for safe air and water.
- Teach avoidance of ultraviolet exposure and use of sunscreen.
- Advocate for reduced waste reduction and effective waste management.
- Support programs for waste reduction and recycling.

Secondary Prevention

- Assess homes, schools, work sites, and communities for environmental hazards.
- Routinely obtain occupational health histories for individuals, counsel about hazard reduction, and refer for diagnosis and treatment.
- Screen children from 6 months to 5 years for blood lead levels.
- Monitor workers for levels of chemical exposure.
- Screen at-risk workers for lung disease, cancer, and hearing loss.
- Participate in data collection regarding the incidence and prevalence of injury and disability in homes, schools, and work sites.

Tertiary Prevention

- Encourage limitation of activity when air pollution is high.
- Support cleanup of toxic waste sites and removal of other hazards.
- Provide appropriate nursing care at work sites or in the home for persons with chronic lung diseases and injury-related disabilities.
- Refer homeowners to approved lead abatement resources.

From Smith, C. Cited in J. Primomo & M. K. Salazar. (1995). Environmental issues: At home, work, and in the community. In C. M. Smith & F. A. Maurer (Eds.), *Community health nursing: Theory and practice.* Philadelphia: W. B. Saunders.

chapter including threats related to housing and living patterns, air pollution, water pollution, food quality, radiation, and solid waste. Nurses like Susan, the pediatric nurse from the chapter-opening case study, must recognize the common environmental threats in their communities and work with other health care providers to identify and intervene in those areas and to take steps to prevent environmental health problems.

By taking a proactive role in health teaching, counseling, and advocacy regarding actual and potential environmental threats, nurses are able to promote health and prevent illness and disability. To further assist in this, a number of resources relevant to each of the issues discussed in this chapter are listed in the Resources box.

Resources

Environmental Health

General Information on Environmental Issues

Centers for Disease Control and Prevention
National Center for Environmental Health
National Institute of Environmental Health Sciences (NIEHS)
Environmental Protection Agency (EPA)
Environmental Defense

Occupational Health and Safety

Department of Labor
Bureau of Labor Statistics
Occupational Safety and Health Administration
National Safety Council
Consumer Product Safety Commission

continued

Resources—cont'd

Food Safety
Food and Drug Administration

Water Safety
EPA—Office of Water

Hazardous Waste
Superfund

Visit the book's website at
www.wbsaunders.com/SIMON/McEwen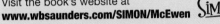
for a direct link to the website for each
organization listed.

KEY POINTS

- Environmental factors have a great impact on human development, health, and disease. Public health efforts have been very successful in reducing threats to health through improving the safety of food and water, management of waste disposal and sewage, and control or elimination of vectorborne illnesses. Contemporary environmental health threats come from toxic and ecological effects associated with the use of fossil fuels and synthetic chemicals and other sources.

- Threats related to housing and living patterns include overcrowding, household chemical exposure, and violence. Indoor air quality may be affected by combustion pollutants (e.g., secondhand smoke, exhausts from space heaters), particles (e.g., asbestos, pollen), and living organisms. Lead may be present in peeling paint and in some water pipes.

- Millions of illnesses and injuries each year are related to workplace risks and hazards. Use of heavy equipment; exposure to chemicals and biohazards, sunlight, cold, and noise; and potential for assault or violence can threaten workers. The OSHA has been given the responsibility for protection of workers and has set and enforces standards to improve worker safety and health.

- Atmospheric quality is threatened by air pollutants that can cause lung damage, inflammatory responses, and respiratory symptoms. Major air pollutants include ozone, CO, nitrogen dioxide, particulates, sulfur dioxide, and lead. The burning of fossil fuels (i.e., gasoline, coal, oil) contributes greatly to air pollution.

- Ensurance of a safe, clean water supply is necessary to health. Sewage, industrial processes and wastes, and agricultural chemicals are the main sources of water pollution. Waterborne diseases can be caused by bacteria, viruses, and protozoa. Common chemical contaminants include pesticides, petrochemicals, lead, and other compounds.

- Food quality may be threatened by both intentional and unintentional food additives (e.g., biological and chemical contaminants). Microbiological contamination is usually caused by improper storage, handling, and/or preparation of food. Intentional food additives include substances added to food during processing to enhance the nutritional content, improve flavor, enhance color, improve consistency, or increase the shelf life. Unintentional food additives are those substances that enter and remain in food as a result of their use as pesticides, after being added to animal food, or from packaging.

- The volume of solid wastes and problems concerning the disposal of toxic and hazardous wastes present threats to the health and well-being of U.S. residents. Effective solid waste management is essential to decrease pathogen transmission through insect and rodent control and to eliminate potential exposure to toxic and infectious materials.

- Radiation threats to health come from several sources—most commonly, radon gas and the sun. Radon is a colorless, odorless gas that causes thousands of deaths each year—most commonly from lung cancer. Radon enters buildings through cracks in solid floors, construction joints, and other ways, and dangerously high levels can be found in many homes. Skin cancer is the most common form of cancer in the United States and exposure to the sun is associated with all three major types of skin cancer.

Learning Activities & Application to Practice

In Class

1. With classmates, discuss each of the areas of environmental health presented. Give examples of health problems they have encountered related to each area. Discuss prevention efforts for each problem discussed including primary, secondary, and tertiary interventions, if possible.

In Clinical

2. Observe for illnesses or health conditions or risks associated with environmental health threats encountered during clinical experiences. For example, in a clinic, you might care for a toddler who is being screened for lead, an adult with carpal tunnel syndrome associated with using a computer, or an elder with skin cancer. Record these in a clinical log or diary and share with other students in the clinical group. How could the risk(s) be prevented or minimized?

3. Be prepared to teach clients about environmental threats to health and safety. Identify times when health education is appropriate (e.g., teaching a new mother not to use hot tap water to make formula, the ABCDs of skin cancer and skin assessment to all adults, and ways to reduce food contamination to high school students).

REFERENCES

American Cancer Society. (1985). *Why you should know about melanoma.* Atlanta: American Cancer Society.

American Cancer Society. (2001). *Cancer facts & figures—2001.* Atlanta: American Cancer Society.

Blumenthal, D. (1990). Red No. 3 and other colorful controversies. *FDA Consumer,* May, 1-4.

Centers for Disease Control and Prevention (CDC). (1991). *Preventing lead poisoning in young children.* Atlanta: Centers for Disease Control and Prevention.

Centers for Disease Control and Prevention (CDC). (1995). Assessing the public health threat associated with waterborne cryptosporidiosis: Report of a workshop. *MMWR Morbidity and Mortality Weekly Report,* 44(RR-6), 1-20.

Centers for Disease Control and Prevention (CDC). (1997). *Screening young children for lead poisoning: Guide for state and offices.* Atlanta: Centers for Disease Control and Prevention.

Centers for Disease Control and Prevention (CDC). (2000a). Recommendations for blood lead screening of young children enrolled in Medicaid. *MMWR Morbidity and Mortality Weekly Report,* 49 (RR-14), 1-13.

Centers for Disease Control and Prevention (CDC). (2000b). Surveillance for waterborne disease outbreaks—United States 1997-1998. *MMWR Morbidity and Mortality Weekly Report,* 49 (SS04), 1-35.

Centers for Disease Control and Prevention/National Center for Environmental Health. (1993). *Radiation studies.* Atlanta: U.S. Department of Health and Human Services, Centers for Disease Control and Prevention.

Clark, R. E. (1994). Cancer of the skin. In R. E. Rakel (Ed.), *Conn's current therapy: 1994* (pp. 742-744). Philadelphia: W. B. Saunders.

Clemen-Stone, S., Eigsti, D. G., & McGuire, S. L. (1995). *Comprehensive community health nursing* (4th ed.). St. Louis: Mosby.

Environmental and Occupational Health Sciences Institute (EOSHI). (1989). Landfills. *INFOletter: Environmental and Occupational Health Briefs,* 3(1), 1-3.

Environmental and Occupational Health Sciences Institute (EOSHI). (1991). The sun and skin: An unhealthy combination. *INFOletter: Environmental and Occupational Health Briefs,* 5(3), 1-5.

Environmental Protection Agency. (EPA). (1991). *Ensuring safe drinking water.* (EPA Publication No. 600-M-91-001). Washington, DC: Government Printing Office.

Environmental Protection Agency. (EPA). (1992). *What you can do to reduce air pollution.* (EPA Publication No. 450-K-92-002). Washington, DC: Government Printing Office.

Environmental Protection Agency. (EPA). (1993a). *Secondhand smoke.* (EPA Publication No. 402-F-93-004). Washington, DC: Government Printing Office.

Environmental Protection Agency. (EPA). (1993b). *Preventing waterborne disease.* (EPA Publication No. 640-K-93-001). Washington, DC: Government Printing Office.

Environmental Protection Agency. (EPA). (1993c). *Lead in your drinking water: Actions you can take to reduce lead in drinking water.* (EPA Publication No. 810-F-93-001). Washington, DC: Government Printing Office.

Environmental Protection Agency. (EPA). (1994). *Protecting the ozone layer: A checklist for citizen action.* (EPA Publication No. 430-94-007). Washington, DC: Government Printing Office.

Environmental Protection Agency. (EPA). (1996). *Protect your family and yourself from carbon monoxide poisoning.* (EPA Publication No. 402-F-96-005). Washington, DC: Government Printing Office.

Environmental Protection Agency. (EPA). (1997a). *Ozone: good up high, bad nearby.* (EPA Publication No. 451-97-002). Washington, DC: Government Printing Office.

Environmental Protection Agency. (EPA). (1997b). *Health and environmental effects of ground-level ozone (fact sheet).* Retrieved 7/13/01 from http://www.epa.gov/ttn/oarpg/naaqsfin/o3health.html.

Environmental Protection Agency. (EPA). (1997c). *Municipal solid waste factbook.* Retrieved 7/12/01 from http://www.epa.gov/epaoswer/non-hw/muncpl/factbook/internet/mswf/gen.htm.

Environmental Protection Agency. (EPA). (1998). *Stay healthy in the sun.* (EPA Publication No. 430-98-004). Washington, DC: Government Printing Office.

Environmental Protection Agency. (EPA). (2000). *Biological pollutants in your home.* Retrieved 7/13/01 from http://www.epa.gov/iaq/pubs/bio_1.html.

Environmental Protection Agency. (EPA). (2001a). *Biological contaminants.* Retrieved 7/13/01 from http://www.epa.gov/iaq/biologic.html.

Environmental Protection Agency. (EPA). (2001b). *About superfund.* Retrieved 7/13/01 from http://www.epa.gov/superfund/about.htm.

Environmental Protection Agency. (EPA). (2001c). *Frequently asked questions about medical waste.* Retrieved 7/18/01 from http://www.epa.gov/epaoswer/other/medical/mwfaqs.htm.

Environmental Protection Agency. (EPA). (2001d). *Radon (Rn).* Retrieved 7/18/01 from http://www.epa.gov/iaq/radon/.

Environmental Protection Agency. (EPA). (2001e). Frequently asked questions about radon. Retrieved 7/17/01 from http://www.epa.gov/iaq/radon/radonqa1.html.

Environmental Protection Agency/U.S. Department of Health and Human Services. (1994a). *Protecting the ozone layer: A checklist for citizen action.* (EPA Publication No. 430-94-007). Washington, DC: Government Printing Office.

Environmental Protection Agency/U.S. Department of Health and Human Services. (1994b). *The Superfund Emergency Response Program.* (EPA Publication No. 450-F-94-041). Washington, DC: Government Printing Office.

Environmental Protection Agency/U.S. Department of Health and Human Services. (1994c). *A citizen's guide to radon* (2nd ed.). (EPA Publication No. 402-K92-001). Washington, DC: Government Printing Office.

Farley, D. (1993). Dietary supplements: Making sure hype doesn't overwhelm science. *FDA Consumer,* 27(9), 1-3.

Food and Drug Administration. (1992). *Foodborne pathogenic microorganisms and natural toxins.* Washington, DC: Government Printing Office.

Foulke, J. E. (1993). FDA reports on pesticides in foods. *FDA Consumer,* 27(5), 29-32.

Foulke, J. E. (1994). Mercury in fish: Cause for concern? *FDA Consumer,* 28(7), 1-3.

Lancaster, J. (1992). Environmental health and safety. In M. Stanhope and J. Lancaster (Eds.), *Community health nursing: Process and practice for promoting health.* St. Louis: Mosby.

McKeown, T. (1995). Determinants of health. In P. R. Lee & C. L. Estes (Eds.), *The nation's health* (4th ed., pp. 9-17). Boston: Jones and Bartlett Publishers.

Neufer, L. (1994). The role of the community health nurse in environmental health. *Public Health Nursing,* 11(3), 1155-1162.

Primomo, J., & Salazar, M. K. (2000). Environmental issues: At home, work, and in the community. In C. M. Smith & F. A. Maurer (Eds.), *Community health nursing: Theory and practice* (2nd ed.). Philadelphia: W. B. Saunders.

Rogers, B. (1994). *Occupational health nursing: Concepts and practice.* Philadelphia: W. B. Saunders.

Segal, M. (1993). Ingredient labeling: What's in a food? *FDA Consumer,* April, 14-18.

Stevens, P. E., & Hall, J. M. (2001). Environmental health. In M. Neis & M. McEwen (Eds.), *Community health nursing: Promoting the health of populations* (3rd ed.). Philadelphia: W. B. Saunders.

Suddeth, M. A. (1993). Genetically engineered foods: Fears & facts. *FDA Consumer,* May, 1993.

U.S. Consumer Product Safety Commission/Environmental Protection Agency. (1994). *A citizen's guide to radon: The guide to protecting yourself and your family* (2nd ed.). (Publication No. 402-K92-001). Washington, DC: Government Printing Office.

U.S. Consumer Product Safety Commission/Environmental Protection Agency and American Lung Association. (1999). *What you should know about combustion appliances and indoor air pollution.* United States: U.S. Consumer Product Safety Commission/Environmental Protection Agency and American Lung Association.

U.S. Department of Health and Human Services/Centers for Disease Control/National Institute for Occupational Health and Safety (1996). *Violence in the Workplace.* Retrieved 7/17/01 from http://www/cdc/gov/niosh/violintr.html.

U.S. Department of Health and Human Services. (2000). *Healthy people 2010: National health promotion and disease prevention objectives.* Washington, DC: Government Printing Office.

U.S. Department of Labor. (1995). *Work injuries and illnesses by selected characteristics, 1993.* Washington, DC: Bureau of Labor Statistics.

U.S. Department of Labor. (2000). *Workplace injuries and illnesses in 1999.* Washington, DC: Bureau of Labor Statistics.

Wagner, B. (1992). FDA keeps antennae out for insect fragments. *FDA Consumer,* November, 19-23.

Cultural Influences on Health

1. Discuss the importance of providing culturally sensitive and culturally competent nursing care.

2. Differentiate among race, ethnicity, and culture and describe characteristics of each.

3. Explain the relationships between socioeconomic levels and culture and socioeconomic status and health.

4. Perform a cultural assessment.

5. Describe cultural variations related to diet, communication patterns, and religion.

6. Discuss variations in health patterns between European Americans, Blacks, Hispanics, Native Americans, and Asian/Pacific Islanders.

key terms

Culture	Racism	*See Glossary for definitions.*
Ethnic group	Subculture	
Race	Transcultural nursing	

case study

Trisha Thomas is a registered nurse working in a city-sponsored pediatric clinic in a large southwestern city. At the clinic, Trisha primarily sees low-income clients, most of whom are eligible for Medicaid or who have no personal health insurance. More than 75% of the clients seen in the clinic are from minority groups and almost half are Hispanic. Other racial and ethnic groups seen include African-Americans; Southeast Asians (Vietnamese, Cambodian, and Laotian); and increasingly, immigrants from Middle-Eastern and African countries (Iraqi Kurds and refugees from Somalia, Ethiopia, and Uganda).

Because Trisha has practiced nursing at the clinic for almost 4 years, she has learned to speak Spanish fairly well. She is able to perform assessments, take health histories, and teach effectively in that language. In addition, the clinic has interpreters for several of the most common languages heard at the clinic.

Trisha's experience working with people from many different cultures has given her an awareness of their health practices, beliefs, diet, and religions. This, in turn, has enabled her to conduct more thorough assessments and provide more effective teaching and anticipatory guidance than most of her colleagues.

On Thursday, Trisha saw Carlos Sepulveda for his well-child visit. Carlos is 5 years old and will begin kindergarten this fall. Because Carlos' health care is financed through Medicaid, Trisha performed an Early and Periodic Screening, Diagnosis, and Treatment (EPSDT) examination (see Chapter 9), which includes a complete physical examination; developmental testing; height and weight measurements; and screenings for vision and hearing, lead, and anemia. Review of Carlos' immunization records showed that he was due for his second diphtheria-pertussis-tetanus and polio boosters and his second measles/mumps/rubella vaccination.

Although Mrs. Sepulveda does not speak English, Trisha was able to gain information about Carlos' diet, sleeping habits, and activity. She learned that the family lives in a subsidized apartment in a safe area. The apartment has smoke detectors and all medications and cleaning products are in cabinets with child-proof latches.

All of the findings from the physical assessment were normal. However, Carlos was small for his age (less than the twentieth percentile). Knowing that because of financial constraints and cultural preferences Carlos' diet might be deficient in protein, calcium, and some vitamins, Trisha directed her health teaching to his nutritional needs. After questioning Mrs. Sepulveda about his daily diet, Trisha gave her information on how to increase these nutrients and referred her to the Women, Infants, and Children (WIC) program (see Chapter 9) located in their building. Before Mrs. Sepulveda and Carlos left to see the WIC counselor, Trisha made an appointment for Carlos to return in 6 months for further evaluation.

The United States is becoming increasingly ethnically diverse. According to U.S. Department of Health and Human Services (USDHHS) reports, members of ethnic minority groups in the United States are disproportionately impoverished and have poorer health outcomes and fewer options for seeking health care (USDHHS, 2000). One of the two broad goals of *Healthy People 2010* is to "Reduce health disparities among Americans" and a number of objectives are specifically directed toward members of various racial and ethnic groups. The *Healthy People 2010* table provides examples of objectives that address the improvement of the health of members of minority groups.

Although the Americas have been a melting pot since colonization began in the 1600s, the makeup of the population is changing. Figures 8-1 and 8-2 depict current and estimated year 2025 population breakdowns by racial and ethnic groups. As these pie charts show, the percentage of whites is declining and the greatest growth is being seen in Hispanics and other immigrants, largely from Southeast Asia.

Many of the objectives from *Healthy People 2010* addressing the disparity between people from various ethnic groups cite health problems that lead to differences in morbidity and mortality. For example, alcoholism is more common in Native Americans, resulting in increases in liver disease and accidental injuries. Diabetes is much more prevalent in Native Americans, Hispanics, and blacks, contributing to related complications and deaths in those groups. To further illustrate some of the differences between health problems found in racial and ethnic groups, Table 8-1 lists the 10 leading causes of death for whites, Hispanics, blacks, Native Americans and Asians.

TRANSCULTURAL NURSING

Nurses who practice in community settings are often in a position to provide nursing care to clients from diverse racial and ethnic groups. To foster understanding and assist those individuals with nursing and health care needs, the Transcultural Nursing Society was established in

healthy people **2010**

Selected Objectives Addressing the Health of Racial and Ethnic Minorities

OBJECTIVE	BASELINE (1998)	TARGET
1.1: Increase the proportion of persons with health insurance (Hispanic or Latino)	70%	100%
1.8 g: Increase nursing degrees awarded to underrepresented populations (black)	6.9%	13%
3.1: Reduce the overall cancer death rate (black)	262.1 per 100,000	158.7 per 100,000
5.3: Reduce the overall rate of diabetes that is clinically diagnosed (Hispanic)	61 per 1000	25 per 1000
8.11: Eliminate elevated blood lead levels in children (black)	11.5%	0%
9.7: Reduce pregnancies among adolescent females (black)	133 per 1000	42 per 1000
15.1: Reduce firearm-related deaths (black)	23.7 per 100,000	4.9 per 100,000
16.1h: Reduce deaths from SIDS (American Indian or Alaska Native)	1.56 per 1000	0.3 per 1000
18.1: Reduce suicide rate (American Indian or Alaska Native)	12.4 per 100,000	6 per 100,000
19.2: Reduce the proportion of adults who are obese (Hispanic)	29%	15%
27.1: Reduce cigarette smoking by adults (American Indian or Alaska Native	34%	12%

SIDS, Sudden infant death syndrome.

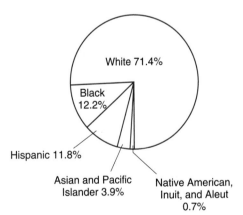

Figure 8-1. Population by race/Hispanic origin, 2000. (Data from the U.S. Bureau of the Census. [2001a]. Projections of the resident population by race, Hispanic origin and nativity: 2000. Retrieved 2/6/02 from http://www.census.gov/population/projections/nation/summary/np-t5-a.txt.)

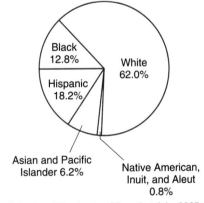

Figure 8-2. Population by race/Hispanic origin, 2025 (estimated). (Data from the U.S. Bureau of the Census. [2001b]. Projections of the resident population by race, Hispanic origin and nativity: 2025-2045. Retrieved 2/6/02 from http://www.census.gov/population/projections/nation/summary/np-t5-f.txt.)

TABLE **8-1** Ten Leading Causes of Death for Whites, Hispanics, and Blacks (1998)

WHITE NON-HISPANICS	BLACKS	HISPANICS	NATIVE AMERICANS	ASIANS/PACIFIC ISLANDERS
Heart disease	Heart disease	Heart disease	Heart disease	Heart disease
Cancer	Cancer	Cancer	Cancer	Cancer
Stroke	Stroke	Injuries	Injuries	Stroke
COPD	Injuries	Stroke	Diabetes	Injuries
Injuries	Diabetes	Diabetes	Stroke	Pneumonia/influenza
Pneumonia/influenza	Homicide	Pneumonia/influenza	Liver disease	Diabetes
Diabetes	Pneumonia/influenza	Homicide	Pneumonia/influenza	COPD
Suicide	COPD	Liver disease	COPD	Suicide
Liver disease	AIDS	COPD	Suicide	Homicide
Kidney disease	Perinatal conditions	Perinatal conditions	Homicide	Kidney disease

From National Center for Health Statistics. (2000). Deaths: Final Data for 1998. *National Vital Statistic Report 48*(11), 1-106. *COPD*, Chronic obstructive pulmonary disease.

1973 by Madeline Leininger (Andrews, 1992; Leininger, 2001a).

According to Herberg, **"Transcultural nursing** is concerned with the provision of nursing care in a manner that is sensitive to the needs of individuals, families and groups" where "a thorough assessment of the cultural aspect of a client's lifestyle, health beliefs and health practices will enhance the nurse's decision making and judgment when providing care" (1995, p. 3). Culturally sensitive nursing interventions show appreciation of and respect for differences and attempt to decrease the possibility of stress or conflict arising from cultural misunderstanding.

In 1992, the American Academy of Nursing published a commitment to quality and "culturally competent" nursing care. Their recommendations included the following:

- Promotion of culturally competent care that is equitable and accessible
- Development and maintenance of a disciplinary knowledge base and expertise in culturally competent care
- Synthesis of existing theoretical and research knowledge regarding nursing care of different ethnic or minority, stigmatized, and disenfranchised populations
- Creation of an interdisciplinary knowledge base that reflects heterogeneous health care practices within various cultural groups

- Identification and examination of methods, theories, and frameworks appropriate for utilization in the development of knowledge related to health care of minority, stigmatized, and disenfranchised populations
- Establishment of ways to teach and guide faculty and nursing students to provide culture-specific care and to support the regulation of content reflecting diversity in nursing curricula

In accordance with these recommendations, nurses—particularly those working in community settings—should be knowledgeable of cultural differences and how they influence health and health practices and be prepared to work within these differences to improve health. Nursing care and interventions to address problems related to cultural, hereditary, social, and other factors that contribute to differences in morbidity and mortality are described in this chapter.

CULTURE AND RELATED CONCEPTS

The terms *race, ethnic group,* and *culture* are frequently confused. They may be erroneously used interchangeably because they refer to different, although sometimes overlapping, concepts. Lack of recognition of the differences and subsequent misuse of the terms may incur confusion or misunderstanding.

RACE

Race refers to classification or grouping of humans primarily based on physical characteristics (e.g., skin color, hair color and texture, eye shape and color, height). Anthropologically, individuals from a given race have a common geographic origin of their ancestors. Early anthropologists recognized three races based largely on skin color: (1) Caucasoid (white), (2) Mongoloid (yellow), and (3) Negroid (black). According to Garn (1985), research studies during the twentieth century led anthropologists to conclude that nine major geographical races exist, roughly based on continental divisions. These races are the following:

- African (Negroid): A collection of related races in sub-Saharan Africa. Members have curly, tightly coiled hair; thick lips; and large amounts of melanin in the skin, hair, and gums. American blacks are mostly of African origin.
- American Indian: The earliest inhabitants of the Western Hemisphere, American Indians are related to Asians, but have different blood groups. Skin color ranges from light to dark brown and hair is black and straight.
- Asian (Mongoloid): Populations are found in continental Asia (except South Asia and the Middle East), including Japan, Taiwan, the Philippines, and parts of Indonesia. Members have straight black hair, inner eyefolds, and pads of fat over their cheekbones. Most have light brown skin and are shorter than Europeans.
- Australian (Australian Aborigine): These groups are native to Australia. Members have large teeth, narrow skulls, and very dark skin coloring.
- European (Caucasoid): Comprised of groups throughout Europe, the Middle East, and northern Africa, group members have lighter skin than do other peoples. The "whites" of Australia, North and South America, and South Africa are members of the European race.
- Indian: Populations in South Asia from the Himalayas to the Indian Ocean. Skin color ranges from light in the north to dark in the south. Blood groups differ somewhat from those of Europeans.
- Melanesian: Comprised of peoples of New Guinea and Solomon Islands, Melanesians resemble Africans in skin color, but have different blood group frequencies.
- Micronesian: Comprised of occupants of islands in the Pacific (e.g., Carolines, Gilberts, Marianas, Marshalls), Micronesians are small and dark skinned and have wavy or woolly hair. They resemble Polynesians somewhat in blood group frequencies.
- Polynesian: Comprised of far southern Pacific Islanders, Polynesians include people from Hawaii, New Zealand, and Easter Island. Members are tall, may be heavy, and have light-to-moderate skin color (Garn, 1985, p. 53).

Although descendants of a given geographical race are similar, variations exist in people from different subgeographical areas and they may differ quite noticeably from other members of the same race. For example, people from Northern Europe usually have very light skin, light hair, and blue eyes, whereas Southern Europeans often have olive skin, dark hair, and dark eyes. Likewise, Alaskan Inuits vary significantly from Southern Native American tribes in height and other characteristics and members of central and eastern African tribes may vary greatly from the Bushmen of South Africa. Race is largely unchanging, although intermarrying between races and subsequent mixing of races does occur. This results in the lessening of some of the distinctive characteristics of each race.

ETHNIC GROUP

An **ethnic group** is a group of people who share common, distinctive characteristics such as race, ancestry, nationality, language, religion, food preferences, literature, and music and a common history. According to Spector (1996), at least 106 ethnic groups are recognized in the United States and more than 170 Native American tribes exist.

Although members of ethnic groups share similar cultural patterns, values, beliefs, customs, behavior, and traditions, intraethnic variations usually exist. For example, in the United States, Hispanic-Americans represent a large ethnic group that varies significantly based on country or area of origin; this ethnic group contains Cuban-Americans, Puerto Ricans, Mexican-Americans, and people from Central America, among others. Likewise, African-Americans differ from Caribbean blacks or sub-Saharan Africans and different tribal groups in Africa may vary greatly from each other.

CULTURE

In 1871, Sir Edward Tylor, an English anthropologist, defined **culture** as "the complex whole which includes knowledge, belief, art, morals, law, custom, and any other capabilities and habits acquired by man as a member of society" (cited by Andrews, 1999a). Other definitions of culture include "nonphysical traits, such as values, beliefs, attitudes and customs that are shared by a group of people and passed from one generation to the next" (Spector, 1996, p. 358) and "a way of perceiving, behaving and evaluating the world… a guide for determining people's values, beliefs and practices" (Andrews, 1999a, p. 3). Culture, therefore, provides the organizational structure or basis for behavior within the group. Culture is not necessarily tied to race because members of a given culture may be from different races. Culture, however, is a component of ethnicity.

To illustrate the differences in these concepts, a second-generation Cuban-American who lives in Miami and whose ancestors were African slaves might be classified as follows:

- Race: African
- Ethnicity: Hispanic
- Cultural group: South Floridian/Cuban-American

Another example would be an immigrant from Korea residing in Houston:

- Race: Asian
- Ethnicity: South Korean
- Cultural group: Korean-American/Texan

Various terms are used in discussing race, ethnicity, and culture. To clarify some of the differences, Box 8-1 gives definitions of terms commonly used in reference to culture and cultural issues.

CHARACTERISTICS OF CULTURE

According to Allender and Spradley (2001), anthropologists and sociologists have identified a number of characteristics common to all cultures. Some characteristics that are particularly pertinent to the practice of nursing are listed in Box 8-2.

A **subculture** is a relatively large subsection of the cultural group that has distinctive characteristics that set it apart from the group as a whole. Teenage gangs, professional football players, members of the military, and nursing students might be considered subcultures. Based on the characteristics described in Table 8-2, members of each of these groups must learn the cultural values, norms, practices, and other characteristics of the group. The soldier must learn terminology, skills, behaviors, and so forth to become a member of the group. In the same way, the beliefs, values, and practices of professional football players are integrated into other aspects of their actions; cultural values, beliefs, and practices of teenage gang members are shared. Nursing students (and other health care providers) do not need to explain thoughts, actions, and beliefs to other health care providers—rationale for actions is largely understood or tacit. Finally, each of the examples listed must remain adaptive and dynamic to subsist and grow.

To illustrate differences in subcultural groups, a white middle-class family from rural Iowa is culturally different from a white middle-class family from Los Angeles. In these two families, variations in values, language, dress, diet, leisure

BOX **8-1** Terms Used in Transcultural Nursing Care

CULTURE SHOCK

"Feelings of bewilderment, confusion, disorganization, frustration, and stupidity, and the inability to adapt to differences in language and word meanings, activities, time, and customs that are part of the new culture" (Murray, Zentner & Samiezade'-Yazd, 2001, p. 46)

CULTURAL BLINDNESS

Failure to acknowledge or respect cultural differences and behaving as though they do not exist

DOMINANT VALUE ORIENTATION

The basic value orientation that is shared by the majority of its members as a result of early common experiences

DISCRIMINATION

The differential treatment of individuals because they belong to a minority group; denying equal opportunity by acting on a prejudice

ENCULTURATION (ACCULTURATION)

The process of becoming a member of a cultural group; adapting to another culture

ETHNICITY

A classification of individuals based on a shared culture or affiliation, values, perceptions, feelings, and assumptions

ETHNOCENTRISM

The belief that one's own group is superior to others

MINORITY GROUP

A segment of the population that differs from the majority based on physical or cultural characteristics

NORMS

The rules by which human behavior is governed that are the result of the cultural values held by the group

PREJUDICE

A hostile attitude toward individuals because they belong to a particular racial or ethnic group presumed to have objectionable qualities; negative beliefs or preferences that are generalized about a group that leads to prejudgment

RACISM

Excessive belief in the superiority of one's own racial group

STEREOTYPING

The belief or notion that all people from a given group are the same

VALUES

Personal perceptions of what is good or useful; desirable beliefs and standards

BOX **8-2** Characteristics of Culture

CULTURE IS LEARNED.

Cultural behaviors are acquired, not inherited; enculturation is learned through socialization and language acquisition.

CULTURE IS INTEGRATED.

The various components of a culture are simultaneously interrelated and independent; they are an integrated web of ideas, beliefs, and practices.

CULTURE IS SHARED.

Cultural values, beliefs, and practices are shared by the members of the culture and identify and stabilize the cultural group.

CULTURE IS TACIT.

Much of culture is outside of awareness; members of a culture know how to act and what to expect without need for discussion.

CULTURE IS DYNAMIC.

Every culture experiences constant change.

Data from Allender, J. A., & Spradley, B. W. (2001). *Community health nursing: Concepts and practice* (5th ed.). Philadelphia: Lippincott.

activities, expectations, and so on would exist. Similarly, a working-class Puerto Rican family living in New York City varies markedly from a Mexican family living in the Rio Grande valley.

CULTURAL ASSESSMENT

Nurses who work in community-based settings must recognize the impact of culture on health and health practices and they should be familiar with the beliefs, values, and practices of the members of cultural groups they may care for. To gain an understanding, pertinent information should be assessed by the nurse; this may be accomplished by using all or part of one of several cultural assessment instruments. One comprehensive cultural assessment instrument, developed by Andrews and Boyle (1999), is presented in Appendix 8-A. As outlined in this assessment guide, some of the components to be considered in cultural assessment are values, socioeconomic status, communication patterns and language, nutrition and dietary habits, religion and religious practices, health beliefs and practices, and biocultural aspects of disease incidence. These are briefly addressed.

CULTURAL VALUES

Values are personal perceptions of what is good or useful and are a universal feature of all cultures (Andrews and Boyle, 1999). Among other purposes, values give meaning to life; provide self-esteem; serve as goals or motivators that direct behaviors; and form the foundation for the individual person on personal, professional, social, political, and philosophical issues.

Much of U.S. culture is shaped by the dominant cultural group (white, middle class), whose values include marriage and family, parental responsibility to children, work ethic, individuality, material wealth, comfort, humanitarianism, physical beauty, democracy, newness, cleanliness, education, science and technology, achievement, free enterprise, punctuality, rationality, independence, respectability, effort and progress,

family unity and stability, pursuit of recreational activities, equality of people, future orientation, economic security for the present and future, sporting events, and cultural arts (Leininger, 2001b; Murray, Zentner, and Samiezade'-Yazd, 2001). Because these values are so entrenched in U.S. culture, often members of the dominant cultural group fail to recognize that these values are not universally shared or even understood by members of other cultural groups.

To assist nurses in understanding differences in values among various cultural groups, Leininger (2001a) and others have researched several different groups. Table 8-2 compares cultural values identified by the research of Leininger (2001b) for several of the most prevalent U.S. cultural groups.

SOCIOECONOMIC STATUS

In addition to variations based on racial or ethnic groups, cultural variations based on socioeconomic levels, or class, are detectable and strongly influence health and health-seeking behaviors. Like other components of culture, socioeconomic class creates a set of values and role expectations regarding factors such as sex, marriage, parenting, birth, education, dress, housing, reading, occupation, and religion. In the United States, health status is more closely linked to income level than to race or ethnicity (USDHHS, 2000). Indeed, poor people, regardless of race or ethnicity, are more likely to experience poor health and poor health care. Murray, Zentner, and Samiezade'-Yazd (2001) describe the following socioeconomic subcultures:

- Upper-upper level: This "affluent, or corporate level" is characterized by a small number of people who have money and power. Values include home, position, lineage, power and prestige, economic achievements, education, possession of art, and philanthropy.
- Lower-upper level: The "new rich" are persons who possess large incomes and lifestyles that flaunt their money. They have and value an abundance of possessions.

TABLE **8-2** Comparison of the Values of Various Cultural Groups

CHARACTERISTIC	ANGLO-AMERICANS	AFRICAN AMERICANS	MEXICAN AMERICANS	NATIVE AMERICANS	ARAB-AMERICAN/ MUSLIMS	JAPANESE AMERICANS
Dependency	Value independence and freedom; focus on self-reliance	Interdependent with other blacks	Extended family valued; interdependent with kin and social activities	Stress harmony between land, people, and environment	Providing family care and support is a responsibility	Duty and obligation to kin and work group
Health and Healing	Value scientific/ medical facts and technology	May employ folk healing and home remedies	May use traditional folk care healers; may believe in hot-cold theory	Folk healers (e.g., Shamans) may be used	Obligation and responsibility to visit and help the sick	Attention to physical complaints; value personal cleanliness; may use folk therapies
Religion/ Spirituality	N/A	Religion valued (many are Baptists)	Religion valued (many are Catholic)	Maintain spiritual inspiration (spirit guidance)	Follow the teaching of the Koran; offering prayers (5 times each day)	N/A
Achievement/ Possessions	Value competition and achievement; materialism	Value technology (e.g., radio, car)	N/A	Value the practice of cultural rituals and taboos	Helping to "save face" and preserve cultural values is important	Ambitious and achievement oriented; maintain high educational standards
Hierarchical Structure/ Authority	Focus on the individual; less respect for authority and elders	Reliance on extended family networks	Patriarchy; respect for authority and elders	Authority of tribal elders; respect and value of children	Respect and protect different gender roles	Patriarchal obligations and respect valued; honor elders
Other	Value youth and beauty; leisure time important	Value music and physical activities	Value native foods; little value for exact time	Pride in cultural heritage and value "Nations"	Value knowing cultural taboos and norms	Futurists; politeness and ritual valued

Data from Leininger, M. M. (2001). *Culture care diversity and universality: A theory of nursing.* Boston: Jones and Bartlett Publishers. N/A, not specifically addressed

- Overclass: This is a new social class comprised of professionals and managers who are upwardly mobile and have earned wealth through hard work. Most are urban singles and couples without children. They tend to be transnational, although many live on the coasts. Values include competitive achievement on the job and in leisure.
- Upper-middle level: This level, which may be described as "well off," includes college-educated "professionals" (e.g., doctors, dentists, engineers, lawyers). Children and family stability are highly valued. Education, hard work, career success, responsibility, honesty, security, materialism, various leisure activities, and travel are also valued.
- Middle level: Included in this level are people who have small or medium-sized businesses, skilled workers, office workers, teachers, and nurses. They are usually educated above the high school level. They live in middle-class neighborhoods and have two cars (often a van). Persons at this level are usually characterized by nuclear families and are child oriented. Education, creativity, hard work, thrift, patience, planning ahead, and postponing immediate rewards are valued.
- Lower-middle level: Often referred to as the "working class," this level includes high school graduates with industrial or "blue-collar" jobs, clerical workers, technicians, semiskilled workers, and waitresses. Chances of advancement are minimal. Persons at this level live in small homes or apartments and possess one or two cars. Their values include patriotism, religion, authority, work ethic, honesty, neatness, respectability, self-reliance, independence, conformity, competition, achievement, education, and saving for the future. Adults are typically less educated and read less. Childrearing is taken for granted and parents often rely heavily on the extended family for support.
- Upper-lower level: Included at this level are those who work at menial tasks (e.g., fast food workers, domestics, gardeners, maintenance, garbage collectors), but are grateful for employment. Persons in this group often did not complete high school, were early parents with a rapid succession of children, and may have an early separation or divorce.
- Underclass: Comprised of those in both acute and chronic poverty, members of the underclass usually have a history of being unemployed or underemployed. Many of the underclass are children (about 45% of poor persons are children). Single-parent (usually mother-headed) families are very common. Other underclass groups are homeless people, migrant workers, immigrants and refugees and their families, and many elders. Low self-esteem, mistrust of others, anger, susceptibility to drug and alcohol abuse, teen pregnancy, and incarceration are not uncommon. Frequently, the poor have not finished high school and are unskilled; they may be employed in temporary or seasonal jobs and/or rely on public assistance.

LANGUAGE AND COMMUNICATION

LANGUAGE

Language barriers are among the most commonly encountered problems in working with members of other cultural groups. Ideally, the nurse speaks the client's language and, in areas of high concentration of a minority group, many nurses are bilingual. For example, in South Florida, Southern California, and South Texas, the percentage of Hispanic and non-Hispanic nurses who can speak Spanish is greater. In areas with many immigrants from China, Japan, and Southeast Asia (e.g., San Francisco), nurses who speak one or more Asian languages or dialects are often found. However, it is becoming increasingly common for the nurse and the client to be unable to speak the same language and nurses need to be prepared and creative to adjust to this challenge (see the Community Application boxes "Overcoming Language Barriers: Use of an Interpreter" and "Overcoming Language Barriers When No Interpreter Is Available").

COMMUNITY APPLICATION
Overcoming Language Barriers: Use of an Interpreter

- Before locating an interpreter, be sure that you know what language the client speaks at home because it may be different from the language spoken publicly (e.g., French is sometimes spoken by aristocratic or well-educated people from certain Asian or Middle Eastern cultures).
- The nurse should avoid interpreters from a rival tribe, state, region, or nation (e.g., a Palestinian who knows Hebrew may not be the best interpreter for a Jewish client).

- The nurse should be aware of gender differences between the interpreter and client to avoid violation of cultural mores related to modesty.
- The nurse should be aware of age differences between interpreter and client.
- The nurse should be aware of socioeconomic differences between interpreter and client.
- The nurse should ask the interpreter to translate as closely to verbatim as possible.
- An interpreter who is not a relative may seek compensation for services rendered.

From Andrews, M. M. (2001). Cultural diversity and community health nursing. In M. A. Nies & M. McEwen (Eds.), *Community health nursing: Promoting the health of populations* (3rd ed., pp. 242-285). Philadelphia: W. B. Saunders.

COMMUNITY APPLICATION
Overcoming Language Barriers When No Interpreter Is Available

- Be polite and formal.
- Greet the client using the last or complete name; gesture to yourself and say your name; offer a handshake or nod; smile.
- Proceed in an unhurried manner; pay attention to any effort by the client or family to communicate.
- Speak in a low, moderate voice. Avoid talking loudly and remember that people tend to raise the volume and pitch of their voice when the listener appears not to understand and the listener may think that you are shouting or angry.
- Use any words known in the client's language. This indicates awareness of and respect for the client's culture.
- Use simple words, such as "pain" instead of "discomfort." Avoid medical jargon, idioms, and slang. Avoid using contractions such as "don't," "can't," and "won't." Use nouns repeatedly instead of pronouns. For example, say "Does Juan take medicine?" instead of "He has been taking his medicine, hasn't he?"
- Pantomime words and simple actions while verbalizing them.

- Give instructions in the proper sequence. For example, say "first wash the bottle; second, rinse the bottle," instead of "Before you rinse the bottle, sterilize it."
- Discuss one topic at a time and avoid using conjunctions. For example, say "Are you cold (while pantomiming)?" and "Are you in pain?" instead of "Are you cold and in pain?"
- Validate if the client understands by having the client repeat instructions, demonstrate the procedure, or act out the meaning.
- Write out several short sentences in English and determine the client's ability to read them.
- Try a third language. Many Indo-Chinese speak French. Europeans often know three or four languages. Try Latin words or phrases.
- Ask who among the client's family and friends could serve as an interpreter.
- Obtain phrase books from a library or bookstore, make or purchase flash cards, contact hospitals for a list of interpreters, and use both formal and informal networking to locate a suitable interpreter.

From Andrews, M. M. (2001). Cultural diversity and community health nursing. In M. A. Nies & M. McEwen (Eds.), *Community health nursing: Promoting the health of populations* (3rd ed., pp. 242-285). Philadelphia: W. B. Saunders.

COMMUNICATION PATTERNS

When caring for clients from culturally diverse backgrounds, the nurse should recognize and identify variations in communication patterns. Communication is transmitted by body cues (e.g., touch, space, distance, position), paralinguistic cues (e.g., voice inflection, intonation, rhythm), and pronunciation and vocabulary (Giger and Davidhizar, 1999). Recognition of variations in communication patterns and familiarity with differences are important to delivering culturally appropriate care.

Nonverbal communication includes pitch, tone, and quality of the voice; use of silence; use of eye contact; posture; facial expression; gestures; object cues (e.g., clothes, jewelry, hair style); touch; and use of territorial space (Andrews and Herberg, 1999). Wide variations may exist in each of these and nurses should recognize and interpret these variations correctly and adapt practice accordingly.

DIET AND NUTRITION

Diet is one of the most significant contributors to health and illness. It is widely known and accepted that excessive intake of certain nutrients (e.g., saturated fats and calories) or lack of nutrients (e.g., protein, vitamins, minerals) adversely affects health. Heart disease, stroke, certain types of cancer, poor outcomes of pregnancy, growth retardation, and other health problems have been linked to diet.

Food preferences are usually developed during childhood and are reflective of cultural heritage, lifestyle, socioeconomic status, religion, education, and lifestyle. In addition, there may be dramatic regional variations in food consumption and preferences (Andrews, 1999b). In most cultures, food is very important. Food brings people together, promotes common interests, and stimulates bonds with other people and society. Andrews (1999b, pp. 345-346) outlined the following cultural functions of food:

- Food enables people to maintain body functions and produce energy.

- Food is used to establish and maintain social and cultural relationships with relatives, friends, strangers, and others.
- Food functions to assess social relationships or interpersonal closeness or distance between people.
- Food helps in coping with emotional stresses, conflicts, and traumatic life events.
- Food is used to reward, punish, and influence the behavior of others.
- Food influences the political and economic status of an individual or group.
- Food is used to assess, treat, and prevent illness or disabilities of people.

Nurses need to be aware of the dietary practices of members of the cultural groups with which they work to recognize potential threats to health and to attempt to modify them as appropriate. Reducing sodium intake for blacks with hypertension; encouraging overweight, middle-class whites with cardiac problems to eat more fruits and vegetables and reduce saturated fats in their diets; modifying the carbohydrate and fat content of diabetic Hispanics; and increasing protein intake in pregnant Asians are examples of frequently encountered dietary challenges.

RELIGION

Having at least a basic understanding of the religious beliefs and practices of clients is extremely important in delivering holistic nursing care. Increasingly, spiritual care is being recognized to be as important as caring for the biological and psychosocial needs of clients. This is particularly evident when working with clients who are very ill or elderly or are at significant developmental stages (e.g., childbirth, puberty, death). Knowledge of religious prohibitions, practices, rules, and rituals can be extremely helpful. For example, awareness of baptism rites, circumcision practices, prayer requirements, and an appropriate religious leader (e.g., priest, minister, rabbi) can assist the nurse in providing the most appropriate assistive care for the client and his or her family.

Almost 60% of U.S. residents are Protestant Christians (e.g., Baptist, Methodist, Presbyterian, Lutheran, Episcopalian). Roman Catholics are the second most common religious group (25% of the general population) and comprise the majority in some areas (e.g., South Louisiana and areas with large concentrations of Hispanics) (Spector, 1996). Other fairly commonly encountered religions, varying greatly by geographic area, include Islam, Judaism, Buddhism, and Hinduism. Table 8-3 describes general information that may affect health and health care for the more commonly encountered religions.

CULTURAL VARIATIONS IN HEALTH AND ILLNESS

When working with clients from a variety of ethnic and racial groups, nurses in community settings must also be familiar with biocultural variations in health and illness. All nurses should recognize these differences and plan care accordingly (e.g., provide anticipatory teaching on signs and symptoms of diabetes to clients in high-risk groups, such as Native Americans or Filipino-Americans). To assist in learning a little about differences in health and illness among different cultural groups, some important characteristics of several groups are described briefly.

AFRICAN-AMERICANS

In the United States, African-Americans comprise about 12% of the total population. The majority of black Americans are direct descendants of West African slaves brought to the United States during the seventeenth century (Spector, 1996). More recently, black immigrants have come to the United States from Caribbean countries (predominately Haiti, the Dominican Republic, and Jamaica). Although blacks live throughout the country, greater percentages live in certain states (predominately the southern states) and urban areas (e.g., Washington, DC, Detroit, and Chicago). About 28% of blacks live below the poverty level (USDHHS, 2000).

Common Health Problems

As mentioned previously, there is significant disparity between health indicators of blacks and other racial groups. For example, the life expectancy for blacks born in 1997 is 71.1 years, whereas for whites, it is 77.2 years. In addition, the difference in life expectancy between male and female whites and blacks is also significant. White women born in 1997 should expect to live 79.9 years as opposed to 74.7 years for black women and white men born in 1997 have a life expectancy of 74.3 years compared with 67.2 years for black men (USDHHS/National Center for Health Statistics [NCHS], 1999).

Although coronary artery disease mortality rates are similar in black and white men, women's rates of heart disease are higher in blacks. Probably the most distinctive difference is in cerebrovascular disease, where stroke accounts for much of the excess mortality in blacks compared with whites. In part, this may be from the prevalence of hypertension in blacks, for whom high blood pressure develops at a younger age and tends to be more severe than in whites. Indeed, it is estimated that some 40% of blacks are hypertensive (USDHHS, 2000).

Although the incidence of cancer is similar between the racial groups, the overall mortality rate for cancer is significantly higher in blacks (268.5 per 100,000 for blacks and 202.2 per 100,000 for whites) (USDHHS, 2000). Additionally, the rates for some of the most common cancers are higher for blacks than for whites as shown in Table 8-4. This possibly is the result of delayed diagnosis and treatment.

Several other significant differences are found in rates of morbidity and mortality. For example, diabetes is one third more common among blacks than among whites. Black babies are more than twice as likely as are white babies to die in their first year of life. Homicide is the most frequent cause of death for black men 15 to 24 years of age, a rate seven times greater than for white men in the same age group (USDHHS, 2000).

TABLE **8-3** Selected Religious Beliefs and Practices and Nursing Implications

RELIGION	TITLE OF RELIGIOUS REPRESENTATIVE	BELIEFS AND PRACTICES	DIETARY PRACTICES	NURSING AND HEALTH CARE ISSUES	ISSUES RELATED TO DEATH AND DYING
Buddhism (Buddhist Churches of America)	Priest	Founded in sixth century B.C. in India by S. Gautama (Buddha). The goal of Buddhism is to attain "Nirvana," in which the mind has supreme tranquility, purity, and stability. Buddha means "enlightened one." Nirvana is attained through "right" views, intention, speech, action, livelihood, effort, mindfulness, and concentration.	No specified restrictions. Extremes of diet are discouraged.	Emphasis is on the person living now. *Reproduction issues:* Birth control is acceptable. Abortion may be acceptable under certain conditions.	*Prolonging life:* If there is hope for recovery and the continuation of the pursuit of enlightenment, all measures of support are encouraged; if the person cannot continue to seek enlightenment, conditions may may permit euthanasia. *Organ donation:* If donation will help another seek enlightenment, it may be encouraged. *Body disposal:* Temple funeral with burial or cremation is common.
Catholicism	Priest	The Roman Catholic Church recognizes seven sacraments: Baptism, Reconciliation, Holy Communion (Eucharist), Confirmation, Matrimony, Holy Orders, and Anointing of the Sick (Extreme Unction).	Fasting and abstaining from meat and meat products may be condoned on certain Holy Days. Alcohol and tobacco may be used in moderation.	*Reproduction issues:* Only natural means of birth control (abstinence, rhythm method) are acceptable. The church teaches the sanctity of life and that abortion is morally wrong.	*Prolonging life:* Ordinary means of preserving life are obligated, but extraordinary means are not. Direct euthanasia is not permitted. *Body disposal:* The body is usually buried following a church service. Cremation may be acceptable in certain circumstances.
Christian (Protestant) Several different denominational groups, with variations in beliefs and practices, based on denomination	Minister Pastor Priest Reverend	Salvation is through faith in the work of Jesus Christ, who was born about 4 B.C. and was crucified about 33 years later.	Usually no dietary restrictions. Many denominations expect abstinence from alcohol and tobacco.	*Reproduction issues:* Birth control is usually permitted and decided on by the family. Abortion is prohibited by some denominations and based on individual decisions in others.	*Prolonging life:* Is based on individual decision. *Body disposal:* Burial following a funeral service is typical. Cremation is usually permitted and based on individual decision.

Continued

Data from Andrews, M. M. and Hanson, P. A. (1999). Religion, culture and nursing. In M. M. Andrews and J. S. Boyle (eds). *Transcultural Concepts in Nursing Care* (3rd ed). Philadelphia: J.B. Lippincott; Carson, V. B. (1989). *Spiritual Dimensions of Nursing Practice.* Philadelphia, W.B. Saunders; Keegan, L. (1993). Spirituality. In J. M. Black and E. Matassarin-Jacobs (eds). *Luckmann and Sorensen's Medical-Surgical Nursing: A Psychophysiologic Approach* (4th ed). Philadelphia, W.B. Saunders; and Martin, W. (1985). *The Kingdom of the Cults.* Minneapolis, MN, Bethany House Publishers.

TABLE 8-3 Selected Religious Beliefs and Practices and Nursing Implications—cont'd

RELIGION	TITLE OF RELIGIOUS REPRESENTATIVE	BELIEFS AND PRACTICES	DIETARY PRACTICES	NURSING AND HEALTH CARE ISSUES	ISSUES RELATED TO DEATH AND DYING
Christian Scientist (Church of Christ, Scientist)	There are no clergy. Practitioners are lay members of the church.	Founded by Mary Baker Eddy in the late 1800s. Christian Scientists believe that God heals through prayer, which results in drawing closer to God in thinking and living.	No dietary restrictions. Alcohol and tobacco are not used. Coffee and tea may also be declined.	Do not normally seek medical care or take medications. A surgeon may be employed to set a broken bone. They seek exemption from immunizations; will allow treatment for minor children if required by law. *Reproduction issues:* Birth control is left to individual judgment. An obstetrician or midwife may be used for delivery.	*Prolonging life:* A Christian Scientist family is unlikely to seek medical care to prolong life. Euthanasia is contrary to the teaching of Christian Science. *Body disposal:* Burial and burial service are decided on by the individual family.
Church of Jesus Christ of Latter-Day Saints (Mormonism)	Elder	Founded in the 1820s by Joseph Smith, whose writings included *The Pearl of Great Price* and *The Book of Mormon*, which were given to him by God through visions. There are two sects, the initial church based in Salt Lake City, Utah and the reorganized church based in Independence, Missouri. Mormons believe salvation is based on faith in Christ, baptism by immersion, obedience to the teaching of the Mormon Church, good works, and keeping the commandments of God.	Abstinence from tobacco, alcohol, and beverages with caffeine (e.g., coffee, tea, colas) is required. Meat is permitted, but dietary intake of fruits, grains, and herbs is encouraged. Fasting one day per month is required.	Cleanliness is very important. A sacred undergarment may be worn at all times and should only be removed in emergencies. *Reproduction issues:* Procreation is one of the major purposes of life, and prevention of conception is contrary to teachings. Abortion is opposed except when the life of the mother is in danger.	*Prolonging life:* When possible, medicine and faith are used to reverse conditions that threaten life. If death is inevitable, efforts to promote peaceful and dignified death are encouraged.
Islam	Imam	Monotheistic religion founded between 610 and 631 A.D. by Mohammed. Followers are called Moslems or Muslims. Islam means subjection to the will of Allah (God). Good deeds will be rewarded at the last judgment and evil deeds will be punished in hell. There are five essential practices: acknowledgment of Allah as the one God and Mohammed as his messenger; praying five times daily (dawn, noon, afternoon, sunset, and night)	No pork is allowed. "Halal" (permissible) meats must be blessed and slaughtered in a directed manner (Zabihah). Alcohol is prohibited. All adults except pregnant women, nursing mothers, the elderly, and the ill are required to fast during Ramadan.	*Reproductive issues:* Contraception is permitted, but many conservative Muslims do not use contraception because it is viewed as interference in God's will. Abortion is objectionable, although there is no official policy. The husband must sign consent forms regarding family planning. Women are very modest and this should be respected during examination.	*Prolonging life:* Any attempt to shorten a life or terminate it is prohibited. *Body disposal:* Donation of body parts or organs is not allowed. Burial of the dead is compulsory and follows a prescribed procedure consisting of ritually washing the body, wrapping of the body in white cloth, special prayers for the dead, burial as soon as possible with the head facing Mecca. A fetus older than 130 days of

	Religious leader	Beliefs	Dietary practices	Birth/Circumcision/Reproductive	Death/Prolonging life
(Islam, continued)		facing Mecca, Saudi Arabia; giving alms to the needy; fasting from dawn until sunset throughout Ramadan (the ninth month of the Islamic calendar); and making one pilgrimage to Mecca if able.		Circumcision is practiced on male children at an early age. For adult converts, it is sometimes practiced, although not required.	gestation is treated as a human and buried in the same manner.
Jehovah's Witnesses	Religious titles are generally not used.	Founded by Charles Taze Russell during the 1870s and 1880s in Pittsburgh, Pennsylvania. He began writing for the Watchtower Bible and Tract Society. Belief that 144,000 servants will rule with Jesus. Every Minister of the Watch Tower Bible and Tract Society devotes approximately 10 hours or more each month to proselytizing.	No dietary restrictions. Alcohol and tobacco are discouraged.	Blood transfusions violate God's laws and are not allowed. Some will accept alternatives to blood transfusions (e.g., nonblood plasma expanders, autologous transfusions, and autotransfusion.) *Reproductive issues:* Birth control is a personal decision, although sterilization is prohibited. Abortion is opposed.	*Prolonging life:* Right to die is a matter of individual choice, but euthanasia is prohibited. *Body disposal:* Burial or cremation is permitted.
Judaism	Rabbi	Judaism is a monotheistic religion that dates to the time of the prophet Abraham around 1900 B.C. The laws of God are contained in the Torah and explained in the Talmud and in oral tradition. There are several divisions (i.e., Orthodox, Conservative, Reform, and fundamentalist [Hasidic]). Each Sabbath (from sunset Friday to just after sunset Saturday) is a holy day and there are a number of other holy days.	Dietary laws are very strict, but the degree to which they are observed depends on the sect. In general, pork, predatory fowl, and milk with meat dishes are not eaten. Only fish with fins and scales are permissible (shellfish are prohibited). All animals should be ritually slaughtered to be kosher (properly prepared). Wine is a part of many religious observances. Alcohol is permitted in moderation. Fasting is required during Yom Kippur.	Medical care is expected according to Jewish law. Circumcision is performed on all Jewish male children on the eighth day following birth. This may be done by a ritual circumciser, by the child's father, or by a pediatrician. *Reproductive issues:* Birth control is permissible, but having children is encouraged. Therapeutic abortion is permitted if the health of the mother is jeopardized.	*Prolonging life:* Death with dignity is a right; euthanasia is strictly prohibited. Jewish beliefs include the need to not be alone when the soul leaves the body, so family or friends should be allowed to stay with dying clients. *Body disposal:* Following death, the body should not be left alone and should not be touched by medical personnel. The body will be ritually washed (usually done at a funeral home). Human remains (including a fetus at any stage of gestation) are to be buried as soon as possible. Cremation is not in keeping with Jewish law.

TABLE **8-4** Comparison of Cancer Death Rates Between Blacks and Whites (1998)

TYPE OF CANCER	DEATH RATES FOR BLACKS (PER 100,000)	DEATH RATES FOR WHITES (PER 100,000)
Lung cancer	69.6	59.9
Breast cancer	37.7	28.0
Cervical cancer	6.7	2.7
Prostate cancer	72.5	31.5
Oropharyngeal cancer	4.8	2.9
Colorectal cancer	29.5	21.4

From U.S. Department of Health and Human Services (USDHHS). (2000). *Healthy people 2010: Conference edition.* Washington DC: USDHHS.

Acquired immunodeficiency syndrome (AIDS) is particularly devastating to blacks because they account for a larger proportion of AIDS cases than do whites. Indeed, the AIDS case rate among blacks in 1998 was 66.4 per 100,000; this is eight times greater than the rate for whites (8.2 per 100,000) (USDHHS, 2000). In addition, almost 80% of AIDS cases in women and children are found in blacks (Spector, 1996).

NATIVE AMERICANS, INCLUDING ALEUTS AND INUITS

Native Americans (including Aleuts and Inuits) comprise just less than 1% of the total U.S. population; they are the smallest minority group. Although many Native Americans (approximately one third) live on reservations, most live in urban areas. Income and educational levels tend to be low. Health problems of Native Americans are often the result of poverty because slightly more than half live below the poverty level.

Common Health Problems

Alcohol abuse and obesity are the two major risk factors affecting Native American populations. Alcohol abuse is a significant health problem that contributes to other health threats, including accidental death, homicide, and suicide. It has been observed that unintentional injuries are the leading cause of death for Native American men younger than 44 years, with 75% of the injuries being alcohol related. Alcohol also contributes to other health problems more commonly found among Native Americans. For example, cirrhosis deaths are 2.5 times greater among American Indians than the total population and fetal alcohol syndrome is 5 times greater among Native Americans.

Diabetes is extremely prevalent among Native Americans. Overall, the incidence rate of diabetes for Native Americans is 8.7 per 1000 (compared with overall incidence of 3.1 per 1000 among all Americans) and in some tribal groups as many as 40% of adults are diabetic (USDHHS, 2000).

ASIANS AND PACIFIC ISLANDERS

A growing number of Americans have ancestors who have immigrated from Korea, China, Japan, Vietnam, Cambodia, Laos, and other countries. Asian and Pacific Islanders now comprise about 3% of the total population. In this group, about 13% live below the poverty level.

Because many Asians are recent immigrants and their health care customs are based on Eastern rather than Western practices, it is helpful to be aware of some of the basics of Eastern health care. Many Asian health practices are based in Chinese tradition. Chinese philosophy of health and illness is holistic in nature and integrated with the external environment. The onset, evolution, and change of diseases are considered in conjunction with geographical, social, and other environmental factors.

Yin and Yang

The terms *yin* and *yang* refer to powers that regulate the universe, with yang representing the male, positive energy, which relates to light, warmth, and fullness. Yin represents the female, negative energy, which relates to darkness, cold, and emptiness (Spector, 1996). Yin and yang regulate themselves to promote normal activities of life and health. Illness is the result of a disharmony of yin and yang.

Acupuncture is an ancient Chinese practice of using needles inserted at specific points of the body to cure disease and relieve pain. The practice and principles of acupuncture are very complex. The basic treatment goal of acupuncture is to restore the balance of yin and yang through insertion of the needles into meridians (the points on the skin corresponding to a network, or channel, of energy that runs longitudinally throughout the body) to treat the condition (Spector, 1996).

Herbology refers to the use of herbs to heal. The Chinese use many herbs and plants for medicinal and healing reasons. Herbal medicines are categorized according to their properties of yin or yang. Ginseng root is an example of an herb used to treat a number of health problems, including anemia, depression, indigestion, and impotence (Spector, 1996). Other herbal remedies include Jen Shen Lu Jung Wan, a general tonic used to improve health and improve digestion; tiger balm, a salve used for relief of minor aches and pains; and white flower, a liquid used to treat colds, influenza, headaches, and coughs (Spector, 1993).

Common Health Problems

Health problems of Asian-Americans vary greatly based on nation of origin, socioeconomic status, and length of time in the United States. In general, however, Asian-Americans have some distinct health problems. For example, liver cancer among Southeast Asians is more than 12 times higher than in whites. This is thought to be the result of endemic hepatitis B, which, in chronic carriers, predisposes to the development of hepatocellular carcinoma. Tuberculosis (TB) is still the leading cause of death in some Asian countries and is a serious threat in the United States, being much more commonly found in Asian-Americans than in white populations (USDHHS, 1990).

WHITES (AMERICANS OF EUROPEAN DESCENT)

Non-Hispanic whites make up about 72% of the U.S. population. Members of this group are descendants of immigrants from Germany, Italy, England, Scotland, Ireland, France, Austria, Russia, and several other countries. About 9% live below the poverty level.

Common Health Problems

The leading causes of deaths for whites are heart disease, cancer, stroke, and chronic obstructive pulmonary disease (COPD); these are, for the most part, diseases of aging. However, health habits and lifestyle choices contribute to morbidity and mortality. Diet and activity levels, in particular, and use of alcohol and tobacco products and unhealthy sex practices contribute to disease and death in whites.

HISPANIC, OR LATINO, AMERICANS (ALL RACES)

Hispanic Americans originate from Cuba (5%), Central and South America (14%), Mexico (60%+), Puerto Rico (11%), and other Spanish-speaking countries of the Caribbean (7.5%) and make up about 11.5% of the total U.S. population. They represent the fastest-growing ethnic group. Although Hispanics live in all states, the greatest concentrations are found in southern border states (i.e., California, Arizona, New Mexico, Texas), Florida, and New York. As a rule, the Hispanic population is very young and has a high birth rate. About 24% of Hispanics live below the poverty level (USDHHS, 2000).

Balance of "Hot" and "Cold"

According to Stasiak (1991), Mexican-Americans consider health to be a state of well-being brought on by eating proper foods and maintaining a "hot/cold" balance in the foods eaten. Illness, to many Hispanic groups, is an imbalance in the body between "hot" and "cold" and "wet" and "dry." The belief is that a hot illness must be treated with a cold substance and vice versa.

Hot or cold does not refer to temperature, but to the substance itself, and foods, beverages, illnesses, and people can be considered hot or cold. Examples of hot conditions are fever, infections, diarrhea, liver problems, and constipation. Cold conditions include cancer, pneumonia, menstrual period, earache, and stomach cramps. Examples of hot foods are chocolate, coffee, corn meal, cheese, eggs, onions, hard liquor, beef, and chili peppers; cold foods include vegetables, fruits, dairy products, fish, chicken, and honey. Hot medicines and herbs include penicillin, tobacco, garlic, cinnamon, vitamins, and aspirin; cold medicines and herbs include sage, milk of magnesia, and bicarbonate of soda (Kuipers, 1999).

Traditional Illness Management and Healers

Although practices vary greatly depending on the ethnic group, traditional or folk healers and religious rituals are sometimes used by Hispanics to treat illness. The use of religious signs, symbols, rituals, and practices is common. The most popular forms of treatment combine Catholic rituals, such as offerings of money, penance, confession, lighting candles, and laying on of hands, with the medicinal use of teas and herbs (Spector, 1996). Examples of Hispanic folk healers are the curandero, the yerbero, and the partera.

A *curandero (curandera)* is a holistic healer, who may be "called" by God or be born with a "gift" of healing and/or may serve an apprenticeship (Spector, 1996). A curandero develops a very personal relationship with the client and the goal of care is to restore harmony with the social, physical, and psychological parts of the person. A central focus of the treatment is relieving clients of their sins, which can cause an imbalance between God and people. Treatment is often provided in a room in the curandero's home that is decorated with religious paraphernalia and may include massage, diet, rest, practical advice, herbs, prayers, magic, and/or supernatural rituals (Kuipers, 1999).

A *yerbero* is a folk healer who specializes in using herbs and spices (Kuipers, 1999) and a *partera* is a Mexican-American midwife (Spector, 1993). Nurses should be aware of common folk treatments, such as herbal teas and roots, used by these traditional healers and question clients decorously and not judgmentally. It should be noted that many traditional health practices have been shown to be beneficial (Stasiak, 1991).

Common Health Problems

Hispanics experience the greatest disparity in health and health problems among American minority groups. Infant mortality rates, for example, vary substantially between cultural groups—Puerto Ricans living in the United States have almost twice the infant mortality rate of Cuban-Americans. Hispanics have a very high birth rate (22.3 births per 1000 women, compared with 15.7 births per 1000 women in the total U.S. population) (USDHHS, 1990). Unintentional injuries, AIDS, and homicide affect Hispanics disproportionately. Diabetes is also very prevalent among Mexican-Americans, as is obesity; this is particularly true for Mexican-American women.

PRINCIPLES FOR NURSING PRACTICE IN COMMUNITY SETTINGS

One of the barriers to provision of culturally sensitive nursing care is the failure to recognize and appreciate the impact of the culture of the health care providers. Health care providers have been socialized into a given culture (usually the dominant cultural group of middle-class white) and then further socialized into the culture of their profession. "Professional socialization teaches the student a set of beliefs, practices, habits, likes, dislikes, norms and rituals...." Therefore "health-care providers can be viewed as a foreign culture or ethnic group" (Spector, 1996, pp. 75-76). As a result, it is very important that all nurses seek to realize the impact of their personal culture and the culture of health care providers on their own behavior, values, and practices.

Following recognition of their own cultural beliefs, values, and biases, nurses can learn to better recognize and appreciate the beliefs, values, and biases of others and to use this information to improve nursing care. Allender and Spradley (2001) succinctly summarized cultural principles for practice for nurses who work in community settings. These principles are the following:

- Develop cultural self-awareness
- Cultivate cultural sensitivity
- Assess client group's culture
- Show respect and patience while learning about other cultures
- Examine culturally derived health practices.

Adherence to these principles promotes culturally competent nursing care. Resources for transcultural nursing and for groups and organizations that encourage culture sensitivity are included in the Resources box at the end of the chapter.

SUMMARY

The United States is comprised of people from many different cultural groups and each of these groups has its own distinctive values, methods of communication, diet, and religious beliefs and practices among other characteristics. In addition, members of different racial, ethnic, and cultural groups have health threats and risks associated with their particular biological, psychological, social, and lifestyle factors.

Like most nurses, Trisha, the nurse from the opening case study, works with clients from various cultures and realizes that culturally competent nursing care should be a priority of all nurses. In the community, however, a recognition of how culture impacts health behaviors, health beliefs and health practices is particularly important. Thus, to practice holistically, nurses should strive to learn about other cultures and to understand and use the information in providing nursing care.

Resources

Cultural Care and Transcultural Nursing

Transcultural Nursing Society
National Association of Hispanic Nurses
National Black Nurses Association
International Council of Nurses
Office of Minority Health
National Center on Minority Health and Health
   Disparities
Indian Health Services

Visit the book's website at
www.wbsaunders.com/SIMON/McEwen
for a direct link to the website for each
organization listed.

KEY POINTS

- The United States is becoming increasingly ethnically diverse and this affects health and health care delivery, particularly for nurses in community-based practice.
- Numerous nursing organizations have recognized the need to provide culturally sensitive and culturally competent nursing care; the Transcultural Nursing Society was established in 1973.
- Race refers to classification of humans based on physical characteristics and there are nine recognized distinct races. An ethnic group is a group of people who share common distinctive characteristics, such as race, ancestry, nationality, language, religion, food preferences, literature, music, and a common history. There are more than 100 ethnic groups in the United States. Culture is closely tied to ethnicity and refers to values, beliefs, attitudes, and customs that provide the organizational structure or basis for behavior within the group. A subculture is a relatively large subsection of a cultural group that has distinctive characteristics that set it apart from the group as a whole.
- Community-based nurses may need to perform a cultural assessment to help recognize the impact of culture on health and health practices. Identification of cultural values should be a component of a cultural assessment.

- Cultural variations based on socioeconomic levels or class can greatly influence health and health-seeking behaviors. Socioeconomic class creates a set of values and role expectations regarding sex, marriage, parenting, birth, education, dress, housing, occupation, and religion.
- Language barriers are frequently encountered when working with members of other cultural groups. Appropriate use of an interpreter and tips for communication without an interpreter can be helpful for nurses working in community-based settings. Familiarity with variations in communication patterns between various cultural groups can also be helpful.
- Cultural factors that also contribute significantly to health and illness include diet and nutrition and religion.
- Cultural variations occur in health, illness, and health practices. Nurses working with significant numbers of persons from a cultural group should be aware of these variations and practices.

Learning Activities & Application to Practice

In Class

1. Talk with classmates from racial or ethnic minorities. Share differences in values, norms, religion, and health beliefs and discuss how these factors influence health practices and might affect health care delivery. Explore ways that nurses can develop sensitivity to other cultural groups.
2. Review *Healthy People 2010* objectives that relate to minority health. Discuss interventions to address the objectives with classmates.
3. Complete a cultural self-assessment and share findings with classmates.

In Clinical

4. Review census data from your area to identify the percentages of persons from non-European origin in the local community. If possible, compare with previous data (e.g., has the percentage increased since 1980? Since 1990?). What are projections for the future?

5. Identify an individual or family from a cultural minority and perform a cultural assessment. Share findings with the clinical group.
6. Outline, in a diary or log, health practices, health problems, and other observations uniquely related to race, culture, or ethnicity encountered in clinical practice. Share these with the clinical group. Were any assessments or interventions performed based on racial, ethnic, or cultural variations?

REFERENCES

Allender, J. A., & Spradley, B. W. (2001). *Community health nursing: Concepts and practice* (5th ed.). Philadelphia: Lippincott.

American Academy of Nursing. (1992). AAN expert panel report: Culturally competent health care. *Nursing Outlook, 40*(6), 277-283.

Andrews, M. M. (1992). Cultural perspectives on nursing in the 21st century. *Journal of Professional Nursing, 8*(1), 1-9.

Andrews, M. M. (1999a). Theoretical foundations of transcultural nursing. In M. M. Andrews & J. S. Boyle (Eds.), *Transcultural concepts in nursing care* (3rd ed., pp. 3-22). Philadelphia: J. B. Lippincott.

Andrews, M. M. (1999b). Culture and nutrition. In M. M. Andrews & J. S. Boyle (Eds.), *Transcultural concepts in nursing care* (3rd ed., pp. 341-377). Philadelphia: J. B. Lippincott.

Andrews, M. M. (2001). Cultural diversity and community health nursing. In M. A. Nies & M. McEwen (Eds.), *Community health nursing: Promoting the health of populations* (3rd ed., pp. 242-285). Philadelphia: W. B. Saunders.

Andrews, M. M., & Boyle, J. S. (1999). *Transcultural concepts in nursing care* (3rd ed.). Philadelphia: J. B. Lippincott.

Andrews, M. M., & Herberg, P. (1999). Transcultural nursing care. In M. M. Andrews & J. S. Boyle (Eds.), *Transcultural concepts in nursing care* (3rd ed., pp. 23-78). Philadelphia: J. B. Lippincott.

Garn, S. M. (1985). Human races. In *World book encyclopedia*. (Vol. 16). Chicago: World Book, Inc.

Giger, J. N., & Davidhizar, R. E. (1999). *Transcultural nursing: Assessment & intervention* (3rd ed.). St. Louis: Mosby.

Herberg, P. (1995). Theoretical foundations of transcultural nursing. In M. M. Andrews & J. S. Boyle (Eds.), *Transcultural concepts in nursing care* (2nd ed., pp. 3-48). Philadelphia: J. B. Lippincott.

Kuipers, J. (1999). Mexican Americans. In J. N. Giger & R. E. Davidhizar (Eds.), *Transcultural nursing:*

Assessment and intervention (3rd ed., pp. 203-236). St. Louis: Mosby.

Leininger, M. M. (2001a). The theory of culture care diversity and universality. In M. M. Leininger (Ed.), *Culture care diversity & universality: A theory of nursing* (pp. 5-71). Boston: Jones and Bartlett Publishers.

Leininger, M. M. (2001b). Selected culture care findings of diverse cultures using culture care theory and ethnomethods. In M. M. Leininger (Ed.), *Culture care diversity & universality: A theory of nursing* (pp. 345-371). Boston: Jones and Bartlett Publishers.

Murray, R. B., Zentner, R. M. J., & Samiezade'-Yazd, C. (2001). Sociocultural influences on the person and family. In R. B. Murray & J. P. Zentner (Eds.), *Nursing assessment and health promotion: Strategies through the life span* (7th ed.). Upper Saddle River, NJ: Prentice Hall.

National Center for Health Statistics. (2000). Deaths: Final Data for 1998. *National Vital Statistic Report 48*(11), 1-106.

Spector, R. E. (1993). Culture, ethnicity and nursing. In P. A. Potter & A. G. Perry (Eds.), *Fundamentals of nursing: Concepts, process & practice* (pp. 94-119). St. Louis: Mosby.

Spector, R. E. (1996). *Cultural diversity in health & illness* (4th ed.). Stamford, CT: Appleton & Lange.

Stasiak, D. B. (1991). Culture care theory with Mexican-Americans in an urban context. In M. M. Leininger (Ed.), *Culture care diversity & universality: A theory of nursing* (pp. 179-202). (Publication No. 15-2402). New York: National League for Nursing Press.

U.S. Bureau of the Census. (2001a). Projections of the resident population by race, Hispanic origin and nativity: 2000. Retrieved 2/6/02 http://www.census.gov/population/projections/nation/summary/np-t5-a.txt.

U.S. Bureau of the Census. (2001b). Projections of the resident population by race, Hispanic origin, and nativity: 2025-2045. Retrieved 2/6/02 http://www.census.gov/population/projections/nation/summary/np-t5-f.txt.

U.S. Department of Health and Human Services (USDHHS). (1990). *Healthy people 2000: National health promotion and disease prevention objectives.* (Publication No. (PHS)91-50212). Washington, DC: Government Printing Office.

U.S. Department of Health and Human Services (USDHHS). (2000). *Healthy people 2010: Conference edition.* Washington DC: Government Printing Office.

U.S. Department of Health and Human Services/ National Center for Health Statistics. (1999). U.S. Life Tables, 1997. *National Vital Statistics Report, 47*(28), 1-38. Hyattsville, MD: U.S. Department of Health and Human Services/National Center for Health Statistics.

Appendix 8-A

Andrews/Boyle Transcultural Nursing Assessment Guide

CULTURAL AFFILIATIONS

With what cultural group(s) does the client report affiliation (e.g., American, Hispanic, Navajo, or combination)? To what degree does the client identify with the cultural group (e.g., "we" concept of solidarity or as a fringe member)?

Where was the client born?

Where has the client lived (country, city) and when (during what years)? Note: If the client has recently relocated to the United States, knowledge of prevalent diseases in the country of origin may be helpful. Current residence? Occupation?

VALUES ORIENTATION

What are the client's attitudes, values, and beliefs about developmental life events such as birth and death, health, illness, and health care providers?

Does culture affect the manner in which the client relates to body image change resulting from illness or surgery (e.g., importance of appearance, beauty, strength, and roles in cultural group)? Is there a cultural stigma associated with the client's illness (i.e., how is the illness or client condition viewed by the larger culture)?

How does the client view work, leisure, and education?

How does the client perceive change?

How does the client perceive changes in lifestyle relating to current illness or surgery?

How does the client value privacy, courtesy, touch, and relationships with individuals of different ages, social class (or caste), and gender?

How does the client view biomedical/scientific health care (e.g., suspiciously, fearfully, acceptingly)? How does the client relate to persons outside of his or her cultural group (e.g., withdrawal, verbally or nonverbally expressive, negatively or positively)?

CULTURAL SANCTIONS AND RESTRICTIONS

How does the client's cultural group regard expression of emotion and feelings, spirituality, and religious beliefs? How are dying, death, and grieving expressed in a culturally appropriate manner?

How is modesty expressed by men and women? Are there culturally defined expectations about male-female relationships, including the nurse-client relationship?

Does the client have any restrictions related to sexuality, exposure of body parts, or certain types of surgery (e.g., amputation, vasectomy, hysterectomy)?

Are there any restrictions against discussion of dead relatives or fears related to the unknown?

COMMUNICATION

What language does the client speak at home? What other languages does the client speak or read? In what language would the client prefer to communicate with you?

What is the fluency level of the client in English—both written and spoken use of the language? Remember that the stress of illness may cause clients to use a more familiar language and to temporarily forget some English.

Does the client need an interpreter? If so, is there a relative or friend whom the client would like to interpret? Is there anyone whom the client would prefer did not serve as an interpreter (e.g., member of the opposite sex, a person younger/older than the client, member of a rival tribe or nation)?

What are the rules (linguistics) and modes (style) of communication? How does the client prefer to be addressed?

Is it necessary to vary the technique of communication during the interview and examination to accommodate the client's cultural background (e.g., tempo of conversation, eye contact, sensitivity to topical taboos, norms of confidentiality, and style of explanation)?

How does the client's nonverbal communication compare with that of individuals from other cultural backgrounds? How does it affect the client's relationship with you and with other members of the health care team?

How does the client feel about health care providers who are not of the same cultural background (e.g., black, middle-class nurse and Hispanic of a different social class)?

Does the client prefer to receive care from a nurse of the same cultural background, gender, and/or age?

What are the overall cultural characteristics of the client's language and communication processes?

HEALTH-RELATED BELIEFS AND PRACTICES

To what cause(s) does the client attribute illness and disease (e.g., divine wrath, imbalance in hot/cold or yin/yang, punishment for moral transgressions, hex, soul loss, pathogenic organism)?

What are the client's cultural beliefs about ideal body size and shape? What is the client's self-image vis-á-vis the ideal?

What name does the client give to his or her health-related condition?

What does the client believe promotes health (e.g., eating certain foods; wearing amulets to bring good luck; sleep; rest; good nutrition; reducing stress; exercise; prayer, rituals to ancestors, saints, or intermediate deities)?

What is the client's religious affiliation (e.g., Judaism, Islam, Pentacostalism, West African voodooism, Seventh-Day Adventism, Catholicism, Mormonism)? How actively involved in the practice of this religion is the client?

Does the client rely on cultural healers (e.g., curandero, shaman, spiritualist, priest, minister, monk)? Who determines when the client is sick and when he or she is healthy? Who influences the choice/type of healer and treatment that should be sought?

In what types of cultural healing practices does the client engage (e.g., use of herbal remedies; potions; massage; wearing of talismans, copper bracelets, or charms to discourage evil spirits; healing rituals; incantations; prayers)?

How are biomedical/scientific health care providers perceived? How does the client and his or her family perceive nurses? What are the expectations of nurses and nursing care?

What comprises appropriate "sick role" behavior? Who determines what symptoms constitute disease/illness? Who decides when the client is no longer sick? Who cares for the client at home?

How does the client's cultural group view mental disorders? Are there differences in acceptable behaviors for physical versus psychological illnesses?

NUTRITION

What nutritional factors are influenced by the client's cultural background? What is the meaning of food and eating to the client?

With whom does the client usually eat? What types of foods are eaten? What is the timing and sequencing of meals?

What does the client define as food? What does the client believe comprises a "healthy" versus an "unhealthy" diet?

Who shops for food? Where are groceries purchased (e.g., special markets or ethnic grocery stores)? Who prepares the client's meals?

How are foods prepared at home (type of food preparation, cooking oil[s] used, length of time foods are cooked [especially vegetables], amount and type of seasoning added to various foods during preparation)?

Has the client chosen a particular nutritional practice such as vegetarianism or abstinence from alcoholic or fermented beverages?

Do religious beliefs and practices influence the client's diet (e.g., amount, type, preparation, or delineation of acceptable food combinations [e.g., kosher diets])? Does the client abstain from certain foods at regular intervals, on specific dates determined by the religious calendar, or at other times?

If the client's religion mandates or encourages fasting, what does the term *fast* mean (e.g., refraining from certain types or quantities of foods, eating only during certain times of the day)? For what period of time is the client expected to fast?

During fasting, does the client refrain from liquids/beverages? Does the religion allow exemption from fasting during illness? If so, does the client believe that an exemption applies to him or her?

SOCIOECONOMIC CONSIDERATIONS

Who comprises the client's social network (e.g., family, friends, peers, and cultural healers)? How do they influence the client's health or illness status?

How do members of the client's social support network define caring (e.g., being con-tinuously present, doing things for the client, providing material support, looking after the client's family)? What is the role of various family members during health and illness?

How does the client's family participate in the promotion of health (e.g., lifestyle changes in diet, activity level) and nursing care (e.g., bathing, feeding, touching, being present) of the client?

Does the cultural family structure influence the client's response to health or illness (e.g., beliefs, strengths, weaknesses, and social class)? Is there a key family member whose role is significant in health-related decisions (e.g., grandmother in many African-American fami-lies or eldest adult son in Asian families)?

Who is the principal wage earner in the client's family? What is the total annual income? (Note: This is a potentially sensitive question.) Is there more than one wage earner? Are there other sources of financial support (extended family, investments)?

What insurance coverage (e.g., health, dental, vision, pregnancy) does the client have?

What impact does economic status have on lifestyle, place of residence, living conditions, and ability to obtain health care? How does the client's home environment (e.g., presence of indoor plumbing, handicap access) influence nursing care?

ORGANIZATIONS PROVIDING CULTURAL SUPPORT

What influence do ethnic/cultural organiza-tions have on the client's receiving health care (e.g., Organization of Migrant Workers; National Association for the Advancement of Colored People [NAACP]; Black Political Caucus; churches such as African-American, Muslim, Jewish, and others; schools, including those that are church-related; Urban League; community-based health care programs and clinics).

EDUCATIONAL BACKGROUND

What is the client's highest education level obtained?

Does the client's educational background affect his or her knowledge level concerning the health care delivery system, how to obtain the needed care, teaching-learning, and any written material that he or she is given in the health care setting (e.g., insurance forms, educational literature, information about diagnostic procedures and laboratory tests, admissions forms)?

Can the client read and write English, or is another language preferred? If English is the client's second language, are materials available in the client's primary language?

What learning style is most comfortable/familiar? Does the client prefer to learn through written materials, oral explanation, or demonstration?

RELIGIOUS AFFILIATION

How does the client's religious affiliation affect health and illness (e.g., life events such as death, chronic illness, body image alteration, cause and effect of illness)?

What is the role of religious beliefs and practices during health and illness? Are there special rites or blessings for those with serious or terminal illnesses?

Are there healing rituals or practices that the client believes can promote well-being or hasten recovery from illness? If so, who performs these?

What is the role of significant religious representatives during health and illness? Are there recognized religious healers (e.g., Islamic imams, Christian Scientist practitioners or nurses, Catholic priests, Mormon elders, Buddhist monks)?

CULTURAL ASPECTS OF DISEASE INCIDENCE

Are any specific genetic or acquired conditions more prevalent for a specific cultural group (e.g.,

hypertension, sickle cell anemia, Tay-Sachs, Glucose-6-phosphate dehydrogenase (G6PD) lactose intolerance)?

Are socioenvironmental diseases more prevalent among a specific cultural group (e.g., lead poisoning, alcoholism, HIV/AIDS, drug abuse, ear infections, family violence)?

Does the client have an increased resistance to any diseases (e.g., skin cancer in darkly pigmented individuals, malaria for those with sickle cell anemia)?

BIOCULTURAL VARIATIONS

Does the client have distinctive physical features characteristic of a particular ethnic or cultural group (e.g., skin color, hair texture)? Does the client have any variations in anatomy characteristic of a particular ethnic or cultural group (e.g., body structure, height, weight, facial shape and structure [nose, eye shape, facial contour], upper and lower extremities)?

How do anatomical and racial variations affect the physical examination?

DEVELOPMENTAL CONSIDERATIONS

Do any distinct growth and development characteristics vary with the client's cultural background (e.g., bone density, psychomotor patterns of development, fat folds)?

What factors are significant in assessing children of various ages from the newborn period through adolescence (e.g., expected growth on standard grid, culturally acceptable age for toilet training, introducing various types of foods, gender differences, discipline, socialization to adult roles)?

What is the cultural perception of aging (e.g., is youthfulness or the wisdom of old age more highly valued)?

How are elderly persons handled culturally (e.g., cared for in the home of adult children, placed in institutions for care)? What are culturally acceptable roles for the elderly?

Does the elderly person expect family members to provide care, including nurturance and other humanistic aspects of care?

Is the elderly person isolated from culturally relevant supportive persons or enmeshed in a caring network of relatives and friends?

Has a culturally appropriate network replaced family members in performing some caring functions for the elderly person?

From Andrews, M. M., & Boyle, J. S. (1999). *Transcultural concepts in nursing care* (3rd ed., pp. 539-544). Philadelphia: J. B. Lippincott.

Three

Community-Based Nursing Care Across the Life Span

Health Promotion and Illness Prevention for Infants, Children, and Adolescents

Upon completion of this chapter, the reader will be able to:

1. Discuss the leading causes of morbidity and mortality for infants, small children, school-aged children, and adolescents.

2. Identify federal and state-sponsored health programs and services for children and explain eligibility requirements and referral processes.

3. Describe recommendations for screening and education for major causes of morbidity and mortality for infants, children, and adolescents.

4. Describe health promotion interventions for infants, children, and adolescents, including nutrition, physical activities, sleep and rest, dental health, and maturation and puberty.

5. Describe prevention interventions for infants, children, and adolescents, focusing on prevention of substance abuse, use of tobacco, and safety issues.

6. Discuss detection, prevention, and management of child abuse.

key terms

Anemia screening
Bottle mouth syndrome
Child abuse
Child safety
Developmental screening

Early and Periodic Screening, Diagnosis and Treatment Program (EPSDT)
Head Start
Hearing screening
Newborn screening

State Children's Health Insurance Program (SCHIP)
Vision screening
Women, Infants and Children Program (WIC)

See Glossary for definitions.

case study

Bonnie Dalton is a registered nurse working in a private pediatric office in a small city. In her position, Bonnie assists the pediatrician and pediatric nurse practitioner (PNP) by taking health histories, weighing and measuring the children, performing health teaching for the children and parents, administering medications, and assisting with some diagnostic and screening procedures (e.g., strep cultures, fingersticks), and performing many other interventions.

Last Monday, Bonnie saw Sally Benson for her 6-month well check. Sally was brought to the clinic by her mother. Bonnie observed that Sally was appropriately dressed, smiling, and responsive. Bonnie asked Mrs. Benson to remove Sally's clothes. While this was being completed, Bonnie questioned her about Sally's eating and sleeping patterns and general health. She learned that Sally is breastfed and nurses six to eight times per day. Currently, she is being given only supplemental apple juice and an occasional bottle of formula when Mrs. Benson leaves her with a babysitter. Sally sleeps 10 to 11 hours at night, occasionally waking, and naps twice daily, for 1 to 2 hours.

Bonnie weighed and measured Sally and plotted the findings on a graphic chart kept in Sally's file. She noted that Sally weighed 17 pounds and measured 27 inches—a gain of 3 pounds and an increase of 1.5 inches since her 4-month visit. According to the chart, Sally's height and weight placed her within the seventy-fifth percentile for girls of her age.

When questioned, Mrs. Benson reported that Sally always rode in her car seat; plugs were on all electrical outlets; and harmful substances and medications were in childproof, latched cabinets. Other safety issues discussed included smoke detectors near the bedrooms and hot water heater temperature.

Bonnie assisted the PNP with a head-to-toe physical examination and Denver II Screening Test. All findings from both the physical and developmental examinations were considered normal for Sally's age.

The PNP instructed Mrs. Benson on slowly adding solid foods to Sally's diet and Bonnie gave her several pamphlets and instruction guides kept in the clinic. The nurses also discussed several other safety issues, including poison control. Mrs. Benson was counseled to buy syrup of ipecac and to keep the number of the local poison control center near her telephone.

Routine neonatal screening tests (phenylketonuria, thyroid function, hemoglobin) had been performed shortly after Sally was born and all results were normal. She was up to date on her immunizations and was scheduled to get her third vaccinations for hepatitis B, diphtheria/tetanus/pertussis, polio, and *Haemophilus influenzae* B. Mrs. Benson reported that the only problem from previous immunizations was a slight fever during the afternoon and evening of the injections, which responded to administration of acetaminophen. Mrs. Benson was counseled again concerning possible side effects of immunizations and how to manage them.

Bonnie gave Sally the immunizations. Sally cried a little, but was consoled by her mother and stopped crying quickly. Mrs. Benson was encouraged to give Sally acetaminophen and to call the office if she developed a temperature higher than 103°F or was crying inconsolably. Finally, Mrs. Benson was instructed to bring Sally back for her next well check when she was 12 to 15 months old.

THE HEALTH OF INFANTS, CHILDREN, AND ADOLESCENTS

Preventative health care for infants and children has had a profound effect on morbidity and mortality. In 1900, 87% of infants lived to age 1 year and only 77% survived to age 20 years. In comparison, in 1997, 99.3% of infants survived until their first birthday and 98.6% could expect to live to age 20 (National Center for Health Statistics [NCHS], 1999). This increase has been attributed to several factors. Improved prenatal and intrapartum care has reduced infant mortality dramatically. Infant mortality declined from approximately 165 per 1000 births in 1900 to 47 per 1000 in 1940 to 29.2 per 1000 in 1950 to 7.2 per 1000 in 1998 (Kovner, 1999; U.S. Department of Health and Human Services [USDHHS], 2000). Additionally, clean water, improved quality and quantity of food, and immunization against communicable diseases have contributed dramatically to infants and children reaching adulthood.

CAUSES OF MORTALITY

As discussed in previous chapters, the overall leading causes of death among adults in the United States are heart disease, cancer, and stroke. These statistics are much different for infants, children, and adolescents, however, as is shown in Table 9-1. Indeed, for infants, congenital anomalies are the leading cause of death and problems related to birth comprise the four leading causes of infant mortality. This trend changes dramatically after the first year of life, however, with accidents claiming the most lives of children and adolescents. Strikingly, homicide and cancer rank high as a cause of child and adolescent mortality and congenital anomalies still contribute to many deaths.

CAUSES OF MORBIDITY

The leading causes of acute illness in children are respiratory conditions (i.e., colds, influenza, acute respiratory infections), other infective and parasitic diseases (e.g., viral infections, intestinal virus), acute ear infections, and injuries. The most common chronic complaints in children are respiratory conditions (e.g., asthma, allergic rhinitis, chronic sinusitis, chronic bronchitis) and skin conditions (e.g., chronic dermatitis and acne). Musculoskeletal conditions (e.g., club foot, hip dysplasia, scoliosis) and vision, speech, and hearing impairments are identified in many children (NCHS, 2000).

Respiratory conditions contribute to the most time lost from school, accounting for more than 50% of days absent. Common childhood diseases (e.g., viral infections) are responsible for almost 22% of school absences. Other common acute complaints that cause school absenteeism include ear infections, injuries (e.g., fractures, sprains), and digestive complaints (e.g., nausea, vomiting) (NCHS, 1994).

Children younger than 5 years see physicians more than any other age group until age 65 and older, averaging 6.9 physician contacts each year. In contrast, children and adolescents 5 to 17 years have 3.5 physician contacts per year (NCHS, 2000). Major reasons for hospitalization of children include respiratory conditions (e.g., asthma, bronchitis, pneumonia), injury and poisoning, digestive disorders (e.g., gastroenteritis, diarrhea), infectious and parasitic diseases, headache and seizures, chemotherapy, and unspecified viral illnesses (Evans and Friedland, 1994; NCHS, 1994).

OTHER INDICATORS OF HEALTH

To prevent, detect, and minimize disease, disability, and death in infants and children, a number of indicators of health and well-being should be assessed and appropriate interventions should be developed and implemented when problems or potential problems are identified. Health indicators to be assessed should include growth and development, vision, and hearing. General strategies for health promotion (e.g., good nutrition, exercise and fitness, dental care) should be taught and encouraged. Finally, identified threats or risk factors, such as threats to safety or substance use (e.g., tobacco, alcohol, drugs), must be addressed.

TABLE **9-1** Leading Causes of Death and Percentage for Infants, Children, and Adolescents

INFANTS (LESS THAN 1 YR)	CHILDREN (1-4 YR)	CHILDREN (5-14 YR)	ADOLESCENTS AND YOUNG ADULTS (15-24 YR)
Congenital anomalies (21%)	Accidents (37%)	Accidents (41.7%)	Accidents (39%)
Short gestation and low birth weight (11%)	Congenital anomalies (10.7%)	Cancer (13%)	Homicide (19%)
Perinatal complications (11%)	Homicide (7.6%)	Homicide (6%)	Suicide (12%)
SIDS and respiratory distress syndrome (7%)	Cancer (7%)	Congenital anomalies (5%)	Cancer (4%)

From the National Center for Health Statistics (NCHS). (2000). *Health United States: 2000.* Hyattsville, MD: USDHHS/NCHS. *SIDS,* Sudden infant death syndrome.

A number of *Healthy People 2010* (USDHHS, 2000) objectives specifically target health-promotion and risk-reduction strategies for infants, children, and adolescents. See the *Healthy People 2010* box for some of these objectives. This chapter describes recommendations for primary health care, health promotion, and illness prevention activities and interventions appropriate for nurses caring for infants, children, and adolescents in community-based settings. Identification and management of common acute and chronic illness and conditions are also described.

SPECIAL HEALTH PROGRAMS AND SERVICES FOR CHILDREN

To meet health care needs of disadvantaged, underserved, and disabled children, a number of federally sponsored programs have been developed over the past three decades. Nurses who practice in community settings, particularly those who care for underserved children, should be aware of services provided by these programs, have an understanding of eligibility requirements, and know how to refer clients. Several of the most commonly encountered programs and services are briefly discussed.

MEDICAID AND THE EARLY AND PERIODIC SCREENING, DIAGNOSIS, AND TREATMENT PROGRAM

Children are overrepresented among those with no health insurance or those covered by public insurance (e.g., Medicaid). Indeed, health care is financed by public sources for 25.5% of all persons 18 years and younger and almost 51% of Medicaid dollars covers children. An additional 14% of all children have no health care insurance.

Most children without health insurance are the dependents of full-time workers whose

healthy people **2010**

Examples of Health-Promotion Objectives for Children and Adolescents

OBJECTIVE		BASELINE (1998)	TARGET
1.4b:	Increase the proportion of children and youth aged 17 years and under who have a specific source of ongoing care	93%	96%
8.11:	Eliminate elevated blood levels in children	4.5% of children aged 1 to 5 years	0%
9.7:	Reduce pregnancies among adolescent females	72 per 1000 females aged 15 to 17 years	46 per 1000 females aged 15 to 17 years
14.4:	Reduce bacterial meningitis in young children	13.0 per 100,000	8.6 per 100,000
15.20:	Increase use of child restraints	92%	100%
16.1a:	Reduce fetal and infant deaths during the perinatal period (i.e., 28 weeks of gestation to 7 days or more after birth)	7.5 per 1000	4.5 per 1000
16.15:	Reduce the occurrence of spina bifida and other NTDs	6 per 10,000 live births	3 per 10,000 live births
18.2:	Reduce the rate of suicide attempts by adolescents	2.6% per year	1% per year
19.3a:	Reduce the proportion of children aged 6 to 11 years who are overweight or obese	11%	5%
24.2a:	Reduce hospitalizations for asthma in children under age 5 years	60.9 per 10,000	25 per 10,000
27.2a:	Reduce tobacco use by adolescents in grades 9 to 12	43%	21%

Data from U.S. Department of Health and Human Services (USDHHS). (2000). *Healthy people 2010: Conference edition.* Washington, DC: Government Printing Office.
NTDs, Neural tube defects.

employers provided no health insurance. Lack of health insurance has a significant effect on children's health, as they are less likely to have a usual source of care, resulting in the use of emergency rooms, hospital outpatient departments, or school health centers as the primary health care provider. As a result, children without health insurance are much less likely to receive preventative health care and are more likely to receive health care after illnesses are advanced and care is more expensive.

As discussed in Chapter 5, Medicaid is a welfare assistance health program jointly sponsored by the federal government and each state. Children with Medicaid coverage are nearly as likely as children with private health insurance to have a usual source of care. This is very important for primary prevention, health education, and early identification and treatment of medical or developmental problems.

The **Early and Periodic Screening, Diagnosis, and Treatment (EPSDT)** program began in 1967 to identify and treat children's health problems before they become complex and costly. The EPSDT is a comprehensive and preventative health care program for Medicaid-eligible individuals up to age 21 (USDHHS/Health Care Financing Association [HCFA], 2001). The program's services may be provided by a public health clinic, community health center, school health program, Head Start program, qualified independent practitioners, and others. Under federal guidelines, all eligible children and their families must be informed about EPSDT services and where to obtain them. Furthermore, assistance with scheduling and transportation and assistance in using health resources effectively are components of EPSDT (USDHHS/HCFA, 2001). Mandatory services of EPSDT are listed in Box 9-1.

STATE CHILDREN'S HEALTH INSURANCE PROGRAM

The **State Children's Health Insurance Program (SCHIP)** was created in 1997 as part of the Balanced Budget Act of 1997 to provide health insurance coverage for uninsured children. Most children covered by SCHIP are from working families with incomes too high to qualify for Medicaid, but too low to afford private health insurance. Like Medicaid, SCHIP is a partnership between the federal and state governments. Most states provide SCHIP coverage for children from families at or above 200% of the poverty level.

States have flexibility in organization of each SCHIP, which may be an expansion of the existing Medicaid program or it may be a separate entity. Mandated covered services include inpatient and outpatient hospital care, physician's surgical and medical care, laboratory and x-ray services, and well baby/child care including

---

BOX 9-1 Required Services—Early and Periodic Screening, Diagnosis, and Treatment

- Screening services
- A comprehensive health and developmental history that includes a physical and mental health assessment
- A comprehensive unclothed physical examination
- Laboratory tests (e.g., blood lead level, hematocrit or hemoglobin, sickle cell test, tuberculosis skin test, as appropriate)
- Appropriate immunizations according to age and health history

- Health education (including anticipatory guidance)
- Dental services
- Hearing services, including hearing aids
- Vision services, including eyeglasses
- Any other necessary health care to correct or ameliorate illnesses and conditions found in screenings

From U.S. Department of Health and Human Services/Health Care Financing Administration (2001). *Medicaid and EPSDT.* Retrieved 7/24/01 from http://www.hcfa.gov/medicaid/epsdthm.htm.

immunizations. Other components that may be offered include prescription drugs, mental health services, vision care, and hearing-related care (USDHHS/HCFA, 2001).

WOMEN, INFANTS, AND CHILDREN PROGRAM

The Special Supplemental Nutrition Program for **Women, Infants, and Children (WIC)** provides food, nutrition counseling, and access to health services for low-income women, infants, and children. The WIC program is a federally funded program that was established in 1972 and is administered by each state. Pregnant or post-partum women, infants, and children up to age 5 who meet income guidelines and residency requirements and who are determined to be at nutritional risk are eligible. All persons receiving Aid to Families with Dependent Children, food stamps, or Medicaid are automatically eligible.

Most WIC programs provide vouchers that participants use at authorized stores to purchase nutritious foods. The foods included are high in protein, calcium, iron, and vitamins A and C. The WIC foods include iron-fortified infant formula and infant cereal, iron-fortified adult cereal, vitamin C-rich fruit or vegetable juice, eggs, milk, cheese, peanut butter, and dried beans. Special infant formulas are provided, if pre-scribed. Participation in WIC has been shown to be effective in increasing gestation periods, raising birth weights, and reducing infant mor-tality. An estimated 45% of the babies born in the United States are served by WIC (U.S. Department of Agriculture/Food and Consumer Service, 2000).

HEAD START

Head Start is a federally funded, comprehensive preschool program for children who are at risk for academic problems associated with poverty and lack of sufficient social stimulation. Head Start was begun in 1965 to incorporate health, nutrition, parent involvement, and children's learning into a comprehensive program for dis-advantaged children. Low-income children 3 to 5

years of age are eligible for Head Start programs. Although programs vary by area, health care is often a component of Head Start programs.

EDUCATION FOR ALL HANDICAPPED CHILDREN ACT

In response to lack of services for handicapped children, the Education for All Handicapped Children Act (Public Law [PL] 94-142) was passed in 1975. The PL 94-142 is important and encom-passing because it mandates a free public edu-cation in the least restrictive environment for all handicapped children. In essence, this law requires public school districts to provide an edu-cational environment that can meet the demands of children with disabilities, including children with physical impairments, learning disabilities, and mental and emotional disabilities.

To encourage early intervention, in a 1986 amendment (PL 99-457), coverage for handi-capped children was ensured from birth until age 21 years. The PL 94-142 and PL 99-457 are now known as the Individuals with Disabilities Education Act. Services mandated by the Indivi-duals with Disabilities Education Act include necessary physical or occupational therapy, speech therapy, transportation to and from school, and counseling or psychiatric services. Periodic health or medical procedures (e.g., inter-mittent catheterization, tube feeding, tracheos-tomy suctioning) may be provided in some areas. Mainstreaming, or normalization (integration of special needs children with other children of the same age in a regular classroom), is encouraged whenever possible (Selekman, 1995).

PRIMARY HEALTH CARE RECOMMENDATIONS: U.S. PREVENTATIVE SERVICES TASK FORCE

The U.S. Preventative Services Task Force (USDHHS/Office of Disease Prevention and Health Promotion [ODPHP], 1998) has developed guidelines to direct health care services for health promotion and illness prevention for individuals in all age groups. These recommendations include frequency of visits, screenings that should be performed (e.g., history, physical examination, laboratory or diagnostic procedures), appropriate parent or client counseling and health teaching, immunization recommendations, and specific guidelines for individuals in high-risk categories. Examples of specific assessment tools, health teaching information, and provider guidelines that address the specific recommendations are included throughout this chapter.

SCREENING RECOMMENDATIONS AND GUIDELINES

The recommendations of the Preventative Services Task Force include screening for a number of genetic, congenital, developmental, maturational, and pathological problems and conditions. Guidelines and examples of tools and teaching tips are described briefly.

Newborn Screenings

Although there is considerable variation between states, all states require that all newborns be tested for congenital diseases. Testing for hypothyroidism and phenylketonuria, for example, is required by all states and screening for galactosemia and hemoglobinopathies (e.g., sickle cell disease, thalassemia) is required by a majority of states. Additionally, some states require newborn screening for maple syrup urine disease, congenital adrenal hyperplasia, cystic fibrosis, and other conditions (USDHHS/ODPHP, 1998). Nurses who care for newborns in community settings should know the newborn screenings required by their state.

Newborn screenings are usually accomplished by collecting drops of blood onto specifically designed filter paper (see the Community Application box "Blood Collection Technique for Infant Screenings"). The blood spot specimens should be obtained from every neonate before discharge or transfer from the nursery, regardless of the status of the infant's feeding or age. For full-term, well infants, the specimen should be obtained as close as possible to discharge from

the nursery and no later than 7 days of age. If the initial specimen is obtained earlier than 24 hours after birth, a second specimen should be obtained at 1 to 2 weeks of age. Premature infants, infants receiving parenteral feeding, and infants receiving treatment for illness should have a specimen obtained for screening at or near the seventh day of life if it has not been done before that time, regardless of feeding status (American Academy of Pediatrics/Committee on Genetics, 1992).

Nurses who work in community settings such as pediatric clinics and health maintenance organizations are frequently in a position to perform repeat testing and to follow up on positive or inconclusive results. They may also be in a position to identify those at risk for not being screened (e.g., premature infants, infants undergoing adoption, infants born at home, children of homeless families, infants born outside the United States) (USDHHS/ODPHP, 1998).

All abnormal results from infant screening tests require confirmatory testing and a thorough physical examination. Counseling should be provided to all parents of children with abnormal results and should include information about the significance of the results, the need for retesting, implications for the child's health, treatment, associated symptoms and complications to watch for, and genetic counseling for future childbearing (USDHHS/ODPHP, 1998).

Body Measurement

Significant childhood conditions, such as growth retardation, malnutrition, eating disorders, and obesity, may be identified by regularly scheduled measurement of height and weight throughout infancy and childhood. In addition, head circumference should be measured at birth; at 2 to 4 weeks; and at 1, 2, 4, 6, 9, 12, 15, 18, and 24 months of age to identify potential abnormalities (e.g., hydrocephalus). General guidelines for body measurement suggested by the ODPHP (USDHHS/ODPHP, 1998) are described here.

HEIGHT. For children younger than 2 years, height should be obtained by measuring recumbent length. A measuring board with a stationary

COMMUNITY APPLICATION
Blood Collection Technique for Infant Screenings

1. The same standards and techniques for collection of blood specimens for neonatal screening should be applied for all of the congenital diseases.
2. Required information should be entered on the specimen collection kit with a ballpoint pen, not a soft-tip pen or typewriter.
3. Universal precautions (e.g., wearing gloves and disposal of used lancets) should be taken.
4. The source of blood must be the most lateral surface of the plantar aspect of the infant's heel. The central area of the newborn's foot (area of the arch) or fingers must not be used.
5. Warming the puncture site can increase blood flow. A warm, moist towel (no hotter than 108°F) may be placed on the site for 3 minutes. Also, holding the infant's leg in a position lower than the heart will increase venous pressure.
6. The infant's heel should be cleaned with 70% isopropyl alcohol. Excess alcohol should be wiped away with a dry sterile gauze or cotton ball and the heel allowed to air dry thoroughly. Failure to remove alcohol may dilute the specimen and affect test results.
7. To ensure that sufficient flow of blood is obtained, the plantar surface of the infant's heel should be punctured with a sterile lancet to a depth of 2.0 to 2.4 mm or with an automated lancet device. The first drop of blood should be wiped away with sterile gauze. The puncture site should not be milked or squeezed because this may cause hemolysis and mixture of tissue fluids with the specimen.
8. Care should be taken to avoid touching the area within the printed circle on the filter paper before collection. The filter paper should be touched gently against a large drop of blood and a sufficient quantity of blood allowed to soak through to fill completely the circle on the filter paper. The paper should not be pressed against the puncture site on the heel and blood should be applied only to one side of the paper. Both sides of the filter paper should be examined to ensure that the blood has penetrated and saturated the paper. Successive drips of blood should not be layered within the circle. If blood flow diminishes so that the circle is not completely filled, the sample should be collected from a different site. The sample should be allowed to dry thoroughly before insertion into the envelope.
9. After the specimen has been collected, the foot should be elevated above the body and a sterile gauze pad or cotton ball pressed against the puncture site until the bleeding stops. It is not advisable to apply adhesive bandages over skin puncture sites in newborns.

Data from National Committee for Clinical Laboratory Standards. (1992). *Blood collection on filter paper for neonatal screening programs* (2nd ed.). Villanova, PA: National Committee for Clinical Laboratory Standards; adapted from U.S. Department of Health and Human Services/Office of Disease Prevention and Health Promotion (USDHHS/ODPHP). (1994). *Clinician's handbook of preventive services.* Washington, DC: Government Printing Office.

headboard and sliding vertical foot piece can be used. If one is not available, a stationary vertical surface (e.g., the wall bordering the examining table) and a yardstick or tape measure may be used. In general, the infant or child should lie flat against the center of the board, with the head held against the headboard and the legs extended. The foot piece, tape measure, or yardstick is positioned to the child's heels and the height should be read to the nearest one-eighth inch.

For children 2 years and older, standing height is measured with a stadiometer or a graduated ruler or tape attached to a wall with a flat surface placed horizontally on top of the head. The child should wear only socks or be barefoot, with the knees straight and feet flat on the floor. While the child looks straight ahead, the flat surface or moveable headboard should be placed on the top of the head, compressing the hair, and the height read and recorded. If height-measuring devices attached to weight scales are used, they should be checked frequently for accuracy.

WEIGHT. To improve accuracy, a balance beam or electronic scale should be used to obtain weights. The scale should be checked to ensure that it reads "0" before each use and should be checked periodically. Infants and small children should be weighed wearing only a dry diaper or

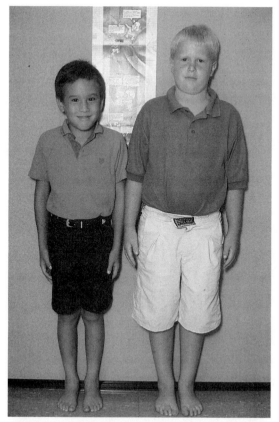

Figure 9-1. These children of identical age (8 years) are markedly different in size. The child on the left, of Asian descent, is at the fifth percentile for height and weight. The child on the right is above the ninety-fifth percentile for height and weight. However, both children demonstrate normal growth patterns. (From Wong, D. [1999]. *Whaley & Wong's nursing care of infants and children* [6th ed., p. 239]. St. Louis: Mosby.)

light underpants. If possible, the same scale should be used for each measurement.

HEAD CIRCUMFERENCE. The circumference of the head should be measured by extending a measuring tape around the most prominent part of the occiput to the middle of the forehead and lightly tightening to compress the hair. Head circumference is usually read to the nearest quarter inch or centimeter. A plastic or disposable paper tape is preferable to a cloth tape, as the latter may stretch.

GENERAL INSTRUCTIONS. All measurements should be plotted on age- and gender-specific growth charts for comparison with reference standards. The NCHS provides growth charts for comparisons with NCHS reference values. Recording serial measurements over time is recommended to detail an accurate growth record. Further, measurements should be interpreted within the context of the individual child's family and growth history (Figure 9-1). If a child's measurements fall within the tenth through twenty-fifth percentile range or the seventy-fifth through ninetieth percentile range, the clinician should assess past growth patterns and genetic and environmental factors to determine if follow-up is necessary. Special growth charts are available for infants born prematurely.

Developmental Screening

Developmental screening is monitoring the progression of infants, children, and adolescents through evaluation of developmental tasks. It is a crucial component of comprehensive health care. Assessment of developmental level can be accomplished by using screening tools, a thorough history, physical assessment, and/or directed observation. To help nurses recognize appropriate developmental tasks, Table 9-2 outlines some common physical, psychosocial, and cognitive developmental tasks.

The Denver II is a revision of the classic tool—the Denver Developmental Screening Test. The Denver II is a screening tool used to assess the overall developmental status of children from birth to age 6 and to alert the health care professional to potential developmental difficulties. Areas covered in the Denver II are personal-social tasks (e.g., getting along with people and caring for personal needs), fine motor-adaptive tasks (e.g., hand-eye coordination, manipulation of small objects), language (e.g., hearing, understanding, using language), and gross motor abilities (e.g., sitting, walking, jumping) (Frankenburg and Dodds, 1990). All persons using this test are urged to participate in a training program to learn

TABLE **9-2** Developmental Tasks for Infants and Children (Includes Physical, Psychosocial, and Cognitive)

AGE	TASK
INFANCY	
3 mo	Experiences decrease in primitive reflexes, except protective and postural reflexes
	Develops social smile (indicates development of memory traces)
4 mo	Laughs
5 mo	Birth weight doubles
	When prone, can push up on arms
	Rolls over
6 mo	Begins teething
	Sits with support
	Exhibits "stranger anxiety" (is wary of strangers and clings to mother)
8 mo	Sits alone
	Crawls
9 mo	Can use pincer grasp
	Holds own bottle
10 mo	Stands with support
12 mo	Birth weight triples
	Takes first steps alone
	Develops trust
	Speaks five words
	Claps hands; waves "bye-bye"
TODDLERHOOD	
13 mo-2.5 yr	Masters walking
	Climbs stairs
	Feeds self (autonomy)
	Uses language (increases to 400 words and two- to three-word phrases)
	Masters toilet training/bowel and bladder control
	Has separation anxiety (screams when the mother leaves)
PRESCHOOL	
2.5-4 yr	Increases vocabulary; uses sentences
	Alternates feet on steps
	Copies circles and lines
	Builds a tower of blocks
	Begins to have concepts of causality, time, and numbers
	Develops body image
	Role plays
	Begins enculturation
	Begins development of conscience
	Has fears of loss of body integrity
SCHOOL AGE	
5-12 yr	Vision matures by age 6 yr
	Loses first baby tooth at age 6 yr; gets all permanent teeth except final molars by age 12 yr
	Develops peer relationships
	Enjoys activities/groups/teams
	Develops morality

From Selekman J. (1993). *Pediatric nursing.* Springhouse, PA: Springhouse.

TABLE **9-2** Developmental Tasks for Infants and Children (Includes Physical, Psychosocial, and Cognitive)—cont'd

AGE	TASK
SCHOOL AGE—cont'd	
5-12 yr	Has cognitive development: concepts of time/space, reversibility, conservation, parts/whole
	Can classify objects in more than one way
	Develops reading/spelling and math concepts
	Begins puberty: age 9 yr for girls; age 11 yr for boys
	Gains sense of industry
ADOLESCENCE	
13-19 yr+	Develops secondary sex characteristics
	Attains adult growth
	Adjusts to body changes
	Begins menses (girls)
	Develops abstract thought
	Develops an identity
	Fantasizes role in different situations
	Has increased heterosexual interests
	Has increased peer influences

to administer and interpret the test correctly. Additional information can be obtained from Denver Developmental Materials, Inc., P.O. Box 6919, Denver, CO 80206-0919; 800-419-4729.

Vision Screening

Vision screening is used to assess children for problems with sight. Refractive errors (myopia, hyperopia, astigmatism) are the most common vision disorders in children, occurring in about 20%. Other visual disorders affecting 2% to 5% of all children include amblyopia (lazy eye), strabismus (ocular misalignment; cross eyes), and anisometropia (difference between the two eyes in nearsightedness, farsightedness, and astigmatism). Each of these conditions usually develop in children between infancy and 5 to 7 years of age. Congenital cataracts, congenital glaucoma, retinoblastoma, and retinopathy of prematurity are other less commonly observed eye conditions occurring in infancy and childhood (USDHHS/ODPHP, 1998).

Normal vision is important for development and failure to treat amblyopia, anisometropia, and strabismus before school age may result in irreversible visual deficits, permanent amblyopia, loss of depth perception and binocularity, cosmetic defects, and educational and occupational restrictions (USDHHS, 1990). Early detection and treatment of vision disorders is essential for normal eye development. A careful history, thorough examination, vision testing, and referral of abnormal or asymmetrical results for further testing and treatment promote normal vision development (see the Community Application box "Guidelines for Vision Screening in Children").

Hearing Screening

Hearing impairment affects all aspects of an individual's life, including developmental, educational, cognitive, emotional, and social components; thus, **hearing screening** is an essential component of a child's health assessment. An estimated 1% to 2% of children in the United States have some degree of hearing impairment. Hearing loss may be congenital or acquired during infancy or childhood. Temporary hearing loss associated with otitis media is fairly common among school-aged children, occurring in 5% to 7% of all children (USDHHS/ODPHP, 1998).

COMMUNITY APPLICATION
Guidelines for Vision Screening in Children

1. The child's health history should include assessment of the child and family for risk factors for vision disorders, including the following:
   Family history of vision or eye problems
   History of maternal, intrapartum, or neonatal conditions that may place the child at risk for visual disorders
   Parental concern about the child's visual function
   Worsening grades and other school difficulties
2. Physical examination of the eye should include inspection of the lids, lashes, tear ducts, orbit, conjunctiva, sclera, cornea, iris, pupillary responsiveness, range of motion, anterior chamber, lens, vitreous, retina, and optic nerve and vessels
3. A comprehensive eye examination should include red reflex examination, corneal light reflex test (to detect strabismus), differential occlusion test (to detect strabismus), fixation (to determine if the eyes are aligned in the same direction without

deviation), cover/uncover test (to detect strabismus), and stereotesting (binocular depth perception); to test for visual acuity, the use of charts such as the Snellen Letters, Tumbling E, or Allen figures is recommended; for children, a distance of 10 feet (using an appropriate chart) may encourage better compliance; a passing score should be given for a line on which the child gives more than 50% correct responses

4. Referral should be made for a child with any abnormalities detected by any test, a visual acuity examination showing a difference in scores of two or more lines between eyes, children younger than 5 years scoring 20/40 or worse in either eye, and children older than 5 years scoring 20/30 or worse in either eye
5. Parents and children should be counseled about eye safety and the use of protective equipment (e.g., safety lenses and frames for science laboratories, shop class, or certain sports)

Adapted from U.S. Department of Health and Human Services (USDHHS). (1994). *Clinician's handbook of preventive services*. Washington, DC: Government Printing Office.

Infants at greatest risk for hearing loss include those with low birth weight; congenital infection (e.g., rubella, toxoplasmosis, syphilis, cytomegalovirus, herpes); craniofacial anomalies; hyperbilirubinemia requiring exchange transfusion; Apgar scores of 0 to 3 at 5 minutes; mechanical ventilation for cardiopulmonary disease for 2 days or more; and neonatal intracranial hemorrhage, prematurity, and hospitalization in the intensive care nursery. Indicators and risk factors for hearing loss in children younger than 2 years include parental concern that a hearing, speech, language, or developmental delay is present; bacterial meningitis; head trauma (particularly in the temporal bone area); infectious diseases known to be associated with sensorineural hearing loss (e.g., mumps, measles); a neurodegenerative disorder associated with hearing loss; and/or ototoxic medications used for more than 5 days (USDHHS/ODPHP, 1998).

Prevention, early detection, and intervention, particularly in infants, are critical in reducing functional limitation and disability from hearing impairment (USDHHS, 2000). Some congenital hearing impairments and some acquired during infancy are preventable. Hearing loss from otitis media and other diseases can be reduced through appropriate primary care. In addition, steps to minimize or manage hearing deficits through employment of assistive devices (e.g., hearing aids and special equipment) should be instituted as soon as possible to minimize developmental delays (see the Community Application box "Guidelines for Hearing Screening in Children").

Lead Screening

The threat of childhood exposure to lead is discussed in Chapter 7. A few key points are repeated here and expanded to include guidelines for screening and treatment.

High blood lead levels have been identified as a very serious threat to children in the United States. This condition disproportionately affects minority and poor children in inner cities,

COMMUNITY APPLICATION
Guidelines for Hearing Screening in Children

1. The health history of each child should assess for risk factors of hearing impairment.
2. Parents should be questioned about the auditory responsiveness and speech and language development of young children; any parental reports of impairment should be seriously evaluated.
3. Clinicians should consider referring all infants and young children with suspected hearing difficulties to an audiologist for evaluation.
4. During physical examinations, clinicians should assess the ear, head, and neck for defects; abnormalities of the ear canal (inflammation, cerumen impaction, tumors, or foreign bodies) and the tympanic membrane (perforation, retraction, or evidence of effusion) should be noted and addressed.
5. Beginning about age 3 years, children may be screened by pure-tone audiometry; the test should be performed in a quiet environment using earphones; each ear should be tested at 500, 1000, 2000, and 4000 Hz.
6. Audiometric evidence of hearing impairment should be substantiated by repeat screening; earphones should be removed and repositioned and instructions carefully repeated to the child; referral to a qualified specialist (e.g., audiologist, otolaryngologist) is recommended if repeat examination suggests impairment.
7. The audiometer should be calibrated yearly and the operator should listen to it each day of use to detect gross abnormalities.

Adapted from U.S. Department of Health and Human Services (USDHHS). (1994). *Clinician's handbook of preventive services*. Washington, DC: Government Printing Office.

where an estimated 3 million children younger than 6 years (about 4.4% of all children in this age group) have blood lead levels high enough to adversely affect their intelligence, behavior, and development (USDHHS/ODPHP, 1998). At greatest risk for lead poisoning are the following:

1. Children who live in a house or regularly visit a day care center, preschool, babysitter, or other house built before 1960
2. Children who live in or regularly visit a house built before 1960 with recent, ongoing, or planned renovation
3. Children who have a brother, sister, or playmate being treated for lead poisoning
4. Children who live with an adult whose job, hobby, or use of ethnic remedies involves lead
5. Children who live near an active lead smelter, battery recycling plant, or other industry likely to release lead

General guidelines for lead screening include initiation of risk assessment and counseling from prenatal visits until the child is 6 years of age. Although some disagreement exists among pediatric health care authorities, in general, recommendations are that children with any risk factors listed here should be tested for lead exposure. Screening should be done at about 6 to 12 months of age and again at about 24 months. Infants at high risk should be screened initially at 6 months and every 6 months. After two consecutive measurements of less than 10 µg/dl, the child should be retested in 1 year. Rescreening should occur at any time when history suggests that exposure has increased, up to about age 6 years, unless otherwise indicated (USDHHS/ODPHP, 1998).

To screen for lead, capillary specimens should be carefully collected to minimize contamination. Recommendations include washing the child's hand (or feet for infants younger than 1 year) with soap and water, then cleansing with alcohol. The first drop of blood should be wiped off with sterile gauze or a cotton ball. Elevated blood lead results (over 15 µg/dl) should be confirmed using venous blood. Finally, all families should be counseled on sources of lead exposure and how to prevent exposure. See Chapter 7 for teaching tips to avoid lead exposure.

Anemia Screening

Iron deficiency anemia is the most common nutritional disorder in the United States, affecting an estimated 25% of low-income children (Wong, 1999). In infants and children, anemia is associated with fatigue, apathy, growth and development impairment, and decreased resistance to infection. Risk of anemia is related to low socioeconomic status, consumption of cow's milk before 6 months of age, consumption of formula not fortified with iron, and low birth weight. Native American and black children and immigrants from developing countries are also at risk. General recommendations are that the hemoglobin or hematocrit levels be checked during infancy (6 to 9 months) and early childhood. **Anemia screening** for adolescent females is also recommended (USDHHS/ODPHP, 1998). Table 9-3 presents standards for diagnosis of anemia in children and adolescents.

Therapeutic management of iron deficiency anemia focuses on increasing the amount of iron that the child receives. Dietary supplementation includes the use of iron-fortified formulas and cereal for infants. Oral supplements may be recommended and the child retested in 3 to

TABLE **9-3** Hemoglobin and Hematocrit Cutpoints for Anemia in Children 1 Year of Age or Older

GENDER	AGE (YR)	HEMOGLOBIN (G/DL)	HEMATOCRIT (%)
Both	1.0-1.9	11.0	33.0
	2.0-4.9	11.2	34.0
	5.0-7.9	11.4	34.5
	8.0-11.9	11.6	35.0
Female	12.0-14.9	11.8	35.5
	15.0-17.9	12.0	36.0
	≥18	12.0	36.0
Male	12.0-14.9	12.3	37.0
	15.0-17.9	12.6	38.0
	≥18	13.6	41.0

From Centers for Disease Control and Prevention (CDC). (1989). CDC criteria for anemia in children and childbearing-aged women. *MMWR Morbidity and Mortality Weekly Report, 38,* 400-404.

4 months if anemia is fairly significant. If anemia does not improve, intramuscular or intravenous iron may be administered. Transfusions are only indicated in severe anemia (Wong, 1999). Prevention of iron deficiency anemia is described later in this chapter.

HEALTH PROMOTION

Health promotion refers to those activities related to individual lifestyle choices that can influence health. Components of health promotion for infants and children that are of particular importance to nurses who practice in community settings are physical activity and fitness, nutrition, and dental health. Basic information for assessment, health teaching, and counseling is presented in the following sections.

Nutrition

Good nutrition is essential for life, health, and well-being. Conversely, poor nutrition can be harmful because dietary factors are associated with 5 of the 10 leading causes of death (i.e., heart disease, some types of cancer, stroke, diabetes, atherosclerosis) (USDHHS, 2000). Malnutrition in the United States is rarely the result of a lack of a sufficient quantity of food, but is more often caused by deficiencies of certain nutrients (e.g., iron, calcium, protein, some vitamins) and excesses of others (e.g., calories, fats, simple sugars).

According to Wong (1999), most food preferences and dietary habits are established during childhood. The importance of good nutritional habits should be taught from an early age. In general, good nutrition for children includes three healthy meals per day and two healthy snacks. Providing nutrition education for children from preschool through high school should be encouraged.

INFANT NUTRITION. As described previously, iron deficiency anemia is the most common nutritional disorder in infants and children. To prevent anemia, the American Academy of Pediatrics recommends use of breast milk or commercial infant formula for the first year of life. Other interventions include the use of iron supplementation (e.g., iron-fortified commercial formula or iron-fortified cereal for breast fed babies) to provide 1 mg/kg/day of iron by 4 to 6 months of age, use of iron (ferrous sulfate) drops (from 2 to 3 mg/kg/day to 15 mg/kg/day) to breastfed preterm infants after 2 months of age, use of iron-fortified infant cereal when solid foods are introduced, and limiting the amount of formula to no more than 1 L/day to encourage the intake of iron-rich solid foods (Wong, 1999).

Addition of solid foods into the infant's diet should be done gradually. Commercially prepared infant cereal (e.g., rice, barley, oatmeal) is usually introduced first. Rice cereal is often suggested because of its easy digestibility and low allergic potential (Wong, 1999). Most often, strained fruits are introduced initially, followed by vegetables and then meats. Crackers or zwieback are offered at about 6 months of age. Small amounts of raw fruits and vegetables can be added gradually. General guidelines for the addition of solid foods is another important consideration in nutrition counseling. Most clinics and physician's offices have pamphlets and brochures to provide parents more detailed information on these topics; the nurse can use these materials to supplement health teaching (see the Health Teaching box "Feeding During the First Year").

Infant nutrition is also discussed in Chapter 11. Included are strategies to encourage breast-feeding, how to choose infant formulas, and techniques for bottle-feeding.

NUTRITIONAL NEEDS OF CHILDREN. Adequate caloric and nutrient intake is critical for supporting growth and development of children. In general, recommended nutrition intake for children includes two to three servings (2 to 3 ounces) per day of meat or meat substitutes (e.g., beans, lentils); 2 to 4 cups of milk or milk equivalent servings, depending on age and size; five or more servings of vegetables and fruits (including a dark green or deep yellow vegetable for vitamin A and fruits or vegetables that contain vitamin C); and four or more servings of breads and cereals. Fats, oils, and sweets should be eaten sparingly (Murray and Zentner, 2001).

NUTRITIONAL NEEDS OF ADOLESCENTS. In general, adolescents should consume more total nutrients than they did as young children. Accelerated physical and emotional development works to increase the metabolic rate and, as a result, nutritional needs. Maximal growth in girls takes place between ages 10 and 12 and approximately 2 years later in boys. Protein, calcium, and calorie needs are higher during this time. In the United States, adolescent girls typically begin menstruating at 12.5 years; menstruation increases the need for iron.

Meal skipping, frequent snacking, eating fast foods, and drinking soft drinks contribute to imbalances in the diet of adolescents. In general, adolescents between 12 and 18 years of age should consume 4 servings of dairy products (low-fat milk is preferred), 2 to 3 servings of meat and meat alternatives, 4 to 5 servings of fruits and vegetables, and 6 to 11 servings of breads and cereals. As with children, fats, oils, and sweets should be used sparingly.

Eating disorders (e.g., anorexia nervosa and bulimia) most often occur in adolescent girls. Teaching adolescents the importance of good nutrition should include discussion of the consequences of eating disorders and how to recognize them. These issues are covered in Chapter 15.

Physical Activity and Exercise

Exercise and physical activity are necessary for muscular development and refinement of coordination and balance, gaining strength, and enhancing other functions, such as circulation and elimination. Toddlers and small children usually have an abundance of energy and rarely need encouragement to promote physical activity. Many school-aged children and adolescents, however, often need to be encouraged to exercise. Several goals of *Healthy People 2010* (USDHHS, 2000) address the importance of physical activity in children 6 years of age through adolescence. In general, all children should engage in light-to-moderate physical activity for at least 30 minutes each day to develop and maintain cardiorespiratory fitness and improve overall physical fitness.

health teaching

Feeding During the First Year

BIRTH TO 6 MONTHS (BREASTFEEDING OR BOTTLE FEEDING)

Breastfeeding

Breastfeeding is the most desirable complete diet for the first half of the year.*

Supplements of fluoride (0.25 mg), regardless of the fluoride content of the local water supply, are required after 6 months of age; iron may be required by 4 to 6 months of age.

Supplements of vitamin D (400 units) are required if the mother's diet is inadequate.

Formula

Iron-fortified commercial formula is a complete food for the first half of the year.†

Requires fluoride supplements (0.25 mg) when the concentration of fluoride in the drinking water is below 0.3 parts per million after 6 months of age.

Evaporated milk formula requires supplements of vitamin C, iron, and fluoride (in accordance with the fluoride content of the local water supply after 6 months of age).

6 TO 12 MONTHS (SOLID FOODS)

Solids may begin to be added by 5 to 6 months of age.

First foods are strained, pureed, or finely mashed.

Finger foods such as teething crackers, raw fruit, or vegetables can be introduced by 6 to 7 months.

Chopped table food or commercially prepared junior foods can be started by 9 to 12 months.

With the exception of cereal, the order of introducing foods is variable; a recommended sequence is weekly introduction of other foods, beginning with fruit, then vegetables, and then meat.

As the quantity of solids increases, the amount of formula should be limited to approximately 900 ml (30 oz) daily and fruit juice to less than 360 ml (12 oz) daily.

Method of Introduction

Introduce solids when infant is hungry.

Begin spoon-feeding by pushing food to back of tongue because of infant's natural tendency to thrust tongue forward.

Use a small spoon with a straight handle; begin with 1 or 2 teaspoons of food and gradually increase to 2 to 3 tablespoons per feeding.

Introduce one food at a time usually at intervals of 4 to 7 days, to identify food allergies.

As the amount of solid food increases, decrease the quantity of milk to prevent overfeeding.

Never introduce foods by mixing them with the formula in the bottle.

Cereal

Introduce commercially prepared iron-fortified infant cereals and administer daily until 18 months.

Rice cereal is usually introduced first because of its low allergenic potential.

Supplemental iron can be discontinued once cereal is given.

Fruits and Vegetables

Applesauce, bananas, and pears are usually well tolerated.

Avoid fruits and vegetables marketed in cans not specifically designed for infants because of variable and sometimes high lead content and addition of salt, sugar, and/or preservatives.

Offer fruit juice only from a cup, not a bottle, to reduce the development of nursing caries.

Meat, Fish, and Poultry

Avoid fatty meats.

Prepare by baking, broiling, steaming, or poaching.

Include organ meats such as liver, which has a high iron, vitamin A, and vitamin B complex content.

If soup is given, be sure all ingredients are familiar to the child's diet.

Avoid commercial meat/vegetable combinations because protein is low.

Eggs and Cheese

Serve egg yolk hard boiled and mashed, soft cooked, or poached.

Introduce egg white in small quantities (1 t) toward end of first year to detect an allergy.

Use cheese as a substitute for meat and as finger food.

From Wong, D. L. (1999). *Whaley & Wong's nursing care of infants and children* (6th ed.). St. Louis: Mosby.
*Breastfeeding or commercial formula feeding for up to 12 months of age is recommended.
†After 1 year, whole cow's milk can be given.

TABLE **9-4** Sleep and Rest Needs of Infants, Children, and Adolescents

AGE GROUP	HOURS OF DAILY REST (NAPS)	NIGHTTIME SLEEP
Neonates	As many as 7 to 8 naps per day*	6-12 hr, interrupted for feedings*
Infants	Morning nap time will shorten, then be eliminated; by 12 mo, one daily nap of 1-4 hr†	9-11 hr; many babies sleep through the night by 7-8 mo†
Toddlers	Daily nap: 1-2 hr	10-12 hr
Younger preschoolers (3 yr of age)	Daily nap: 1-2 hr; nap time may diminish, but a rest time (1-2 hr) should be encouraged	10-12 hr
Older preschoolers (4-5 yr of age)	Often will refuse to nap; afternoon "rest" times should be encouraged	10-11 hr
Younger school-aged (6-9 yr)		10-11 hr
Older school-aged (10-12 yr)		9-10 hr
Adolescents (13 yr of age and older)	May occasionally nap or sleep in to catch up on rest needs	8-10 hr (variable): sleep and rest needs may increase because of rapid growth and energy expenditure

Data from Murray, R. B., & Zenter, J. P. (2001). *Nursing assessment and health promotion: Strategies through the life span* (7th ed.). Norwalk, CT: Appleton & Lange; Wong, D. L. (1999). *Whaley & Wong's nursing care of infants and children* (6th ed.). St. Louis: Mosby.
*Total of 16-20 hr of sleep/day during the first few weeks.
†Total of 14-15 hr of sleep/day by 3-4 mo of age.

In addition to exercises that improve heart and lung functioning, physical activities that enhance and maintain muscular strength, muscular endurance, and flexibility are recommended.

School-based physical education programs, and nonschool-related activities such as sports (e.g., soccer, baseball, basketball, hockey) and recreational activities (e.g., skating, swimming, bicycling), can be good sources of exercise. The use of appropriate safety equipment (e.g., helmets, pads, mouth protectors), however, must be stressed. Activities that can be easily incorporated into a child's daily routine and enjoyed all year should be encouraged because activity levels tend to decrease in the winter.

Sleep and Rest

Sleep and rest are essential to good health. Sleep needs vary dramatically with age, ranging from 20 hours or more per day for neonates to 8 hours per day for older teenagers. Table 9-4 outlines sleep and rest needs for infants, children, and adolescents.

The positioning of infants for sleep is very important because sleeping in a prone position has been associated with sudden infant death syndrome (SIDS). In 1992, the American Academy of Pediatrics recommended that almost all infants up to 6 months of age sleep on their sides or backs (exceptions are infants with gastroesophageal reflux and some infants with upper airway problems) (Wong, 1999). Placing the infant on a firm mattress, rather than a pillow or soft bedding, is also suggested. Widespread adherence to these recommendations has resulted in an almost 40% decrease in SIDS during the past few years. All parents should be informed of these recommendations and taught to position infants on their backs, rather than prone, and to avoid overly soft bedding.

Dental Health

Dental caries have been described as the most prevalent disease known. In recent years, however, the oral health of children in the United States has improved dramatically, largely because of community water fluoridation, use of preventative services (e.g., sealants, topical fluoride treatment), and appropriate tooth care (e.g., brushing, flossing). Despite these improvements in oral health, more than half of all children have caries by the second grade and about 80% by the time they finish high school (USDHHS, 2000). *Healthy People 2010* objectives to promote oral health include increasing the percentage of communities with fluoridated water, encouraging the use of dental sealants, and increasing the use of topical or systemic fluorides (e.g., tooth pastes, mouth rinses, fluoride drops) (USDHHS, 2000). Prevention of baby bottle tooth decay and screening of all preschool children for tooth decay are also encouraged.

It has been observed that community water fluoridation is the most effective and efficient means of preventing dental caries in children. Furthermore widespread exposure to fluorides through drinking water and dental products has led to a 68% decline in the amount of decayed, missing, or filled teeth in the U.S. population (Centers for Disease Control and Prevention [CDC], 1999).

According to Ripa (1993), approximately 62% of U.S. residents have drinking water containing optimal levels of fluoride, with the highest levels (73%) being in the Midwestern states (i.e., Minnesota, Michigan, Wisconsin, Iowa, Missouri, Illinois, Indiana, Ohio) and the lowest (17.9%), in the Pacific states (i.e., Washington, Oregon, California).

Dental care of infants and young children may include fluoride supplementation. If the infant is fed with formula concentrate or powdered formula prepared with fluoridated water, supplements are not necessary. If the community does not have fluoridated water, supplemental fluoride drops should be used. The amount of supplementation depends on the amount of fluoride in the drinking water. If no fluoride is in the drinking water, the recommendations of the American Dental Association (ADA) are 0.25 mg/day for chil-

dren 6 months to 3 years of age, 0.50 mg/day for children 3 to 6 years, and 1.0 mg/day for children 6 to 16 years. For older children, dentists often recommend using fluoride tablets, fluoride application in the dental office, or use of fluoride toothpaste or mouthwash (ADA, 1999).

Dental sealants are thin plastic coatings painted on the chewing surfaces of the back teeth and are applied in the dentist's office or clinic and sometimes in schools. The process is simple, painless, and effective in preventing tooth decay. The process lasts up to 10 years and is fairly inexpensive (National Institutes of Health, 1994). All parents should be encouraged to discuss dental sealants with their child's dentist.

Bottle mouth syndrome, or baby bottle tooth decay, occurs in older infants and toddlers who are allowed to fall asleep with a bottle of formula or milk or another sweetened fluid in their mouth. These fluids pool in the mouth, particularly around the upper front teeth. Bacteria normally present in the mouth consume the carbohydrates from the milk or juice and, as a by-product, the bacteria produce metabolic acids. These acids decalcify the tooth enamel, resulting in destruction of the tooth. All parents should be taught to prevent baby bottle tooth decay by using only plain water in naptime and bedtime bottles.

The primary teeth (deciduous teeth or baby teeth) begin erupting at about 6 months of age and continue until 2 years of age; they start shedding at about 6 years of age. The permanent teeth begin erupting at about 6 to 7 years of age and continue into adulthood. Figure 9-2 depicts normal tooth formation.

To promote oral health, the ADA (2001) offers the following recommendations:

- Take children to the dentist regularly, beginning within 6 months of the eruption of the first tooth, but no later than the child's first birthday.
- Encourage children to drink from a cup by their first birthday.

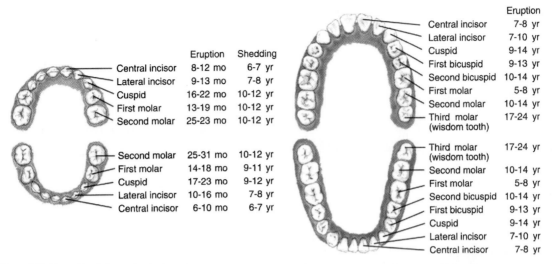

Figure 9-2 Normal tooth formation in the child. (From Ashwill, J. W., & Droske, S. C. [1997]. *Nursing care of children* [p. 244]. Philadelphia: W. B. Saunders.)

- Begin brushing the child's teeth with water as soon as the first tooth appears.
- Start flossing when two of the child's teeth begin to touch.
- Brush and floss the child's teeth daily until the child can be taught to do it alone; then encourage the child to brush and floss.
- Ensure that children get adequate fluoride for decay-resistant teeth (this varies based on the community—consult a dentist).
- Ask the dentist about dental sealants.

Thumb sucking or use of a pacifier generally does not cause permanent dental problems for children younger than 4 years of age. However, alignment problems in the permanent teeth may develop if thumb sucking persists beyond age 5 years. Observation of thumb sucking or use of pacifiers in small children should alert the nurse to inform the parents of potential problems. If thumb sucking persists, the child should be referred to a dentist.

Oral injuries are common during childhood. Children should be encouraged to wear mouth protectors or mouthguards when participating in activities that may involve falls, head contact, tooth clenching, or flying equipment (e.g.,

gymnastics, football, skateboarding, soccer, basketball). In addition to protecting teeth, mouthguards also prevent injury to lips, cheeks, and tongue and may reduce the severity and incidence of concussions (ADA, 2000). Mouth protectors are available at sporting goods stores or may be custom made by the dentist.

If a dental injury occurs, the child should be taken to the dentist immediately. If a permanent tooth is knocked out, it should be rinsed gently with cool water without removing any attached tissue and immediately reinserted into the socket. If that is not possible, the tooth should be placed in cool water or milk and the child should see a dentist as soon as possible, bringing the tooth along.

Maturation and Puberty

Like infancy, adolescence is a period of accelerated growth and development. When caring for older children and young teenagers in community settings, nurses are frequently in a position to teach adolescents and their parents about growth and development changes associated with puberty.

Puberty is the time of physical development in which individuals develop sexual maturity. In

9-2 Physical Changes in Girls During Preadolescence*

- Increase in transverse diameter of the pelvis
- Broadening of hips
- Tenderness in developing breast tissue and enlargement of areolar diameter
- Axillary and body sweating
- Change in vaginal secretions from alkaline to acid pH
- Change in vaginal layer to thick, gray, mucoid lining
- Change in vaginal flora from mixed to Döderlein's lactic acid-producing bacilli
- Appearance of pubic hair from 8 to 14 years (hair first appears on labia and then spreads to mons; adult triangular distribution does not occur for approximately 2 years after initial appearance of pubic hair)

From Murray, R. B., & Zentner, J. P. (2001). *Nursing assessment and health promotion: Strategies through the life span* (7th ed.). Norwalk, CT: Appleton & Lange.
*These physical changes for girls are listed in the approximate sequence of their occurrence.

9-3 Physical Changes in Boys During Preadolescence*

- Axillary and body sweating
- Increased testicular sensitivity to pressure
- Increase in size of testes
- Changes in color of scrotum
- Temporary enlargement of breasts
- Increase in height and shoulder breadth
- Appearance of lightly pigmented hair at base of penis
- Increase in length and width of penis

From Murray, R. B., & Zentner, J. P. (2001). *Nursing assessment and health promotion: Strategies through the life span* (7th ed.). Norwalk, CT: Appleton & Lange.
*These physical changes for boys are listed in the approximate sequence of their occurrence.

girls, puberty begins between 10 and 14 years of age; menarche marks puberty and sexual maturity. Age at menarche ranges from 10 to 16, with a mean of about 12.5 years. During puberty, the breasts enlarge, and axillary and pubic hair grows thicker and darker (Murray and Zentner, 2001). Early instruction on menstruation should be provided. Box 9-2 describes physical changes in girls during preadolescence.

In boys, puberty begins between 12 and 16 years. At that time, hair begins to grow at the axilla and the pubis. Also, body hair, particularly facial hair, increases, and the voice deepens. Additionally, the penis, scrotum, and testes enlarge; the scrotum reddens; and the scrotal skin changes texture. Penile development occurs between 10 and 16 years and testicular development occurs between 9 and 17 years. Spermatogenesis and seminal emissions designate puberty and sexual maturity in boys. Nocturnal emissions occur approximately at age 14 (Murray and Zentner, 2001). Box 9-3 gives additional information on physical changes in boys during puberty.

ILLNESS PREVENTION AND HEALTH PROTECTION

When working in community settings, nurses can dramatically affect the health of infants, children, and adolescents through measures to prevent illness and protect health and safety. Illness prevention and health protection strategies for children include prevention of communicable diseases; prevention of initiation of tobacco, alcohol, and drug use; promoting safety; and prevention and detection of child abuse. Prevention of communicable disease in children is addressed at length in Chapter 16. Interventions to improve safety; prevent alcohol, tobacco, and drug use; and detect and prevent child abuse are described in the following sections.

Prevention of Substance Use

DRUGS AND ALCOHOL. Alcohol use contributes dramatically to the three leading causes of adolescent deaths. As stated earlier, injuries are the leading cause of death in adolescents and an estimated 40% of injury deaths in this age group are related to the use of alcohol. Alcohol use also contributes significantly to adolescent homicide and suicide (the second and third leading causes of death in this age group) (USDHHS/ODPHP, 1998). School-based alcohol and drug education programs have been somewhat successful because alcohol and marijuana use among adolescents (aged 12 to 17 years) declined between 1988 and 1992. Rates of alcohol and drug use, however, began to increase slowly beginning in 1992 and have fluctuated somewhat since that time. To assist in reducing alcohol and drug use, health care providers are encouraged to screen and counsel adolescents for alcohol and other drug use. Components of alcohol and drug abuse counseling suggested by the USDHHS/ODPHP (1998) include the following:

- Begin education on alcohol and drug use during the preteen years. All children and adolescents should be informed of the dangers of alcohol and other drugs, emphasizing associated dangers of human immunodeficiency virus (HIV) exposure and motor vehicle accidents while under the influence of alcohol and other drugs.
- Ask parents about their own use of alcohol and other drugs and whether they discuss the use of alcohol and drugs with their children. Assessment for a family history of alcoholism or drug use should be made.
- Establish a caring and confidential relationship with adolescents; however, the adolescent must be informed of the limits of confidentiality.
- As nonthreateningly as possible, question children and adolescents about drug and alcohol use in their environment (e.g., home, school, work). Suggested questions to be asked include "Do most of your friends drink alcohol or smoke marijuana at parties?" "Have you ever tried alcohol, marijuana, or other drugs?" "Do your parents know that you've used alcohol or drugs?" "Have you ever been drunk or stoned and driven a car?"
- If alcohol or drug use is determined, assess the type of drugs used and the quantity, frequency, and setting of use.
- Evaluate the extent to which alcohol or other drugs are affecting the adolescent's life (e.g., school performance, peer relationships, family relationships, work).

- Be aware of signs and symptoms of dependence, addiction, and withdrawal and teach them to parents and adolescents.
- Refer for evaluation and treatment if evidence of significant psychosocial impairment or physiological dependence is present. Familiarity with available treatment options in the community is essential.

TOBACCO. Use of tobacco products is the leading preventable cause of death in the United States, accounting for more than 430,000 deaths each year (about one out of every five deaths) (USDHHS, 2000). Initiation of smoking occurs almost entirely during adolescence, as surveys have indicated that 82% of those who have ever smoked started by the twelfth grade (USDHHS, 2000). Approximately 22% of high school students report smoking cigarettes daily and the average age of initial cigarette use is 12 years (USDHHS/ODPHP, 1998).

In addition to the direct health problems associated with tobacco use, concern arises because cigarettes are considered to be a gateway drug and their use often leads to abuse of alcohol and illicit drugs. Indeed, teens who smoke are 3 times more likely than nonsmokers to use alcohol, 8 times more likely to use marijuana, and 22 times more likely to use cocaine (Pourciau & Vallette, 2001). Because of the health problems associated with tobacco use, reduction of the initiation of cigarette smoking by teenagers has been termed a national priority. Strategies to prevent tobacco use among children and teenagers include enforcement of youth access laws, establishment of tobacco-free environments, and ongoing prevention programs in schools and the community.

Surveillance and enforcement of retail restriction of sale of tobacco to nonadults is essential to reduce the prevalence of smoking among teenagers. Most states have a minimum age of 18 years for purchasing cigarettes; however, almost 58% of teenage smokers report that they usually buy their own cigarettes. Small stores are the most commonly mentioned site for purchase of cigarettes: almost 80% of youths 12 to 15 and 87%

of youths 16 to 17 years of age reported buying cigarettes from small stores. Interestingly, vending machines were the source of cigarettes for fewer than 20% of adolescents ages 12 to 15 and less than 12% of older youths (CDC, 1992).

The establishment of tobacco-free environments and tobacco use prevention education programs is an important component in decreasing the initiation of tobacco use among youth. The Pro-Children Act of 1994 requires that federally funded facilities that provide services to children (e.g., schools and libraries) be smoke free (USDHHS, 1995). Increasingly, state and city ordinances and laws are being enacted that prohibit smoking in public places. These efforts should be supported by all health care workers.

Health education and counseling strategies developed by the USDHHS/ODPHP (1998) to encourage teenagers to prevent initiation of or to stop tobacco use include the following:

- Maintain a smoke-free environment in the health care office or clinic; do not permit smoking by staff, clients, or their parents. Post no-smoking signs and provide literature about the importance of smoking cessation and avoiding tobacco use.
- If parents or other family members smoke, stress the importance of stopping; emphasize the negative health consequences for children.
- Provide counseling or referral to those who want to quit smoking.
- Begin in elementary school to discuss tobacco use and its negative effects; emphasize the unattractive cosmetic consequences of tobacco use (i.e., stained teeth, oral sores, bad breath) and negative athletic consequences of tobacco use. Also emphasize the negative social consequences (e.g., disapproval by peers) because this is generally more effective with children and adolescents than discussing the long-term health consequences.
- Elicit information in a nonthreatening manner; have parents leave the room or ask adolescents to complete a previsit questionnaire discussing tobacco use and other sensitive issues.

Safety

In the United States, injuries are the leading cause of mortality in children and adolescents, accounting for about 20,000 deaths each year. Almost half (47%) of fatal accidents involve motor vehicle crashes. Injuries cause 43% of deaths of children aged 1 through 4 and for ages 15 to 24, injury deaths exceed deaths from all other causes combined (USDHHS, 2000). In addition to motor vehicle accidents, significant risks are associated with other sources. Homicide accounts for about 13% of injury deaths; suicide, 10%; drowning, 9.2%; fire or burns, 7.2%; and "other" (e.g., choking, falls, poisoning, sports, accidents involving firearms), 14% (CDC, 1990). Childhood injuries also cause an estimated 16 million emergency room visits and 600,000 hospitalizations (USDHHS, 2000). Interventions for childhood injury prevention are discussed in each of the following subsections.

VEHICLE SAFETY. As mentioned, motor vehicles are involved in almost half of all injury deaths and contribute to numerous hospitalizations in children and adolescents. More than 42,000 people are killed annually in motor vehicle accidents (USDHHS, 2000), including those who are an occupant in a vehicle and those struck while riding a bicycle or as a pedestrian. Motorcycle (11% of total), bicycle (4.5% of the total), and pedestrian (14.5% of total) casualties account for almost 30% of motor vehicle deaths each year.

Motor vehicle safety begins with the ride home from the hospital. Although some variation exists in specific regulations, all states require the use of child safety seats. Other interventions that have been suggested include adoption and enforcement of seat belt laws and ordinances, enforcement of strict penalties for operating a vehicle under the influence of drugs or alcohol, adoption and enforcement of laws and ordinances requiring motorcyclists and bicyclists to wear helmets, enforcement of speed limits, enforcement of minimum drinking age laws, and enforcement of laws and ordinances requiring child safety seat use and the extension of these laws and ordinances to cover all passengers sitting in all vehicles (CDC, 1990). Equipping vehicles with both driver and passenger airbags, improving vehicle designs to better protect both occupants (e.g., side impact protection, improved door design, roof crush resistance, and restraint system), and developing community-based pedestrian and bicycle

safety programs are other safety measures (see the Health Teaching box "Basic Safety Counseling").

POISONING. Each year almost 700,000 children younger than 5 years are exposed to some type of poison, and more than 107,000 children are

---

health teaching

Basic Safety Counseling

GENERAL INFORMATION

Encourage parents and others to learn basic life-saving skills (e.g., CPR).

Teach children to dial 911 and other local emergency numbers.

Encourage parents and others to teach children how to manage peer pressure that might result in risk-taking behavior that may interfere with making good safety decisions.

Encourage parents to be good role models for safe behavior (i.e., avoid drinking alcohol before driving, always wear a seat belt and bicycle helmet, drive within the posted speed limit).

Be aware of community resources and programs related to safety.

CHOKING AND SUFFOCATION

Advise parents and other caregivers to keep objects that can cause suffocation (e.g., plastic bags) and choking (e.g., coins, small toy parts, and certain foods such as grapes, gum, peanuts, hot dogs) away from small children.

DROWNING

Never leave infants and small children in the bathtub without supervision.

Do not allow children to swim alone.

Advise that fences around swimming pools/spas should be at least 4 feet high with completely self-closing gates.

ELECTRICAL SAFETY

Keep unused electrical outlets covered with plastic guards or install breaker outlets.

Ground fault interrupter circuits should be used in bathrooms and other areas where water is likely to touch bare skin.

FALL PREVENTION

Those caring for small children should use safety gates on both top and bottom of stairways,

install window guards above the first floor, and move furniture away from upper-story windows so children cannot climb onto the window sill.

Baby walkers should be used under supervision, particularly to avoid falls down stairs.

FIRE AND BURN PREVENTION

To avoid scalding burns, reduce the temperature setting on the water heater to 49°C (120°F) or install antiscald devices on bathroom and kitchen faucets.

Smoke alarms should be installed properly in sleeping areas and in the kitchen; batteries should be changed at least twice yearly. The family should have a fire escape plan and practice fire drills.

FIREARMS

Parents and other caregivers should be advised about the dangers of keeping a firearm in the home. If a gun is kept in the home, it should be unloaded and locked up separately from the ammunition.

MOTOR VEHICLE SAFETY

Use car seats for all children, based on state laws. Child safety seats should be in the rear seat of the car and should be used every time the children ride. Safety seats should face backward until child weighs at least 20 pounds or reaches 1 year of age.

Booster seats should be used until children grow tall enough so the lap belt stays low on their hips. Children should never ride in the cargo areas of pickup trucks, vans, or station wagons. Infants and children should never be placed in the front seat of a vehicle equipped with a passenger-side air bag. If a vehicle does not have a rear seat, children riding in the front seat should be positioned as far back as possible from the air bag.

U.S. Department of Health and Human Services/Public Health Service (USDHHS/PHS) (1999). *Clinician's hand book of preventive service* (2nd ed.). Mclean, V. A.: International Medical Publishing, Inc.

health teaching

Protection of Children from Accidental Poisoning

1. Request safety-lock tops on all prescription drugs.
2. Keep household cleaners, bug sprays, medicines, and garage products out of reach and out of sight of children; lock them up if possible.
3. Never store food and household cleaners together.
4. Always store medicines in their original containers and throw out medicine when old or no longer in use; rinse out empty containers.
5. Do not take medicines in front of your child because children love to imitate.
6. Never call medicine "candy."
7. Read the label before taking medicine; turn on the light when giving or taking medicine.
8. If you leave the room when using a medicine or a household product, take it or the child with you; a child can get into it in only a few seconds.
9. Anticipate your child's curiosity and abilities; for example, if you have a crawling infant, keep household products locked up, not under the kitchen sink or on the refrigerator.
10. Never put products like kerosene, gasoline, insecticides, or household cleaning agents in another container, such as a soft drink bottle, cup, or bowl.
11. If you need potentially poisonous products, buy them only when needed and only enough to do the specific job.
12. Always prepare and use products according to label directions.
13. Place "Mr. Yuk" stickers (available from many pharmacies or health departments) on all poisons in the home if children are older than 3 years of age and teach them that this means danger.
14. Be alert for repeat poisoning; a child who has swallowed a poison is more likely to become poisoned again within a year.
15. The child's life may depend on how fast you get expert emergency information and treatment—be prepared.

Post the poison control center number for your area near the phone; tell all babysitters it is there.
Have the following products on hand (use only on the advice of the Poison Control Center, emergency center, or a physician):
   1-ounce bottle of syrup of ipecac for each child in the house
   Epsom salt
   Activated charcoal

From Texas Department of Health. (1990). *Protect your child against accidental poisoning.* Austin: Texas Department of Health.

treated in hospital emergency rooms for poisoning (USDHHS, 2000). Most poisoning accidents take place in the home and involve children younger than 5 years. Any nonfood item is a potential poison and many children die or are injured from swallowing medicines, polishes, insecticides, antifreeze, drain cleaners, and other household products. Parents of small children should be given information on how to protect their children from potential poisoning (see the Health Teaching box "Protection of Children from Accidental Poisoning"). Additionally, instruction on emergency actions to be taken in the event of accidental poisoning should be a priority (Box 9-4).

HEAD INJURY. Head injuries are the most common severe disabling injuries in the United States, with an estimated half million new cases occurring annually. The most common causes of head injury include motor vehicle (including bicycles and motorcycles) crashes, falls, diving and other water-related accidents, and violence. Recently, efforts to prevent head injuries in children have targeted laws and ordinances requiring bicycle helmets.

Each year nearly 1000 bicyclists are killed in the United States and more than 550,000 persons are treated in emergency departments for bicycle-related injuries. More than 87% of bicyclist fatalities occur in males and more than one

BOX 9-4 Emergency Action for Poisoning

SWALLOWED MEDICINE

1. Call the poison control center—if not available, call 911; do not give anything to drink by mouth until you call; do not wait for symptoms to develop.
2. If emergency personnel tell you to make the child vomit, give 1 T of syrup of ipecac; keep the child moving; if the child does not vomit within 15 minutes, give a second tablespoon; do not give a third.
3. If you go to an emergency treatment center, take the medicine container.

SWALLOWED CHEMICAL OR HOUSEHOLD PRODUCTS

1. If child is conscious, immediately give one or two glasses of milk (give water if milk is not available).
2. Call the poison control center—if not available, call 911.
3. Do not make the child vomit for acid, alkali, or petroleum poisoning.

INHALED POISON

1. Immediately get the child to fresh air; avoid breathing fumes; open doors and windows wide.
2. If victim is not breathing, start artificial respiration.
3. Call 911.

POISON ON THE SKIN

1. Remove contaminated clothing and flood skin with water for 10 minutes.
2. Wash gently with soap and water; rinse.
3. Call the Poison Control Center.

POISON IN THE EYE

1. Flood the eye with lukewarm (not hot) water, poured from a large glass held 2 to 3 inches from the eye.
2. Repeat for 15 minutes.
3. Have the child blink as much as possible while flooding the eye; do not force the eyelid open.
4. Call a physician or the Poison Control Center.

From Texas Department of Health. (1990). *Protect your child against accidental poisoning.* Austin, TX: Texas Department of Health.

third occur in boys between the ages of 5 and 15 years (CDC, 1995). The majority of bicycle fatalities are caused by bicyclist error (e.g., failure to yield right of way, improper crossing of an intersection or road, failure to obey traffic signs and lights) and alcohol is involved in many bicycle fatalities.

Head injury accounts for 62% of bicycle-related deaths and 67% of bicycle-related hospital admissions. Based on evidence that 74% to 85% of the risk of head injury can be reduced by the use of bicycle helmets, the CDC (1995) has recommended that state and local agencies and organizations develop programs to increase their use. These recommendations are as follows:

- Bicycle helmets should be worn by all persons (i.e., bicycle operators and passengers) at any age when bicycling.
- Bicycle riders should wear helmets whenever and wherever they ride a bicycle (Figure 9-3).
- Bicycle helmets should meet the standards of the American National Standards Institute, the Snell Memorial Foundation, or the American Society for Testing and Material.

- To effectively increase helmet use rates, states and communities must implement programs that include legislation, education and promotion, enforcement, and program evaluation.

Other measures to improve bicycle safety include education and training to improve knowledge of and adherence to traffic laws, use of appropriate clothing (light colored and marked with reflective materials) when riding at night, and bicycle maintenance. Bicycle safety programs are available in most communities.

Head injury is also the most commonly recorded cause of deaths for motorcycle drivers and passengers who die in crashes. Nonhelmeted riders are two and a half times more likely than helmeted riders to sustain a fatal head injury. Further, helmet use is the single most important factor in preventing death and head injuries (Advocates for Highway and Auto Safety, 1994). All motorcycle riders should be informed of these statistics and helmet laws should be encouraged in those states where they do not exist and strongly enforced in all other states. Nurses and other health care providers should consistently

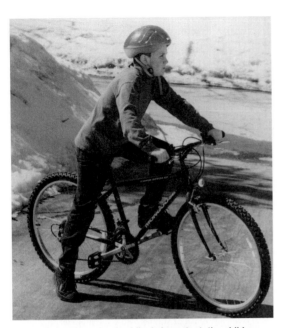

Figure 9-3. The right-size bike is important; the child should be able to sit on the bike and place the balls of both feet on the ground. The foot should comfortably reach and manipulate the pedal in the down position. Wearing a protective helmet is mandatory for safe cycling. The helmet should sit on top of the head in a level position and should not rock back and forth or from side to side. The strap should always be fastened securely under the chin. (From Wong, D. L. [1999]. *Whaley & Wong's nursing care of infants and children* [6th ed., p. 239]. St. Louis: Mosby.

encourage parents, adolescents, and children to use protective helmets whenever using a bicycle or motorcycle.

FIRE AND BURNS. Fire and burns are the fifth leading cause of childhood deaths from injury, but they are the second leading cause of deaths from injury in children 1 to 9 years of age (CDC/National Center for Injury Prevention and Control [NCIPC], unpublished data, 1994). Indeed, 73% of burn deaths in children occurred in those younger than 9 years. Overall, 80% of deaths from fire or burns resulted from house fires, 9% from electrical burns, and 2% from scalding (CDC, 1990).

According to the USDHHS (2000), those who live in substandard housing without smoke detectors are at the highest risk for fire death. Improved public awareness of home fire safety, including use of functional smoke detectors in all sleeping areas and establishment of home evacuation plans, can help reduce home fire deaths and disabilities. The most common sources of fire and burns are wood stoves, space heaters, cooking equipment, cigarettes, matches and lighters.

Many fire deaths and injuries are caused by smoke and gases because the victims inhale smoke that occurs ahead of the flames. Early warning and having an escape plan can dramatically diminish injury and death. General recommendations for fire safety from the U.S. Consumer Products Safety Commission (1994) include the following:

- Read the manufacturer's instructions on installation and location of fire detectors.
- Install smoke detectors on each floor of the house, near all sleeping areas, and in the kitchen.
- Follow the manufacturer's instructions for cleaning and maintenance; replace the battery annually or when a chirping sound is heard.
- Develop an escape plan and an alternate escape plan for the family and practice the escape routes periodically. The escape plan should include choosing a place outside the house where the family will meet to be sure that everyone got out safely.
- Ensure that there are at least two exits from each part of the house.

DROWNING. Drowning is the third leading cause of deaths from injury in children 1 to 4 years and the fourth for children 5 to 14 years. In Arizona, California, and Florida, drowning was the leading cause of fatal injury for children younger than 4 years (CDC/NCIPC, unpublished data, Atlanta, 1994). Those at highest risk for drowning are men and boys, children younger than 5 years, African-Americans, and Native Americans. The highest drowning rates are among children 4 years and younger and males 15 to 19 years of age. The drowning rate for African-American children (4.5/100,000) is almost twice that for white children (2.6/100,000). For adolescents, drownings are most often associated with water activities (e.g., boating, skiing). Alcohol is a factor in an estimated 40% to 50% of adolescent drownings (CDC, 1990; USDHHS/ODPHP, 1994).

As many as 90% of drownings occur in residential swimming pools. Fencing of all pools, use of pool alarms and pool covers, and safety regulations can prevent pool drowning by preschool children and should be encouraged. Counseling of parents should include admonishment to never leave infants, toddlers, and small children in or near the bathtub, wading pool, or swimming pool without supervision.

To prevent deaths in adolescents, all states have laws prohibiting operating a boat under the influence of alcohol or drugs. Enforcement of these laws and increasing public awareness of safe operating practices and discouraging alcohol use can be helpful (USDHHS/ODPHP, 1994).

VIOLENT BEHAVIOR. Violence in the United States is pervasive and claims many lives and threatens the health and well-being of many more. On an average day in the United States, 53 people die from homicide and at least 18,000 others survive interpersonal assaults. In addition, 84 people commit suicide each day and 3000 others attempt suicide (USDHHS, 2000). Homicide was the cause of death of almost 20,000 Americans in 1997. It is the second leading cause of death for young persons 15 to 24 and the leading cause of death for blacks in this age group. Indeed, the homicide rate in the United States is 10 times higher than in Canada, 15 times higher than in Australia, and 28 times higher than in France or Germany (USDHHS, 2000).

Homicide most often affects men, teenagers, and minority group members—particularly blacks and Hispanics. To assist in the detection and prevention of violence, Box 9-5 lists sociological, developmental, and familial risk factors.

Firearms, particularly handguns, have been implicated in an alarming number of homicides and suicides. Firearms accounted for 75% of the

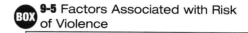

BOX 9-5 Factors Associated with Risk of Violence

SOCIOLOGICAL

Low socioeconomic status
Involvement with gangs
Drug dealing
Access to guns
Media exposure to violence
Community exposure to violence

DEVELOPMENTAL/PSYCHOLOGICAL

Alcohol or drug abuse
Rigid sex role expectations
Peer pressure, especially for adolescents
Poor impulse control
History of mental health problems
High individual stress level
Manual laborer, unemployed, or employed part time
Younger than 30 years

FAMILY

History of intergenerational abuse
Social isolation
Parents verbally threaten children
High levels of family stress
Two or more children

From Maurer, F. A. (2000). Violence: A social and family problem. In C. M. Smith & F. A. Mauer (Eds.), *Community health nursing: Theory and practice* (2nd ed., pp. 571-606). Philadelphia: W. B. Saunders.

suicide/homicide deaths for the 15- to 24-year-old age group and 66% of deaths in those 10 to 14 years of age. All parents, children, and adolescents should receive information and counseling to prevent violence. Information on the danger of guns is particularly important (see the Health Teaching box "Strategies for Prevention of Gun-Related Injuries and Violent Behaviors").

OTHER SAFETY HAZARDS. Additional hazards threaten the safety of infants, children, and adolescents. These include participation in hazardous sports and recreational activities, choking or aspiration, suffocation, and other concerns.

To prevent injuries from sports and recreational activities, all children should be taught to wear appropriate protective gear at all times when participating. For example, batting helmets, catcher's gear, and athletic supporters and protective cups for all boys should be required when playing baseball; helmets, wrist guards, knee pads, and elbow pads should be worn for in-line skating and skateboarding; and hockey and football players should wear the full complement of pads, helmets, and mouthguards whenever they play. Parents should be counseled to ensure that children are properly supervised when engaging in activities that are associated with injury risk. Finally, many organized athletic organizations require a yearly physical examination by a health care professional before participation. A physical examination may identify undetected problems

---

health teaching

Strategies for Prevention of Gun-Related Injuries and Violent Behaviors

1. Every child and family should be assessed for the potential for injury from violence; areas to assess include the following:
   - Is there a history of violent injury to the child or other family members?
   - Is there a history of alcohol or other drug abuse by the child or the other family members?
   - Are there guns or other weapons in the home?
   - Is violent injury a prevalent problem in the community?
2. All parents should be advised about the danger of keeping a gun in the home; basic rules of safety include the following:
   - Never keep a loaded gun in the house or car.
   - Keep guns and ammunition locked in separate places.
   - Always treat a gun as if it were loaded and ready to fire.
   - Never allow children access to guns.
   - Have a gunsmith check antique and souvenir guns to ensure that they are not loaded and fix them so they cannot be fired.
3. Parents should be advised to inquire about the availability of guns in places where their children spend time, such as at friends' houses, schools, and recreational facilities. Parents should be encouraged to take an active role in limiting the availability of guns in their children's environment.
4. When treating clients with injuries that have been or may have been caused by violence, ask questions about the cause of the injury. If the injury has been caused by violence, attempt to determine if the conflict has been settled or may lead to further violence. The following questions might be addressed:
   - Has the argument been settled?
   - Do you have a place to go if this is not settled?
   - Are you safe?
   - Is there anyone who can help settle the argument?
5. Despite the desirability of maintaining confidentiality, it may be necessary to consult with parents, police, and other authorities to protect the safety of children and adolescents involved in potentially violent situations.
6. Parents and children should be given the facts about violence through various media in classes, offices, or clinics; posters, videotapes, lectures, and brochures may be helpful.
7. Children and adolescents should be encouraged to discuss how they deal with anger and to develop positive ways to manage anger and arguments; one suggested strategy for anger management is termed CALM:
   - C—Cool down and count to 10; consider the cause and consequences
   - A—Accept responsibility for your actions and reactions
   - L—Listen to all sides and talk it over
   - M—Move away and move on to something else

Adapted from U.S. Department of Health and Human Services/Office of Disease Prevention and Health Promotion (USDHHS/ODPHP). (1994). Counseling: Violent behavior and firearms. In *Clinician's handbook of preventive services* (pp. 126-128). Washington, DC: Government Printing Office; data from American Academy of Pediatrics/Center to Prevent Handgun Violence. (1992). *Rx for safety: Preventing firearms injuries among children and adolescents.* Washington, DC: Center to Prevent Handgun Violence; American Academy of Pediatrics/Committee on Injury Control for Children and Youth. (1987). *Injury control for children and youth.* Elk Grove Village, IL: American Academy of Pediatrics; Violence Prevention Project. (1992). *Identification and prevention of youth violence: A protocol of health care providers.* Boston: Violence Prevention Project.

that might threaten health (e.g., asthma, heart problems, musculoskeletal problems).

Each year, many children suffer serious injury or death through inappropriate use of objects or toys (e.g., beanbags, plastic bags, balloons), misuse of equipment (e.g., highchairs, baby walkers), and lack of close supervision or precautions (e.g., leaving the side rail down on the crib, giving a toddler food that might cause choking, not covering electric outlets). Box 9-6 presents general guidelines for **child safety** that are essential components of health teaching for all parents.

BOX **9-6** Child Safety Home Checklist

SAFETY: FIRE, ELECTRICAL, BURNS

Guards in front of or around any heating appliance, fireplace, or furnace (including floor furnace)*
Electrical wires hidden or out of reach*
No frayed or broken wires; no overloaded sockets
Plastic guards or caps over electrical outlets; furniture in front of outlets*
Hanging tablecloths out of reach, away from open fires*
Smoke detectors tested and operating properly
Kitchen matches stored out of child's reach*
Large, deep ashtrays throughout house (if used)
Small stoves, heaters, and other hot objects (e.g., cigarettes, candles, coffee pots, slow cookers) placed where they cannot be tipped over or reached by children
Hot water heater set at 49°C (120°F) or lower
Pot handles turned toward back of stove, center of table
No loose clothing worn near stove
No cooking or eating hot foods or liquids with child standing nearby or sitting in lap
All small appliances, such as iron, turned off, disconnected, and placed out of reach when not in use
Cool, not hot, mist vaporizer used
Fire extinguisher available on each floor and checked periodically
Electrical fuse box and gas outlet accessible
Family escape plan in case of a fire practiced periodically; fire escape ladder available on upper-level floors
Telephone number of fire or rescue squad and address of home with nearest cross-street posted near phone

SAFETY: SUFFOCATION AND ASPIRATION

Small objects stored out of reach*
Toys inspected for small removable parts or long strings*
Hanging crib toys and mobiles placed out of reach

Plastic bags stored away from young child's reach, large plastic garment bags discarded after tying in knots*
Mattress or pillow not covered with plastic or in manner accessible to child*
Crib design according to federal regulations with snug-fitting mattress*†
Crib positioned away from other furniture or windows*
Portable playpen gates up at all times while in use*
Accordion-style gates not used*
Bathroom doors kept closed and toilet seats down*
Faucets turned off firmly*
Pool fenced with locked gate
Proper safety equipment at poolside
Electric garage door openers stored safely and garage door adjusted to rise when door strikes object
Doors of ovens, trunks, dishwashers, refrigerators, and front-loading clothes washers and dryers kept closed*
Unused appliance, such as a refrigerator, securely closed with lock or doors removed*
Food served in small noncylindric pieces*
Toy chests without lids or with lids that securely lock in open position*
Buckets and wading pools kept empty when not in use*
Clothesline above head level
At least one member of household trained in basic life support (cardiopulmonary resuscitation [CPR]) including first aid for choking‡

SAFETY: POISONING

Toxic substances, including batteries, placed on a high shelf, preferably in locked cabinet
Toxic plants hung or placed out of reach*
Excess quantities of cleaning fluids, paints, pesticides, drugs, and other toxic substances not stored in home
Used containers of poisonous substances discarded where child cannot obtain access
Telephone number of local poison control center and address of home with nearest cross-street posted near phone

---

From Wong, D. L. (1999). *Whaley & Wong's nursing care of infants and children* (6th ed.). St. Louis: Mosby.
*Safety measures are specific for homes with young children. All safety measures should be implemented in homes where children reside and visit frequently, such as those of grandparents or babysitters.
†Federal regulations are available from U.S. Consumer Product Safety Commission, 800-638-CPSC.
‡Home care instructions for infant CPR and infant/child choking are available in Wong and Whaley's *Clinical Manual of Pediatric Nursing*.

9-6 Child Safety Home Checklist—cont'd

Syrup of ipecac in home containing two doses per child

Medicines clearly labeled in childproof containers and stored out of reach

Household cleaners, disinfectants, and insecticides kept in their original containers, separate from food and out of reach

Smoking in areas away from children

SAFETY: FALLS

Nonskid mats, strips, or surfaces in tubs and showers

Exits, halls, and passageways in rooms kept clear of toys, furniture, boxes, or other items that could be obstructive

Stairs and halls well lighted, with switches at both top and bottom

Sturdy handrails for all steps and stairways

Nothing stored on stairways

Treads, risers, and carpeting in good repair

Glass doors and walls marked with decals

Safety glass used in doors, windows, and walls

Gates on top and bottom of staircases and elevated areas, such as porch or fire escape*

Guardrails on upstairs windows with locks that limit height of window opening and access to areas such as fire escape*

Crib side rails raised to full height; mattress lowered as child grows*

Restraints used in high chairs, walkers, or other baby furniture; preferably walkers not used*

Scatter rugs secured in place or used with nonskid back

Walks, patios, and driveways in good repair

SAFETY: BODILY INJURY

Knives, power tools, and unloaded firearms stored safely or placed in locked cabinet

Garden tools returned to storage racks after use

Pets properly restrained and immunized for rabies

Swings, slides, and other outdoor play equipment kept in safe condition

Yard free of broken glass, nail-studded boards, other litter

Cement birdbaths placed where young child cannot tip them over*

Child Abuse: Detection and Prevention

Child abuse and neglect refers to any physical or mental injury, sexual abuse or exploitation, negligent treatment, or maltreatment of a child by a person who is responsible for the child's welfare. The incidence of child abuse appears to be rising. It is estimated that about 1 million children suffer abuse and neglect each year and these numbers appear to be increasing. Child abuse results in an estimated 1200 deaths each year—about half from physical abuse and half from neglect (USDHHS, 2000).

Although child abuse and neglect cases cross all age, race, education, and socioeconomic lines, reported cases show individuals who are poor, young, black, and who have little education are more frequent abusers (Maurer, 2000). It is important to realize that reported data may be biased and observation for and reporting of suspected cases should consider suspicious cases from any social class, race, or age.

Nurses who practice in community settings are sometimes in a position to recognize and intervene in cases of suspected child abuse. To assist in recognizing individuals at risk to be abusive parents, Box 9-7 lists characteristics of abusive parents and Table 9-5 details physical and behavioral indicators of child abuse and neglect.

Child abuse and neglect are crimes in all 50 states and nurses have a legal responsibility to report suspected or actual cases of child abuse. Most institutions providing care to children have a written policy regarding the reporting of suspected child abuse. These policies need to be reviewed periodically (see the Community Application box "Typical Procedure for Notification and Investigation of Child Abuse and Neglect Cases"). Finally, to assist in the reduction of family violence, see the Community Application box "Components of a Comprehensive Program to Reduce Family Violence."

BOX 9-7 Characteristics and Behaviors of Abusive Parents

CHARACTERISTICS

At or below poverty level
History of abuse or neglect as a child
Poor parenting skills
Poor coping skills
Involved in a crisis situation (e.g., unemployment, divorce, financial difficulties)
Does not understand normal growth and development patterns
Unrealistic expectations of their child's behavior
Looking to child for satisfaction of needs of love, support, and reassurance
Poor impulse control
Low tolerance for frustration
Poor or inadequate role models
Socially isolated from support systems
Women more frequently physically abuse children

Men more frequently sexually abuse children
Stepfathers are five to eight times more likely to engage in sexual abuse of their children than are birth fathers

BEHAVIORS

Frequent use of harsh punishment
Projection of blame onto the child
History of drug or alcohol abuse
Delay getting medical attention for child
Respond inappropriately to child during treatment (e.g., ignore, show no concern or overinvolved with attention)
Use different facilities for treatment of child
Blame siblings, babysitters, or others without substantiation or place blame on child's clumsiness
Tell contradictory stories to explain injury
Vague about cause of the injury

Data from Grant, C. (1995). Physical and sexual abuse. In D. Antai-Otong (Ed.), *Psychiatric nursing: Biological and behavioral concepts* (pp. 407-426). Philadelphia: W. B. Saunders; Maurer, F. A. (2000). Violence: A social and family problem. In C. M. Smith & F. A. Maurer (Eds.), *Community health nursing: Theory and practice* (2nd ed., pp. 571-606). Philadelphia: W. B. Saunders; Pappas, A., & Hakala, K. L. D. (2001). Violence in the community. In M. A. Nies & M. McEwen (Eds.), *Community health nursing: Promoting the health of populations* (3rd ed., pp. 596-623). Philadelphia: W. B. Saunders; Smith-DiJulio, K., & Holzapfel, S. K. (1994). Families in crisis: Family violence. In E. M. Varcarolis (Ed.), *Foundations of psychiatric mental health nursing* (2nd ed.). Philadelphia: W. B. Saunders.

TABLE **9-5** Physical and Behavioral Indicators of Child Abuse and Neglect

PHYSICAL INDICATORS	BEHAVIORAL INDICATORS
PHYSICAL ABUSE	
Unexplained bruises and welts in various stages of healing that may form patterns	Wariness of adult contacts
Unexplained burns by cigars or cigarettes or immersion burns (e.g., socklike, glovelike, or on buttocks or genitalia)	Apprehensive when other children cry
	Constantly on the alert
Rope burns	Exhibiting extremes of behavior; aggressiveness or passive and withdrawn or overly friendly to strangers
Unexplained lacerations or abrasions	Frightened of parents
Unexplained fractures in various stages of healing; multiple or spiral fractures	Afraid to go home
Unexplained injuries to mouth, lips, gums, eyes, or external genitalia	Reporting injury by parents
PHYSICAL NEGLECT	
Hunger	Begging or stealing food
Poor hygiene	Alone at inappropriate times or for prolonged periods
Poor or inappropriate dress	Delinquent

From Pappas, A., & Hakala, K. L. D. (2001). Violence in the community. In M. A. Nies & M. McEwen (Eds.), *Community health nursing: Promoting the health of populations* (3rd ed., pp. 596-623). Philadelphia: W. B. Saunders.

continued

TABLE **9-5** Physical and Behavioral Indicators of Child Abuse and Neglect—cont'd

PHYSICAL INDICATORS	BEHAVIORAL INDICATORS
Lack of supervision for prolonged periods	Stealing
Lack of medical or dental care	Arriving early to and departing late from school
Constant fatigue, listlessness, or falling asleep in class	Reporting having no caretaker
SEXUAL ABUSE	
Difficulty in walking or sitting	Exhibiting negative self-esteem
Torn, stained, or bloody underwear	Exhibiting inability to trust and function in intimate relationships
Genital pain or itching	Exhibiting cognitive and motor dysfunctions
Bruises or bleeding from the external genitalia, vaginal, or anal areas	Exhibiting deficits in personal and social skills
Venereal disease	Exhibiting bizarre, sophisticated, or unusual sexual behavior or knowledge
Drug and alcohol abuse	Delinquency or a runaway
Developmental delays	Exhibiting suicide ideation
	Reporting sexual assault
EMOTIONAL MALTREATMENT	
Failure to thrive	Exhibiting behavior extremes from passivity to aggression
Lags in physical development	Exhibiting habit and conduct disorders (e.g., antisocial behavior and destructiveness)
Speech disorders	Exhibiting neurotic traits
Developmental delays	Attempting suicide

COMMUNITY APPLICATION
Typical Procedure for Notification and Investigation of Child Abuse and Neglect Cases

Actions Taken by Community Health Nurse
Identify suspected case abuse/neglect
Verbally report to:
1. Child protection agency
or
2. Local law enforcement
Send written report to child protection agency within 48 hours of initiating complaint and send a copy to the state's attorney's office

Actions Taken by Designated Child Protection Agency
Prompt investigation within 24 hours if abuse, usually longer—perhaps as much as 5 days—if neglect

Completed investigation within 10 days and report of findings to state's attorney's office
Dispensation of case
1. No evidence found
2. Inconclusive, file kept open
3. Evidence exists, action taken
Possible actions include:
1. Mandated supervision in home
2. Conditions imposed on parents to continue custody (e.g., attend parenting classes, drug rehabilitation)
3. Temporary removal of children to foster care or other relatives' homes
4. Permanent removal of child from home
5. Court action to cease parental rights to clear for adoption

From Maurer, F. A. (2000). Violence: A social and family problem. In C. M. Smith & F. A. Maurer (Eds.), *Community health nursing: Theory and practice* (2nd ed., pp. 571-606). Philadelphia: W. B. Saunders.

COMMUNITY APPLICATION
Components of a Comprehensive Program to Reduce Family Violence

Primary Prevention—Goal: Promotion of Optimal Parenting and Family Wellness

Individuals

Family life education in schools, churches, and communities

Education of children on methods of conflict resolution

Birth control services for sexually active teens

Child care education for teenagers who babysit

Preventative mental services for adults and children

Training for professionals in early detection of violence

Family

Parenting classes in hospitals, schools, and other community agencies

Provision of bonding opportunities for new parents

Referral of new families to community health nurses after early discharge from the hospital for follow-up services

Social services for families

Community

Community education concerning family violence

Reduction of media violence

Development of community services such as crisis lines, respite placement for children, respite care for families with dependent older adult members, shelters for battered women and their children

Handgun control

Secondary Prevention—Goal: Diagnosis of and Service for Families in Stress

Individuals

Nursing assessment for evidence of family violence in all health care settings

A well thought out safety plan for victims

Knowledge of legal options to help ensure safety

Shelter or foster home placement for victims

Family

Social services for individuals or families

Referral to self-help groups in the community

Referral to community agencies that provide services for victims

Community

All health professionals skilled in assessment of violence and equipped with protocols for dealing with the victims to help ensure their safety

Hospital emergency rooms and trauma centers with 24-hour reporting, response, case intake, coordination with legal and medical authorities, coordination with voluntary agencies that have services, coordination with social services departments for provision of services

Death review teams to review deaths from injury, especially for infants and children

Public authority involvement by police, district attorneys, and courts

Epidemiological tracking and evaluation of violence

Handgun control

Tertiary Prevention—Goal: Reeducation and Rehabilitation of Violent Families

Individuals

Empowerment strategies for battered women

Professional counseling services for individuals

Family

Parenting reeducation (i.e., formal training in child rearing)

Professional counseling services for families

Self-help groups

Community

Foster homes, shelters, and care for older adults

Public authority involvement

Follow-up care for known cases of abuse

Gun control

From Pappas, A., & Hakala, K. L. D. (2001). Violence in the community. In M. A. Nies & M. McEwen (Eds.), *Community health nursing: Promoting the health of populations* (3rd ed., pp. 596-623). Philadelphia: W. B. Saunders.

NURSING CARE FOR COMMON HEALTH PROBLEMS

Nurses who care for infants and children in community settings should be aware of common illnesses and conditions. Table 9-6 describes some of the more frequently encountered acute and episodic illnesses and chronic conditions in infants and children, including prevention strategies, identification, and treatment.

Text continued on p. 230

TABLE 9-6 Common Health Problems in Infants and Children

DISEASE/CONDITION	DEFINITION/ETIOLOGY	PREVENTION STRATEGIES	SIGNS AND SYMPTOMS/COMPLICATIONS	MANAGEMENT/TREATMENT
		Acute Respiratory/Ear, Nose, and Throat Conditions		
Viral infection (e.g., cold, influenza)	*Cold:* caused by up to 200 virus strains. *Incubation:* 1-7 days (usually 2-3 days). Children have 6-10 colds/year, decreasing with age.	Avoid exposure. Wash hands carefully; avoid touching nose or eyes with contaminated fingers. Influenza may be prevented or lessened with vaccination. Those in high-risk groups should be immunized yearly. Amantadine and remantadine may be used prophylactically in high-risk groups and during epidemics of influenza A.	*Cold:* nasal stuffiness, sneezing, scratchy throat, coughing, malaise, headache, slight fever. *Influenza:* sudden onset of moderate-to-high fever (102°F or higher), chills, headache, anorexia, malaise, muscle aches, cough, runny nose, sore throat, cervical lymphadenopathy, hoarseness, possible abdominal pain, vomiting, nausea, diarrhea. *Complications:* otitis media, pneumonia, bronchitis, and sinusitis are most common.	*Medications:* analgesics and antipyretics (avoid aspirin), decongestants, antitussives. *Symptom management:* bed rest, oral hydration. Observe for complications.
Bacterial pharyngitis (e.g., strep throat, tonsillitis)	*Strep throat:* caused by group A betahemolytic streptococci bacteria. Greatest incidence in children 5-18 years of age.	Avoid contact with respiratory secretions. Children should not return to school until after 24 hours of antibiotic therapy.	Sore throat, reddened throat, enlarged tonsils, soft palate petechia, cervical adenopathy, fever (moderate-to-high), anorexia, chills, malaise, headache. Abdominal pain and vomiting may occur. *Complications:* Scarlet fever (red, papular rash beginning in the axilla and chest, spreading to the abdomen and extremities.) *Progressive complications:* rheumatic fever, glomerulonephritis, myocarditis.	Throat culture for suspected infection. For streptococcal pharyngitis, a 10-day course of penicillin is the standard. Erythromycin or cephalexin may be used for penicillin-allergic children. Teach parents the importance of completing the 10-day course of therapy. Monitor for complications.
Otitis media	Inflammation of the middle ear, usually bacterial. Almost 93% of children have one or more cases of otitis media by age	*Risk factors:* upper respiratory infection, smoking in household, family history of middle ear infections.	Ear pain, decreased hearing, may have accompanying nasal discharge and cough, fever. *Infants:* irritability, may have slight fever. Otoscopic examination reveals decreased eardrum mobility, bulging eardrum redness.	*Medications:* Amoxicillin, cephalosporin. Antihistamines and decongestants may be used, but not always effective.

	7 years; 36% of children have six or more cases of otitis. Peak incidence is at 6-12 months; declines after age 7 years.	*Complications:* perforation of eardrum, hearing loss, scarring of eardrum, mastoiditis.	Referral for tympanostomy tubes and adenoidectomy for multiple infections, middle ear fluid that persists for 4-6 months, and/or hearing loss. *Medications:* antibiotics for bacterial bronchitis or pneumonia. Analgesics, antipyretics, cough suppressant.
Respiratory infections: bronchitis and pneumonia	Inflammation and infection of the respiratory tract, usually as a secondary infection. May be caused by a virus or bacteria. *Viral pneumonia:* most common cause of lower respiratory tract infections in young children and often follows an upper respiratory infection. About 90% of pneumonia in children is viral. *Bacterial pneumonia:* usually caused by pneumonococci, streptococci, and staphylococci.	Coughing—may be dry and hacking; nonproductive cough is common in bronchitis. Fever (may be mild to severe), chills, dyspnea, pulmonary rales and rhonchi, altered breath sounds, pleurisy, friction rub, headache. Tachypnea, malaise, wheezing.	Vaccine is now recommended for all children to protect against bacterial pneumonia Monitor colds and influenza for complications and secondary infection.

Chronic Respiratory Diseases

Asthma	Reversible airway disease characterized by bronchial constriction, mucosal edema, and increased mucous production.	Abnormal pulmonary function tests, wheezing, cough, prolonged expiration, hyperresonance, decreased breath sounds, nocturnal dyspnea, cyanosis, use of accessory respiratory muscles.	*Avoidance of triggers:* allergens (e.g., pollens, molds, dust mites, animal dander, smoke and other pollutants, viral infections. Use of medications to prevent inflammation and exacerbation. *Medication:* steroids, beta-agonists, anticholinergics, theophylline; monitoring of peak expiratory flow rates (PEFR); identify and eliminate irritants.

continued

Data from Betz, C. L., Hunsberger, M. M., & Wright, S. (1994). *Family-centered nursing care of children* (2nd ed.). Philadelphia: W. B. Saunders; Dambro, M. R. (1996). *Griffith's 5-minute clinical consult.* Baltimore: Williams & Wilkins; Jackson, D. B., & Saunders, R. B. (1994). *Child health nursing: A comprehensive approach to the care of children and their families.* Philadelphia: J. B. Lippincott.

TABLE 9-6 Common Health Problems in Infants and Children—cont'd

DISEASE/CONDITION	DEFINITION/ETIOLOGY	PREVENTION STRATEGIES	SIGNS AND SYMPTOMS/COMPLICATIONS	MANAGEMENT/TREATMENT
Vaccine-Preventable Diseases				
Measles (rubeola)	Highly contagious, acute viral infection; incubation 8-12 days postexposure. Contagious from 1-2 days before symptoms to 4 days after onset of rash.	Vaccine preventable. Postexposure prophylaxis-vaccine is protective if given within 72 hours postexposure; immune globulin prevents/modifies illness if given within 6 days postexposure.	*Prodromal phase:* fever and cold-like symptoms, conjunctivitis, photophobia, nasal congestion, cough, Koplik spots (small white spots circumscribed in red, opposite lower molars). *Acute phase:* rash begins as fever peaks; dark red, maculopapular rash begins behind ears and at hairline and spreads from head to feet and lasts 10-15 days. Rash turns brown and scaly after 5-6 days. *Complications:* otitis media, bronchitis, and pneumonia are most common.	Bed rest, antitussives, antipyretics (avoid aspirin). *Notify Health Department.*
Mumps	Acute viral infection presenting with unilateral or bilateral parotitis. Incubation period 14-24 days; 85% of cases occur before age 15 years.	Vaccine preventable.	Parotid pain and swelling in one or both glands. Swelling peaks in 1-3 days and lasts 3-7 days. Mild-to-moderate fever.	Analgesics for pain (avoid aspirin). Liquid or soft diet, warm or cold compresses for swelling. *Complications:* orchitis or epididymitis are fairly common in postpubertal boys. *Less common:* meningoencephalitis, nephritis, pancreatitis, and oophoritis.
Chicken pox	Highly contagious infections caused by the varicella zoster virus. Most commonly affects children age 5-9 years of age, but can develop in any age. *Incubation period:* 13-17 days postexposure.	Vaccine preventable. Postexposure varicella zoster immune globulin may be given to high-risk children. Avoidance of exposure (communicability—1 day before eruption of lesions until all vesicles have crusted).	*Prodromal stage:* slight fever, malaise, mild headache, and anorexia for first 24 hours. Rash begins on the trunk, spreads to face and then extremities. Lesions may develop on oral and vaginal mucous membranes. Lesions begin as macules and rapidly progress to papule, then vesicle and present in varying degrees at one time.	Isolate child in home until vesicles have dried (usually 1 week after onset); decrease itching with antipruritic agent (e.g., calamine lotion), antihistamines, and oatmeal baths. Use mild antipyretics for fever, but *avoid aspirin.*

Genitourinary Conditions

Urinary tract infection (UTI)	Inflammation or infection of the urethra, bladder, or kidney. In neonates, UTIs are more common in boys; by 4 months, they are *much* more common in girls and this continues throughout childhood. *Escherichia coli* causes 75%-90% of UTIs in children.	Good toileting hygiene (e.g., teaching girls to wipe from front to back); encourage frequent emptying of bladder; use cotton underpants. Avoid bubble baths.	Urinary urgency and frequency, burning, lower abdominal pain and cramping, hematuria, foul-smelling urine, fever. High fever and flank pain may indicate kidney infection. Recurrent infections may indicate renal anomalies and referral for diagnostic evaluation is very important.	*Medications:* antibiotics based on culture/sensitivity. A 7- to 10-day course of trimethoprim-sulfamethoxazole (TMP/SMZ) or amoxicillin is usually given. Stress the importance of completing all medications.
Enuresis	Nocturnal enuresis is involuntary urination during sleep more than once a month in girls over 5 years and boys over 6 years of age. Enuresis affects about 10% of children (40% of 3-year-olds, 10% of six-year-olds, and 3% of 12-year-olds), with boys more commonly affected than girls.	More common if one or both parents report being enuretic as a child. Associated with reduced bladder capacity and/or frequent uninhibited bladder contractions.	Inability to keep from urinating while asleep at least once per month. Some children may be withdrawn and shy.	Encourage daytime fluids and less frequent urination to increase bladder size. Discourage any fluids 2 hours before bedtime; void just before bedtime; protect bed by having the child wear extra-thick underwear (not diaper) and put towel under the child; encourage the child to get up to urinate during the night, but parents should not awaken the child to urinate; do not punish the child for a wet night; praise dry nights. Bed-wetting alarms may help.

continued

TABLE **9-6** Common Health Problems in Infants and Children—cont'd

DISEASE/CONDITION	DEFINITION/ETIOLOGY	PREVENTION STRATEGIES	SIGNS AND SYMPTOMS/COMPLICATIONS	MANAGEMENT/TREATMENT
				Medications: Imipramine may be used. Intranasally administered desmopressin helps reduce nighttime production of urine and assists about 70% of children. Relapse is common after medications are discontinued. Emotional support of the child and parents is important.
Gastrointestinal Problems				
Colic	Excessive crying seen in young infants who are otherwise well. Believed to be caused by paroxysmal abdominal cramping. Colic affects 10%-25% of infants age 3 weeks to 3 months.	Milk allergy may contribute to some cases.	Inconsolable crying, often more than 3 hours per day; fist clenching, arching back, and drawing up of legs; excessive flatus.	Use of a pacifier, gentle rhythmic motions (e.g., rocking, car rides), music. Usually subsides by 3 months of age. Changing the baby's formula or removing dairy products from the diet of lactating mother may help. Give smaller, frequent feedings; burp during and after feedings; and place infant upright after feeding; place prone over a warm towel, hot water bottle, recovered heating pad. Emotional support and respite care for the primary caregiver is very important.

| Gastroenteritis/ stomach flu | In the United States, most cases of nausea, vomiting, and diarrhea are caused by viruses (rotavirus, parvovirus, adenovirus, and coronavirus). Symptoms usually occur 1-2 days after exposure. | Good handwashing, avoidance of exposure. | Nausea, vomiting, diarrhea, abdominal pain and distention, anorexia, malaise. Usually self-limiting, lasting 1-3 days. Dehydration in infants and small children may occur rapidly, however, and parents need to observe for fever, increasing thirst; decreasing urine production, sunken eyes or fontanel, diminished skin turgor, lethargy, cool extremities. | Replacement of fluids and electrolytes by encouraging consumption of clear liquids, such as uncaffeinated beverages, broth, flavored gelatin, water, or rehydration fluids (e.g., Pedialyte, Gatorade). As nausea and diarrhea decrease, slowly add mild foods, such as saltines, dry toast, rice, baked potato; avoid dairy products, most fruits, vegetables, meats. Hospitalization for intravenous rehydration may be necessary in severe cases. |
| Appendicitis | Acute inflammation of the vermiform appendix. Affects about 7% of all persons; children, adolescents, and young adults (10-30 years of age) are most commonly infected, although persons of any age may be affected. | Familial tendency is possible. High-fiber diets may help prevent appendicitis. | Constant abdominal pain—initially periumbilical then right-lower quadrant; guarding of the abdomen; anorexia, nausea; vomiting; slight fever. Leukocytosis (10,000 to 18,000/mm³); ultrasound usually reveals appendix inflammation. *Complications:* perforation with abscess, peritonitis, bowel obstruction, gangrene. | *Surgery:* emergency appendectomy. If uncomplicated, broad-spectrum antibiotic given postoperatively. |

continued

TABLE **9-6** Common Health Problems in Infants and Children—cont'd

DISEASE/CONDITION	DEFINITION/ETIOLOGY	PREVENTION STRATEGIES	SIGNS AND SYMPTOMS/COMPLICATIONS	MANAGEMENT/TREATMENT
Hepatitis A	Hepatitis A (infectious hepatitis) is the most common form of acute viral hepatitis. The virus is spread directly through the fecal-oral route directly or indirectly through ingestion of contaminated food or water. The highest incidence occurs among preschool and school-aged children. Incubation is approximately 4 weeks.	Vaccine is available. Immune globulin for postexposure (given 1-2 weeks after exposure prevents illness in 80%-90% of individuals). Use proper handwashing.	Usually rapid onset of fever, malaise, nausea, anorexia, jaundice, dark urine, abdominal pain. *Complications:* rare.	*Supportive/ symptomatic care:* children should not return to school until jaundice has resolved and serum enzyme levels are no more than twice normal. Household contacts should be given immune globulin.
Pinworms (*Enterobium vermicularis*)	The most common helminthic infection in the United States, infecting about one third of all U.S. children at any one time. Predominant age is 5-14 years, with girls being more frequently infected than are boys. More common in warm climates and crowded living conditions.	Prevention of reinfection includes treating all family members with two doses of medication 2 weeks apart. Washing all sleeping garments and bed linen in hot water and vacuuming around the beds may be helpful. Careful, thorough handwashing after toileting and before eating and daily showering may also help.	Intense perianal itching, particularly nocturnal, poor sleep, restlessness, enuresis, and distractibility.	*Tape test:* to diagnose, parents must press transparent tape firmly against the child's perianal area as soon as the child awakens in the morning. The tape is placed in a container and taken to a clinic for microscopic examination. *Medication:* Mebendazole (Vermox) is used to treat all family members (not recommended for children under 2 years or pregnant women).
Infectious diarrhea	Diarrhea and related symptoms are frequently caused by	Etiology is typically contaminated food or water. Symptoms usually	Symptoms vary somewhat based on causative organism. Severe, watery diarrhea;	*Medication:* antibiotics appropriate for the organism. Symptomatic

	bacteria or parasites, in addition to viral gastrointestinal conditions described above. Bacteria include *E. coli*; *Staphylococcus*, *Salmonella*, and *Shigella* species; *Campylobacter jejuni*; *Vibrio cholerae*; and *Yersinia enterocolitica*. Parasitic organisms include *Giardia* species, *Cryptosporidium* species.	occur within a few hours of exposure. See Chapter 7 for information on food preparation and clean water. Good handwashing (particularly following toileting and changing diapers) is essential.	abdominal cramps; nausea; vomiting; headache; anorexia; malaise. Stools may contain blood or mucus. With *Giardia* species, pale, greasy stools; fatigue; and weight loss are seen. Observe for signs and symptoms of dehydration (see above).	treatment (see above).
Constipation	Stool is passed infrequently or consists of hard, small masses. Etiology is usually dietary, such as too much milk or insufficient fluids or bulk-forming foods. More common in boys 1-5 years of age, although not uncommon in infants.	Good dietary practices, including recommended servings of fruits, vegetables, and grain products. Prunes or prune juice may help infants and small children who have hard stools. Encourage drinking noncaffeinated, noncarbonated fluid and good elimination patterns.	Infrequent, hard stools, pain or difficulty during defecation. Chronic constipation may be caused by underlying conditions (e.g., anorectal malformation, Hirschsprung's disease, endocrine disorder or side effect of medication [e.g., iron]). Referral for evaluation may be indicated.	Occasional constipation in infants may be treated with glycerin suppositories, but caution parents not to overuse. Stool softener, such as docusate sodium (Colace), may be prescribed. Laxatives and cathartics are generally not recommended. Promote good toileting and dietary changes.

Dermatologic Disorders

Diaper dermatitis	Caused by irritation in the diaper area.	Change diapers frequently; use of ointments and exposing the diaper area to air periodically may help prevent. Wash cloth diapers in mild soap and rinse thoroughly. Avoid commercial wipes.	Redness and irritation in the diaper area.

continued

TABLE 9-6 Common Health Problems in Infants and Children—cont'd

DISEASE/CONDITION	DEFINITION/ETIOLOGY	PREVENTION STRATEGIES	SIGNS AND SYMPTOMS/COMPLICATIONS	MANAGEMENT/TREATMENT
Impetigo	A superficial skin infection usually caused by *Staphylococcus aureus* or *Group A streptococci*. Most common bacterial skin infection in children. Predominate age, 2-5 years. Most often occurring in hot, humid climates.	Good hygiene. Discourage children from scratching scabs or insect bites. Keep fingernails short and clean.	Begins as an erythematous papule, which progresses to a vesicle and crusts over. Pustules most frequently occur on face (around mouth or nose) or at a site of skin breakage (scratch or insect bite). Often multiple sites or satellite lesions occur. May be a complication of scabies, chicken pox, pediculosis, or eczema.	*Medication:* erythromycin, cephalosporins, topical antibiotic ointments. Encourage cleanliness; wash areas two or three times per day with diluted antibacterial soap; wash linens and clothing separately from other family members' (this may need to be done daily until lesions have resolved). Exclude from school or day care until after antibiotics have been administered for 24 hours. Monitor for signs of spread.
Pediculosis	Infestation of lice—*Pediculus humanus capititis* (head lice)—is the most common type of lice found in children. Whites, Asians, Hispanics, and Native Americans are most commonly affected and girls are more commonly affected than boys.	Lice are transmitted by close personal contact. Encourage children to avoid sharing objects such as combs, brushes, hats, and clothing with other children. May also be transmitted through bed linen and upholstered chairs.	Nits (egg cases) are white spheres on the hair shaft. Nits are found most often on the back of the head and neck and behind the ears and are "glued" to the shaft and thus cannot be moved (distinguishing them from dandruff). Adult lice are small black specks that move and jump on the scalp and hair. Itching is very common. Eyelashes may be involved.	*Medication:* Lindane (Kwell) or permethrin (Nix) shampoo. Treat the entire family. After treatment, remove nits with a nit comb. Wash all linens, brushes, combs, and hats in hot water. (Infants and pregnant women should not use Lindane.) Exclude from school or day care until treated.
Scabies	Skin infestation by the mite *Sarcoptes scabiei*. Most common in children and young adults.	Good general hygiene.	Generalized itching, which is often worse at night. Burrows are commonly found in finger webs, wrists, hands, feet, penis, scrotum, buttocks, and waistline. Vesicle and pustules may be evident if infection occurs.	*Medication:* Permethrin (Elimite cream), Lindane (Kwell), or Crotamiton (Eurax) cream or lotions are applied into the skin from

			the head to the soles of feet and left on for 8-14 hours, then thoroughly washed off. A second application 48 hours later is usually recommended. Treat all family members. Wash clothing, bed linen, and towels. *Medications:* Topical administration of antifungal agents. Encourage good hygienic practices.
Ringworm (fungal infections of the skin)	Refers to several related fungi infections. Commonly infected are the scalp (*Tinea capitis*), body (*Tinea pedis*), and groin (*Tinea cruris*—jock itch)	Associated with confined living quarters, poor hygiene. May become epidemic in schools and day care centers. Good personal hygiene and avoidance of sharing clothing, shoes, brushes, and combs can stop the spread. Identification and treatment of infected individuals and household pets are important.	Although some variation occurs depending on the site, lesions usually appear as round patches of scale that spread. Itching is very common.
Acne	The most common skin disorder, Acne is an inflammatory disorder of the sebaceous glands resulting in progression of comedones (whiteheads, blackheads), to papules, inflammatory pustules. Scarring occasionally occurs. Acne most commonly affects adolescents during early to later puberty.	Diet probably has little effect on acne. Good nutrition and adequate sleep and exercise are beneficial.	Presence of comedones (whitehead and blackheads). Inflammatory lesions, including papules, pustules, and nodules occur. Most often affected are the face, upper chest, and upper back. *Medications:* Topical medications such as benzoyl peroxide and topical erythromycin are helpful for milder cases. Low-dose oral tetracycline, erythromycin, and oral contraceptives can be effective in more severe acne. Isotretinoin (Accutane) may also help. Good skin care should include daily washing with a mild soap.

SUMMARY

Nurses who practice in community settings are uniquely able to affect the health and well-being of children through appropriate assessment, counseling, health teaching, and providing other interventions as needed. Early detection of congenital, developmental, or acquired health problems and referral for treatment can dramatically influence the child's health and development.

Pediatric nurses like Bonnie, from the opening case study, recognize that preventative measures, such as encouraging appropriate, consistent use of safety devices (e.g., car seats, helmets, smoke detectors) and advance preparation (e.g., keeping poisons and matches away from children, having ipecac available), can be life saving. Furthermore, they understand that establishing healthy habits (e.g., good nutrition, dental hygiene, regular exercise) and failure to establish poor habits (e.g., smoking, drug and alcohol use) while in childhood can improve the quality and length of the individual's life.

This chapter has presented a great deal of information regarding health promotion and illness prevention for infants, children, and adolescents. Some of the many agencies and organizations that assist in providing care and information to promote the health of children are listed in the accompanying Resources box.

Resources

Infants, Children, and Adolescents

Governmental Programs

Medicaid
State Children's Health Insurance Program
Women, Infants and Children Program

Safety

National SAFE KIDS Campaign
National Highway Traffic Safety Administration
Consumer Product Safety Commission

Injury and Violence

Childabuse.org
Children's Defense Fund

Parents Anonymous 800-421-0353
National Abuse Hotline 800-422-4453

Dental Care

American Dental Association

Miscellaneous

Easter Seal Society for Crippled Children and Adults
March of Dimes Birth Defects Foundation
Mothers Against Drunk Driving
Students Against Driving Drunk

Visit the book's website at
www.wbsaunders.com/SIMON/McEwen
for a direct link to the website for each organization listed.

KEY POINTS

- The leading causes of mortality for infants are congenital anomalies, low birth weight, SIDS, and respiratory distress syndrome. After 1 year of age and through adolescence, the leading causes of death are unintentional injury, cancer, and homicide. In teenagers, suicide is added to the list.

- The leading causes of acute illness in children are respiratory conditions (e.g., colds, influenza, respiratory infections), other infections (e.g., viral infections, intestinal virus), acute ear infection, and injuries. Major chronic conditions are respiratory conditions (e.g., allergic rhinitis, asthma, chronic bronchitis); skin conditions (e.g., acne, dermatitis); musculoskeletal conditions; and vision, speech, and hearing impairment.

- Several federal- and state-sponsored health programs and services are available for disadvantaged, underserved, and disabled children. These include Medicaid, EPSDT, SCHIP, WIC, Head Start, and PL 94-142 (Education for All Handicapped Children Act).

- The Preventative Services Task Force has issued screening guidelines for infants and children to test for genetic, congenital, developmental, and pathological problems and conditions. These include routine infant screenings (e.g., testing of newborns for phenylketonuria, congenital hypothyroidism), body measurement (height, weight, and head circumference), developmental screening, vision screening, hearing screening, lead screening, and screening for anemia.

- Health-promotion activities for infants, children, and adolescents include nutrition education and counseling on nutrition, physical activity, and exercise; sleep and rest patterns; dental health; and maturation and puberty.
- Illness prevention should include information on prevention of substance (drugs and alcohol) use and abuse, prevention of use of tobacco products, and safety issues (e.g., vehicle safety, poisoning, head injury prevention, drowning prevention, and prevention of fire and burns).
- Detection and prevention of child abuse are very important in community-based nursing practice and nurses should be informed regarding patterns of abuse and how to identify suspected abuse and how and when to intervene.

Learning Activities & Application to Practice

In Class

1. Discuss the *Healthy People 2010* objectives for infants, preschool children, school-aged children, and adolescents. What can nurses in communities do to help meet the objectives?

In Clinical

2. Observe and assist in completion of an EPSDT screening.
3. Observe and assist in collecting blood samples for routine infant screenings. Ensure that agency protocols are carefully followed.
4. Complete a developmental screening, such as the Denver II, on two or three children of differing ages. Share results with the clinical group.
5. Complete a "child safety home checklist" for a family encountered during clinical or for a

neighbor or friend. Share findings and suggestions or recommendations for change with the clinical group.

REFERENCES

Advocates for Highway and Auto Safety. (1994). *Motorcycle helmet laws: Questions & answers.* Washington, DC: Advocates for Highway and Auto Safety.

American Academy of Pediatrics/Center to Prevent Handgun Violence. (1992). *Rx for safety: Preventing firearms injuries among children and adolescents.* Washington, DC: Center to Prevent Handgun Violence.

American Academy of Pediatrics/Committee on Genetics. (1992). Issues in newborn screening. *Pediatrics, 89,* 345-349.

American Academy of Pediatrics/Committee on Injury Control for Children and Youth. (1987). *Injury control for children and youth.* Elk Grove Village, IL: American Academy of Pediatrics.

American Dental Association (ADA). (1999). *Facts about fluoride.* Retrieved 7/25/01 from http://www.ada.org/public/topics/fluoride/artcl-01.html.

American Dental Association (ADA). (2000). *Mouthguards can help protect your child from mouth injuries.* Retrieved 7/25/01 from http://www.ada.org/public/media/newsrel/0002/nr-02.html.

American Dental Association (ADA). (2001). *Good oral health practices should begin in infancy.* Retrieved 7/25/01 from http://www.ada.org/public/media/newsrel/0101/nr-01.html.

Ashwill, J. W., & Droske, S. C. (1997). *Nursing care of children* (p. 244). Philadelphia: W. B. Saunders.

Betz, C. L., Hunsberger, M. M., & Wright, S. (1994). *Family-centered nursing care of children* (2nd ed.). Philadelphia: W. B. Saunders.

Centers for Disease Control and Prevention (CDC). (1989). Criteria for anemia in children and childbearing-aged women. *MMWR Morbidity and Mortality Weekly Report, 38*(22), 400-404.

Centers for Disease Control and Prevention (CDC). (1990). Fatal injuries to children—United States, *MMWR Morbidity and Mortality Weekly Report, 39*(26), 442-445.

Centers for Disease Control and Prevention (CDC). (1992). Accessibility of cigarettes to youths aged 12-17 years—United States, 1989. *MMWR Morbidity and Mortality Weekly Report, 41*(27), 485-488.

Centers for Disease Control and Prevention (CDC). (1995). Injury-control recommendations: Bicycle helmets. *MMWR Morbidity and Mortality Weekly Report, 44*(RR-1), 1-18.

Centers for Disease Control and Prevention (CDC). (1999). Achievements in public health, 1900-1999: Fluoridation of drinking water to prevent dental caries. *MMWR Morbidity and Mortality Weekly Report, 48*(41), 933-940.

Centers for Disease Control and Prevention/National Center for Injury Prevention and Control (CDC/NCIPC). (1994). Ten leading causes of deaths due to injury—1991, Unpublished data, Atlanta, 1994.

Dambro, M. R. (1996). *Griffith's 5-minute clinical consult.* Baltimore: Williams & Wilkins.

Evans, A., & Friedland, R. B. (1994). *Financing and delivery of health care for children.* Washington, DC: National Academy of Social Insurance.

Frankenburg, W. K., & Dodds, J. B. (1990). *DENVER II: Training manual.* Denver: Denver Developmental Materials, Inc.

Grant, C. (1995). Physical and sexual abuse. In D. Antai-Otong (Ed.), *Psychiatric nursing: Biological and behavioral concepts* (pp. 407-426). Philadelphia: W. B. Saunders.

Kovner, A. R. (1999). *Jonas and Kovner's health care delivery in the United States* (6th ed.). New York: Springer Publishing Co.

Maurer, F. A. (2000). Violence: A social and family problem. In C. M. Smith & F. A. Maurer (Eds.), *Community health nursing: Theory and practice* (2nd ed., pp. 571-606). Philadelphia: W. B. Saunders.

Murray, R. B., & Zentner, J. P. (2001). *Nursing assessment and health promotion: Strategies through the life span* (7th ed.). Norwalk, CT: Appleton & Lange.

National Center for Health Statistics (NCHS). (1994). *Advance data from the National Ambulatory Medical Care Survey: 1992 summary.* (DHHS Publication No. [PHS] 94-1250). Hyattsville, MD: National Center for Health Statistics.

National Center for Health Statistics (NCHS). (1999). United States Life Tables—1997. *National Vital Statistics Report 47*(28), 1-38. Washington, DC: Public Health Service.

National Center for Health Statistics (NCHS). (2000). *Health United States: 2000.* Hyattsville, MD: USDHHS/NCHS.

National Committee for Clinical Laboratory Standards. (1992). *Blood collection on filter paper for neonatal screening programs* (2nd ed.). Villanova, PA: National Committee for Clinical Laboratory Standards.

National Institutes of Health (NIH). (1994). *Seal out dental decay.* (NIH Publication No. 94-489). Washington, DC: National Institutes of Health.

Pappas, A., & Hakala, K. L. D. (2001). Violence in the community. In M. A. Nies & M. McEwen (Eds.), *Community health nursing: Promoting the health of populations* (3rd ed., pp. 596-623). Philadelphia: W. B. Saunders.

Pourciau, C. A., & Vallette, E. C. (2001). School health. In M. A. Nies & M. McEwen (Eds.), *Community health nursing: Promoting the health of populations* (3rd ed., pp. 702-729). Philadelphia: W. B. Saunders.

Ripa, L. W. (1993). A half-century of community water fluoridation in the United States: Review and commentary. *Journal of Public Health Dentistry, 53*(1), 17-44.

Selekman, J. (1993). *Pediatric nursing.* Springhouse, PA, Springhouse.

Selekman, J. (1995). Children in the community. In C. Smith & F. A. Maurer (Eds.), *Community health nursing: Theory and practice* (pp. 693-718). Philadelphia: W. B. Saunders.

Smith-DiJulio, K., & Holzapfel, S. K. (1994). Families in crisis: Family violence. In E. M. Varcarolis (Ed.), *Foundations of psychiatric mental health nursing* (2nd ed.). Philadelphia: W. B. Saunders.

Texas Department of Health. (1990). *Protect your child against accidental poisoning.* Austin, TX: Texas Department of Health.

U.S. Department of Agriculture/Food and Consumer Service. (2000). *Women, infants, and children, program basics: WIC at a glance.* Retrieved 7/25/01 from http://www.fns.usda.gov/wic/CONTENT/glanc/basic.htm.

U.S. Department of Health and Human Services (USDHHS). (1990). *Healthy people 2000: National health promotion and disease prevention objectives.* Washington, DC: Government Printing Office.

U.S. Department of Health and Human Services (USDHHS). (1995). *Healthy people 2000: Midcourse review and 1995 revisions.* Washington, DC: Government Printing Office.

U.S. Department of Health and Human Services (USDHHS). (2000). *Healthy people 2010: Conference edition.* Washington, DC: Government Printing Office.

U.S. Department of Health and Human Services/Health Care Financing Administration (USDHHS/HCFA). (2001). *The state children's health insurance program (SCHIP). HHS fact sheet.* U.S. Department of Health and Human Services. Retrieved 7/25/01 from http://www.hhs.gov/news/press/2001/pres/01fsschip.html.

U.S. Department of Health and Human Services/Office of Disease Prevention and Health Promotion (USDHHS/ODPHP). (1994). *Clinician's handbook of preventive services.* Washington, DC: Government Printing Office.

U.S. Department of Health and Human Services/Office of Disease Prevention and Health Promotion (USDHHS/ODPHP). (1997). *Guide to clinical preventive services* (2nd ed.). Washington DC: Government Printing Office.

U.S. Department of Health and Human Services/ Office of Disease Prevention and Health Promotion (USDHHS/ODPHP). (1998). *Clinician's handbook of preventive services* (2nd ed.). Washington, DC: Government Printing Office.

U.S. Department of Health and Human Service/Public Health Service (USDHHS/PHS) (1999). *Clinician's hand book of preventive service* (2nd ed.). Mclean, V. A.: International Medical Publishing Inc.

Violence Prevention Project. (1992). *Identification and prevention of youth violence: A protocol of health care providers.* Boston: Violence Prevention Project.

Wong, D. L. (1999). *Whaley & Wong's nursing care of infants and children* (6th ed.). St. Louis: Mosby.

Health Promotion and Illness Prevention for Adults

objectives

1. Discuss the importance of health-promotion activities in positively influencing the health of adults.

2. Describe the health benefits of regular exercise and give an example of a recommended exercise program.

3. Discuss problems related to being overweight and obese and explain basic components of a healthy diet.

4. Describe problems associated with tobacco use and cite ways to avoid smoking initiation and tips for smoking cessation.

5. Discuss risk factors for heart disease and stroke and provide ways to minimize them.

6. Discuss risk factors, screening recommendations, and treatment options for the most common types of cancer.

7. Discuss risk factors for diabetes and describe prevention and management strategies.

key terms

Health promotion	**Obesity**	**Smoking cessation**
Illness prevention	**Physical activity and fitness**	
Nutrition guidelines	**Screening**	*See Glossary for definitions.*

case study

Ben Rogers is a staff nurse at a cardiac rehabilitation center in an urban area. The cardiac center provides comprehensive care to clients with heart disease and services to prevent heart disease. At the center, Ben's responsibilities involve assisting in prevention, diagnosis, monitoring, and rehabilitation of cardiovascular disease in adults.

On Monday, Ben saw Mr. Ryan, a 50-year-old bank vice president. Although he has never had symptoms indicating a heart condition, Mr. Ryan was referred to the center by his internist because he was determined to be at risk for developing coronary artery disease during a recent physical examination.

At the cardiac center, each client initially completes a health history and questionnaires that assess known risk factors for heart disease. Among the findings from Mr. Ryan's completed assessments are that he is approximately 30 pounds heavier than the ideal for his height, smokes one to one and a half packs of cigarettes a day (he has cut down from more than two packs a day during the past year), rarely engages in strenuous physical activity, drinks alcohol occasionally, and reports moderate stress in his life. He eats a variety of foods, but admits that he probably eats too many snacks and prefers sweets and bread to fruits and vegetables. He has no history of hypertension or diabetes and his serum cholesterol results over the past 5 years have remained steady, ranging from 200 to 220. He has a positive family history for heart disease. At age 65, his mother died from a heart attack, as did both grandfathers (ages at death unknown). His older brother has had no symptoms of heart disease. His father died in an automobile accident at age 45.

At the cardiac rehab center, additional laboratory tests and diagnostic studies were performed to assess risk and determine if Mr. Ryan has evidence of coronary artery disease. Laboratory tests included a lipid profile to assess high-density and low-density lipoprotein values and ratios, an electrocardiogram, and a cardiac stress test. Ben assisted the physicians and technicians with these tests.

Fortunately, Mr. Ryan's tests showed no evidence of previous myocardial infarction and no angina. Following the examinations, Ben worked with a team composed of a cardiologist, a dietitian, and an exercise therapist to develop a plan of action for Mr. Ryan to reduce his risk of developing heart disease. Their recommendations follow:

1. Stop smoking: Written information on methods to stop smoking was provided and discussed.
2. Dietary changes: Detailed literature on methods to lose weight and reduce dietary fat intake was provided and reviewed.
3. Increase physical activity: A program to improve physical fitness was presented. Detailed instructions to gradually increase daily exercise to at least 40 minutes, 3 to 4 days a week while increasing his heart rate to between 85 and 127 beats per minute were outlined.
4. Reduce stress: Stress management literature was provided. Stress avoidance, relaxation techniques, building supportive relationships, fatigue avoidance, and use of support groups, where indicated and were discussed.
5. Medications: It was determined that Mr. Ryan would not be put on medication to reduce his cholesterol at this time because it is hoped that dietary management will be sufficient to reduce his cholesterol levels. His lipid profile will be reassessed in 3 months to see if his total cholesterol and low-density versus high-density lipoprotein ratios are improved. Aspirin, 325 mg/day, was prescribed following determination that Mr. Ryan had no allergies or history of bleeding tendencies.

Mr. Ryan agreed to these recommendations and reasonable goals for each area were set. Finally, he made an appointment to return to the cardiac center in 3 months to assess progress toward his goals.

Health promotion refers to those activities or actions related to encouraging individual lifestyles or personal choices that positively influence health. Physical activity and fitness, nutrition, and substance (e.g., tobacco, alcohol) use and abuse are examples of controllable behaviors or actions that ultimately affect health. In their practice, all nurses, particularly those working in community settings, should be prepared for opportunities to assist clients (whether individuals, families, or groups) by providing information, counseling, advocacy, referral, or other interventions that allow the client to make informed choices to promote health.

Primary and secondary prevention refer to those interventions, such as counseling, **screening**, immunization, and education, that directly affect health to prevent acute or chronic disease

TABLE **10-1** Estimated Deaths, Death Rates, and Percentage of Total Deaths for the 10 Leading Causes of Death: United States, 1998

RANK	CAUSE OF DEATH	NUMBER	DEATH RATE (PER 100,000)	TOTAL DEATHS (%)
	All Causes	2,337,256	864.7	100.0
1	Diseases of the heart	724,859	268.2	31.0
2	Malignant neoplasms	541,532	200.3	23.2
3	Cerebrovascular diseases	158,448	58.6	6.8
4	Chronic obstructive pulmonary diseases and allied conditions	112,584	41.7	4.8
5	Accidents and adverse effects	97,835	36.2	4.2
6	Pneumonia and influenza	91,871	34.0	3.9
7	Diabetes	64,751	24.0	2.8
8	Suicide	30,575	11.3	1.3
9	Nephritis, nephritic syndrome, and nephrosis	26,182	9.7	1.1
10	Chronic liver disease and cirrhosis	25,192	9.3	1.1
—	All other causes	463,427	171.5	19.8

From National Center for Health Statistics (NCHS). (2000). Deaths: Final Data for 1998. *National Vital Statistics Reports*, *48*(11), 1-106. Washington, DC: National Center for Health Statistics.

or disability. This chapter contains assessment and teaching tools and information specific to these concepts. Initially, general health-promotion strategies such as assessment of health risks, promotion of exercise and physical fitness, improving nutrition, and reduction or elimination of harmful substances are described in the discussion of health promotion. Primary and secondary prevention, specifically with regard to several of the leading causes of death and disability (i.e., heart disease and stroke, cancer, and diabetes), are then considered.

CAUSES OF DEATH

Table 10-1 shows the leading causes of death in the United States. As depicted in this table, heart disease, cancer, cerebrovascular disease, and chronic obstructive pulmonary disease are the top four causes of death. Smoking—particularly cigarette smoking—is a risk factor strongly associated with each of these conditions. Indeed, according to McGinnis and Foege (1993), tobacco is implicated in almost 20% of the annual deaths in the United States—approximately 400,000 individuals. Additionally, diet and activity patterns were deemed to account for 14% of deaths (about 300,000 per year); alcohol contributes to about 5% of all deaths because it is associated with a significant percentage of accidents, suicides, homicides, and cirrhosis and chronic liver disease. The Community Application box "Recommendations for Preventing Motor Vehicle Deaths" presents recommendations from a national panel on preventing motor vehicle deaths.

HEALTH PROMOTION AND ILLNESS PREVENTION

Health promotion consists of activities directed toward increasing the level of well-being and actualizing the health potential of individuals, families, communities, and society (Pender, 1996). *Healthy People 2010* (U.S. Department of Health and Human Services [USDHHS], 2000a) identifies health-promotion strategies as those that relate to promoting positive individual lifestyles choices, including physical fitness, nutrition, and tobacco and alcohol use. Likewise, **illness prevention** strategies involve lessening or removal of risk factors for specific diseases

COMMUNITY APPLICATION
Recommendations for Preventing Motor Vehicle Deaths

Motor vehicle-related injuries are the leading cause of death for Americans 1 to 34 years of age, resulting in approximately 41,000 deaths each year. A national panel of community health experts reviewed available information on motor vehicle injuries and made the following recommendations on how to prevent them:

- Pass laws requiring the use of child safety seats
- Encourage distribution of and education programs for child safety seats
- Enhance safety belt laws
- Pass seat belt enforcement laws that allow a police officer to stop a vehicle solely for an observed belt law violation

- Enhance safety belt enforcement programs
- Lower the illegal blood alcohol concentration for adult drivers to 0.08%
- Maintain the minimum legal drinking age at 21 years
- Provide sobriety checkpoints
- Provide information and enforcement campaigns to promote use of child safety seats
- Offer incentives and education programs to promote the use of child safety seats
- Maintain a lower legal blood alcohol concentration for young or inexperienced drivers

From Centers for Disease Control and Prevention (CDC). (2001b). Recommendations for preventing motor vehicle deaths. *MMWR Morbidity and Mortality Weekly Report, 50*, RR-7, 1-13.

and early identification of diseases through screening and prompt remediation. Examples of goals in *Healthy People 2010* for health promotion and illness prevention are included in the *Healthy People 2010* box.

ASSESSMENT OF HEALTH RISKS AND HEALTH HABITS

To apply the nursing process to health promotion and illness prevention, nurses should begin with assessment. In addition to individual physical, functional, and cognitive assessments that are routinely accomplished, an assessment of behaviors and habits that influence health is also important. An understanding of the client's health beliefs and knowledge and health habits (both positive and negative) will help the nurse plan appropriate interventions. Found at the end of the chapter, Appendix 10-A is an example of a tool for general assessment of health risks, lifestyles, and beliefs.

As positive health practices and potential threats to health are identified, nurses can assist individuals, families, and groups by developing plans and programs to promote health and prevent illness. Areas to target should relate to

the most common, preventable causes of morbidity and mortality, based on risk factors and identified and potential health threats. This includes such areas as diet, tobacco use, exercise, obesity, substance use, and others. Table 10-2 depicts the relationships among various risk factors and the 10 leading causes of death. The remainder of this chapter describes specific assessments and risk-reduction techniques and provides educational materials and tools to equip nurses to assist clients in reducing risks and promoting health.

PHYSICAL ACTIVITY AND FITNESS

Physical activity and fitness are important to good health. The health benefits of regular exercise and physical activity have been thoroughly researched and documented. Indeed, it has been observed that moderate, regular exercise for about half an hour each day, three times a week, can significantly lower death rates for many causes, including cancer and cardiovascular disease (The President's Council on Physical Fitness & Sports, 1993).

healthy people 2010

Examples of Objectives for General Health Promotion for Adults

OBJECTIVE	BASELINE (1998)	TARGET
1.5: Increase the proportion of persons with a usual primary care provider	77%	85%
3.10a: Increase the proportion of physicians (interns) who counsel their at-risk patients about tobacco use cessation	50%	85%
3.13: Increase the proportion of women aged 40 years and older who have received a mammogram within the preceding 2 years	68%	70%
5.4: Increase the proportion of adults with diabetes whose condition has been diagnosed	65%	80%
7.6: Increase the proportion of employees who participate in employer-sponsored health-promotion activities	28%	50%
11.2: Improve the health literacy of persons with inadequate or marginal literacy skills	NA	NA
12.12: Increase the proportion of adults who have had their blood pressure measured within the preceding 2 years and can state whether their blood pressure was normal or high	90%	95%
12.15: Increase the proportion of adults who have had their blood cholesterol checked within the preceding 5 years	68%	80%
15.19: Increase use of safety belts	69%	92%
19.2: Reduce the proportion of adults who are obese	23%	15%
19.8: Increase the proportion of persons aged 2 years and older who consume less than 10% of calories from saturated fat	36%	75%
20.3: Reduce the rate of injury and illness cases involving days away from work from overexertion or repetitive motion	675 injuries per 100,000 workers	338 injuries per 100,000 workers
21.7: Increase the proportion of adults who, in the past 12 months, report having had an examination to detect oral and pharyngeal cancer	14%	35%
22.2: Increase the proportion of adults who engage regularly, preferably daily, in moderate physical activity for at least 30 minutes per day	15%	30%
22.5: Increase the proportion of adults who perform physical activities that enhance and maintain flexibility	30%	40%
26.13: Reduce the proportion of adults who exceed guidelines for low-risk drinking	73%	50%
27.1a: Reduce tobacco use (cigarette smoking) by adults	24%	12%

SIDS, Sudden infant death syndrome.

Exercise training positively affects health by increasing cardiovascular functional capacity and decreasing myocardial oxygen demand. Exercise helps control blood lipid abnormalities, diabetes, and obesity and can help lower blood pressure. Potential protective benefits from regular physical activity include lowered resting heart rate, more blood pumped with each beat, reduced blood pressure, increased high-density lipoprotein, and improved carbohydrate metab-olism (American Heart Association [AHA], 1996). In addition, regular activity helps control weight, increases lean body mass, decreases body fat percentage, produces relief from some symptoms of depression, improves flexibility, increases muscle strength and endurance, and increases bone density. These benefits help reduce or minimize other health threats such as arthritis, diabetes, and osteoporosis (AHA, 1996).

TABLE 10-2 Relationship Between Risk Factors and 10 Leading Causes of Death

CAUSE OF DEATH	PERCENT OF TOTAL DEATHS	SMOKING	HIGH-FAT, LOW-FIBER DIET	SEDENTARY LIFESTYLE	HIGH BLOOD PRESSURE	ELEVATED CHOLESTEROL	OBESITY	DIABETES	ALCOHOL ABUSE
Heart disease	31.0	X	X	X	X	X	X	X	X
Cancer	23.2	X	X	X			X		X
Stroke	6.8	X	X		X	X	X		
COPD	4.8	X							
Unintentional injury	4.2	X							X
Pneumonia and influenza	3.9	X							
Diabetes	2.8		X	X			X	X	
Suicide	1.3								X
Kidney disease	1.1	X			X	X	X	X	X
Liver disease	1.1								X
All other causes	19.8								

Despite the known benefits, levels of physical activity among Americans remain low. Indeed, it is estimated that more than 60% of adults are not regularly physically active and 25% report no physical activity at all. Women tend to be less active than men and members of racial and ethnic minorities are more inactive than whites (USDHHS/Office of Disease Prevention and Health Promotion [ODPHP], 1998).

The AHA (1996) states that persons of all ages should include physical activity as part of a comprehensive health program. A health care provider should be consulted, however, before starting an exercise program if an individual meets any of the following conditions:

• Has been diagnosed with a heart condition and the doctor recommends only medically supervised physical activity
• Has pain or pressure in the left or midchest area, left neck area, shoulder, or arm during or following exercise
• Has developed chest pain within the past month
• Has a tendency to lose consciousness or suffers from dizziness
• Feels extremely breathless after mild exertion
• Takes medication for blood pressure or a heart condition

• Has bone or joint problems that could be worsened by physical activity
• Has a medical condition that might need special attention during an exercise program (e.g., type 2 diabetes)
• Is middle aged or older and has not been physically active (AHA/National Heart, Lung, and Blood Institute, 1993).

An exercise program should be vigorous enough to increase the heart rate to 50% to 75% of the maximum heart rate (220 minus your age). This is termed the target heart rate zone. The AHA (1996) suggests a combination of low-intensity activities, which increase the heart rate to 40% to 60% of maximum capacity, and moderate intensity activities, which increase the heart rate to 60% to 75% of maximum capacity, totaling 30 minutes or longer on most days (4 to 5 times per week). Activities such as walking, hiking, stair climbing, aerobic exercise, jogging, running, bicycling, rowing, swimming, and sports such as tennis, racquetball, soccer, and basketball are particularly beneficial in improving cardiac fitness. In addition to using aerobic exercises to enhance cardiac fitness, the AHA suggests adding resistance weight training for a minimum of 2 days per week. Recommendations are to use 8 to 10 different exercise sets targeting arms, shoulders, chest, trunk, back, hips and legs, with 10 to 15 repetitions each performed at a moderate-to-high intensity. Additionally, the ODPHP (1998) suggests that physical activity programs should be the following:

1. Medically safe (e.g., following physician's advice if one of the risk factors listed previously is a possibility; increasing activities gradually; use of stretching exercise to decrease the risk of musculoskeletal injuries)
2. Enjoyable (e.g., varying activities, exercising with friends or family)
3. Convenient (e.g., flexible, nearby, requiring a minimum of special preparation)
4. Realistic (e.g., gradual increases in intensity, frequency, and duration)
5. Minimally structured (schedules and goals should be set and maintained when possible, but some flexibility is important because very structured programs may reduce compliance)

NUTRITION AND WEIGHT CONTROL

Good nutritional practices and maintenance of a desirable weight are essential for good health. However, maintenance of a desirable weight is becoming a problem in the United States, where overweight and obesity are rapidly growing problems. It is estimated that nearly 55% of the U.S. adult population is overweight or obese. The rate of obesity has increased more than 50% in the last two decades and approximately 25% of U.S. adult females and 20% of adult males are obese.

As a risk factor, **obesity** (weight 20% or more above desirable weight) is associated with hypertension, type 2 diabetes, hypercholesterolemia, coronary artery disease, some types of cancer, gallbladder disease, arthritis, sleep apnea, and stroke (USDHHS, 2000a). Overweight or obese adults are found in all population groups, but obesity is particularly common among Hispanic, black, Native American, and Pacific Islander women. People residing in the south Atlantic states (West Virginia, North and South Carolina, and Georgia), the east south central region (Kentucky, Tennessee, Alabama, and Mississippi), and the south central region (Arkansas, Louisiana, Oklahoma, and Texas) of the United States have the highest rates of obesity (Centers for Disease Control and Prevention [CDC], 2001).

Nurses who work in community settings are frequently in a position to counsel adults on matters related to weight (see the Community

---

COMMUNITY APPLICATION
Fighting Obesity

In the United States, obesity (which is defined as having a body mass index of 30 or higher) is growing at an alarming rate. Between 1998 and 1999 alone, obesity rose 6%. Since 1991, obesity among adults has increased by nearly 60% nationally (from 12% to 19.8% of the population).

There is significant concern that as obesity rates continue to grow, the effect will be dramatic increases in related chronic health conditions such as diabetes and cardiovascular disease. Indeed, diabetes increased by 33% during the 1990s. This is widely attributed to the surge in obesity during that same period. To control the obesity epidemic, the CDC makes the following recommendations:

- Health care providers must counsel their obese clients on nutrition and weight reduction.
- Workplaces should offer healthy food choices in their cafeterias and provide opportunities for employees to be physically active on site.
- Schools should offer more physical education that encourages lifelong physical activity.
- Urban policymakers should provide more sidewalks, bike paths, and other alternatives to cars.
- Parents should reduce their children's TV and computer time and encourage outdoor play.

From Centers for Disease Control and Prevention/National Center for Chronic Disease Prevention and Health Promotion (2001). *Obesity continues climb in 1999 among American adults*. Retrieved 7/30/01 from http://www.cdc.gov/nccdphp/dnpa/pr-obesity.htm.

TABLE **10-3** Height and Weight Tables for Men 25 Years and Older

HEIGHT (FEET, INCHES)*	WEIGHT (POUNDS)†			
	SMALL FRAME	MEDIUM FRAME	LARGE FRAME	20% OVERWEIGHT‡
5,1	105-113	111-122	119-134	140
5,2	108-116	114-126	122-137	144
5,3	111-119	117-129	125-141	148
5,4	114-122	120-132	128-145	151
5,5	117-126	123-136	131-149	155
5,6	121-130	127-140	135-154	160
5,7	125-134	131-145	140-159	166
5,8	129-138	135-149	144-163	170
5,9	133-143	139-153	148-167	175
5,10	137-147	143-158	152-172	181
5,11	141-151	147-163	157-177	186
6,0	145-155	151-168	161-182	191
6,1	149-160	155-173	168-187	197
6,2	153-164	160-178	171-192	203
6,3	157-168	165-183	175-197	209

Adapted from Metropolitan Life Insurance Company. (1983). New weight standards for men and women. *Statistical Bulletin Metropolitan Life Insurance Company, 64,* 2-9.
*Without shoes
†Without clothing
‡Twenty percent over midpoint of medium frame; not in original Metropolitan table

TABLE **10-4** Height and Weight Tables for Women 25 Years and Older

HEIGHT (FEET, INCHES)*	WEIGHT (POUNDS)†			
	SMALL FRAME	MEDIUM FRAME	LARGE FRAME	20% OVERWEIGHT‡
4,9	90-97	94-106	102-118	120
4,10	92-100	91-109	106-121	124
4,11	95-103	100-112	108-124	127
5,0	98-106	103-116	111-127	131
5,1	101-109	106-118	114-130	134
5,2	104-112	109-122	117-134	139
5,3	107-115	112-126	121-138	141
5,4	110-119	116-131	125-142	148
5,5	114-123	120-136	129-146	154
5,6	118-127	124-139	133-150	158
5,7	122-131	128-143	137-154	163
5,8	126-136	132-147	141-159	167
5,9	130-140	136-151	145-164	172
5,10	134-144	140-155	149-169	177

Adapted from Metropolitan Life Insurance Company. (1983). New weight standards for men and women. *Statistical Bulletin Metropolitan Life Insurance Company, 64,* 2-9.
*Without shoes
†Without clothing
‡Twenty percent over midpoint of medium frame; not in original Metropolitan table

Application box "Fighting Obesity"). Tables 10-3 and 10-4 present recommended height and weight tables for men and women, respectively. The tables are easy reference guides to identify "20% overweight," the recognized point at which negative health consequences occur (USDHHS/ODPHP, 1994).

To help clients achieve and maintain a healthy weight, nurses can share several recommendations with them. General **nutrition guidelines** for a healthy diet are as follows:

- Eat a variety of foods.
- Balance the food you eat with physical activity; maintain or improve your weight.
- Choose a diet low in fat (less than 30% of calories), saturated fat (less than 10% of calories), and cholesterol.
- Choose a diet moderate in sugars.
- Choose a diet moderate in salt and sodium (less than 2400 mg per day).
- Drink only in moderation (no more than one drink daily for women or 2 drinks daily for men). (One drink is 12 oz of regular beer, 5 oz of wine, or 1.5 oz of 80-proof distilled spirits.)
- Women should consume adequate calcium and folic acid (USDHHS/ODPHP, 1998).

Also, Table 10-5 provides basic information on types and amounts of foods recommended for daily consumption for women, men, teens, and children. Specific information should also be given to address lowering fat and cholesterol intake and ensuring adequate vitamin and mineral intake.

LOWERING FAT AND CHOLESTEROL INTAKE

Because of the association of dietary fat and cholesterol with heart disease, stroke, obesity and other problems, limitation of these nutrients is one of the main objectives when counseling on nutrition. Dietary guidelines for fat and cholesterol intake are as follows:

- Reduce total dietary fat to 30% or less of total calories.
- Reduce saturated fat intake to less than 10% of calories.
- Reduce cholesterol intake to less than 300 mg per day (U.S. Department of Health and Human Services [USDHHS], 2000a).

VITAMINS AND MINERALS

Adequate intake of vitamins and minerals is essential for good heath, but misinformation is common. Nutrition counseling should include information on essential nutrients, including vitamins and minerals. Table 10-6 provides general data on vitamins and Box 10-1 gives general information on minerals. These can be

TABLE 10-5 How Many Servings Each Day

	MOST WOMEN, OLDER ADULTS	CHILDREN, TEEN GIRLS, ACTIVE WOMEN, MOST MEN	TEEN BOYS, ACTIVE MEN
Calories*	About 1600	About 2200	About 2800
Bread group servings (whole grain products are recommended)	6	9	11
Vegetable group servings	3	4	5
Fruit group servings	2	3	4
Milk group servings	2-3†	2-3†	2-3†
Meat group servings	2 (total of 5 oz)	2 (total of 6 oz)	3 (total of 7 oz)
Total fat (g)	53	73	93

From Human Nutrition Information Service. (1992). *The food guide pyramid: Beyond the basic 4.* Washington, DC: U.S. Department of Agriculture.
*These are the calorie levels if you choose low-fat, lean foods from the five major food groups and use foods from the fats, oils, and sweets group sparingly.
†Women who are pregnant or breastfeeding, teenagers, and young adults to age 24 need three servings.

TABLE **10-6** Facts About Vitamins

VITAMIN	FOOD SOURCES	BENEFITS TO WELLNESS	DEFICIENCY SIGNS AND SYMPTOMS
Water-Soluble Vitamins			
B complex	Meat products (beef, pork, poultry, eggs, fish), milk, cheese, grains, dried beans, nuts, starchy vegetables	Facilitates release of energy from other nutrients Aids in formation of red blood cells, growth and function of the nervous system, and formation of hormones Contributes to good vision and healthy skin Assists in the metabolism of proteins, fats, and carbohydrates	Fatigue, nausea, weakness, irritability, depression, weight loss, inflamed skin, cracked lips, muscle pain, cramps or twitching, low blood sugar, decreased resistance to disease, nerve dysfunction
C (ascorbic acid)	Citrus fruits, strawberries, cantaloupe, honeydew melons, broccoli, brussel sprouts, green peppers, cauliflower, spinach	Contributes to production of collagen Aids in protection against infection Contributes to tooth and bone formation and repair and wound healing Aids in absorption of iron and calcium	Dry, rough, and scaly skin; bleeding gums; slowly healing wounds; listlessness; fatigue; low glucose tolerance
Fat-Soluble Vitamins			
A	Milk; cheese; butter; fat; eggs; liver; dark-green, leafy vegetables; carrots; cantaloupe; yellow squash; sweet potatoes	Essential for growth of epithelial cells such as hair, skin, and mucous membranes Aids in vision in dim light Contributes to bone growth and tooth development Plays a role in reproduction (sperm production and estrogen synthesis) Increases resistance to infection	Decreased resistance to infection, skin changes, alteration of tooth enamel, night blindness, corneal deterioration
D*	Milk (fortified), butter, cheese, eggs, clams, fish, salmon, tuna	Is essential for bones and teeth Contributes to calcium and phosphorus absorption	Bone softening and fractures, muscle spasms, tooth malformation
E	Vegetable oils; green, leafy vegetables; liver; eggs; whole-grain cereals and breads	Assists in formation of red blood cells and muscle tissue Aids in absorption of vitamin A Serves as an antioxidant, which preserves vitamins and unsaturated fatty acids Aids in normal formation of the liver	Destruction of cell membrane of red blood cells
K	Green, leafy vegetables; liver; cabbage; cauliflower; eggs; tomatoes; peas; potatoes; milk	Contributes to normal blood clotting	Severe bleeding, prolonged coagulation, bruising

From Anspaugh, D. J., Hamrick, M. H., & Rosato, F. D. (1994). *Wellness: Concepts and applications* (2nd ed.). St. Louis: Mosby.
*Sunlight also stimulates vitamin D production.

BOX 10-1 Facts About Minerals

MAJOR (MACRO) MINERALS

Calcium, phosphorus, potassium, sulfur, sodium chloride, and magnesium

Trace (Micro) Minerals

Iron, iodine, zinc, selenium, manganese, copper, molybdenum, cobalt, chromium, fluorine, silicon, vanadium, nickel, tin, cadmium

MINERALS OF SPECIAL CONCERN*

Calcium

Wellness benefits: Contributes to bone and tooth formation, general body growth, maintenance of good muscle tone, nerve function, cell membrane function, and regulation of normal heart beat

Food sources: Dairy products, dark-green vegetables, dried beans, shellfish

Deficiency signs and symptoms: Bone pain and fractures, muscle cramps, osteoporosis

Iron

Wellness benefits: Facilitates oxygen and carbon dioxide transport, formation of red blood cells, production of antibodies, synthesis of collagen, and use of energy

Food sources: Red meat (lean), seafoods, eggs, dried beans, nuts, grains, green leafy vegetables

Deficiency signs and symptoms: Fatigue, weakness

Sodium

Wellness benefits: Is essential for maintenance of proper acid-base balance and body fluid regulation, aids in formation of digestive secretions, assists in nerve transmission

Food sources: Processed foods, meats, table salt

Deficiency signs and symptoms: Rare

From Anspaugh, D. J., Hamrick, M. H., & Rosato, F. D. (1994). *Wellness: Concepts and applications* (2nd ed.). St. Louis: Mosby.
*Calcium and iron are of special concern because deficiencies are likely to exist, especially among women and children.

---

used as teaching tools and to encourage good dietary habits.

TOBACCO USE

"Smoking is the most preventable cause of death in our society. Tobacco use is responsible for nearly one in five deaths in the United States" (American Cancer Society [ACS], 1995, p. 22). It is estimated that about 430,000 deaths each year in the United States and approximately 3 million deaths worldwide are attributable to smoking (USDHHS, 2000b). Furthermore, almost half of all smokers die from diseases caused by smoking, losing an average of 20 to 25 years of life expectancy. Lung cancer mortality is particularly strongly associated with tobacco use because tobacco contributes to 87% of all lung cancers. It is important to realize that lung cancer mortality rates are more than 20 times higher for current male smokers and 12 times higher for current female smokers compared with persons who have never smoked (ACS, 2001).

In addition to heart disease, lung cancer, and chronic respiratory diseases (e.g., chronic bronchitis and chronic obstructive pulmonary disease), tobacco use is associated with cancers of the mouth, pharynx, larynx, esophagus, pancreas, uterine cervix, kidney, and bladder, and intrauterine growth retardation, low birth weight, and birth defects (ACS, 2001). To put the impact of smoking in perspective, the U.S. Surgeon General estimates that cigarettes cost Americans $130 billion annually in tobacco-related health care costs and lost productivity (AHA, 2000). From a different perspective, the cost of treating smoking-related diseases and lost productivity amounts to $2.59 for each pack of cigarettes sold in the United States (ACS, 1995). The impact of tobacco on the health and the economy of U.S. residents cannot be overstated.

Per capita cigarette consumption increased annually from 1901 until 1964, when more than 42% of adults were daily smokers. A gradual decline began following the publication of the Surgeon General's Advisory Committee Report on Smoking and Health in the mid-1960s. Consumption varied somewhat over the next decade (1964 to 1974), but has declined steadily since the mid-1970s before tapering off in the

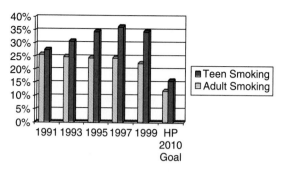

	1991	1993	1995	1997	1999	2010
Data: Teen	27.5	30.5	34.8	36.4	34.8	16
Adult	25.7	25.0	24.7	24.7	22.7	12

Figure 10-1. Prevalence of adult and teen smoking, 1990s. (From U.S. Department of Health and Human Services. [USDHHS]. [2000a]. *Healthy people 2010: Conference edition.* Washington, DC: USDHHS.)

1990s (USDHHS, 2000b). Figure 10-1 shows trends in smoking for both teens and adults during the 1990s.

About 80% of smokers begin smoking before 18 years of age, with the most common age for initiation being 14 to 15 years (CDC, 1999). Despite knowledge of related health problems, approximately 3000 young persons (mostly children and teenagers) begin smoking each day in the United States. Reportedly, 63.5% of high school students have tried cigarette smoking and 20% state that they have smoked cigarettes during the past 30 days (CDC, 2000). School-based smoking prevention programs have been encouraged to combat the alarming statistics described here. The USDHHS (2000b) supports the following recommendations to reduce smoking initiation by adolescents:

1. Develop and enforce a school policy on tobacco use.
2. Provide instruction about the short-term and long-term negative physiological and social consequences of tobacco use, social influences on tobacco use, peer norms regarding tobacco use, and refusal skills.
3. Provide tobacco use prevention education in kindergarten through twelfth grade; this instruction should be especially intensive in junior high or middle school and should be reinforced in high school.
4. Provide program-specific training for teachers.
5. Involve parents or families in support of school-based programs to prevent tobacco use.
6. Support cessation efforts among students and all school staff who use tobacco.
7. Assess the tobacco use prevention program at regular intervals.

SMOKING CESSATION

The CDC (2000) reports that 70% of adults who smoke want to quit, but only about 2.5% per year succeed in quitting smoking permanently. Positively, however, almost half of all living adults who have ever smoked have quit. Programs, tools, medications, and various interventions abound to help with **smoking cessation**. Recognized interventions include self-help groups, videos, and written materials; nicotine chewing gum; nicotine patches; hypnosis; and acupuncture. However, most people who stop (about 90%) do so on their own. The National Cancer Institute has developed a list of tips for smokers to help them quit, which are presented in the Health Teaching box "Tips to Help Smokers Quit."

HEALTH TASK FORCE RECOMMENDATIONS— ILLNESS PREVENTION

In the early 1990s, the U.S. Preventative Services Task Force (USDHHS/ODPHP,1994) published general guidelines or recommendations for periodic individual health examinations based on age. These were updated a few years later (USDHHS/ODPHP, 1998). Included in the guidelines is information on the leading causes of death, appropriate screenings, counseling, and immunizations. Special guidelines and frequencies were detailed for those who are identified as being at high risk for a particular health threat or problem. Table 10-7 gives an overview of the recommendations specifically for adults younger than 65 years. General screening principles are presented in the Community Application box "Screening

health teaching

Tips to Help Smokers Quit

TIPS FOR PREPARING TO STOP

- Decide positively that you want to stop. Try to avoid negative thoughts about possible difficulties.
- List all the reasons why you want to stop. Every night before going to bed, repeat one of the reasons 10 times.
- Develop strong personalized reasons for stopping. For example, think of all of the time you waste taking cigarette breaks, rushing out to buy a pack, or hunting for a lighter.
- Begin to condition yourself physically: Start a moderate exercise program, drink more fluids, get plenty of rest, and avoid fatigue.
- Know what to expect: Have realistic expectations—stopping isn't easy, but it is not impossible either. More than 3 million people in the United States stop each year. Understand that withdrawal symptoms are temporary and are healthy signs that the body is repairing itself from its long exposure to nicotine. Know that most relapses occur in the first week or two after stopping. At this time, withdrawal symptoms are strongest and your body is still most dependent on nicotine.
- Involve someone else: Make a bet with a friend, ask your spouse or a friend to stop smoking with you and make a buddy system, tell your family and friends that you are stopping.

TIPS FOR JUST BEFORE STOPPING

- Practice going without tobacco.
- Do not dwell on the fact that you will never use tobacco again: Think of being tobacco free in terms of 1 day at a time.
- Stop carrying tobacco with you at all times.
- Do not empty your ashtrays or the container that you spit into. This will remind you how much you have used each day and the sight and smell will be very unpleasant.
- Collect all your cigarette butts into one large glass container as a visual reminder of the mess that smoking represents. Occasionally screw off the lid to smell the foul butt and ash odors.

TIPS FOR THE DAY YOU STOP

- Throw away all of your tobacco, lighters, ashtrays, spittoons, and other tobacco-related paraphernalia.

- Clean your clothes to rid them of the smell of smoke.
- Develop a clean, fresh, smoke-free environment around yourself—at work and at home.
- Schedule an appointment to have your teeth cleaned.
- Make a list of things you would like to buy for yourself or someone else. Estimate your cost of using tobacco and put the money aside to buy yourself a present.
- Keep very busy during the big day. Go to the movies, exercise, take long walks, or go bike riding.
- Buy yourself a treat or do something to celebrate.
- Stay away from other tobacco users.
- Remember that one cigarette or one chew could ruin a successful attempt.
- Remember that alcohol will weaken your willpower. Avoid it.
- Refuse to allow anything to change your mind.

TIPS TO HELP YOU COPE WITH THE PERIODIC URGE TO USE TOBACCO

- First remind yourself that you have stopped and you are a nonuser. Look closely at your urge to use tobacco and ask yourself: "Where was I when I got the urge?" "What was I doing at the time?" "Who was I with?" "What was I thinking?"
- Think about why you stopped. Repeat to yourself your three main reasons for stopping.
- Anticipate triggers and prepare to avoid them. Keep your hands busy, avoid people who smoke or chew, find activities that make smoking difficult, put something other than tobacco in your mouth (e.g., carrots, sunflower seeds, apples, celery, or sugarless gum), and avoid places where smoking is permitted.
- Change your daily routine to break old habits and patterns. After meals, immediately get up from the table, brush your teeth or take a walk, change your morning routine, do not sit in your favorite chair, eat lunch at a different location.
- Use positive thoughts. Remind yourself that you are a nonuser; observe people who do not smoke and remind yourself that they feel normal and healthy without using tobacco and so can you.
- Use relaxation techniques. Breathe in deeply and slowly while you count to five; breathe out slowly, counting to five again.

health teaching

Tips to Help Smokers Quit—cont'd

TIPS FOR COPING WITH RELAPSE

- Stop using tobacco immediately.
- Get rid of any tobacco products that you may have.
- Recognize that you have had a slip or small setback and that a small setback does not make you a smoker or a chewer again.
- Do not be too hard on yourself. One slip does not mean that you are a failure or cannot be a

nonuser, but it is important to get yourself back on the nonuser track immediately.

- Realize that many successful former tobacco users stop for good only after more than one attempt.
- Identify triggers. Exactly what was it that prompted you to use tobacco? Be aware of your triggers and decide how you will cope with them when they come up again.
- Sign a contract with yourself to remain a nonuser.

Adapted from U.S. Department of Health and Human Services/National Institutes of Health/National Cancer Institute. (1991). *Clearing the air: How to quit smoking and quit for keeps.* (NIH Publication No. 92-1647). Washington, DC: U.S. Department of Health and Human Services/National Institutes of Health/National Cancer Institute.

TABLE **10-7** Preventative Services Task Force Risk Factors Screening, Referral, and Service for Adults

RISK FACTOR OR GROUP	PREVENTION TARGET CONDITION	PREVENTION SERVICE AND/OR REFERRAL
All adults	Obesity	Obesity screening
	Hypertension	Blood pressure screening
	Coronary heart disease	Cholesterol screening, nutritional counseling, exercise counseling, smoking cessation counseling, aspirin therapy (if indicated)
	Diabetes	Plasma glucose
	Malnutrition	Nutritional counseling
	Dental Disease	Dental check-ups
	Alcohol-related problems	Assess for problem drinking
	Injuries	Counsel about various preventative measures
	Measles, mumps (persons born after 1956 only)	Serology for immune status if no record of vaccination and MMR vaccine if nonimmune
Men 35-65 years and women 45-65 years	Elevated cholesterol	Cholesterol screening, nutritional counseling, exercise counseling, and aspirin therapy (if indicated)
Women ≥40 years of age	Breast cancer	Mammography and clinical breast exam
Men ≥40 years of age	Prostate cancer	Digital rectal exam and prostate specific antigen (should be offered)
Persons who are obese	Coronary heart disease and hypertension	Obesity screening, blood pressure screening, cholesterol screening, nutritional counseling, exercise counseling, aspirin therapy (if indicated)
	Diabetes	Fasting glucose

continued

TABLE **10-7** Preventative Services Task Force Risk Factors Screening, Referral, and Service for Adults—cont'd

RISK FACTOR OR GROUP	PREVENTION TARGET CONDITION	PREVENTION SERVICE AND/OR REFERRAL
Persons undergoing recent divorce or separation, unemployment, or bereavement	Depression	Mental health counseling, possible referral, and hospitalization
	Suicide	Question regarding preparatory actions
Persons who received radiation exposure to head and neck during infancy or childhood	Thyroid cancer and hypothyroidism	Palpation of thyroid
		Thyroid function tests
Persons with history of dysplastic or congenital nevi; history of immunosuppression; history of severe sunburn in childhood; poor tanning ability, light skin, hair or eyes, or freckles	Skin cancer	Counseling to avoid sun exposure between 10 AM and 3 PM; use protective clothing and sunscreen; consider dermatology referral for those at highest risk
Persons with severe myopia	Glaucoma	Ophthalmology referral for screening

COMMUNITY APPLICATION
Screening Principles

Screening for signs and symptoms of disease should be based on age and risk factors and the following guidelines or principles for screening should be followed:

- The condition must have a significant effect on longevity and the quality of life.
- Acceptable methods of treatment must be available.
- The condition must have an asymptomatic period during which detection and treatment significantly reduce morbidity or mortality.
- Treatment in the asymptomatic phase must yield a therapeutic result superior to that obtained by delaying treatment until symptoms appear.

- Tests that are acceptable to clients must be available, at a reasonable cost, to detect the condition in the asymptomatic period.
- The incidence of the condition must be sufficient to justify the cost of the screening.
- The screening test performed must be reliable and valid (i.e., the test should have good sensitivity and specificity).
- Methods for follow-up tracking for client referrals should be available.
- Clients should be clearly informed of the potential cost and morbidity of necessary follow-up testing and treatment.

Principles." The Research Highlight box presents information about a study that examined preventative health services.

PRIMARY AND SECONDARY PREVENTION OF SELECTED CONDITIONS

HEART DISEASE AND STROKE

As discussed earlier and presented in Table 10-1, heart disease and stroke are the number one and number three leading causes of death, respectively, in the United States each year. Indeed, each year as many as 1.5 million U.S. residents have a heart attack and about one third of these die. It is important to note that although heart disease is associated with aging, about 5% of all heart attacks occur in people younger than 40 years and 34% occur in people younger than 75

Research Highlight

Americans Not Receiving Valuable Health Care Services

Recently, a large-scale research study examined 30 preventative health services recommended for average-risk clients and prioritized them based on the services' health benefits and cost effectiveness. The researchers then looked at thousands of Americans to see if they had received the recommended services and reported on their findings. In this study, it was learned that five of the top-ranked services—childhood vaccinations, cervical cancer screening, hypertension screening, cholesterol screening, and vaccinating older adults against influenza—are delivered to more than half of Americans.

On the other hand, several highly ranked preventative health services are not offered to most people. These highly ranked services are tobacco cessation counseling for adults, screening older adults for undetected vision impairments, screening adults older than 50 years for colorectal cancer, screening young women for chlamydia, screening and counseling adults for problem drinking, and vaccinating older adults against pneumococcal disease. Furthermore, the researchers learned that counseling adolescents to avoid or quit using tobacco products and counseling them to avoid alcohol and drugs are two additional high-ranking, low-delivery services. In the conclusions, health care providers were encouraged to focus increased efforts toward addressing these and other recommended preventative services.

Fom Centers for Disease Control and Prevention (CDC). (2001a). *Fewer than half of Americans receive some of the most valuable health care services: Colorectal cancer screening and tobacco counseling top the list.* Retrieved 7/30/01 from http://www.cdc.gov/od/oc/media/pressrel/r010622.htm.

BOX 10-2 Risk Factors Associated with Heart Disease and Stroke

Age: Risk of heart disease and stroke increases steadily with age (about 80% of people who die from heart disease are 65 or older).

Gender: Men have three to four times greater risk of heart disease then premenopausal women; after menopause, women's rate of heart disease increases sharply, although elderly men have roughly twice the risk as elderly women.

Heredity (including race): Risk increases if a parent or sibling has had a heart attack or stroke or died of heart disease before age 55; blacks have more severe high blood pressure and a higher risk of heart disease. Heart disease is also higher among Mexican Americans, Native Americans, Native Hawaiians, and some Asian Americans.

Smoking: Smoking more than doubles the risk of heart attack and stroke; smokers who have a heart attack are more likely to die and to die suddenly than are nonsmokers.

High blood cholesterol: High blood cholesterol causes narrowing in the arterial walls, thus increasing the possibility of occlusion in the brain or heart.

Hypertension: High blood pressure is a major risk factor in heart attack and is the most important risk factor in stroke.

Physical inactivity: Regular exercise helps prevent heart disease and arteriosclerosis, lessens the development of diabetes and obesity, and helps lower blood pressure in some people.

Obesity: Obesity increases the risk of heart disease, particularly in individuals more than 30% above ideal body weight.

Diabetes: Diabetes is linked with increased risk of both heart disease and stroke.

Data from American Heart Association. (2001). *Risk factors and coronary heart disease: AHA scientific position.* Retrieved 7/30/01 from http://216.185.112.5/presenter.jhtml?identifier=539.

(AHA, 2000). Strokes afflict more than 500,000 U.S. residents each year and stroke is the leading cause of serious disability in the United States. Risk factors associated with heart disease and stroke are listed in Box 10-2.

Assessment tools for identification of an individual's risk of heart disease can be helpful. Many such tools describe how risks can be lowered or managed and can be useful in addressing the problem of heart disease. Appendix 10-B shows one example. Nurses and others may use these

---

health teaching

Warning Signs of Heart Attack and Stroke

If you or someone you are with has chest discomfort, especially with one or more of the other signs, or has any of the warning signs of stroke, call for help or get to a hospital immediately.

HEART ATTACK WARNING SIGNS
- Chest Discomfort: Most have discomfort in the center of the chest. The discomfort lasts more than a few minutes or goes away and comes back; it typically feels like uncomfortable pressure, squeezing, fullness, or pain.
- Discomfort in Other Areas of the Upper Body: Discomfort can radiate to one or both arms, the back, neck, jaw, or stomach.

- Shortness of Breath: Shortness of breath often accompanies the chest discomfort, but it can occur before.
- Other signs: Additional indicators are breaking out in a cold sweat, nausea, or lightheadedness.

STROKE WARNING SIGNS
- Sudden numbness or weakness of the face, arm, or leg (especially on one side of the body)
- Sudden confusion, trouble speaking, or understanding
- Sudden trouble seeing in one or both eyes
- Sudden trouble with walking, dizziness, loss of balance, or coordination
- Sudden, severe headache with no known cause

From American Heart Association (1998). *Warning signs.* Retrieved 7/30/01 from http://www.americanheart.org/presenter.jhtml?identifier=3053.

tools as part of a comprehensive program that includes health teaching and counseling on nutrition, exercise, and smoking cessation, if applicable, to lower risk for all individuals (see the Health Teaching box "Warning Signs of Heart Attack and Stroke").

CANCER

Cancer, as has been discussed, is the second leading cause of death in the United States, accounting for about one of every four deaths. The ACS estimates that about 1,200,000 new cancer cases are diagnosed each year (excluding basal and squamous cell skin cancers), resulting in more than 550,000 deaths (1500 people each day) (ACS, 2000). Figures 10-2 and 10-3 graphically illustrate trends in cancer death rates for men and women in the United States and Figure 10-4 shows estimates of newly diagnosed cases and deaths for different types of cancer.

These figures demonstrate the dramatic increase in lung cancer deaths that began during the mid-1950s for men and the mid-1960s for women. As stated earlier, these increases are the direct result of smoking and although they have started to decline slightly for men, they are expected to remain high through the next several decades.

Prevention and Diagnosis of Selected Cancers

Early detection and treatment of cancer has resulted in improved survival rates for most cancers. For example, cancer of the uterus for women and stomach cancer for men have declined considerably over the decades. In addition, death rates for male lung cancer, female breast cancer, prostate cancer, and colorectal cancers all decreased significantly during the 1990s.

Prevention interventions have thus proven to be effective, but more can be done. Indeed, it is estimated that as much as 50% of cancers can be prevented through smoking cessation and improved dietary habits (i.e., such as reducing fat consumption and increasing fruit and vegetable consumption). Physical activity and weight control can also contribute to cancer prevention (USDHHS, 2000a). To assist nurses in teaching and counseling regarding cancer prevention, detection, and treatment, Table 10-8 lists

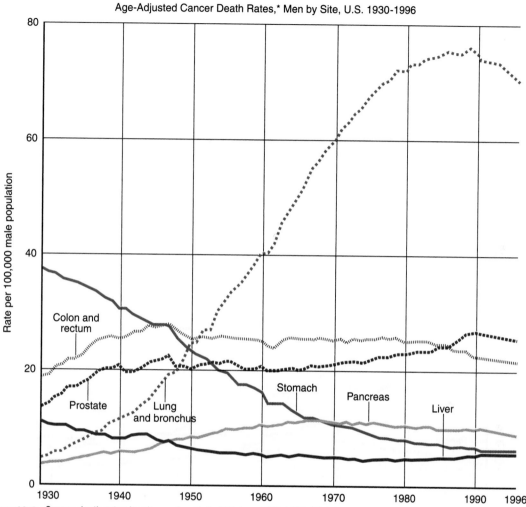

Figure 10-2. Cancer death rates by site, males, United States, 1930-1996. *Rates are per 100,000 and are age-adjusted to the 1970 U.S. standard population. Note: Because of changes in ICD coding, numerator information has changed over time. Rates for cancers of the liver, lung, and bronchus and colon and rectum are affected by these coding changes. (From American Cancer Society. [2001]. *Cancer facts & figures. 2001.* Atlanta: American Cancer Society.)

incidence, symptoms, risk factors, and treatment options for several of the most common cancers.

Compliance with screening recommendations for cancers of the breast, cervix, and colon/rectum could dramatically reduce deaths from these cancers. For example, reduction in colon/rectal cancer can be achieved through biennial screen-ing with fecal occult blood tests and detection and removal of precancerous polyps.

DIABETES

Approximately 16 million U.S. residents (about 6% of the total population) have diabetes and it is estimated that about one third are not aware of

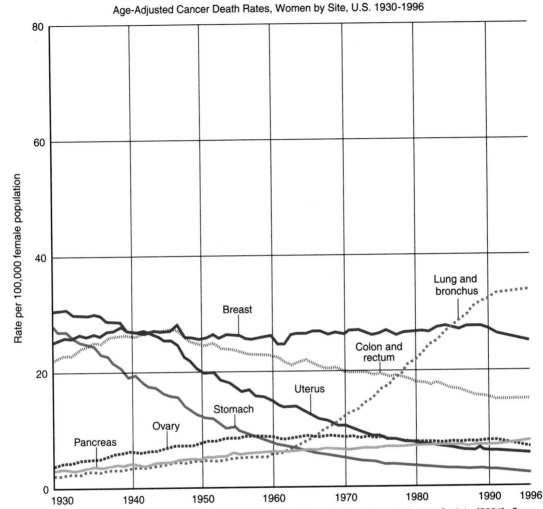

Figure 10-3. Cancer death rates by site, females, United States, 1930-1996. (From American Cancer Society. [2001]. *Cancer facts & figures. 2001.* Atlanta: American Cancer Society.)

it. Each year, some 800,000 people are diagnosed with diabetes (2200 per day). Many people with diabetes (90% to 95%) have type 2 diabetes, which usually develops in adults older than 40 years. The remainder (5% to 10%) of clients have type 1 diabetes, which most often develops in children and young adults (USDHHS, 2000a). Additionally, gestational diabetes develops in 2% to 5% of all pregnancies, but disappears

when the pregnancy is over. Women who have had gestational diabetes are at increased risk for developing type 2 diabetes later in life (American Diabetes Association, 2000).

Diabetes is one of the leading causes of death and disability in the United States, contributing to almost 200,000 deaths each year. Additionally, diabetes is associated with many severe illnesses and conditions, including blindness, heart

Leading Sites of New Cancer Cases and Deaths— 2001 Estimates*

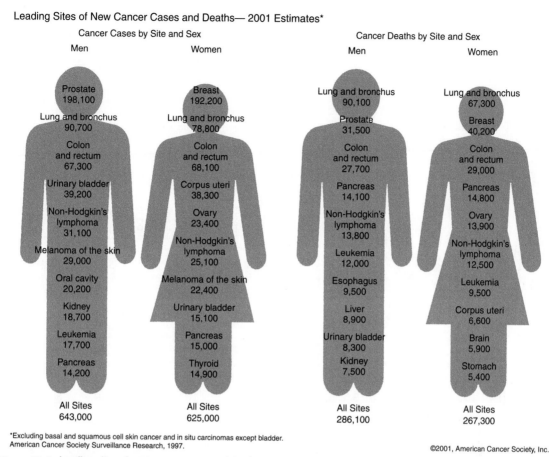

Figure 10-4. Leading sites of new cancer cases and deaths—2001 estimates. (From American Cancer Society. [2000]. *Cancer facts & figures. 2001.* Atlanta: American Cancer Society.)

disease, stroke, kidney failure, nerve damage, amputations, and birth defects in babies born to women with diabetes (CDC, 1998).

Several major risk factors are associated with diabetes. Type 2 diabetes is strongly associated with age. Those 65 years of age or older are the most affected and 18.4% of all persons in that age group are diabetic. Being Hispanic, black, or Native American strongly predisposes many to type 2 diabetes. Indeed, blacks are 1.7 times as likely to have diabetes as are whites and almost 11% of blacks are diabetic. Likewise, Hispanics are almost twice as likely as are whites to have

diabetes and American Indians and Alaska Natives are 2.8 times as likely to have diabetes as are non-Hispanic whites. Other significant risk factors for type 2 diabetes include obesity (about 80% of people with type 2 diabetes are overweight) and/or strong family history (CDC, 1998).

Most groups recommend screening of high-risk groups (blacks, Hispanics, and Native Americans) and obese men and women over 40 and those with a strong family history of diabetes (USDHHS/ODPHP, 1998). In addition, individuals, particularly those in high-risk groups, should

TABLE **10-8** Incidence, Risk Factors, Symptoms, Early Detection, and Treatment of Selected Cancers

CANCER SITE	INCIDENCE	RISK FACTORS	SYMPTOMS	SCREENING/EARLY DETECTION	TREATMENT
Lung	170,000 cases with 157,000 deaths	Cigarette smoking; exposure to radiation, asbestos, and other substances	Persistent cough, sputum streaked with blood, chest pain, recurring pneumonia or bronchitis	Very difficult to detect; chest x-ray, sputum analysis, and fiberoptic examination of the bronchial passages when indicated	Usually a combination of surgery, radiation therapy, and chemotherapy
Colon and rectum	135,400 new cases, with 56,700 deaths	Personal or family history of cancer or polyps of the colon or rectum; inflammatory bowel disease, high-fat diet	Rectal bleeding, blood in the stool, change in bowel habits	Digital rectal examination, stool occult blood examination, proctosigmoidoscopy	Surgery; surgery and radiation therapy
Breast	193,700 new cases, with an estimated 41,000 deaths (less than 0.1% occur in men)	Increasing age, family history, early menarche, late menopause, never had children or late age at first birth, high-fat diet	Changes on mammogram, lump, thickening, swelling, dimpling, skin irritation, distortion, retraction, pain, nipple discharge	Screening mammogram by age 40; women 40-49 should have a mammogram every 1-2 years, and women 50 years or older, each year; clinical examination of the breast every 3 years to age 40 and every year thereafter; monthly breast self-examination for all women age 20 and older	Lumpectomy, mastectomy, radiation therapy, chemotherapy, hormone manipulation therapy, or a combination of the above
Prostate	198,000 new cases each year, with 31,500 deaths	Age (over 80% are diagnosed in men over age 65); possibly family history; possibly high-fat diet	Weak or interrupted urine flow, inability to urinate, need to urinate frequently, blood in the urine, pain or burning on urination, lower back or pelvic pain	Somewhat controversial. All men should be counseled on screening. A digital rectal examination for all men 40 years or older and prostate specific antigen (PSA) test for all men over age 50 should be offered.	Surgery, radiation, and/or hormone treatment
Cervix	12,900 invasive and 65,000 carcinoma in situ cases annually, with 4400 deaths	Early age at first intercourse, multiple sex partners, cigarette smoking, infection with human papillomavirus	Abnormal uterine bleeding or spotting, abnormal vaginal discharge	Papanicolaou test and pelvic examination should be performed annually for women who are sexually active and those age 18 or older	Surgery and or radiation; precancerous (in situ) cases may be treated by cryotherapy or electrocoagulation

Skin cancer	1.3 million+ cases of basal cell or squamous cell cancer each year; 51,400 cases and 7800 deaths each year from melanoma	Excessive exposure to ultraviolet radiation, fair complexion	Change in size or color of a mole or spot; scaliness, oozing, bleeding, or change in appearance of a bump	Skin self-examination once a month and reporting of changes to a physician	Surgery, radiation, cryosurgery, and electrodessication; for melanoma, wide margin excision and possible lymph node excision
Ovary	Estimated 23,400 new cases and 13,900 deaths each year	Increase with age, never having had children, family history	Asymptomatic in early stages; enlargement of the abdomen, vague digestive disturbances	Pelvic examination, including palpation each year	Surgery, radiation therapy, and chemotherapy
Oral	Estimated 30,100 new cases and 7800 annual deaths	Cigarette, cigar, or pipe smoking; use of smokeless tobacco; excess use of alcohol	Sore that bleeds easily and does not heal; lump or thickening or red or white patch that persists on the mouth, tongue, or gums	Examination of the mouth, lips, tongue, and throat annually by a dentist or primary care provider	Radiation therapy and surgery

Data from American Cancer Society (ACS). (2000). *Cancer facts & figures—2001.* Atlanta: American Cancer Society. Reprinted by the permission of the American Cancer Society, Inc.

be taught the following symptoms of diabetes (USDHHS/Public Health Service/CDC, 1992):

- Excessive thirst
- Excessive urination
- Blurred vision
- Sensory nerve damage, particularly in the extremities
- Fatigue
- Weight loss
- Slow healing of skin
- Gum infection
- Urinary tract infection

Whereas type 1 diabetes is managed with strict adherence to a prescribed diet, intensive monitoring of blood glucose levels, and administration of insulin (often two to four times daily), type 2 diabetes is primarily controlled through diet and other lifestyle changes. Weight loss is strongly encouraged, as is avoidance of alcohol and smoking when indicated. Frequently, people with type 2 diabetes must take medication to control blood glucose levels. Usually, oral medications (e.g., oral hypoglycemic/sulfonylureas such as tolbutamide, chlorpropamide, and tolazamide) are sufficient, but many type 2 diabetics eventually need to take insulin to better control serum glucose levels.

Health teaching and counseling for all individuals with diabetes should focus on closely following the recommended diet; monitoring blood glucose levels as directed by their physician; taking medications, including insulin, as prescribed; and carefully observing for complications. Some relatively common complications, prevention methods, and teaching principles include the following:

- Diabetic ketoacidosis (insulin deficiency resulting in hyperglycemia, osmotic diuresis, and acidosis): Ketoacidosis is usually caused by failure to adhere to a program for insulin management or failure to alter insulin intake during intercurrent illnesses. Clients should be taught the importance of compliance with the prescribed medication regimen and how to manage serum glucose levels during illness.

- Hypoglycemia: A low blood glucose level often results from delay or decrease in food intake, vigorous physical activity, or alcohol consumption. Clients should be taught to recognize symptoms of low blood glucose (e.g., apprehension, tremors, sweating, palpitations, fatigue, confusion, headache) and treat with rapidly absorbable carbohydrates (e.g., three to five pieces of hard candy, two to three packets of sugar, or 4 ounces of fruit juice). A family member or friend should be taught to administer oral carbohydrates if the client is unable to treat himself or herself. If this is not possible, the Emergency Medical Service should be notified.

- Periodontal disease: Gingivitis and periodontitis are common in diabetics. Instruction on proper brushing and flossing is essential and preventive dental care, ideally every 6 months, should be encouraged.

- Eye disease: Diabetes is a major cause of blindness in the United States. Roughly 70% of people with type 1 diabetes develop diabetic retinopathy and 40% develop macular edema. Clients with diabetes should be taught to report any changes in vision (e.g., blurred vision, "floaters," and flashing lights) immediately. A yearly eye examination is very important because early detection of ophthalmic complications and prompt treatment with laser surgery can reduce visual loss significantly.

- Kidney disease: Diabetic nephropathy is characterized by albuminuria, hypertension, and progressive renal insufficiency. As a result of chronic renal insufficiency, end-stage renal disease may occur (about a third of end-stage renal disease cases in the United States are attributed to diabetes). To prevent kidney disease, diabetics must be taught to monitor blood pressure and adhere to treatment of hypertension when indicated; closely monitor blood glucose levels; avoid excessive protein intake; and observe for symptoms of urinary tract infection.

- Cardiovascular disease: Clients should be told that diabetes increases the risk of developing cardiovascular disease. Maintaining a low-fat, low-sodium diet is very important and should be encouraged. Signs and symptoms of cardiovascular disease can be discussed and the client told to report possible symptoms immediately.
- Neuropathy: Clients should be informed about the relationship between poor glycemic control and development of diabetic neuropathy. Complications of neuropathy include orthostatic hypotension, constipation, diabetic diarrhea and fecal incontinence, diabetic bladder dysfunction, and sexual dysfunction. Careful monitoring and maintenance of glucose levels can help reduce neuropathy.
- Foot problems: Persons with diabetes account for approximately 50% of all nontraumatic amputations performed each year. To prevent foot ulcers and potential complications, diabetics should be taught meticulous foot care. Principles include to wash and inspect feet daily, use foot creams or oils, cut toenails correctly and never cut corns or calluses, avoid extremes of temperature, never walk barefooted, wear appropriate shoes, inspect the inside of shoes daily, and seek medical care for all skin lesions (USDHHS/Public Health Service/CDC, 1992).

To prevent these and other complications, it is vitally important that all diabetics maintain their diets and treatment regimens, monitor illnesses carefully, and report any complications immediately to their primary care providers. Many organizations and resources are available for clients with diabetes. Health care providers should be aware of these resources and refer clients appropriately.

SUMMARY

Nursing interventions focused on health promotion and illness prevention are largely conducted in community-based settings such as primary health care offices, occupational health settings, clinics, and rehabilitations settings, as illustrated in the opening case study. Like Ben, the nurse from the case study, nurses who practice in these settings should be familiar with current recommendations and guidelines to promote and improve the health of adults.

This chapter describes many issues related to health promotion and illness prevention for

---

Resources

Adult Health Promotion and Illness Prevention
Office of Disease Prevention and Health Promotion
Bureau of Primary Health Care

Physical Fitness/Sports
President's Council on Physical Fitness and Sports
American Heart Association

Nutrition
U.S. Department of Agriculture Food, Nutrition, and Consumer Services
Food and Drug Administration

Tobacco Use/Smoking Cessation
CDC Office on Smoking and Health
National Heart, Lung, and Blood Institute
National Cancer Institute
American Lung Association

Heart Disease and Stroke
National Institute of Neurological Disorders and Stroke
American Heart Association
National Stroke Association

Cancer
National Cancer Institute
American Cancer Society

Diabetes
National Institute of Diabetes and Digestive and Kidney Disorders
American Diabetes Association

Visit the book's website at
www.wbsaunders.com/SIMON/McEwen $\mathcal{S}$iMoN
for a direct link to the website for each organization listed.

adults. For more information on the topics presented here, see the Resources box at the end of the chapter. Additionally, the reader is referred to Chapter 9 to study health-promotion and illness-prevention strategies for children, Chapter 11 for a discussion of women's health issues, and Chapter 12 for health promotion and illness prevention for older adults.

KEY POINTS

- Health promotion refers to activities or actions related to encouraging individual lifestyles or personal choices that positively influence health (e.g., encouraging physical activity and fitness, good nutrition, substance abuse prevention).
- Health benefits of regular exercise and physical activity are well documented. Individuals should work up to moderate-level activities (50% to 75% of maximum heart rate) for a minimum of 30 minutes, three to four times per week, depending on age and presence of existing physical problems. Walking, aerobic dancing, bicycling, jogging, and swimming are examples of recommended activities.
- Good nutritional practices and maintenance of a desirable weight are essential for good health. In the United States, it is estimated that 20% of men and 25% of women are obese. Obesity is associated with hypertension, type 2 diabetes, hypercholesterolemia, coronary artery disease, some types of cancer, and stroke. Nutrition guidelines for a healthy diet include eating a variety of foods; maintaining healthy weight; choosing a diet low in fat, saturated fat, and cholesterol; eating five or more servings daily of vegetables, fruits, and grains; using sugar, salt, and sodium in moderation; and drinking alcoholic beverages in moderation, if at all.
- In the United States, tobacco use is associated with more than 430,000 deaths annually from heart disease; lung cancer; chronic respiratory diseases; cancers of the mouth, pharynx, larynx, pancreas, and other sites; intrauterine growth retardation; low birth weight; and birth defects. More than 80% of smokers began before 18 years of age and more than 60% of high school students have reportedly tried cigarette smoking. A number of programs, tools, medications, and other interventions are available for clients who want to stop smoking.
- Primary and secondary prevention interventions for heart disease and stroke are essential because these diseases account for the number one and three causes of death and disability in the United States. Risk factors for heart disease and stroke include smoking, hypertension, hypercholesterolemia, diabetes, obesity, age, sex, and genetic predisposition. Prevention efforts to reduce or eliminate these risk factors include teaching and counseling on nutrition, exercise, and smoking cessation (if applicable).
- Cancer is the second leading cause of death in the United States, resulting in about 540,000 deaths each year. Early detection and treatment of cancer has improved survival rates for most cancers.
- Diabetes affects about 16 million U.S. residents, about half of whom are not aware of it. Diabetes is one of the leading causes of death and disability and is associated with many health conditions, including blindness, heart disease, stroke, renal failure, nerve damage, amputations, and birth defects. Risk factors for noninsulin-dependent diabetes mellitus include obesity, increasing age, family history, and being a member of certain minority groups (blacks, Hispanics, and Native Americans).

Learning Activities & Application to Practice
In Class

1. With classmates, discuss objectives of *Healthy People 2010* related to health promotion and illness prevention of adults (e.g., improving physical activity and nutrition; quitting use of tobacco; and reducing rates of heart disease, stroke, cancer, and diabetes). Analyze baselines and variations in special populations. What objectives should nurses working in

community-based settings address? What health education and anticipatory guidance should be provided?

2. Complete one of the assessment tools presented in the appendices. Share results with classmates. What are areas of strength and weakness? How can tools of this type be used in community settings to help improve the individual's health?

In Clinical

3. Observe for opportunities to share health-promotion and illness-prevention strategies in all settings, particularly as they relate to the leading causes of morbidity and mortality. For example, if you are working with heart disease, stroke, or diabetes patients, provide instruction on minimization and elimination of risk factors and management of the disease process. How can this be accomplished effectively? How might health teaching be enhanced?

REFERENCES

American Cancer Society (ACS). (1995). *Cancer facts & figures— 1995*. Atlanta: American Cancer Society.

American Cancer Society (ACS). (2000). *Cancer facts & figures—2001*. Atlanta: American Cancer Society.

American Cancer Society. (2001). *Cancer facts & figures—2001*. Atlanta: American Cancer Society.

American Diabetes Association. (2000). *Basic diabetes information*. Retrieved 7/31/01 from http://www.diabetes.org/main/application/commercewf?origin=*.jsp&event=link(B).

American Heart Association (AHA). (1994). *RISKO: A heart health appraisal*. Dallas, TX: American Heart Association.

American Heart Association (AHA). (1996). *Statement on exercise: Benefits and recommendations for physical activity programs for all Americans*. Dallas, TX: American Heart Association. Retrieved 7/30/01 from http://216.185.112.5/presenter.jhtml?identifier=1249.

American Heart Association. (1998). *Warning signs*. Retrieved 7/30/01 from http://www.americanheart.org/presenter.jhtml?identifier=3053.

American Heart Association (AHA). (2000). *2001 heart and stroke statistical update*. Dallas, TX: American Heart Association.

American Heart Association. (2001). *Risk factors and coronary heart disease: AHA scientific position*. Retrieved 7/30/01 from http://www.americanheart.org/presenter.jhtml?identifier=4726.

American Heart Association and National Heart, Lung and Blood Institute. (1993). *Exercise and your heart: A guide to physical activity*. Dallas, TX: American Heart Association.

Anspaugh, D. J., Hamrick, M. H., & Rosato, F. D. (1994). *Wellness: Concepts and applications* (2nd ed.). St. Louis: Mosby.

Centers for Disease Control and Prevention (CDC). (1998). *National diabetes fact sheet 1998*. Retrieved 7/31/01 from http://www.cdc.gov/diabetes/pubs/facts98.htm.

Centers for Disease Control and Prevention (CDC). (1999). Cigarette smoking among high school students—11 states 1991-1997. *MMWR Morbidity and Mortality Weekly Report, 48*(31), 686-692.

Centers for Disease Control and Prevention (CDC). (2000). Youth tobacco surveillance, U.S. 1998-1999. *MMWR Morbidity and Mortality Weekly Report, 49* (SS-10), 1-93.

Centers for Disease Control and Prevention (CDC). (2001a). *Fewer than half of Americans receive some of the most valuable health care services: Colorectal cancer screening and tobacco counseling top the list*. Retrieved 7/30/01 from http://www.cdc.gov/od/oc/media/pressrel/r010622.htm.

Centers for Disease Control and Prevention (CDC). (2001b). Recommendations for preventing motor vehicle deaths. *MMWR Morbidity and Mortality Weekly Report, 50*, RR-7, 1-13.

Centers for Disease Control and Prevention/National Center for Chronic Disease Prevention and Health Promotion. (2001). *Obesity continues climb in 1999 among American adults*. Retrieved 7/30/01 from www.cdc.gov/nccdphp/dnpa/pr-obesity.htm.

Human Nutrition Information Service. (1992). *The food guide pyramid: Beyond the basic 4*. Washington, DC: U.S. Department of Agriculture.

McGinnis, M. J., & Foege, W. (1993). Actual causes of death in the United States. *Journal of the American Medical Association, 270*(18), 2207-2212.

Metropolitan Life Insurance Company. (1983). New weight standards for men and women. *Statistical Bulletin of Metropolitan Life Insurance Company, 64*, 2-9.

National Center for Health Statistics (NCHS). (2000). Deaths: Final Data for 1998. *National Vital Statistics Reports, 48*(11), 1-106. Washington, DC: National Center for Health Statistics.

National Heart, Lung and Blood Institute. (1992). *Healthy heart I.Q.* (NIH Publication No. 92-2724).

Washington, DC: National Heart, Lung and Blood Institute.

Office of Disease Prevention and Health Promotion. (1981). *Healthstyle: A self-test.* (Publication No. H0012). Washington, DC: National Health Information Clearinghouse.

Pender, N. J. (1996). *Health promotion in nursing practice* (3rd ed.). Stamford, CT: Appleton & Lange.

President's Council on Physical Fitness & Sports. (1993). The health benefits of physical activity. *Physical activity and fitness research digest.* Vol. 1. Issue 1. Washington, DC: USDHHS/President's Council on Physical Fitness and Sports.

U.S. Department of Health and Human Services. (2000a). *Healthy people 2010: Conference edition.* Washington, DC: Government Printing Office.

U.S. Department of Health and Human Services. (2000b). *Reducing tobacco use: A report of the surgeon general.* Atlanta: USDHHS/CDC.

U.S. Department of Health and Human Services/ National Institutes of Health/National Cancer Institute. (1991). *Clearing the air: How to quit smoking and quit for keeps.* (NIH Publication No. 92-1647). Washington DC: U.S. Department of Health and Human Services/National Institutes of Health/ National Cancer Institute.

U.S. Department of Health and Human Services/Office of Disease Prevention and Health Promotion. (1994). *Clinician's handbook of preventive services.* Washington, DC: Government Printing Office.

U.S. Department of Health and Human Services/ Office of Disease Prevention and Health Promotion. (1998). *Clinician's handbook of preventive services* (2nd ed.). Washington, DC: Government Printing Office.

U.S. Department of Health and Human Services/Public Health Service/Centers for Disease Control. (1992). *The prevention and treatment of complications of diabetes mellitus: A guide for primary care practitioners.* Atlanta: U.S. Department of Health and Human Services.

Appendix 10-A

Healthstyle: A Self-test

All of us want good health. But many of us do not know how to be as healthy as possible. Health experts now describe *lifestyle* as one of the most important factors affecting health. In fact, it is estimated that as many as seven of the ten leading causes of death could be reduced through common-sense changes in lifestyle. That's what this brief test, developed by the Public Health Service, is all about. Its purpose is simply to tell you how well you are doing to stay healthy. The behaviors covered in the test are recommended for most Americans. Some of them may not apply to persons with certain chronic diseases or handicaps, or to pregnant women. Such persons may require special instructions from their physicians.

Cigarette Smoking

	Almost Always	Sometimes	Almost Never
If you *never smoke*, enter a score of 10 for this section and go to the next section on *Alcohol and Drugs*.			
1. I avoid smoking cigarettes.	2	1	0
2. I smoke only low-tar and nicotine cigarettes *or* I smoke a pipe or cigars.	2	1	0

Smoking Score:_____

Alcohol and Drugs

	Almost Always	Sometimes	Almost Never
1. I avoid drinking alcoholic beverages *or* I drink no more than one or two drinks a day.	4	1	0
2. I avoid using alcohol or other drugs (especially illegal drugs) as a way of handling stressful situations or the problems in my life.	2	1	0
3. I am careful not to drink alcohol when taking certain medicines (for example, medicine for sleeping, pain, colds, and allergies), or when pregnant.	2	1	0
4. I read and follow the label directions when using prescribed and over-the-counter drugs.	2	1	0

Alcohol and Drugs Score:_____

	Almost Always	Sometimes	Almost Never

Eating Habits

1. I eat a variety of foods each day, such as fruits and vegetables, whole grain breads and cereals, lean meats, dairy products, dry peas and beans, and nuts and seeds.   4   1   0
2. I limit the amount of fat, saturated fat, and cholesterol I eat (including fat on meats, eggs, butter, cream, shortenings, and organ meats such as liver).   2   1   0
3. I limit the amount of salt I eat by cooking with only small amounts, not adding salt at the table, and avoiding salty snacks.   2   1   0
4. I avoid eating too much sugar (especially frequent snacks of sticky candy or soft drinks).   2   1   0

          Eating Habits Score:_____

Exercise/Fitness

1. I maintain a desired weight, avoiding overweight and underweight.   3   1   0
2. I do vigorous exercises for 15–30 minutes at least three times a week (examples include running, swimming, brisk walking).   3   1   0
3. I do exercises that enhance my muscle tone for 15–30 minutes at least three times a week (examples include yoga and calisthenics).   2   1   0
4. I use part of my leisure time participating in individual, family, or team activities that increase my level of fitness (such as gardening, bowling, golf, and baseball).   2   1   0

          Exercise/Fitness Score:_____

Stress Control

1. I have a job or do other work that I enjoy.   2   1   0
2. I find it easy to relax and express my feelings freely.   2   1   0
3. I recognize early, and prepare for, events or situations likely to be stressful for me.   2   1   0
4. I have close friends, relatives, or others whom I can talk to about personal matters and call on for help when needed.   2   1   0
5. I participate in group activities (such as church and community organizations) or hobbies that I enjoy.   2   1   0

          Stress Control Score:_____

Safety

1. I wear a seat belt while riding in a car.   2   1   0
2. I avoid driving while under the influence of alcohol and other drugs.   2   1   0
3. I obey traffic rules and the speed limit when driving.   2   1   0
4. I am careful when using potentially harmful products or substances (such as household cleaners, poisons, and electrical devices).   2   1   0
5. I avoid smoking in bed.   2   1   0

          Safety Score:_____

WHAT YOUR SCORES MEAN TO YOU

Scores of 9 and 10

Excellent! Your answers show that you are aware of the importance of this area to your health. More important, you are putting your knowledge to work for you by practicing good health habits. As long as you continue to do so, this area should not pose a serious health risk. It's likely that you are setting an example for your family and friends to follow. Since you got a very high test score on this part of the test, you may want to consider other areas where your scores indicate room for improvement.

Scores of 6 to 8

Your health practices in this area are good, but there is room for improvement. Look again at the items you answered with a "Sometimes" or "Almost Never." What changes can you make to improve your score? Even a small change can often help you achieve better health.

Scores of 3 to 5

Your health risks are showing! Would you like more information about the risks you are facing and about why it is important for you to change these behaviors? Perhaps you need help in deciding how to successfully make the changes you desire. In either case, help is available.

Scores of 0 to 2

Obviously, you were concerned enough about your health to take the test, but your answers show that you may be taking serious and unnecessary risks with your health.

Perhaps you are not aware of the risks and what to do about them. You can easily get the information and help you need to improve, if you wish. The next step is up to you.

YOU CAN START RIGHT NOW!

In the test you just completed were numerous suggestions to help you reduce your risk of disease and premature death. Here are some of the most significant:

AVOID CIGARETTES. Cigarette smoking is the single most important preventable cause of illness and early death. It is especially risky for pregnant women and their unborn babies. Persons who stop smoking reduce their risk of getting heart disease and cancer. So if you're a cigarette smoker, think twice about lighting that next cigarette. If you choose to continue smoking, try decreasing the number of cigarettes you smoke and switching to a low tar and nicotine brand.

FOLLOW SENSIBLE DRINKING HABITS. Alcohol produces changes in mood and behavior. Most people who drink are able to control their intake of alcohol and to avoid undesired, and often harmful, effects. Heavy, regular use of alcohol can lead to cirrhosis of the liver, a leading cause of death. Also, statistics clearly show that mixing drinking and driving is often the cause of fatal or crippling accidents. So if you drink, do it wisely and in moderation. **Use care in taking drugs**. Today's greater use of drugs—both legal and illegal—is one of our most serious health risks. Even some drugs prescribed by your doctor can be dangerous if taken when drinking alcohol or before driving. Excessive or continued use of tranquilizers (or "pep pills") can cause physical and mental problems. Using or experimenting with illicit drugs such as marijuana, heroin, cocaine, and PCP may lead to a number of damaging effects or even death.

EAT SENSIBLY. Overweight individuals are at greater risk for diabetes, gall bladder disease, and high blood pressure. So it makes good sense to maintain proper weight. But good eating habits also mean holding down the amount of fat (especially saturated fat), cholesterol, sugar and salt in your diet. If you must snack, try nibbling on fresh fruits and vegetables. You'll feel better—and look better, too.

EXERCISE REGULARLY. Almost everyone can benefit from exercise—and there's some form of exercise almost everyone can do. (If you have any doubt, check first with your doctor.) Usually, as little as 15 to 30 minutes of vigorous exercise three times a week will help you have a healthier heart, eliminate excess weight, tone up sagging muscles, and sleep better. Think how much difference all these improvements could make in the way you feel!

LEARN TO HANDLE STRESS. Stress is a normal part of living; everyone faces it to some degree. The causes of stress can be good or bad, desirable or undesirable (such as a promotion on the job or the loss of a spouse). Properly handled, stress need not be a problem. But unhealthy responses to stress—such as driving too fast or erratically, drinking too much, or prolonged anger or grief—can cause a variety of physical and mental problems. Even on a very busy day, find a few minutes to slow down and relax. Talking over a problem with someone you trust can often help you find a satisfactory solution. Learn to distinguish between things that are "worth fighting about" and things that are less important.

BE SAFETY CONSCIOUS. Think "safety first" at home, at work, at school, at play, and on the highway. Buckle seat belts and obey traffic rules. Keep poisons and weapons out of the reach of children and keep emergency numbers by your telephone. When the unexpected happens, you'll be prepared.

Where Do You Go From Here?

Start by asking yourself a few frank questions: "Am I really doing all I can to be as healthy as possible?" "What steps can I take to feel better?" "Am I willing to begin now?" If you scored low in one or more sections of the test, decide what changes you want to make for improvement. You might pick that aspect of your lifestyle where you feel you have the best chance for success and tackle that one first. Once you have improved your score there, go on to other areas.

If you already have tried to change your health habits (to stop smoking or exercise regularly, for example), don't be discouraged if you haven't yet succeeded. The difficulty you have encountered may be due to influences you've never really thought about—such as advertising—or to a lack of support and encouragement. Understanding these influences is an important step toward changing the way they affect you.

THERE'S HELP AVAILABLE. In addition to personal actions you can take on your own, there are community programs and groups (such as the YMCA or the local chapter of the American Heart Association) that can assist you and your family to make the changes you want to make. If you want to know more about these groups or about health risks, contact your local health department or the National Health Information Clearinghouse. There's a lot you can do to stay healthy or to improve your health—and there are organizations that can help you. Start a new HEALTHSTYLE today!

For assistance in locating specific information on these and other health topics, write to the National Health Information Clearinghouse: National Health Information Clearinghouse, P.O. Box 1133, Washington, DC 20013.

From Office of Disease Prevention and Health Promotion. (1981). *Healthstyle: A self-test.* (Publication No. H0012). Washington, DC: National Health Information Clearinghouse.

Appendix 10-B

Healthy Heart I.Q.

Please answer "true" or "false" to the following questions to test your knowledge of heart disease and its risk factors. Then check the answers and explanations that follow to see how well you do.

1. The risk factors for heart disease that you *can do something about* are high blood pressure, high blood cholesterol, smoking, obesity, and physical inactivity. T F
2. A stroke is often the first symptom of high blood pressure and a heart attack is often the first symptom of high blood cholesterol. T F
3. A blood pressure greater than or equal to 140/90 mm Hg is generally considered to be high. T F
4. High blood pressure affects the same number of blacks as it does whites. T F
5. The best ways to treat and control high blood pressure are to control your weight, exercise, eat less salt (sodium), restrict your intake of alcohol, and take your high blood pressure medicine, if prescribed by your doctor. T F
6. A blood cholesterol level of 240 mg/dl is desirable for adults. T F
7. The most effective dietary way to lower the level of your blood cholesterol is to eat foods low in cholesterol. T F
8. Lowering blood cholesterol levels can help people who have already had a heart attack. T F
9. Only children from families at high risk of heart disease need to have their blood cholesterol levels checked. T F
10. Smoking is a major risk factor for four of the five leading causes of death including heart attack, stroke, cancer, and lung diseases such as emphysema and bronchitis. T F
11. If you have had a heart attack, quitting smoking can help reduce your chances of having a second attack. T F
12. Someone who has smoked for 30 to 40 years probably will not be able to quit smoking. T F
13. The best way to lose weight is to increase physical activity and eat fewer calories. T F
14. Heart disease is the leading killer of men **and** women in the United States. T F

1. TRUE High blood pressure, smoking, and high blood cholesterol are the three most important risk factors for heart disease. On the average, each one doubles your chance of developing heart disease. So a person who has all three of these risk factors is eight times more likely to develop heart disease than someone who has none. Obesity increases the likelihood of developing high blood cholesterol and high blood pressure, which increase your risk for heart disease. Physical inactivity increases your risk of heart attack.

Regular exercise and good nutrition are essential to reducing high blood pressure, high blood cholesterol, and overweight. People who exercise are also more likely to cut down or stop smoking.

2. TRUE A person with high blood pressure or high blood cholesterol may feel fine and look great; there are often no signs that anything is wrong until a stroke or heart attack occurs. To find out if you have high blood pressure or high blood cholesterol, you should be tested by a doctor, nurse, or other health professional.

3. TRUE A blood pressure of 140/90 mm Hg or greater is generally classified as high blood pressure. However, blood pressures that fall below 140/90 mm Hg can sometimes be a problem. If the diastolic pressure, the second or lower number, is between 85 and 89, a person is at increased risk for heart disease or stroke and should have his/her blood pressure checked at least once a year by a health professional. The higher your blood pressure, the greater your risk of developing heart disease or stroke. Controlling high blood pressure reduces your risk.

4. FALSE High blood pressure is more common in blacks than in whites. It affects 29 of every 100 black adults compared to 26 of every 100 white adults. Also, with aging, high blood pressure is generally more severe among blacks than among whites and therefore causes more strokes, heart disease, and kidney failure.

5. TRUE Recent studies show that lifestyle changes can help keep blood pressure levels normal even into advanced age and are important in treating and preventing high blood pressure. Limit high-salt foods, which include many snack foods, such as potato chips, salted pretzels, and salted crackers; processed foods, such as canned soups; and condiments, such as ketchup and soy sauce. Also, it is **extremely important** to take blood pressure medication, if prescribed by your doctor, to make sure your blood pressure stays under control.

6. FALSE A total blood cholesterol level of under 200 mg/dl is **desirable** and usually puts you at a lower risk for heart disease. A blood cholesterol level of 240 mg/dl or above is **high** and increases your risk of heart disease. If your cholesterol level is high, your doctor will want to check your levels of LDL cholesterol ("bad" cholesterol) and HDL cholesterol ("good" cholesterol). A HIGH level of LDL cholesterol increases your risk of heart disease, as does a LOW level of HDL cholesterol. A cholesterol level of 200–239 mg/dl is considered **borderline-high** and usually increases your risk for heart disease. If your cholesterol is borderline-high, you should speak to your doctor to see if additional cholesterol tests are needed. All adults 20 years of age or older should have their blood cholesterol level checked at least once every 5 years.

7. FALSE Reducing the amount of cholesterol in your diet is important; however, eating foods **low in saturated fat** is the most effective dietary way to lower blood cholesterol levels, along with eating less total fat and cholesterol. Choose low-saturated fat foods, such as grains, fruits, and vegetables; low-fat or skim milk and milk products; lean cuts of meat; fish; and chicken. Trim fat from meat before cooking; bake or broil meat rather than fry; use less fat and oil; and take the skin off chicken and turkey. Reducing overweight will also help lower your level of LDL cholesterol as well as increase your level of HDL cholesterol.

8. TRUE People who have had one heart attack are at much higher risk for a second attack. Reducing blood cholesterol levels can greatly slow down (and, in

some people, even reverse) the buildup of cholesterol and fat in the walls of the coronary arteries and significantly reduce the chances of a second heart attack.

9. TRUE   Children from "high risk" families, in which a parent has high blood cholesterol (240 mg/dl or above) or in which a parent or grandparent has had heart disease at an early age (at 55 years of age or younger), should have their cholesterol levels tested. If a child from such a family has a cholesterol level that is high, it should be lowered under medical supervision, primarily with diet, to reduce the risk of developing heart disease as an adult. For most children, who are not from high-risk families, the best way to reduce the risk of adult heart disease is to follow a low-saturated fat, low cholesterol eating pattern. All children over the age of 2 years and all adults should adopt a heart-healthy eating pattern as a principal way of reducing coronary heart disease.

10. TRUE   Heavy smokers are two to four times more likely to have a heart attack than nonsmokers and the heart attack death rate among all smokers is 70% greater than that of nonsmokers. Older male smokers are also nearly twice as likely to die from stroke than older men who do not smoke and these odds are nearly as high for older female smokers. Further, the risk of dying of lung cancer is 22 times higher for male smokers than male nonsmokers and 12 times higher for female smokers than female nonsmokers. Finally, 80% of all deaths from emphysema and bronchitis are directly because smoking.

11. TRUE   One year after quitting, exsmokers cut their extra risk for heart attack by about half or more, and eventually the risk will return to normal in healthy exsmokers. Even if you have already had a heart attack, you can reduce your chances of having a second attack if you quit smoking. Exsmokers can also reduce their risk of stroke and cancer, improve blood flow and lung function, and help stop diseases like emphysema and bronchitis from getting worse.

12. FALSE   Older smokers are more likely to succeed at quitting smoking than younger smokers. Quitting helps relieve smoking-related symptoms like shortness of breath, coughing, and chest pain. Many quit to avoid further health problems and take control of their lives.

13. TRUE   Weight control is a question of balance. You get calories from the food you eat. You burn off calories by exercising. Cutting down on calories, especially calories from fat, is key to losing weight. Combining this with a regular physical activity, like walking, cycling, jogging, or swimming, not only can help in losing weight, but also in maintaining weight loss. A steady weight loss of 0.5 to 1 pound a week is safe for most adults and the weight is more likely to stay off over the long run. Losing weight, if you are overweight, may also help reduce your blood pressure, lower your LDL cholesterol, and raise your HDL cholesterol. Being physically active and eating fewer calories will also help you control your weight if you quit smoking.

14. TRUE   Coronary heart disease is the number one killer in the United States. Approximately 489,000 Americans died of coronary heart disease in 1990 and approximately half of these deaths were women.

From National Heart, Lung and Blood Institute. (1992). *Healthy Heart I. Q.* (NIH Publication No. 92-2724). Washington, DC: National Heart, Lung and Blood Institute.

Issues in Women's Health Care

Upon completion of this chapter, the reader will be able to:

1. Discuss issues related to family planning, including contraception options, treatment of infertility, preconception counseling, and prenatal care.

2. Describe the care of an infant focusing on nutrition (breastfeeding and bottle-feeding), sleeping positions and patterns, basics of bathing and cord care, dressing and diapering, and stooling and voiding patterns.

3. Explain the issue of teen pregnancy and suggest ways to decrease problems associated with it.

4. Discuss prevention efforts related to common women's health problems, including breast and gynecological cancers, osteoporosis, and domestic violence.

Assisted reproductive technology	Domestic violence	Osteoporosis
Breast cancer	Emergency contraception	Prenatal care
Breastfeeding	Family planning services	Teenage pregnancy
Contraception	Infant care	
	Infertility	*See Glossary for definitions.*

Lisa Lewis is a registered nurse (RN) practicing in a public-sponsored, comprehensive obstetrical and family clinic in an urban area. The clinic is staffed by physicians, gynecological nurse practitioners (NPs), certified nurse-midwives, RNs, and social workers. In her role, Lisa performs various services, including health teaching, obtaining health histories, taking vital signs (including fetal heart rate assessment and measuring fundal height), counseling, performing screenings and skilled tasks (e.g., injections, venipuncture), and assisting the primary care providers in other services (e.g., insertion of intrauterine devices [IUDs] and performance of Papanicolaou [Pap] smears, colposcopy, ultrasonography, and biopsies).

On a recent Friday, Lisa cared for Patty Smith, a 25-year-old mother of two who was being seen for her yearly gynecological examination and to discuss family planning options. Because Lisa completed Patty's health history, she learned that Patty's last Pap test was 2 years ago while she was pregnant with her second child. That Pap test and all previous tests have been normal. Since the birth of her last child, Patty reports that she and her husband have been using condoms and foam to prevent pregnancy, but she would like to explore other forms of contraception. Her vital signs were: blood pressure, 110/68; pulse, 76; and respirations, 16, and her weight was appropriate for her height. Patty stated that she smokes approximately one pack of cigarettes each day and has for the past 8 years (except during her pregnancies). She reports no serious health problems and states that both of her parents are living and in good health.

Lisa briefly explained the contraceptive options available, including the effectiveness and pros and cons of each. Lisa explained that because Patty smokes, hormonal contraceptives (e.g., birth control pills, medroxyprogesterone acetate [Depo-Provera] injections, and levonorgestrel implants [Norplant]) are contraindicated. Other options would be a diaphragm, IUD, cervical cap, or continuation with condoms and spermicidal preparations. Surgical sterilization for Patty or her husband was also discussed. Patty reported that she and her husband have not yet decided whether they want any more children, so sterilization was not considered. After learning about benefits and potential side effects of each of her options, Patty decided to be fitted for a diaphragm.

Lisa assisted the NP with the general physical examination, breast examination (including instruction on breast self-examination [BSE]), and Pap test. No abnormalities were noted. The NP carefully fitted Patty for a diaphragm and instructed her on how to insert it properly. The NP allowed Patty to practice insertion and removal several times and checked to ensure that Patty could perform the procedure properly. Lisa gave Patty several informational pamphlets on the diaphragm and reminded Patty of the necessity of using spermicidal jelly or cream with each act of intercourse.

Before leaving, Lisa informed Patty that she would receive the results of her Pap test in the mail in about 2 weeks. She was reminded to come back in 2 years if she did not have problems.

Nursing practice in community settings encompasses diverse areas of women's health, including family planning, pregnancy, childbearing and infant care, cancer detection, detection and prevention of domestic violence, and prevention of osteoporosis. *Healthy People 2010* (U.S. Department of Health and Human Services [USDHHS], 2000) lists several objectives related to women's health, including specific objectives to encourage breastfeeding, discourage smoking, reduce unplanned pregnancies, and improve access to prenatal care. Reducing domestic violence and complications arising from osteoporosis are also among the stated objectives. The *Healthy People 2010* table presents some examples of objectives related to women's health.

This chapter discusses a number of topics related to women's health. Presented here is information on family planning, including avail-able contraception options; women's health care (e.g., screening for reproductive diseases, breast care); prenatal care; infant care; and infertility. Finally, prevention and intervention in teenage pregnancy and domestic violence are discussed.

FAMILY PLANNING

Approximately one half (49%) of pregnancies in the United States are unintended (mistimed or unwanted). This is attributed to lack of knowledge, failure to translate knowledge into behavior, or lack of family planning services and information (USDHHS, 2000). **Family planning services** offer health and medical care and counseling that provide women with the information and care they need to make informed choices about whether and when to become parents. Comprehensive family planning includes con-

healthy people **2010**

Examples of Objectives for Family Planning, Maternal/Infant/Child Health, Domestic Violence, and Women's Health

OBJECTIVE	BASELINE (1998)	TARGET
Family Planning		
9.1: Increase the proportion of pregnancies that are intended	51%	70%
9.3: Increase the proportion of females at risk of unintended pregnancy (and their partners) who use contraception	93%	100%
9.7: Reduce pregnancies among adolescent females	72 pregnancies per per 1000 females 15-17 years	46 pregnancies per 1000 females 15-17 years
9.12: Reduce the proportion of married couples whose ability to conceive or maintain a pregnancy is impaired	13%	10%
Maternal/Infant/Child Health		
16.4: Reduce maternal deaths	8.4 per 100,000 live births	3.3 per 100,000 live births
16.5a: Reduce maternal complications during labor and delivery	32.1 per 100 deliveries	20 per 100 deliveries
16.6b: Increase the proportion of pregnant women who receive early and adequate prenatal care	83%	90%
16.9a: Reduce cesarean deliveries among low-risk women (no prior cesarean delivery)	17.8%	15.5%
16.11a: Reduce preterm births	11.4%	7.6%
16.13: Increase the percentage of healthy full-term infants who are put down to sleep on their backs	35%	70%
Intimate Partner Violence		
15.34: Reduce the rate of physical assault by current or former intimate partners	4.5 physical assaults per 1000 persons	3.6 physical assaults per 1000 persons
Women's Health		
2.9: Reduce the number of cases of osteoporosis	16% of females	8% of adults
3.3: Reduce breast cancer death rate	27.7 deaths per 100,000	22.2 deaths per 100,000
3.4: Reduce death rate from cervical cancer	3 deaths per 100,000	2 deaths per 100,000
3.11b: Increase the proportion of women 18 years of age and older who have received a PAP test within the preceding 3 years	79%	90%

From U.S. Department of Health and Human Services (USDHHS). (2000). *Healthy people 2010: Conference edition.* Washington, DC: Government Printing Office.

sideration of factors regarding childbearing, adoption, abstinence from sexual activity outside of a monogamous relationship, use of contraceptives, natural family planning, treatment of infertility, and preconception counseling (USDHHS, 1995).

Without effective contraception, 85% to 89% of couples who regularly engage in sexual intercourse will conceive within 1 year (USDHHS, 2000). As stated earlier, an estimated 49% of all pregnancies in the United States are unintended. Black women experience much higher rates of unplanned pregnancy, with 72% of their pregnancies being unplanned (USDHHS, 2000). Several suggestions have been made to reduce rates of unintended pregnancy. These include encouraging the postponement of sexual activity (particularly in adolescents) and providing health education to improve the understanding of fertility and to promote the appropriate use of available family planning options. Improved access to providers of family planning services is also essential.

Abstinence education has been promoted since the mid-1980s to help cut down on initiation of sexual activity among adolescents. The "Just Say 'No'" and related campaigns have been somewhat successful in abstinence education. According to the USDHHS (1995), the number of both adolescent males and females reporting that they have never engaged in sexual intercourse has increased slightly. Counselors and educators who work with adolescents and teenagers should continue to provide abstinence education and to help young people who choose abstinence sustain their choice. Use of educational materials, counseling, and peer group support should be encouraged.

CONTRACEPTION

At present, several methods are available to prevent pregnancy. Abstinence is the most effective means of avoiding unintended pregnancy and is certainly a key method of contraception for many (e.g., teenagers). Other methods of **contraception** include barriers (e.g., condoms, diaphragm), hormonal methods (e.g., oral contraceptives, Depo-Provera, Norplant), IUDs, sterilization, and natural family planning. These methods vary in effectiveness and each has positive and negative consequences. Table 11-1 compares available contraceptives.

Emergency Contraception

In 1997, the Food and Drug Administration (FDA) recommended approval of the use of high doses of standard birth control pills as postcoital contraception or "morning after pills." Depending on the stage in the woman's reproductive cycle, **emergency contraception** prevents pregnancy by prevention of ovulation or prevention of fertilization of the egg or transportation of the egg to the uterus. Additionally, it may render the uterine lining unfavorable to implantation (Jaroff, 1996; USDHHS/Office of Disease Prevention and Health Promotion [ODPHP], 1998).

For emergency contraception, the recommended dose is two to four oral contraceptive pills (depending on the brand) taken up to 72 hours after sex, followed by a repeat of the same dose 12 hours later. If initiated within 72 hours following intercourse, this regimen reduces the risk of pregnancy by 55% to 95% (USDHHS/ODPHP, 1998). Nausea and vomiting are the most common side effects.

PRENATAL CARE

A country's infant mortality rates and maternal mortality rates are often cited as an indicator of the overall health of the country and the efficacy of its health care system. Although U.S. infant and maternal mortality rates have improved during the past several decades, the United States ranks an astonishingly poor twenty-fifth among industrialized countries (USDHHS, 2000).

In 1997, the overall infant mortality rate in the United States was 7.2 per 1000, which although relatively high, demonstrates steady improvement over the past several decades. The infant mortality rate for black infants, however, remains problematic because it is more than double the rate for white infants (Jonas, 1999; USDHHS, 2000). The higher rate for black infants has long been attributed to lack of access to health care, poverty, teen pregnancy, and several other factors. Indeed, black babies have twice the risk of having a low birth weight (LBW) as do white babies. In 1997, 13% of black infants were born with LBW compared with 6.5% of white infants (USDHHS, 2000). Risk factors associated with LBW are younger or older maternal age, high parity, poor reproductive history, low socioeconomic status, low level of education, late entry into prenatal

TABLE **11-1** Methods of Contraception—Effectiveness, Risks, Benefits, Convenience, and Availability

METHOD	EFFECTIVENESS (TYPICAL USE)	POTENTIAL COMPLICATIONS AND SIDE EFFECTS	POTENTIAL BENEFITS	CONVENIENCE/USE	AVAILABILITY AND COST
Oral contraceptive pills	97-99%	*Side effects:* water retention, nausea, headaches, spotting, missed periods, breast tenderness, depression, mood changes *Complications:* blood clots, heart attack, stroke (associated with smoking), hypertension, gallbladder disease, liver tumors; may increase risk of ovarian tumors	May reduce volume and pain associated with menstruation; periods are regular; may protect women from cancer of the ovary and endometrium and benign breast disease; protects against anemia and ectopic pregnancy	Must be taken daily; effectiveness declines when pills are missed	Prescription required; costs vary depending on source—retail, approximately $20 per month
Condom	85-88%	Decreases sensation, loss of spontaneity; a few people are allergic to latex or to spermicide; condoms may break	Helps protect both partners against transmission of STDs and HIV if used properly	Must be put onto the erect penis before the penis comes into contact with the vagina; use a new condom for each act of intercourse	Easy availability; minimal costs
IUD	94-98%	*Side effects:* cramping, bleeding, anemia *Complications:* pelvic inflammatory disease, infertility, perforation of the uterus (rare)	IUDs with progestin decrease menstrual cramping in some users	Requires no preparation for intercourse; at least once a month (usually after menstruation), user must check in vagina for strings to ensure IUD is in place	Requires insertion by a trained health professional
Implant (Norplant)	99%	*Side effects:* menstrual irregularity, headaches, nervousness, depression, nausea, dizziness, breast	May decrease menstrual cramps, pain, and blood loss	Effective 24 hours after implantation; effectiveness	Requires a prescription and a minor outpatient surgical procedure

Method	Effectiveness	Side Effects/Complications	Benefits	Directions	Availability
		tenderness, weight gain, enlargement of ovaries and/or fallopian tubes, excessive growth of body and facial hair; (side effects may decrease after first year) *Complications:* infection at insertion site			lasts approximately 5 years; can be removed by a trained health care professional at any time
Injectables (Depo-Provera)	99%	*Side effects:* amenorrhea, weight gain, headaches, and others (similar to with implant)	May be used when lactating; may have protective effects against endometrial cancer	Effective almost immediately; require no preparation for intercourse	Requires prescription; one injection every 3 months
Barriers (diaphragms, cervical caps, sponges)	82% for women who have never had a baby; 64% for women who have borne children	*Side effects:* cervical, vaginal irritation; pelvic pressure; vaginal discharge if left in too long; difficulty in removal *Complications:* cervical, vaginal, or bladder infection; toxic shock syndrome (very rare)	Provides some protection against STDs	Require preparation to insert devices before intercourse (diaphragm and cervical cap, up to 6 hours before intercourse; sponge up to 24 hours before intercourse); should be left in place for 6-8 (but not more than 24) hours after intercourse; should not be used by women who have recently given birth	Diaphragm and cervical cap require a prescription and fitting by a trained health care provider; sponge is available without prescription
Periodic abstinence (natural family planning)	Very variable 53-86%	None	Careful monitoring can help determine timing for a planned pregnancy; requires no drugs or devices	Requires frequent monitoring of body functions and periods of abstinence	No prescription; obtain instructions from a trained health care provider; basal

Data from Goldberg, M. S. (1994). *Choosing a contraceptive. Current issues in women's health* (2nd ed.). Washington, DC: Food and Drug Administration; U.S. Department of Health and Human Services (USDHHS). (1989). *Your contraceptive choices for now, for later.* Bethesda, MD: U.S. Department of Health and Human Services; and U.S. Department of Health and Human Services (USDHHS). (1994). *Clinician's handbook of preventive services.* Washington, DC: Government Printing Office.

HIV, Human immunodeficiency virus; *IUD,* intrauterine device; *STD,* sexually transmitted disease.

TABLE 11-1 Methods of Contraception—Effectiveness, Risks, Benefits, Convenience, and Availability—cont'd

METHOD	EFFECTIVENESS (TYPICAL USE)	POTENTIAL COMPLICATIONS AND SIDE EFFECTS	POTENTIAL BENEFITS	CONVENIENCE/USE	AVAILABILITY AND COST
					thermometers and charts available at drugstores and family planning clinics
Spermicides (foam, gel, cream)	70-80%	*Side effects:* allergic reaction	Provides some protection against STDs	Must be inserted immediately before intercourse; some find the products messy; no douching for 6-8 hours after intercourse	No prescription necessary; relatively inexpensive
Sterilization	99+%	*Side effects:* pain at surgical site, psychological reactions *Complications:* infection, regret that the procedure was performed	No interference with sex drive or sexual functioning	Must be certain there is no desire for future pregnancies; surgery must be done by a trained doctor and must follow postsurgery instructions; men must return for sperm checks until all sperm have been cleared from the system	Vasectomy: minor surgical procedure for men; usually performed in a physician's office under local anesthesia; tubal ligation: minor procedure for women, under general anesthesia (fairly expensive); most health insurance plans cover sterilization
Abstinence	100%	None	Prevention of STDs and HIV; avoids drugs and devices; safest method of contraception	May be hard to avoid pressure to have intercourse	Prepare responses; talk about decision with partner

care, low pregnancy weight gain, and smoking and other substance abuse.

Prenatal care is particularly important for women at increased medical and/or social risk. Prenatal care dramatically reduces the likelihood of having a baby with LBW; an expectant mother with no prenatal care is three times more likely to have a baby with LBW than an expectant mother who begins prenatal care during the first trimester (USDHHS, 2000). Despite this, nearly one fourth of all pregnant women do not receive early and adequate prenatal care. Most of the women who receive delayed or no prenatal care are poor, lack a high school education, or are very young. Box 11-1 outlines barriers to prenatal care.

In addition to LBW, lack of prenatal care has been associated with prematurity, maternal complications, and infant mortality (USDHHS, 2000). Comprehensive and early prenatal care reduces rates of infant death and LBW. Improving prenatal care beginning in the first trimester of pregnancy is one of the objectives cited in *Healthy People 2010*. This can best be accomplished through removing or lessening barriers.

To reduce the incidence of infants with LBW and other complications, prenatal care should include (Sherwen, Scoloveno, and Weingarten, 1995):

1. Initial and ongoing risk assessment
2. Individualized care based on case management principles

BOX 11-1 Barriers to Use of Prenatal Care

I. SOCIODEMOGRAPHIC

Poverty
Residence: inner city or rural
Minority status
Age: <18 or >39
High parity
Non-English speaking
Unmarried
Less than high school education

II. SYSTEM-RELATED

Inadequacies in private insurance policies (waiting periods, coverage limitations, coinsurance and deductibles, requirements for up-front payments)
Absence of either Medicaid or private insurance coverage of maternity services
Inadequate or no maternity care providers for Medicaid-enrolled, uninsured, and other low-income women (long wait to get appointment)
Complicated, time-consuming process to enroll in Medicaid
Availability of Medicaid poorly advertised
Inadequate transportation services, long travel time to service sites, or both
Difficulty obtaining childcare
Weak links between prenatal services and pregnancy testing
Inadequate coordination among such services as Women, Infants, and Children (WIC) and prenatal care

Inconvenient clinic hours, especially for working women
Long waits to see physician
Language and cultural incompatibility between providers and clients
Poor communication between clients and providers exacerbated by short interactions with providers
Negative attributes of clinics, including rude personnel, uncomfortable surroundings, and complicated registration procedures
Limited information on exactly where to get care (phone numbers and addresses)

III. ATTITUDINAL

Pregnancy unplanned, viewed negatively, or both
Ambivalence
Signs of pregnancy not known or recognized
Prenatal care not valued or understood
Fear of doctors, hospitals, procedures
Fear of parental discovery
Fear of deportation or problems with the Immigration and Naturalization Service
Fear that certain health habits will be discovered and criticized (smoking, eating disorders, drug or alcohol abuse)
Selected lifestyles (drug abuse, homelessness)
Inadequate social supports and personal resources
Excessive stress
Denial or apathy
Concealment

Reproduced with the permission of The Alan Guttmacher Institute from Brown, S. S. (1989). Drawing women into prenatal care. *Family Planning Perspectives, 21*(2), 73-78, Table 4.

3. Nutritional counseling
4. Education to reduce or eliminate unhealthy habits
5. Stress reduction
6. Social support services
7. Health education

These are discussed briefly in the following sections.

RISK IDENTIFICATION AND CASE MANAGEMENT

Routine health care visits should monitor normal progression of the pregnancy (Figure 11-1). This would include assessment of fetal growth and development (e.g., measurement of fundal height, listening to fetal heart tones, assessing fetal movement); of maternal response to the pregnancy; and of possible complications such as hypertension, gestational diabetes, or multiple fetuses. Identification of risk factors and developing and implementing interventions to eliminate, reduce, or manage the risk factors is essential in producing good pregnancy outcomes. To help nurses who work with women of childbearing age identify women at risk, Box 11-2 lists some factors that contribute to high-risk pregnancy.

Once a possible risk or complication has been identified, a comprehensive plan of care should be outlined to monitor and minimize risks. This plan or program may include detailed case man-

agement if the risk factors are significant. For example, if gestational diabetes is diagnosed, the pregnant woman should receive comprehensive education on this condition and receive ongoing monitoring and intervention as indicated. Likewise, if other complications, such as pregnancy-induced hypertension, multifetal pregnancy, or preexisting maternal health problems dictate the need, a case management plan should be implemented. For pregnant teenagers, a structured case management program should be encouraged to help minimize the risks associated with teenage pregnancy. These are described later in this chapter.

NUTRITION COUNSELING

Maintenance of good nutrition during pregnancy is vital to the health of both the mother and developing baby. In general, pregnant women need to increase their caloric intake by about 15% above their normal intake. Basic recommendations include four servings of dairy products, four servings of meat or other protein source, six or more servings of breads and cereals, one serving of dark green or orange/yellow vegetables, two or more servings of other vegetables, and at least one serving of fruit high in vitamin C. Of particular concern in pregnant women is ensuring adequate iron and folic acid (see the Community Application "Folic Acid Recommendations"). To obtain sufficient vitamins and minerals, most pregnant women are encouraged to take a multivitamin/multimineral supplement.

Iron supplementation is recommended for virtually all pregnant women. According to Boyne (1995), "iron is the one nutrient that cannot be obtained in adequate amounts from dietary sources during pregnancy" (p. 183). Iron is needed to promote fetal and placental growth, increase maternal red blood cell mass, and compensate for basal losses. However, the use of iron supplements may produce unwanted side effects and abdominal discomfort and constipation are the most common. Nurses who care for pregnant women should counsel them on minimizing these side effects. Suggestions may

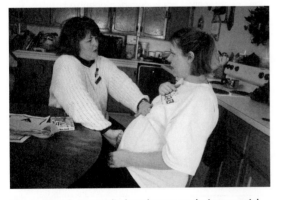

Figure 11-1 A community-based nurse conducts a prenatal evaluation during a home visit. (Courtesy of Caroline E. Brown.)

BOX 11-2 Factors Associated with High-Risk Pregnancy

I. Demographic Factors
   a. Lower socioeconomic status
   b. Disadvantaged ethnic groups
   c. Marital status: unwed mothers
   d. Maternal age
      1. Gravida less than 16 years of age
      2. Primigravida 35 years of age or older
      3. Gravida 40 years of age or older
   e. Maternal weight: nonpregnant weight less than 100 pounds or more than 200 pounds
   f. Stature: height less than 62 inches (1.57 m)
   g. Malnutrition
   h. Poor physical fitness

II. Past Pregnancy History
   a. Grand multiparity: six previous pregnancies terminating beyond 20 weeks of gestation
   b. Antepartum bleeding after 12 weeks of gestation
   c. Premature rupture of membranes, premature onset of labor, premature delivery
   d. Previous cesarean section or mid- or high-forceps delivery
   e. Prolonged labor
   f. Infant with cerebral palsy, mental retardation, birth trauma, central nervous system disorder, or congenital anomaly
   g. Reproductive failure: infertility, repetitive abortion, fetal loss, stillbirth, or neonatal death
   h. Delivery of preterm (less than 37 weeks) or post-term (more than 42 weeks) infant

III. Past or Present Medical History
   a. Hypertension or renal disease or both
   b. Diabetes mellitus (overt or gestational)
   c. Cardiovascular disease (rheumatic, congenital, or peripheral vascular)
   d. Pulmonary disease producing hypoxemia and hypercapnia
   e. Thyroid, parathyroid, and endocrine disorders
   f. Idiopathic thrombocytopenic purpura
   g. Neoplastic disease
   h. Hereditary disorders
   i. Collagen diseases
   j. Epilepsy

IV. Additional Obstetrical and Medical Conditions
   a. Toxemia
   b. Asymptomatic bacteriuria
   c. Anemia or hemoglobinopathy
   d. Rh sensitization
   e. Habitual smoking
   f. Drug addiction or habituation
   g. Chronic exposure to any pharmacological or chemical agent
   h. Multiple pregnancy
   i. Rubella or other viral infection
   j. Intercurrent surgery and anesthesia
   k. Placental abnormalities and uterine bleeding
   l. Abnormal fetal lie or presentation, fetal anomalies, oligohydramnios, polyhydramnios
   m. Abnormalities of fetal or uterine growth or both
   n. Maternal trauma during pregnancy
   o. Maternal emotional crisis during pregnancy

Adapted from Clemen-Stone, S., Eigsti, D. G., & McGuire, S. L. (1995). *Comprehensive community health nursing* (4th ed.). St. Louis: Mosby; data from Vaughn, V. C., McKay, R. J., & Behrman R. E. (Eds.), and Nelson, W. E. (Senior Ed.), (1979). *Textbook of pediatrics* (11th ed.). Philadelphia: W. B. Saunders.

COMMUNITY APPLICATION
Folic Acid Recommendations

For almost 10 years, the Centers for Disease Control and Prevention (CDC) and the U.S. Public Health Service (USPHS) have recommended that all women of childbearing age consume 400 µg of folic acid each day to decrease the risk of neural tube defects (NTDs) such as spina bifida and anencephaly. In 1996, the FDA authorized the addition of folic acid to enriched grain products; this became mandatory in 1998. Fortification of grain products is estimated to provide an additional 100 µg of folic acid to the diet of reproductive-aged women.

Recently, the CDC reported that since folic acid fortification became common in the U.S. food supply, NTDs have decreased by 19%. As a result, according to the researcher's report, about 800 more healthy babies are born in the United States each year.

From Centers for Disease Control and Prevention (CDC). (2001). *Neural tube birth defects down by 19% since food fortification.* Retrieved 07/24/01 from www.cdc.gov/od/oc/media/pressrel/r010619.htm.

include taking the supplements at bedtime to decrease nausea, increasing fluids and daily exercise, and eating high-fiber foods to reduce constipation.

Research has shown that folic acid is essential to the developing baby and that supplementation is effective in reducing fetal abnormalities, particularly NTDs. Consequently, the benefits of ensuring adequate dietary intake of folic acid should be presented to all women, even before pregnancy. All women of childbearing age should maintain a daily intake of 0.4 mg of folic acid. This may be obtained through the diet or through supplementation. In addition to vitamin and mineral supplements, foods high in folic acid include dark green leafy vegetables (e.g., broccoli, spinach), oranges, bananas, whole wheat products, liver, black beans, pinto beans, peanuts, potatoes, and fortified breads and cereals. Pregnant women should be encouraged to eat these foods in addition to taking their daily vitamins.

Weight gain during pregnancy and the birth weight of the infant are strongly correlated and low maternal weight gain is a risk factor for having an infant with LBW. An estimated one third of all mothers gain inadequate weight during their pregnancies, a complication particularly common in teenagers and black women (USDHHS, 2000). Because of this, pregnant women should be taught the importance of sufficient weight gain. Weight gain should be measured with each prenatal visit and monitored closely for signs that might indicate complications (e.g., sudden weight gain suggestive of pregnancy-induced hypertension or failure to gain) (Boyne, 1995).

General recommendations on total weight gain for pregnant women are 25 to 35 pounds for women whose prepregnancy weight is low to normal for height and 15 to 25 pounds for women whose weight for height is high or who are obese. The rate of weight gain should be 2 to 4 pounds during the first trimester and about 0.8 pounds per week thereafter (Moore, 2000).

ELIMINATION OF UNHEALTHY HABITS

The detrimental effects of smoking, alcohol consumption, and use of recreational drugs on the developing fetus have been definitively established. Smoking alone is associated with 20% to 30% of all LBW births in the United States (USDHHS, 2000). In addition to LBW, smoking during pregnancy is associated with delayed neurological and intellectual development, spontaneous abortion, premature rupture of membranes, placenta previa, abruptio placentae, bacterial infection, and infant mortality (Saunders, 2000; Sherwen et al., 1995). Therefore maternal smoking should be strongly discouraged throughout pregnancy.

Consumption of alcohol is known to cause defects in developing infants. One of the most serious complications of alcohol use during pregnancy is fetal alcohol syndrome, which is characterized by growth retardation, facial malformations, and central nervous system dysfunction (USDHHS, 2000). Even as little as two drinks per day is associated with developmental delays. As a result, it is recommended that women consume no alcohol during pregnancy.

Recreational or illegal drug use during pregnancy can cause a number of problems for the infant and the mother. The potential effects depend on the substance used and the amount. In general, illicit drug use may cause growth retardation, withdrawal symptoms, and physical anomalies (Sherwen et al., 1995). In addition, maternal use of intravenous drugs is associated with human immunodeficiency virus (HIV) infection, which may, in turn, be transmitted to the developing fetus. To eliminate these potential problems, all women who are planning on becoming pregnant or who are pregnant should be counseled to avoid illicit drug use before and during pregnancy. Furthermore, testing for HIV is now recommended for all pregnant women.

The effect of caffeine on the developing baby has not been determined. Heavy maternal caffeine consumption may be associated with intrauterine growth retardation. Therefore pregnant women should be encouraged to limit their intake of caffeine (Saunders, 2000; Sherwen et al., 1995).

STRESS REDUCTION

Pregnancy and childbirth are stressful for all concerned because the expectant mother and father must face new experiences and pressures that may produce anxiety. Stress is often higher near the end of pregnancy and many pregnancy-related concerns are shared with the nurse during the third trimester. Fear of childbirth; effects of birth on the baby, finances, and family; future pregnancies; negative self-concept; previous loss of a fetus; terminating work; major life changes; and apprehension about pain in labor and delivery are common concerns. Other stressors more commonly seen in multiparous women include increased fears for the unborn baby with each successive pregnancy, stress from too much company or interfering relatives, concerns about weight reduction following delivery, concern about housework and family routines, fatigue during the postpartum period, increased depression, fear of not having enough time for self and others, disillusionment with parenting and child care, and concern about her own emotional ability to meet the needs of all family members (Sherwen et al., 1995).

Nurses who work with pregnant women and their families should be alert to signs and comments indicating increased stress. Adaptive changes related to the pregnancy and impending birth can be promoted. To this end, the nurse should provide information on childbirth and referral to prepared childbirth classes and provide literature on recognizing and managing postpartum depression and other potential problems. Encouraging healthful behaviors, such as getting adequate rest and good nutrition, can help reduce stress. A referral to a psychologist, counselor, or social worker might be necessary to assist with more serious problems (e.g., depression, financial difficulties, or abuse). Nurses should be prepared in advance to provide these referrals by maintaining a list of providers, with their addresses and telephone numbers.

SOCIAL SUPPORT SERVICES

Serving as an advocate and referral source for social programs for eligible mothers and children is one of the most important roles of nurses in community-based practice. Almost 40% of expectant mothers are eligible for at least one social program such as WIC, Medicaid, Aid to Families with Dependent Children, and food stamps. Nurses caring for expectant mothers and infants should be aware of social programs in the area for pregnant clients and be prepared to refer those who might need social services.

HEALTH EDUCATION

General health education for pregnant women includes providing anticipatory guidance and health teaching about the normal course of pregnancy, labor and delivery, and the postpartum period. Management of common discomforts associated with pregnancy (e.g., nausea and vomiting, constipation, heartburn, urinary frequency, sleep pattern disturbances) should be discussed. The pregnant woman should be encouraged to get adequate rest and regular exercise. Preparation for labor and delivery should include several discussions on signs and symptoms indicating that labor has begun and when to go to the hospital or birthing center for delivery. Finally, signs and symptoms of possible complications (e.g., vaginal bleeding, abdominal cramping, severe headache) should be described and the mother-to-be should know when to call her physician or clinic and when to seek emergency care.

PRENATAL SCREENING

The U.S. Preventative Services Task Force has developed specific guidelines for periodic health examinations for pregnant women.

TABLE **11-2** Preventative Services Task Force Risk Factors Screening, Referral, and Service for Pregnant Women

RISK FACTOR OR GROUP	PREVENTION TARGET CONDITION	PREVENTION SERVICE AND/OR REFERRAL
All pregnant women	Asymptomatic bacteriuria, pyelonephritis	Urinalysis and culture
	Anemia	CBC
	Rh incompatibility	Blood typing and antibody testing
	Preeclampsia	Periodic blood pressure measurement
	Domestic violence	Direct questioning about abuse, using screening instrument; referral for counseling; referral to crisis center, shelter, and social services; notify protective authorities
	Problems related to substance abuse including alcohol, tobacco, and illicit drugs	Screen for use and counsel regarding personal hazards, effects on fetus, and potential to transmit drugs through breast milk
	Nutritional and immunological deficiencies	Counsel regarding adequate calcium intake and breast feeding
	Vertical transmission of hepatitis B and HIV	Hepatitis B surface antigen and HIV serology
	Obstetric complications related to STDs	STD/HIV screening and counseling
	Hemoglobinopathy	Hemoglobin electrophoresis and counseling
Periconception period with prior pregnancy affected by NTD	NTD	Referral for amniocentesis with alpha-fetoprotein measurement; folic acid supplementation
Pregnant women <35 years of age with no prior pregnancy affected with Down syndrome	Down syndrome	Serum multiple-marker screening and counseling
Pregnant women >35 years of age or prior pregnancy affected with Down syndrome	Down syndrome	Referral for amniocentesis or chorionic villus sampling or multiple-marker screening and counseling
Pregnant women >35 years of age, with obesity or glucosuria on screening urinalysis	Gestational diabetes, fetal macrosomia, birth trauma	Glucose tolerance test
Postpartum period	Thyroid dysfunction	Thyroid screening

From U.S. Department of Health and Human Services/Office of Disease Prevention and Health Promotion (USDHHS/ODPHP). (1998). *Clinician's handbook of preventive services* (2nd ed.). McLean, VA: International Medical Publishing.

These recommendations are summarized in Table 11-2. In addition, prenatal screening and counseling for prenatal detection of fetal abnormalities is sometimes warranted. These screenings allow for initiation of interventions to ameliorate the consequences of disorders through counseling and specialized obstetrical and neonatal care (USDHHS, 1990). Table 11-3 lists some prenatal screening and diagnostic tests.

TABLE **11-3** Types of Prenatal Genetic Testing

TEST	PURPOSE	ADVANTAGES	DISADVANTAGES	RISKS
Maternal serum alpha-fetoprotein (MS-AFP)	Screening test for NTDs, ventral wall defects	Identifies women at higher risk for further testing who would not otherwise receive it	Is not diagnostic; only indicates need for further testing	Venipuncture Minimal risk
Ultrasonography	Assesses gestational age, fetal growth, placental sufficiency Detects multiple gestation and structural anomalies Screening and diagnostic test	Detects structural anomalies and effects of intrauterine environment that may not be detected by chromosome analysis	Accuracy depends on skill of ultra-sonographer, quality of equipment, and size of defect	Noninvasive
Amniocentesis	Chromosome analysis of fetal cells DNA analysis AFP analysis, other biochemical analyses	Diagnostic for chromosome abnormalities Provides DNA for direct and indirect testing for single-gene disorder High accuracy for detection of NTDs by biochemical analysis	Does not detect structural anomalies not caused by chromosome abnormalities except for neural tube or ventral wall defects Usually not performed until second trimester (14-16 wk) Results are usually available in 2-3 wk Relatively expensive	Invasive 0.5% risk of spontaneous abortion Nongrowth of fetal cells requires repeat procedure
Chorionic villus sampling (CVS)	Chromosome analysis of chorionic (fetal) cells DNA analysis	Diagnostic for chromosome abnormalities Provides DNA for direct and indirect testing for single-gene disorders Test is done earlier than amniocentesis (9-12 wk); therefore results are available earlier	Diagnostic accuracy may be less because of greater risk of maternal cell contamination and false evidence of mosaicism, which may require subsequent amniocentesis	Invasive Risk of spontaneous abortion about 2% Controversial evidence of limb-reduction defects

From Wong, D. L. (1995). *Whaley & Wong's nursing care of infants and children* (5th ed.). St. Louis: Mosby.

INFANT CARE

Caring for a newborn can be a very frightening and confusing experience for new parents. Nurses who work in community settings, such as pediatric clinics, are often in a position to teach parents about **infant care**, including feeding, bathing, cord care, stooling and voiding patterns, dressing and diapering, sleeping, and observing for problems. These issues are described briefly in the following sections.

INFANT NUTRITION

Nutrition education for new parents should begin during the prenatal period and include information on the choice of breastfeeding versus bottle-feeding. Basic information on both forms of infant feeding is provided and infant feeding is also discussed in Chapter 9.

Breastfeeding

Breastfeeding is the recommended sole form of feeding for the first 5 to 6 months and should be encouraged by all health care providers. Indeed, one of the objectives of *Healthy People 2010* is to encourage breastfeeding in the early postpartum period. Women most likely to breastfeed their infants are mothers who are older, well educated, relatively affluent, and/or who live in the western United States. Those least likely to breastfeed are women who are low income, black, younger (younger than 20 years), and/or who live in the southeastern United States (USDHHS, 2000). Several barriers to breastfeeding have been identified. One barrier is the high number of women in the workforce who must leave their infants for extended periods each day, making breastfeeding more difficult. Likewise, teenage mothers (who rarely breastfeed their infants) who continue schooling are not usually able to nurse their infants during the day. Cultural and social preferences and acceptance that bottle-feeding is the norm also reduce breastfeeding rates.

Health care providers should instruct all pregnant women on the benefits and advantages of breastfeeding. For example, breastfeeding is more economical and convenient and provides a number of health benefits to both mother and infant. Breast milk is the ideal food for infants, supplying all nutrient needs, and immunological enhancement is a very important benefit for the baby. Furthermore, breastfeeding has psychological benefits of enhancing bonding between the infant and mother during feeding (Wong, 1999).

However, breastfeeding should be discouraged in a few cases. Breastfeeding is contraindicated for women who use illegal drugs (e.g., cocaine, marijuana), have untreated tuberculosis, or are taking certain medications or chemotherapy. Also, women who are HIV positive should not breastfeed their babies (USDHHS, 2000).

Although breastfeeding is natural and relatively simple, women who plan on breastfeeding their infants need both instruction and support. Ideally, instruction and support begin during the prenatal period and continue throughout the time the mother nurses the baby. Numerous booklets and pamphlets supporting breastfeeding and providing instruction are available and should be given to the mother-to-be during early prenatal visits. The Health Teaching box "Guidelines for Breastfeeding" presents general breastfeeding procedures. Women who desire more information or who are experiencing problems should be referred to local, regional, or national support groups or organizations for more assistance (see the Resources box at the end of the chapter).

Bottle-Feeding

If the mother chooses to bottle-feed her baby, she will need information on selection of a formula and instruction on formula preparation and cleaning of equipment. Commercial infant formulas are available in ready-to-use cans or bottles, concentrated liquid form that is to be diluted with an equal amount of water, and powdered form that must be prepared according to the manufacturer's directions.

For infants with no special nutritional requirements, modified cow's milk-based formulas (e.g.,

health teaching

Guidelines for Breastfeeding

1. Wash hands. Wash nipples with warm water, no soap.
2. There are three basic positions:
   a. The cradle position is achieved by cradling the infant in one arm, head resting in the bend of the elbows. The infant's lower arm is tucked out of the way and the infant's mouth is close to the breast. The mother can be sitting up in bed with pillows supporting the back or sitting in a chair.
   b. The lying down position is attained by having the mother lie on her side in bed with the infant lying on his or her side also.
   c. A pillow is needed to be successful with the football hold. The mother is seated in a chair and a pillow placed next to her on the nursing side. The pillow supports the elbow and the infant's buttocks, and should bring the infant's head up to the level of the breast.
3. Stroke the infant's cheek with the nipple.
4. The infant's mouth should be opened wide, as with a yawn, and should cover the entire areola or a large amount of the areola. If necessary, apply pressure to the infant's chin with your

index finger to open the infant's mouth more widely. The breast needs to be placed far back into the infant's mouth to drain the breast adequately. Your hand position is important. Hold your hand in a "C" position around your breast with the thumb on top behind the areola and the fingers against the chest wall, supporting the underside of the breast.

5. Both breasts are used—the first breast for about 10 minutes, the other breast for about 6 minutes. At the next feeding, the infant starts to feed on the breast used to finish the preceding feeding.
6. Retract breast tissue from the infant's nose during sucking. Break suction by placing a finger in a corner of the infant's mouth.
7. The neonate is nursed shortly after birth and approximately every 2 to 3 hours thereafter.
8. Infants should be burped after each breast and at the end of the feeding.
9. Nipples often become tender during the first week of nursing, but should not become sore. Soreness and prolonged feedings are most often the result of a baby who is not latched onto the breast properly.

From Ashwill, J. W., & Droske, S. C. (1997). *Nursing care of children: Principles and practice.* Philadelphia: W. B. Saunders.

Enfamil, Similac) may be used. These are available both fortified with iron and without extra iron. Soy protein formulas (e.g., Prosobee, Isomil, Nursoy) are used for infants who are sensitive to milk protein or who are lactose intolerant. Hydrolysate formulas (e.g., Portagen, Ross Carbohydrate Free, Alimentum) are available for infants with malabsorption syndromes or milk allergy. Other special formulas are available for children who have special nutritional needs (e.g., to reduce sodium intake or to increase calories, protein, fat, or calcium) and for infants with phenylketonuria (Wong, 1999). In addition to selection of formula, parents who choose to bottle-feed their infants need instruction on formula preparation, washing the bottles, and techniques for feeding. See the Health Teaching box "Guidelines for Bottle-Feeding."

SLEEPING

The positioning of infants for sleep is very important because sleeping in a prone position has been associated with sudden infant death syndrome (SIDS). In 1992, the American Academy of Pediatrics recommended that almost all infants up to 6 months of age sleep on their sides or backs (exceptions are infants with gastroesophageal reflux, premature infants with respiratory distress, and some infants with upper airway problems) (Wong, 1999). Placing the infant on a firm mattress, rather than on a pillow or soft bedding, is also suggested. Widespread adherence to these recommendations has resulted in a reported 30% decrease in SIDS during the past few years. All parents should be informed of these recommendations and taught to position infants on their sides or

---

health teaching

Guidelines for Bottle-Feeding

SUPPLIES

- Six bottles and 12 nipples. The type does not matter, but all should be the same to avoid frustrating the infant.
- Bottle brush (used to reach all crevices).
- Dishwasher basket (for securing the pieces in the dishwasher).

PREPARATION

- Use commercial formula rather than cow, goat, or soy milk. These types of milk lack the nutrients necessary for growth.
- Do not use raw or unpasteurized milk. This type of milk contains bacteria that can make the infant ill.
- Tap water does not need to be boiled before it is mixed with formula. Boiling can concentrate the minerals that are found in the water supply.
- If well water is used to mix formula, it should be checked for safety before use.
- Formula does not need to be sterilized. It is sterilized during the manufacturing process. It needs to be refrigerated.
- It is not necessary to heat bottles before feeding them to the infant.
- Bottles should never be heated in a microwave oven. Hot spots can occur in the formula and cause burns. Heating also changes the nutritional composition of the formula.

FEEDING

- Hold the infant close, with the head elevated.
- A quivering motion during sucking indicates that the nipple has collapsed. Remove the bottle from the infant's mouth to break the vacuum.
- Low flow despite vigorous sucking indicates that the nipple opening is clogged or the screw cap is too tight. Loosen the cap and see if the flow improves. If not, inspect the nipple opening.
- Do not prop the bottle or put the infant to bed with a bottle in his or her mouth. Bottle propping prevents close contact and increases chances of aspiration and middle ear infections. These practices also allow sugar to accumulate around the teeth and may lead to milk bottle caries.

STORING INFANT FORMULA

- Unopened formula should be stored in a cool, dry place and used before the expiration date printed on the can.
- Refrigerate opened cans of formula. If unrefrigerated formula is not used within 2 hours, discard it.
- Opened cans of formula (ready-to-feed or concentrate) should be used within 24 hours.
- Do not save the remainder of a bottle for later. Formula becomes contaminated with bacteria from the infant's mouth and using it later could lead to illness.
- Formula should not be frozen.

From Ashwill, J. W., & Droske, S. C. (1997). *Nursing care of children: Principles and practice.* Philadelphia: W. B. Saunders; data from Heslin, J. A. (1988). *No-nonsense nutrition for your baby's first year.* Englewood Cliffs, NJ: Prentice-Hall; and Heslin, J. (1992). *If you bottlefeed. American Baby, 54*(5), B10-B14.

---

back, rather than prone, and to avoid overly soft bedding.

Choice of the infant's bed or crib is also very important to ensure safety. Federal regulations require that there should be no more than $2\frac{3}{8}$ inches between the slats on infant beds and no slats should be missing. Mattresses and bumper pads should fit snugly against the slats, so that the infant cannot fall between the mattress and the side of the bed. The crib should not be placed near a window where the child could reach cords for blinds or drapes and so the bed is free of drafts. Finally, plastic bags or plastic covering should not be used as mattress protectors. If a mattress protector is desired, parents should purchase zip-on covers specifically designed for crib mattresses (Jackson and Saunders, 1994).

BATHING AND CORD CARE

Care of the umbilical cord frequently concerns new parents. In anticipation of these concerns, parents should be taught that the umbilical stump

health teaching

Bathing a Newborn

- Parents should be taught to assemble all necessary items before beginning the bath (e.g., soap, shampoo, washcloth, towel).
- The infant's, eyes are washed with a washcloth and clear water from the inner to outer corner, using a different part of the washcloth for each eye.
- The face, including the nose and ears, is then washed with clear water.
- The scalp and hair is cleansed with water or shampooed with mild shampoo and rinsed with warm water. The hair is then towel dried.
- The shirt can then be removed and the folds of the neck, the arms, axillae, chest, back, and abdomen may be washed with mild soap, then rinsed and dried. Careful attention should be made to keep the cord area dry.
- The upper part of the baby can be wrapped in the towel to prevent chilling and the legs and feet are unwrapped and washed with mild soap and water and dried thoroughly.

- The genitalia and buttocks are washed last. The female genitalia are cleansed from front to back to avoid contamination of the urethra and vagina with fecal material. The scrotum and the penis in the boy are washed with soap and water. The foreskin on uncircumcised boys does not need to be retracted. If the male infant is circumcised, the penis should also be washed gently with soap and water and dried. Observation for signs of infection is important.
- Unscented lotions, vitamin A and D ointment, and petroleum jelly may be used to help prevent or heal skin irritations.
- Powders and oils are not recommended because oils may clog the pores, and the neonate may inhale powders, causing respiratory problems

Data from Sherwen, L. N., Scoloveno, M. A., & Weingarten, C. T. (1995). *Nursing care of the childbearing family* (2nd ed.). Norwalk, CT: Appleton & Lange.

will deteriorate in 5 to 10 days and the cord base will heal completely about 2 weeks later. Care of the cord usually includes instruction on application of alcohol to the umbilical area two to three times per day to help it dry. Also, diapers should be folded away from the cord to prevent rubbing and to expose the cord to air (Delahoussaye, 1994). Sponge bathing the newborn is recommended until the cord falls off. See the Health Teaching box "Bathing a Newborn."

After the cord area has healed, tub baths are allowed. A sink or a special infant tub should be used to bathe newborns. As with the sponge bath, the bath should begin with clear water on the eyes and face and progress from head to toe, finishing with the diaper area. Care should be taken to ensure that the temperature of the bath water is neither too hot nor too cold. Two or three inches of water is sufficient and parents should be admonished to never leave the baby alone in the bath to prevent drowning.

DRESSING AND DIAPERING

A number of factors, such as cost, convenience, skin care, infection control, and environmental concerns, influence the parent's choice of cloth versus disposable diapers. Wong (1999) reports that "in general, home-laundered diapers are the least expensive when home labor cost is not included. Once home labor cost is included, the price difference between disposable diapers, diaper service reusable diapers, and home-laundered diapers is quite small, although paper diapers tend to cost the most" (p. 332).

Diapers should be the appropriate size and positioned to fit snugly, but not tightly. Soiled diapers should be changed immediately to avoid prolonged exposure of the diaper area to stools. Wet diapers should be changed frequently to minimize exposure to dampness. The genitalia, buttocks, and anal area should be washed after each diaper change to prevent skin irritation.

Clothing should be appropriate for the temperature of the room or outdoors, as warranted. During cold weather, it is important to dress and wrap the baby appropriately to maintain body temperature. A bonnet, hat, or other head covering should be used when taking the infant outside during cold weather. Overdressing during warm temperatures and underdressing during cold weather can cause discomfort.

Whenever possible, a newborn's clothing should be laundered separately from the rest of the family. A mild detergent should be used and the clothing, linens, and diapers should be double rinsed to remove all soap residue (Sherwen et al., 1995).

STOOLING AND VOIDING PATTERNS

Parents should be taught about the progression of the infant's first stools from meconium to normal. Most normal-term infants pass meconium within 12 to 24 hours of birth (Hammond, 2000). Meconium is composed of amniotic fluid, intestinal secretions, shed mucosal cells, and possibly blood and is greenish-black, viscous, and odorless. Transitional stools usually begin by the third day and are greenish-brown to yellowish-brown and are thinner and less sticky than meconium. Transitional stools last 2 to 3 days, and milk stools usually appear by 4 to 5 days. In breast-fed infants, stools are yellow to golden and pasty in consistency and smell somewhat like sour milk. The stools of formula-fed infants are pale yellow to light brown, are firmer in consistency, and have a more offensive odor (Wong, 1999).

Frequency of bowel movements for newborns varies from one with each feeding to one every 3 to 4 days. In general, the number of stools decreases in the first 2 weeks from five to six daily to one or two per day (Hammond, 2000). Most newborn infants void during the first few hours of life and neonates may void up to 20 times per day (Sherwen et al., 1995).

OBSERVING FOR COMPLICATIONS

New parents should be taught to observe their babies for relatively common problems that may arise, how to manage these problems, and when to contact their pediatrician or pediatric NP. Examples of relatively common concerns include hyperbilirubinemia, problems with temperature regulation (particularly in infants with LBW), and concerns over respiratory patterns. Parents should also be instructed on possible signs of infection (e.g., increased temperature, decreased feeding, lethargy, inconsolable crying) and taught how to take the baby's temperature.

INFERTILITY

Infertility refers to the inability to conceive after 1 year of regular sexual intercourse without contraception (Nichols and Lowdermilk, 2000). Approximately 13% of married couples experience problems with conception (USDHHS, 2000).

Factors related to the female partner account for 40% to 50% of infertility problems and factors related to the male account for about 30%; a combination of factors of both partners accounts for another 20% to 30% (Sherwen et al., 1995). In women, the most common causes of infertility are problems in ovulation, blocked or scarred fallopian tubes, and endometriosis. Delay of childbirth until after the optimal age for fertility has also been identified as contributing to problems with conception.

In men, abnormal or too few sperm is the most frequent cause of infertility. Factors that contribute to problems with sperm and thus male infertility include underlying disease processes, structural disorders such as undescended testes, trauma, poor nutrition, prolonged exposure to high temperature in the scrotal area (e.g., associated with wearing tight briefs, use of hot tubs), low testosterone levels, and varicocele (Nichols and Lowdermilk, 2000).

Complications (e.g., pelvic inflammatory disease) of sexually transmitted diseases—primarily gonorrhea and chlamydia—contribute to about 20% of cases of infertility. Other factors that may affect fertility of U.S. residents include previous abortion, the use of IUDs, stress, and exposure to environmental factors (e.g., radiation, pollution, and toxic chemicals) (USDHHS, 2000).

The process of trying to discover the cause of infertility can be expensive, painful, embarrassing, and emotionally draining. To diagnose infertility, both partners must undergo testing, including complete health history and physical examination. A detailed sexual history of both partners is also necessary. Based on information from the histories and physical examination, one or more diagnostic tests may be performed. Table 11-4 lists some tests that may be conducted to diagnose the cause of infertility. Following identification of the reason for infertility, the couple is counseled on treatment options. Treatment of infertility can be very expensive and outcomes are far from certain.

If the problem is related to ovulation, medications such as clomiphene citrate (Clomid) may be given to increase or regulate ovulation. Endometriosis may be treated medically, through use of hormones, or, in more severe cases, surgical repair of the uterus or fallopian tubes (Sherwen et al., 1995). Similarly, treatment of male infertility may involve use of drug therapy and lifestyle changes (e.g., improved nutrition, wearing boxer shorts, no hot baths or hot tubs, stopping smoking). Surgery may be required if a varicocele is detected.

If initial therapies are unsuccessful, several other options are available for infertile couples. Again, the possible treatments depend on the identified cause of the problem. For example, if the cervical mucus is not supportive of sperm, artificial insemination with the partner's sperm is an option. Artificial insemination with donor sperm is an option if the male's sperm are insufficient in number or motility.

TABLE **11-4** Tests for Impaired Fertility

TEST/EXAMINATION	TIMING (MENSTRUAL CYCLE DAYS)	RATIONALE
Hysterosalpingogram	7-10	Late follicular, early proliferative phase will not disrupt a fertilized ovum; may open uterine tubes before time of ovulation
Postcoital test	1-2 days before ovulation	Ovulatory late proliferative phase—look for normal motile sperm in cervical mucus
Sperm immobilization antigen-antibody reaction	Variable, ovulation	Immunological test to determine sperm and cervical mucus interaction
Assessment of cervical mucus	Variable, ovulation	Cervical mucus should have low viscosity, high spinnbarkheit
Ultrasound observation of follicular collapse	Ovulation	Collapsed follicle is seen after ovulation
Serum assay of plasma progesterone	20-25	Midluteal midsecretory phase—check adequacy of corpus luteal production of progesterone
Basal body temperature (BBT)	Chart entire cycle	Elevation occurs in response to progesterone
Endometrial biopsy	21-27	Late luteal, late secretory phase—check endometrial response to progesterone and adequacy of luteal phase
Sperm penetration assay	After 2 days but no more than 1 week of abstinence	Evaluation of ability of sperm to penetrate an egg

From Nichols, A. N., & Lowdermilk, D. L. (2000). Infertility. In D. L. Lowdermilk, S. E. Perry, & I. M. Bobak (Eds.), *Maternity and women's health care* (7th ed.). St. Louis: Mosby.

Assisted reproductive technology refers to several therapies that have been developed to treat infertility. Some of the available options cited by Nichols and Lowdermilk (2000) and Sherwen et al. (1995) include the following:

- In vitro fertilization (IVF; "test tube" fertilization): the woman's eggs are laparoscopically collected from her ovaries and fertilized in the laboratory, then transferred back to her uterus after normal embryo development has begun. Success rate is about 20%.
- Gamete intrafallopian transfer (GIFT): the eggs are harvested from the ovary and placed in a catheter with washed, motile sperm and immediately transferred into the end of the fallopian tube(s). Fertilization occurs in the fallopian tube rather than in the laboratory. Success rates are 20% to 30%.
- Zygote intrafallopian transfer: a combination of IVF and GIFT in which the ova are fertilized in the laboratory and then transferred to the fallopian tube for development and transport to the uterus. Success rates are comparable with those of GIFT and IVF.
- Donor ovum transfer: ova from a donor are fertilized in the laboratory by the male partner's sperm and then transferred into the recipient's uterus, which has been hormonally prepared with estrogen and progesterone therapy.
- Donor embryo (embryo adoption): a donated embryo is transferred to the uterus of an infertile woman at the appropriate time (normal or induced) of the menstrual cycle.
- Gestational carrier (embryo host): the infertile couple undergoes IVF, but the embryo(s) are transferred to another woman's uterus (the carrier) who will carry the baby to term. The carrier does not provide ova.
- Therapeutic donor insemination: donor sperm are used to inseminate the female partner.

Nurses who work with couples experiencing problems with fertility should be prepared to discuss their options. Information on these options and resources for referral should be made available.

TEENAGE PREGNANCY

"Pregnancy and childbearing rates for teenagers remain high in the United States despite well-documented associated adverse health, social, and economic consequences for many of these teenagers and their children" (Centers for Disease Control and Prevention [CDC], 1995, p. 677). In the United States, **teenage pregnancy** is one of the most serious, complicated, and far reaching of all public health problems. The statistics are astonishing. Consider the following (CDC, 1995; USDHHS, 2000; USDHHS/ODPHP, 1998):

- The United States has the highest rate of teenage pregnancy among developed countries.
- Each year, about 10% of teenage girls (approximately 1 million girls) 15 to 19 years of age become pregnant and more than 500,000 give birth.
- By age 18, 24% of teenage girls have become pregnant at least once.
- Ninety-five percent of teenage pregnancies are unintended.
- Almost 78% of all births to teenagers and more than 92% of births to black teenagers are to unmarried girls.
- Approximately 75% of teenagers report that they use no contraception or use contraception inconsistently.
- Nearly two thirds of pregnancies among girls 15 years of age or younger end in abortion or fetal loss.

CONSEQUENCES

Teenage pregnancy is associated with serious problems. Teenage mothers are more likely to experience complications of pregnancy largely because of delayed or no prenatal care, poor nutrition, and other lifestyle factors. They are more likely to experience maternal complications, including pregnancy-induced hypertension, toxemia, anemia, nutritional deficiencies, and urinary tract infections. They are more prone to deliver prematurely, experience rapid or prolonged labor, and have fetal and maternal infections. Infants born to teenage mothers are more likely to have LBW and suffer associated problems (e.g., respiratory problems, neurological defects) and are more likely to be stillborn (Maurer, 2000a).

Probably the most significant factor, however, is the socioeconomic impact of teenage pregnancy. Indeed, "teenage pregnancy is viewed as the hub of the poverty cycle in the United States, because teenage mothers are likely to rear children who repeat the cycle" (Maurer, 2000a, p. 642). Many pregnant girls and teenage mothers fail to complete high school. This, in turn, is associated with unemployment and underemployment, resulting in living below the poverty level and reliance on welfare programs.

CONTRIBUTING FACTORS

Higher teenage pregnancy rates are directly tied to reports that teenagers are becoming sexually active at younger ages. In 1970, 28.6% of adolescent women (15 to 19 years) were sexually active. By 1995, the rate of sexually active adolescent females had increased to 50% (USDHHS/ODPHP, 1998).

Several factors contribute to early engagement in sexual activity. These include peer pressure; pervasive sexually explicit media (e.g., television, movies, music, music videos, information on the Internet); need for love, acceptance, and approval; efforts to gain independence; increased acceptance of unmarried mothers; present, rather than future, orientation; and lack of maturity (Aretakis, 1996; Maurer, 2000a).

COUNSELING TEENAGERS ON ISSUES OF SEXUALITY

The benefits of practicing sexual abstinence should be stressed by health care providers to all teenagers. Providing information on reasons to avoid initiation of sexual intercourse and how to say "no" has been shown to be helpful. Resources that provide materials on sexuality issues for adolescents are available for health care providers and educators who work with teenagers. Several are listed in the Resources box at the end of this chapter. To assist nurses working with

teenagers, the Health Teaching box "Counseling Guidelines to Prevent Adolescent Pregnancy" offers suggestions by the Preventative Services Task Force (USDHHS/ODPHP, 1998).

In addition to these guidelines, nurses who care for sexually active and pregnant teenagers should be aware of their state's laws regarding age of consent for engaging in sexual activity and statutory rape. Although there is no firm consensus on how and when to notify child protective services or other authorities, agencies that work with sexually active and pregnant minors should have or should develop policies describing circumstances under which to notify authorities and the process that is involved. For example, in some states, girls younger than 15 years cannot legally consent to sex and adults who engage in sexual intercourse with these teenagers are subject to prosecution. Other states base age of consent on age differences between the girl and her partner (e.g., the older partner cannot be more than 3 years older than the younger one). It may be legally permissible for a 15-year-old girl to have intercourse with a 17-year-old boy, but not with a 24-year-old man. Finally, the nurse should always consider the possibility of sexual child abuse and assess appropriately—particularly when caring for younger girls.

PRENATAL CARE FOR PREGNANT TEENS

For all of the reasons cited, pregnant teenagers need early and comprehensive prenatal care. Case management is preferred. It is particularly important that teenagers be counseled on good nutritional practices, getting plenty of rest, and recognition of signs and symptoms of complications. Pregnant teenagers should be encouraged to stay in school. Because of the extent of this problem, as described earlier, many school districts have developed special programs designed to meet the educational, developmental, maturational, and social needs of the pregnant teenager. On-site health care is frequently a component of school programs. Additionally, many programs offer childbirth education, parenting classes, and after-delivery childcare (Figure 11-2).

---

health teaching

Counseling Guidelines to Prevent Adolescent Pregnancy

1. All adolescents should be asked about their sexual experiences and use of contraceptives. The clinician should maintain a nonjudgmental, empathetic manner and should be willing to answer questions and provide contraceptive advice or refer to another clinician for prescriptions, as appropriate. Information should include consequences of pregnancy and STDs and effective methods to prevent them.

2. State laws vary regarding minimum age for consenting to treatment and receiving contraceptives for minors. Clinicians should familiarize themselves with the laws in their state regarding these issues. Adolescents should be informed about issues of confidentiality regarding pregnancy prevention, STD testing, and treatment, as directed by state regulations and agency policy.

3. Parents should be counseled about the emerging sexuality in teenagers' lives and options for contraception. Clinicians should encourage effective communication between adolescents and their families regarding responsible sexual behavior.

4. Adolescents who are sexually abstinent should be supported in remaining abstinent and should be counseled in methods to resist unwelcome or coercive sexual relationships.

5. Within the parameters set by the state and the agency, adolescents who are sexually active should be assisted in choosing an effective, appropriate method of contraception. Considerations include their personal preferences and motivation, religious beliefs, cultural norms, and relationship with their partner(s). The most popular contraceptive methods among adolescents are birth control pills and condoms; implants or injectable contraceptives may be appropriate choices for teens. Diaphragms, cervical caps, and periodic abstinence are difficult for teens to use effectively and IUDs are not recommended for adolescents.

6. All sexually active adolescents should be taught that hormonal contraception (e.g., pills, injections, implants) *does not* protect against STDs and HIV. The use of condoms, in addition to these contraceptives, should be encouraged to reduce STDs in sexually active individuals. It should be stressed that condoms are *not* 100% effective.

7. Adolescents of both genders should be encouraged to talk frankly with their partners about STDs, HIV, and use of contraceptives. Assertiveness with partners about the use of contraception and protective measures against STDs should be supported. *It should be stressed that saying "no" is every person's right.*

8. Boys should be provided with as much counseling as girls about contraception and STD prevention. Young adolescent males should be taught the benefits of abstinence, the importance of responsible sexual behavior, and the importance of condom use if engaging in sexual intercourse, at an early age.

9. Adolescents using prescribed contraceptives should be followed closely to determine proper use and to monitor for side effects.

Adapted from U.S. Department of Health and Human Services (USDHHS). (1998). *Clinician's handbook of preventive services.* Washington, DC: Government Printing Office.

HIV, Human immunodeficiency virus; *IUD,* intrauterine device; *STD,* sexually transmitted disease.

POSTDELIVERY NEEDS

After delivery, teenagers need ongoing social support and encouragement to complete their education. Financial assistance is also frequently a need and nurses who practice in community-based settings should know how to refer new mothers to obtain social services such as Aid to Families with Dependent Children, WIC, and food stamps.

Finally, all pregnant teenagers should be counseled regarding sexual activity and contraception choices following delivery. Somewhat surprisingly, repeat pregnancy is frequently a problem. Maurer (2000a) reports that 25% of teenage girls are pregnant again within 2 years of their first pregnancy. All teenagers who have experienced one pregnancy should be emphati-

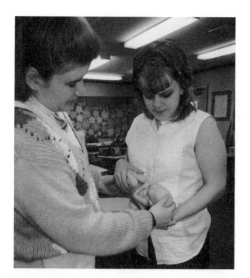

Figure 11-2 A teacher and student in a school-based childbirth and parenting class for pregnant teenage girls. (From Matteson, P. S. [2001]. *Women's health during the childbearing years: A community-based approach.* St. Louis: Mosby.)

cally encouraged to avoid another pregnancy and supported in their contraceptive choices.

WOMEN'S HEALTH CARE

In addition to health needs related to child-bearing and family planning, several health promotion- and illness-prevention issues should be addressed by health care professionals who care for women of all ages in community settings.

The Research Highlight details statistics about women's use of health care services. The following sections discuss screening recommendations for breast cancer and diseases of the reproductive organs, prevention of osteoporosis, and prevention and identification of and interventions for domestic violence.

SCREENING RECOMMENDATIONS FOR BREAST CANCER

Breast cancer is the most common cancer among women in the United States (excluding skin cancer) and the second leading cause of cancer deaths in women. In the United States, a woman's average lifetime risk for developing breast cancer is approximately one in eight (USDHHS/ODPHP, 1998).

Risk factors for breast cancer are age (over 50); personal or family history (e.g., mother, sister); first pregnancy after 30 years of age; having had no children; menarche before age 12; menopause after age 50; postmenopausal obesity; high socioeconomic status; heavy alcohol consumption (2 to 5 drinks per day); and a personal history of breast, ovarian, or endometrial cancer (American Cancer Society [ACS], 2000; USDHHS/ODPHP, 1998). Mortality from breast cancer is strongly influenced by its stage at detection; therefore early detection is critical to promoting a good outcome. A BSE, examination by a trained clinician, and mammography are the most commonly used tools to screen women for breast cancer.

Research Highlight

Women's Use of Health Care

Excluding pregnancy-related visits, women are 33% more likely than men to visit a doctor. On average, women make about 4.6 visits a year to the doctor, ranging from 3.8 for those 15 to 44 to about 7.5 for those 65 and older. Visits by younger women are more likely to be to a primary care provider and older women are more likely to see specialists.

Women also use more prescription drugs than do men. Women are more likely to receive hormones and are dramatically more likely to have an antidepressant prescribed. The most frequently prescribed drugs for women are nonnarcotic analgesics, antidepressants, and estrogen/progestin.

From Centers for Disease Control and Prevention (CDC). (2001). *New study profiles women's use of health care.* Retrieved 07/24/01 from http://www.cdc.gov/od/oc/media/pressrel/r010725.htm.

Most authorities agree that all women should be taught how to perform BSE and encouraged to practice BSE monthly (about 1 week after the end of the menstrual period). In addition, all women 20 to 39 years of age should have a breast examination performed by a health professional at least every 3 years and every year beginning at age 40 (ACS, 2000).

The ACS and other groups have excellent teaching materials, educational pamphlets, and reminders available to help instruct women on performing BSE. Nurses who care for women in community settings are in an excellent position to teach this important skill and should provide literature and other materials to help instruct their clients.

Mammography is the most effective means of early detection for breast cancer (USDHHS/ODPHP, 1998). There is some debate on the benefit of routinely screening women younger than 50, but most authorities agree that potential benefits are much greater than any potential harm from routine screening of younger women. In general, mammography screening recommendations are as follows (ACS, 2000; USDHHS/ ODPHP, 1998):

- Women 40 to 49 years of age should have screening mammograms every 1 to 2 years.
- Women 50 years or older should have screening mammograms every year.
- High-risk women (women with a family history of premenopausally diagnosed breast cancer in a first-degree relative) should have mammograms beginning at 35 years of age.
- Any palpable breast lump, even if not detected on a mammogram, should be carefully evaluated.

When breast cancer is suspected, a surgical biopsy or needle biopsy is performed. If the lump is confirmed as breast cancer, treatment is typically a combination of surgery (e.g., lumpectomy, simple mastectomy, modified radical mastectomy) and radiation and/or chemotherapy or hormone therapy. All treatment options should be discussed thoroughly with the client, including potential outcomes, side effects, benefits, and negative consequences. Again, the nurse should assist in informed decision making by providing literature on breast cancer and referral to organizations and agencies (e.g., ACS, Reach for Recovery) that provide information on the treatment of breast cancer.

SCREENING RECOMMENDATIONS FOR CANCERS OF THE FEMALE REPRODUCTIVE TRACT

Cancers of the cervix, ovary, and endometrium are relatively common and are successfully treatable if caught early. Screening recommendations for each are described briefly here.

Cancer of the endometrium is the most common gynecological malignancy and the fourth most common malignancy in women (after breast, colorectal, and lung cancer) (ACS, 2000). Endometrial cancer most often occurs in postmenopausal women between the ages of 50 and 65 years (average age at diagnosis is 58 years). Risk factors include nulliparity, infertility, late menopause, early menarche, obesity, a family history of breast cancer, higher socioeconomic status, pelvic irradiation, and endometrial hyperplasia (Jones and Trabeaux, 1996; Lowdermilk, 2000). Hormone replacement therapy also strongly increases the risk of uterine cancer. Abnormal vaginal bleeding and an enlarged uterus are the most common symptoms of endometrial cancer. If postmenopausal bleeding occurs, an endometrial biopsy is usually performed.

Total abdominal hysterectomy and bilateral salpingo-oophorectomy is the treatment of choice for cases of endometrial cancer. If staging determines metastases, radiation and/or chemotherapy or hormone therapy may be considered (Lowdermilk, 2000).

Cancer of the cervix is one of the most common cancers in women, but is highly treatable if caught early. The major risk factor for cervical cancers is infection with human papillomavirous (HPV) (USDHHS/ODPHP, 1998). Other risk factors for cervical cancer are early age at first intercourse, having had multiple sexual partners, a history of exposure to diethylstilbestrol, long-term use of oral contraceptives (longer than 5 years) and smoking (Sherwen et al., 1995; USDHHS/

ODPHP, 1998). Cervical carcinoma in situ is most commonly seen in women between 20 and 30 years of age and invasive cervical carcinoma increases with age. Indeed, 40% to 50% of all women who die of cervical cancer are older than 65 years of age. Also, black women have dramatically higher incidences of invasive cancer than white women (USDHHS/ODPHP, 1998).

Symptoms of cervical cancer include vaginal bleeding or discharge, often associated with douching or sexual intercourse. The widespread use of the Pap test for early detection of cervical cancer has contributed greatly to the decline in deaths from cervical cancer. Recommendations for routine Pap testing are as follow:

- Sexually active women 18 years of age or older should have Pap tests at least every 3 years
- Frequency of Pap tests should be based on risk factors and performed at the discretion of the physician and the client, but not less frequently than every 3 years (USDHHS/ODPHP, 1998)

Results of Pap tests are described as (Lowdermilk, 2000)

- "Within normal limits"—minimal inflammation; no malignant cells
- "Inflammatory atypia"—mild atypical inflammation
- "Cervical intraepithelial neoplasia (CIN) grade I"—mild dysplasia, abnormal nucleus, normal cytoplasm
- "CIN grade II"—moderate dysplasia, abnormal nucleus, minimal cytoplasm abnormalities
- "CIN grade III"—abnormal chromosome and cytoplasm, abnormal cells predominate, many undifferentiated cells, severe dysplasia

For cervical changes and abnormal Pap results, one of several diagnostic examinations and treatment options may be chosen. Colposcopy and directed cervical biopsies, cone biopsy (by cold knife, laser, or loop excision), endocervical curettage, and/or loop electrosurgical procedure may be performed. Following treatment, Pap tests every 4 months for the first year and every 6 months thereafter are recommended. If invasive cervical cancer is detected, a total abdominal hysterectomy is usually performed. Additional therapy (e.g., radiation and/or chemotherapy) may be recommended for advanced disease (Dambro, 1996).

Cancer of the ovary is quite rare, affecting 1 out of 70, or 1.4%, of women; however, it is the most deadly of the cancers of the reproductive organs (ACS, 2000). The high death rate is largely attributable to delay in diagnosis because ovarian cancer rarely produces symptoms until it reaches advanced stages. Risk factors for ovarian cancer include family history; nulliparity; older age at the first pregnancy; fewer pregnancies; and a personal history of breast, endometrial, or colorectal cancer (USDHHS/ODPHP, 1998). The pelvic examination is the most common screening examination for ovarian cancer. Treatment is usually a combination of surgery and radiation and/or chemotherapy.

PREVENTION OF OSTEOPOROSIS

Osteoporosis is a very common skeletal disease characterized by decreased bone mass, which leads to increased skeletal fragility and subsequent tendency to fracture. Osteoporosis affects about 8 million U.S. residents, including an estimated 18% of women older than 50 years and 90% of women older than 75 (USDHHS, 2000). Of those individuals, over half have fractures related to osteoporosis. Indeed, each year approximately 1.5 million fractures in the United States are related to osteoporosis (Jones and Trabeaux, 1996). The most common sites of atraumatic fractures are the vertebral column, upper femur, distal radius, and proximal humerus. The most serious fractures are hip fractures, which affect about 250,000 U.S. residents each year. It is estimated that about 17% of women and 6% of men experience a hip fracture by the time they reach 90 years of age (USDHHS, 2000). As the population of the United States ages, the incidence of osteoporosis-related fractures is expected to increase.

Risk factors for osteoporosis include age, female gender, family history, diet (inadequate calcium and vitamin D and excessive protein and phosphate), decreased activity, sedentary lifestyle, use of alcohol and caffeine, smoking, some medications (corticosteroids, excess thyroid replacement, long-term heparin therapy, chemotherapy, and anticonvulsants), and radiation therapy (Dambro, 1996; USDHHS/ODPHP, 1998). At greatest risk for osteoporosis-related fractures are women who are older, white, and slender and who have had a bilateral oophorectomy or early menopause. In addition to increased risk of fractures, osteoporosis is associated with both acute and chronic back pain, kyphosis, and loss of height.

Postmenopausal estrogen replacement has proven effective in reducing osteoporosis-related fractures. In addition, estrogen replacement helps decrease vasomotor symptoms associated with menopause (e.g., hot flashes) and may improve genitourinary symptoms (urgency, incontinence, frequency, and vaginal dryness) and reduce cardiovascular mortality in postmenopausal women (USDHHS/ODPHP, 1998). Significant concern, however, is associated with possible complications and side effects related to hormone replacement therapy. Estrogen replacement therapy is strongly associated with increased risk of endometrial cancer and the use of estrogen and progestin combinations may increase the risk of breast cancer. See the Health Teaching box "Counseling Guidelines for Hormone Replacement Therapy."

Other preventative measures to reduce osteoporosis include increased calcium intake (1500 mg/day), adequate vitamin D intake (400 to 800 IU/day), and avoiding excess meat and phosphoric acid-containing beverages (Dambro, 1996). Premenopausal women, particularly those in high-risk groups, should be taught the benefits of calcium supplementation, with the recommended dosage being 1000 mg/day. Encouragement of weight-bearing exercise is also very important.

DOMESTIC VIOLENCE

Studies indicate that between 2 and 4 million women in the United States are physically abused by an intimate partner each year (Grant, 1995). As a result, "battering of women is the foremost cause of injury to women" and "40 to 60 percent of battered women are abused during pregnancy" (Grant, 1995, p. 411). Maurer (2000b) reports that 30% to 50% of police investigations involve domestic violence, as many as 70% of emergency room assault victims are women attacked at home, and around 25% of abused women require hospitalization for their injuries.

Once the pattern of **domestic violence** begins in a relationship, it tends to recur and become more severe over time. Furthermore, intrafamilial homicide accounts for almost one of six homicides and is often preceded by a history of physical and emotional abuse. Therefore prevention of homicide among spouses and intimates should be linked to the prevention of abuse of women.

Nurses working in community settings are often in a position to identify and intervene in cases of domestic violence. Although there may be considerable variation, there are commonalities in the characteristics of the abuser and the victim. For example, the abuser often has poor impulse control, an unpredictable temper, and an inability to tolerate frustration. He is typically egocentric, emotionally dependent, has poor social skills, and a need to dominate. The batterer may also be excessively jealous and may have unrealistic expectations. Frequently, he has been a victim of child abuse and is often unemployed or underemployed. Finally, alcohol use may facilitate aggression or may be used as an excuse for aggression (Grant, 1995; Maurer, 2000b; Pappas and Hakala, 2001).

In general, victims of domestic violence have low self-esteem. They are typically poorly educated and economically and emotionally dependent on the abuser. They generally marry young and have children early; risk increases during pregnancy. They may experience constant fear and gradual isolation from friends and family. Many were victims of child abuse. They often report a hope that "things will get better," but many have a history of suicide attempts (Grant, 1995; Maurer, 2000b; Pappas and Hakala, 2001).

To help nurses identify suspected cases of domestic violence, Box 11-3 lists physical and

health teaching

Counseling Guidelines for Hormone Replacement Therapy

- All women should be counseled about the probable risks and benefits of hormone replacement therapy and participate with their physician in deciding whether to take preventative hormone therapy.
- Women and clinicians should consider risk factors in determining whether to institute hormone replacement therapy. Risk factors include coronary heart disease risk factors (family history, blood pressure, weight, smoking status, cholesterol), osteoporosis risk factors (race, body build, physical activity level, bone mineral density), breast cancer risk factors (personal and family history, later parity, early menarche, late menopause), client's desire for quality-of-life benefits (e.g., decreased vasomotor and genitourinary tract symptoms), client's tolerance of side effects (e.g., endometrial bleeding and breast tenderness), and client's willingness to participate in follow-up monitoring (endometrial sampling and mammography).
- If hormone replacement therapy is used, it may be desirable to begin estrogen replacement soon after the onset of menopause. Upper age limit for estrogen replacement has not been established.

- The concurrent use of progestin or careful endometrial monitoring is recommended for women with intact uteri.
- Contraindications for estrogen replacement include unexplained vaginal bleeding, active liver disease, impaired liver function, recent vascular thrombosis, breast cancer, and endometrial cancer.
- Other conditions that may be considered as contraindications include seizure disorders, hypertension, uterine leiomyoma, familial hyperlipidemia, migraines, endometriosis, gallbladder disease, and thrombophlebitis.
- For women choosing estrogen therapy, a pelvic examination should be performed at initiation of therapy and yearly thereafter. Endometrial evaluation should be accomplished for women with uteri taking only estrogen. Follow-up evaluation of any vaginal bleeding should be made.
- Breast cancer screening should be the same as for women not taking hormone replacement therapy.

Adapted from U.S. Department of Health and Human Services. (1998). *Clinician's handbook of preventive services.* Washington, DC: Government Printing Office.

behavioral signs and symptoms that might indicate abuse. See the Community Application box "Nursing Interventions for Victims of Domestic Violence."

SUMMARY

Lisa, the nurse from the opening case study, worked in a women's health clinic; she was familiar with the many health issues commonly encountered in this group. However, all nurses who work with women of any age in community-based settings, including worksites, schools, practitioner offices, and clinics, should understand the scope of women's health care and be prepared to intervene as appropriate to prevent health problems and promote health.

Health care for women goes beyond issues related to reproduction and encompasses a variety of issues. This chapter covers several areas related to the unique health care needs of women. Primary and secondary prevention strategies and health education for diverse topics of family planning, prenatal care, infant care, teenage pregnancy, early detection of cancers, and prevention of osteoporosis are described. The chapter concludes with information on detection and prevention of domestic violence. For further information on any of these topics, see the Resources box at the end of the chapter. Nurses in community-based practice should maintain a list of local resources related to women's health and be prepared to refer their clients as needed.

BOX 11-3 Injuries, Signs, and Symptoms Suggestive of Domestic Violence

IN AN OFFICE OR CLINIC

- Presenting complaints related to chronic stress or anxiety (e.g., hyperventilation, gastrointestinal disturbances, hypertension, panic attack, headache, chest pain, choking sensation)
- Depression or stress-related conditions (e.g., insomnia, anxiety, fatigue)
- Evidence of fear, embarrassment, or humiliation
- Poor grooming or inappropriate attire
- Any suspicious physical injuries (e.g., bruises, lacerations, scars, burns, swelling, fractures, ear or eye problems secondary to injury, clumps of hair missing)
- Any evidence of physical injury during pregnancy

IN AN EMERGENCY ROOM

- Bleeding injuries, particularly to the head and face
- Perforated eardrum, eye injuries (e.g., black eye, orbital fracture)
- Broken or fractured jaw, arms, ribs, and legs
- Internal injuries; concussion
- Severe bruising, particularly on the back, buttocks, breasts, abdomen, and upper extremities

- Genital/urinary or rectal trauma
- Strangulation marks on the neck
- Burns from cigarettes, liquids, or acids
- Evidence of psychological trauma (e.g., anxiety, panic attacks, heart palpitations)
- Suicide attempt
- Miscarriage

IN ANY SETTING

- Reports domestic problems; reports being trapped or powerless
- History of hospitalization for traumatic injuries
- Increased anxiety in presence of spouse/partner
- Inappropriate or anxious nonverbal behavior; uncontrolled crying
- Injuries in various stages of healing
- Injuries indicating failure to seek immediate care
- Timid and evasive behavior
- Inconsistent description of the cause of the injury
- Accompanied by male partner who does not wish to leave her alone

Data from Grant, C. (1995). Physical and sexual abuse. In D. Antiai-Otong (Ed.), *Psychiatric nursing: Biological and behavioral concepts.* Philadelphia: W. B. Saunders; Maurer, F. A. (2000b). Violence: A social and family problem. In C. M. Smith & F. A. Maurer (Eds.), *Community health nursing theory and practice* (2nd ed.). Philadelphia: W. B. Saunders; Pappas, A., & Hakala, K. L. D. (2001). Family violence. In M. A. Nies & M. McEwen (Eds.), *Community health nursing: Promoting the health of populations* (3rd ed.). Philadelphia: W. B. Saunders.

Resources

Women's Health

Family Planning

National Institute of Child Health and Human Development
Office of Population Affairs/Office of Adolescent Pregnancy Programs
The Alan Guttmacher Institute
Planned Parenthood Federation of America, Inc.
Catholic Charities (adoption and foster care services)
American College of Obstetricians and Gynecologists
National Association of Nurse Practitioners in Reproductive Health
National Organization on Adolescent Pregnancy, Parenting, and Prevention

Maternal and Child Health

U.S. Department of Agriculture/Food and Nutrition Service
Women, Infants, and Children Program

National Institute of Child Health and Human Development
March of Dimes Birth Defects Foundation
La Leche League

Specific Illnesses

National Cancer Institute
American Cancer Society
Cancer Survivors Network
National Osteoporosis Foundation

Domestic Violence

National Coalition Against Domestic Violence
American Bar Association Commission on Domestic Violence
Department of Justice Program/Violence Against Women Office
Domestic Violence Hotlines and Resources
Shelter Aid Hotline 1-800-799-SAFE

Visit the book's website at
www.wbsaunders.com/SIMON/McEwen
for a direct link to the website for each organization listed.

COMMUNITY APPLICATION
Nursing Interventions for Victims of Domestic Violence

1. Interview women with suspicious symptoms or injuries to confirm or refute abuse.

   Talk with the woman in a quiet, private area.

   Be professional, direct, and honest in questioning.

   Be understanding; do not express anger, shock, or disapproval.
2. If abuse is confirmed, assess safety and explore the victim's options to reduce danger.

   Affirm to the woman that battering is unacceptable.

   Assess the seriousness of the circumstances.

   Assist in calling and explaining the situation to friends or family when appropriate.

   Assure the victim that disclosed information will be kept confidential to the maximal extent possible.

   Counsel the victim about the dynamics of domestic violence and provide information on potential danger to the woman and her children.
3. If the woman wants to leave the situation and if no other options are feasible, provide information on shelters or safe houses.

   Obtain information (telephone numbers, criteria, and process for admittance to the shelter) in advance.

   Offer to contact the shelter and make arrangements for transportation.

   Offer to contact legal authorities to report the abuse and press charges.
4. If the woman chooses to stay in the relationship, encourage and assist her to develop a safety plan for fast escape should violence recur. Include ways to identify the signs of escalation of violence and select a sign that will be a cue to leave.

   Suggest that she keep a bag packed for herself and her children (include clothing, toiletries, medications, money) and ask a friend or neighbor to store the bag.

   Save money if possible.

   Take important financial records, such as rent or mortgage receipts and/or the car title.

   Provide a list of shelters and the appropriate telephone numbers—know exactly where to go and how to get there.
5. Encourage follow-up care; individual and family therapy should be encouraged, when possible.

Data from U.S. Department of Health and Human Services/Office of Disease Prevention and Health Promotion (USDHHS/ODPHP). (1998). *Clinician's handbook of preventive services.* Washington, DC: Government Printing Office.

KEY POINTS

- Nursing practice in community settings includes several issues pertaining to women's health. These are family planning, prenatal care, infertility, general health care (e.g., screening for reproductive diseases, breast care, prevention of osteoporosis), detection and prevention of domestic violence, and prevention and intervention in teenage pregnancy.
- More than half of all pregnancies in the United States are unintended; therefore comprehensive family planning is an important component of health care. Family planning includes consideration of factors regarding childbearing, such as abstinence from sexual activity, use of contraceptives, treatment of infertility, and preconception counseling.

- Several methods can be used to prevent pregnancy. Contraception options include barriers (e.g., condoms, diaphragm), hormonal methods (e.g., oral contraceptives, Depo-Provera, Norplant), sterilization, natural family planning, and abstinence. Each method has positive and negative consequences, which should be discussed and considered.
- Prenatal care is important for good pregnancy outcomes. Lack of prenatal care is associated with babies with LBW, prematurity, maternal complications, and infant mortality. Removing or lessening barriers to early and comprehensive prenatal care is important in improving infant mortality rates.
- Education regarding infant care should include infant nutrition, recommending breastfeeding. If the mother chooses to bottle-feed the baby,

information on formula selection and preparation and cleaning of equipment should be provided. Crib selection, sleeping position, and sleeping patterns should be discussed with parents. Basics of bathing, cord care, dressing and diapering, stooling and voiding patterns, and observing for problems or complications are also important.

- Infertility affects between 8% and 15% of married couples. Diagnosis of infertility should include testing of both partners to determine the cause of infertility. Following identification of the reason(s) for infertility, the couple is counseled on treatment options, which may include medications, surgery, lifestyle changes, artificial insemination, and more dramatic interventions, such as variations of IVF.

- Teenage pregnancy rates in the United States remain higher than in most industrialized countries and contribute to a number of health and social problems. Teenage pregnancy is associated with complications of pregnancy (both fetal and maternal), failure of the mother to complete high school, unemployment, poverty, and reliance on government assistance.

- Health promotion and illness prevention for women should also include various screenings and health education. Routine screenings for breast cancer include monthly BSE, periodic examination by a health care provider, and routine mammography for women older than 40. Screening for cancer of the cervix through yearly or biyearly Pap tests is important.

- Osteoporosis affects about 18% of all women older than 45 years and 90% older than 75 and many develop complications such as atraumatic fractures. Postmenopausal estrogen replacement therapy has been shown to be effective in reducing osteoporosis-related fractures and all women should be counseled regarding estrogen therapy.

- Domestic violence is a major cause of injury to women. Nurses working in community settings are often in a position to identify and intervene in cases of domestic violence and should be aware of characteristics of the victim, the batterer, and the family; recognize injuries and signs suggestive of domestic violence; and be prepared to intervene.

Learning Activities & Application to Practice
In Class

1. Research one of the issues described in this chapter (e.g., infertility, osteoporosis, domestic violence, contraception, cancer screening). What additional information were you able to identify and how should the information be used in providing care to women in community-based settings?

2. Examine the problem of teenage pregnancy in your area. How does it compare with other areas? What efforts have been made to reduce teenage pregnancy and to minimize the long-term associated problems?

In Clinical

3. Provide care in a prenatal/postpartum clinic or private practice for several days. Prepare by reviewing relevant material (e.g., nutrition, developmental milestones in pregnancy, breastfeeding) to be ready for opportunities for health promotion and education.

4. Observe contraception counseling. What issues are discussed between the counselor and the client? What factors appear to determine the woman's choice? Are all relevant factors (e.g., effectiveness of method, possible complications and side effects, cost, proper use) presented and discussed?

5. Participate in screening activities for women. Opportunities include teaching BSE, assisting with Pap smears, and observing for signs of domestic violence. Record impressions in a log or diary and share with other members of the clinical group.

REFERENCES

American Cancer Society. (2000). *Cancer facts & figures—2001.* Atlanta: American Cancer Society.

Aretakis, D. (1996). Teen pregnancy. In M. Stanhope & J. Lancaster (Eds.), *Community health nursing: Promoting health of aggregates, families and individuals* (4th ed., pp. 665-680). St. Louis: Mosby.

Ashwill, J. W., & Droske, S. C. (1997). *Nursing care of children: Principles and practice.* Philadelphia: W. B. Saunders.

Boyne, L. J. (1995). Maternal and fetal nutrition. In I. M. Bobak, D. L. Lowdermilk, & M. D. Jensen (Eds.), *Maternity nursing* (4th ed., pp. 172-204). St. Louis: Mosby.

Brown, S. S. (1989). Drawing women into prenatal care. *Family Planning Perspectives, 21*(2), 73-78.

Centers for Disease Control and Prevention (CDC). (1995). State-specific pregnancy and birth rates among teenagers—United States, 1991-1992. *MMWR Morbidity and Mortality Weekly Report, 44*(37), 677-683.

Centers for Disease Control and Prevention (CDC). (2001a). *Neural tube birth defects down by 19% since food fortification.* Retrieved 07/24/01 from www.cdc.gov/od/oc/media/pressrel/r010619.htm.

Centers for Disease Control and Prevention (CDC). (2001b). *New study profiles women's use of health care.* Retrieved 07/24/01 from http://www.cdc.gov/od/oc/media/pressrel/r010725.htm.

Clemen-Stone, S., Eigsti, D. G., & McGuire, S. L. (1995). *Comprehensive community health nursing* (4th ed.). St. Louis: Mosby.

Dambro, M. R. (1996). *Griffith's 5-minute clinical consult.* Baltimore: Williams & Wilkins.

Delahoussaye, C. P. (1994). Families with neonates. In C. L. Betz, M. M. Hunsberger, & S. Wright (Eds.), *Family-centered nursing care of children* (2nd ed., pp. 107-141). Philadelphia: W. B. Saunders.

Goldberg, M. S. (1994). *Choosing a contraceptive. Current issues in women's health* (2nd ed.). Washington, DC: Food and Drug Administration.

Grant, C. (1995). Physical and sexual abuse. In D. Antai-Otong (Ed.) *Psychiatric nursing: Biological and behavioral concepts* (pp. 407-426). Philadelphia: W. B. Saunders,.

Hammond, B. B. (2000). Physiology and physical adaptations of the newborn. In D. L. Lowdermilk, S. E. Perry, & I. M. Bobak (Eds.), *Maternity & women's health care* (7th ed., pp. 671-715). St. Louis: Mosby.

Heslin, J. (1992). If you bottlefeed. *American Baby, 54*(5), B10-B14.

Heslin, J. A. (1988). *No-nonsense nutrition for your baby's first year.* Englewood Cliffs, NJ: Prentice-Hall.

Jackson, D. B., & Saunders, R. B. (1994). *Child health nursing: A comprehensive approach to the care of children and their families.* Philadelphia: J. B. Lippincott.

Jaroff, L. (1996). Rx: "Morning after" pills. *Time,* July 15, 59.

Jonas, S. (1999). Population data for health and health care. In A. R. Kovner & S. Jonas (Eds.), *Jonas's health care delivery in the United States* (6th ed., pp. 7-31). New York: Springer Publishing Co.

Jones, L. C., & Trabeaux, S. (1996). Women's health. In M. Stanhope & J. Lancaster (Eds.), *Community health nursing: Promoting health of aggregates, families and individuals* (4th ed., pp. 545-564). St. Louis: Mosby.

Lowdermilk, D. L. (2000). Structural disorders and neoplasms of the reproductive system. In D. L. Lowdermilk, S. E. Perry, & I. M. Bobak (Eds.), *Maternity & women's health care* (7th ed., pp. 268-302). St Louis: Mosby.

Maurer, F. A. (2000a). Teenage pregnancy. In C. M. Smith & F. A. Maurer (Eds.), *Community health nursing: Theory and practice* (2nd ed., pp. 641-671), Philadelphia: W. B. Saunders.

Maurer, F. A. (2000b). Violence: A social and family problem. In C. M. Smith & F. A. Maurer (Eds.), *Community health nursing: Theory and practice* (2nd ed., pp. 571-606). Philadelphia: W. B. Saunders.

Moore, M. C. (2000). Maternal and fetal nutrition. In D. L. Lowdermilk, S. E. Perry, & I. M. Bobak (Eds.), *Maternity & women's health care* (7th ed., pp. 353-379). St. Louis: Mosby.

Nichols, A. N., & Lowdermilk, D. L. (2000). Infertility. In D. L. Lowdermilk, S. E. Perry, & I. M. Bobak (Eds.), *Maternity & women's health care* (7th ed., pp. 206-224). St. Louis: Mosby.

Pappas, A., & Hakala, K. L. D. (2001). Violence in the community. In M. A. Nies & M. McEwen (Eds.), *Community health nursing: Promoting the health of populations* (3rd ed., pp. 596-623). Philadelphia: W. B. Saunders.

Saunders, R. B. (2000). Nursing care during pregnancy. In D. L. Lowdermilk, S. E. Perry, & I. M. Bobak (Eds.), *Maternity & women's health care* (7th ed., pp. 380-428). St. Louis: Mosby.

Sherwen, L. N., Scoloveno, M. A., & Weingarten, C. T. (1995). *Nursing care of the childbearing family* (2nd ed.). Norwalk, CT: Appleton & Lange.

U.S. Department of Health and Human Services (USDHHS). (1990). *Healthy people 2000: National health promotion and disease prevention objectives.* Washington, DC: Government Printing Office.

U.S. Department of Health and Human Services (USDHHS). (1995). *Healthy people 2000: Midcourse review and 1995 revisions.* Washington, DC: Government Printing Office.

U.S. Department of Health and Human Services (USDHHS). (2000). *Healthy people 2010: Conference edition.* Washington, DC: Government Printing Office.

U.S. Department of Health and Human Services/ Office of Disease Prevention and Health Promotion (USDHHS/ODPHP). (1998). *Clinician's handbook of preventive services* (2nd ed.). Washington, DC: Government Printing Office.

Vaughn, V. C., McKay, R. J., & Behrman R. E. (Eds.), and Nelson, W. E. (Senior Ed.), (1979). *Textbook of pediatrics* (11th ed.). Philadelphia: W. B. Saunders.

Wong, D. L. (1999). *Whaley & Wong's nursing care of infants and children* (6th ed.). St. Louis: Mosby.

www.wbsaunders.com/SIMON/McEwen **SIMON**

Health Promotion and Illness Prevention for Elders

objectives

Upon completion of this chapter, the reader will be able to:

1. Discuss the impact of changing demographics and the "Aging of America" on the health care delivery system and explain why it is important to promote the health of this population.

2. Describe the parameters to be assessed in older adults, including assessment of physical health, health history, functional ability, cognitive and mental state, and nutritional status.

3. Explain the importance of promoting functional independence and give examples of related interventions.

4. Discuss health-promotion and illness-prevention guidelines for older adults including recommendations on immunizations, safety concerns, and elder abuse.

5. Recognize common health problems in older adults and give examples of interventions for each.

6. Discuss care assistance arrangements for older adults, including nursing homes, home health agencies, adult day care, and respite care.

key terms

Activities of daily living (ADL)
Adult immunization
Alzheimer's disease
Care assistance

Cognitive impairment
Elder abuse
Functional independence
Hearing deficit
Incontinence

Instrumental activities of daily living (IADL)
Polypharmacy
Vision deficit

See Glossary for definitions.

case study

Frank Jefferson is a registered nurse (RN) working in a senior health clinic in a small city. The clinic provides comprehensive, integrated, and systematic care for individuals aged 65 years and older. In addition to three RNs, the clinic employs two physicians, two nurse practitioners, a dietitian, a pharmacist who specializes in geriatrics, laboratory and radiology technicians, and a social worker. Services are individualized and clients are seen in the clinic, at home, or in the hospital, as warranted.

On Friday, Frank sees Mr. Peterson, a 75-year-old retired postal worker, for his annual physical examination. Mr. Peterson lives with his wife in a small house not far from the clinic. Five years earlier, Mr. Peterson had a mild heart attack and was hospitalized for several days. He has been hospitalized on two other occasions: 10 years previously for a cholecystectomy and a year ago for prostate surgery. He takes daily medication for hypertension, a multivitamin, and 325 mg of aspirin. He has occasional bouts of constipation that he states are relieved with over-the-counter laxatives. Mr. Peterson has no physical limitations, drives without difficulty, and wears glasses.

Physical findings show that his weight is unchanged from 1 year ago, blood pressure is 138/86, pulse rate is 76 beats per minute and regular, and respiration rate is 20 breaths per minute. In accordance with guidelines from the U.S. Preventative Services Task Force, Mr. Peterson is given a complete physical examination, including a complete blood count with a blood lipid profile, an electrocardiogram (ECG), and test for fecal occult blood. Mr. Peterson reports no problems with depression and, because his mental and cognitive states are appropriate, no formal assessments are performed. According to clinic records, Mr. Peterson had received a pneumococcal immunization 3 years earlier. Because it was the beginning of the influenza season, he is offered a flu shot, for which he consents.

Physical examination reveals a relatively healthy older adult. Blood pressure appears controlled, the ECG shows no new changes, and the fecal occult blood test is negative. The eye examination, however, shows some degree of cataract formation and Mr. Peterson is referred to an ophthalmologist. In addition, several small lesions are detected on his hands and face, so he is referred to a dermatologist for evaluation.

Health teaching performed by Frank and other members of the clinic staff focuses on diet and physical activity, prevention of falls, signs and symptoms of heart attack, and warning signs of cancer. Before Mr. Peterson left, Frank gave him a flu shot, informing him that the results of the blood tests would be available early the next week and that he would call with the results.

In 1900, people over 65 years of age constituted 4% of the population; by 2000, that proportion increased to 12.65%. With the increasing number of baby boomers, it is projected that by the year 2030, the proportion of those over age 65 may reach 22%. Additionally, the most rapid population increase over the next decade is expected to be among those over age 85 years (U.S. Department of Health and Human Services [USDHHS], 2000).

A major goal for the health of the nation is to increase the years of healthy life for all Americans. For older adults, achievement of *Healthy People 2010* objectives will be confirmed by the visibility of active elders who continue to make a valuable contribution to all aspects of community life. Seeking to improve the health and limiting disabilities of older Americans

are key components of *Healthy People 2010*. The *Healthy People 2010* table presents examples of related objectives.

Because of the complex and unique health needs of the aging population and the anticipated growth in this aggregate and the resulting impact on the health care delivery system, all nurses should be knowledgeable about health care needs of elders. To offer a better understanding of this population, Box 12-1 presents some facts about older Americans.

Chronic health problems are common among older persons. Indeed, almost 80% of those 70 years of age and older have at least one chronic health problem and most have multiple problems (National Center for Health Statistics [NCHS], 1999). Arthritis and other orthopedic impairments, hypertension, hearing loss, heart

healthy people **2010**

Examples of Objectives for Older Adults

OBJECTIVE	BASELINE (1998)	TARGET
2.9: Reduce the overall number of cases of osteoporosis	10%	8%
3.12a: Increase the proportion of adults 65 years of age and older who have received a fecal occult blood test within the preceding 2 years	34%	60%
6.11: Reduce the proportion of people with disabilities who report not having the assistive devices and technology needed	NA	NA
7.12: Increase the proportion of older adults who have participated during the preceding year in at least one organized health-promotion activity	12%	90%
12.6b: Reduce hospitalizations of adults between 75 and 84 years of age with heart failure as the principal diagnosis	26.9 per 1000	13.5 per 1000
14.5b: Reduce invasive pneumococcal infections in adults 65 years of age and older	62 per 100,000	42 per 100,000
14.29a: Increase the proportion of adults aged 65 years and older who are vaccinated annually against influenza	63%	90%
15.28a: Reduce hip fractures among females 65 years of age and older	1121 per 100,000	491 per 100,000
18.14: Increase the number of states, territories, and the District of Columbia with an operational mental health plan that addresses mental health crisis interventions, ongoing screening, and treatment services for elderly persons	24 states	50 states and the District of Columbia
21.4: Reduce the proportion of older adults (aged 65 to 74 years) who have had all their natural teeth extracted	26%	20%
24.2c: Reduce hospitalizations for asthma among adults aged 65 years and older	19.3 per 10,000	10 per 10,000
28.15: Increase the number of people who are referred by their primary care physician for hearing evaluation and treatment	NA	NA

From Department of Health and Human Services (2000). *Healthy people 2010: Conference edition.* Washington, DC: Government Printing Office.

conditions, and visual impairments are the most common chronic conditions among older adults. The extent of chronic conditions associated with aging is illustrated in Table 12-1. These conditions, in turn, are often accompanied by functional disabilities.

Improving functional independence through prevention or control of chronic illnesses, such as heart disease, cancer, stroke, chronic obstructive pulmonary disease, arthritis, and osteoporosis, and conditions associated with aging (i.e., vision and hearing impairments, incontinence, dementia), is a goal for all older adults. Promoting regular, moderate physical activity (e.g., walking,

gardening, swimming) can help control or limit chronic conditions. Enhanced clinical services directed at prevention of illnesses, such as immunization against pneumonia and influenza, and screening for cancer and heart disease can help prevent serious conditions and may provide early diagnosis and referral for prompt treatment when they are detected. In addition, enhanced primary care can assist in the management of chronic problems such as hypertension, arthritis, and diabetes. See the Research Highlight "Physician Visits and Prescription Medications Increase for Elders." Improving social networks can promote independence and reduce social isolation, thereby

BOX 12-1 Facts About the Elderly

LIFE EXPECTANCY AND POPULATION TRENDS

The life expectancy at birth for Americans is almost 79 years.

Persons 65 years of age can expect to live for 18 more years.

Persons aged 85+ years, America's "oldest old," increased almost 38% and constitute the most rapidly growing segment of the population.

By 2040, the United States may have more persons aged 65 and older than persons younger than 20 years of age.

LIVING PATTERNS

Most men older than 65 years live with their wives (75%).

Many women older than 65 years are widows (45%).

Less than 5% of the older population is institutionalized at any given time; however, about one in four older adults will spend some time in a nursing home during the last years of their lives.

California, New York, Florida, Pennsylvania, and Texas have the greatest numbers of older adults. Florida, Iowa, West Virginia, and Arkansas have the greatest percentages of older adults, and populations are rising most dramatically in Nevada, Alaska, Hawaii, and Arizona.

More than 66% of the elderly live in a family setting; about 31% live alone.

RETIREMENT AND INCOME

About two thirds of American workers retire before age 65 and spend more than 20% of their lives in retirement.

Social Security benefits are the major source of income for the elderly, providing more than half of the monthly income for the majority of recipients.

HEALTH AND HEALTH CARE

The leading causes of death for persons aged 65 years and older are (in order): heart disease, cancer, cerebrovascular accident, chronic obstructive pulmo-nary disease, pneumonia/influenza, diabetes, and accidents.

Elderly persons use 32% of all prescription medications.

Adults over 65 years of age average about 6.5 visits to a physician annually.

Medicare is the major source of payment for health care of the elderly and pays approximately 93% of hospital costs for this population.

Data from McEwen, M., & Davis, L. (2001). Senior health. In M. A. Nies & M. McEwen (Eds.), *Community health nursing: Promoting the health of populations* (3rd ed.). Philadelphia: W. B. Saunders.

TABLE **12-1** Most Prevalent Chronic Conditions Among Older Americans: Prevalence per 1000 People

CONDITION	AGE 65 TO 74 YEARS	AGE 75+ YEARS
Arthritis/gout	477	562
Hypertension	361	352
Heart conditions (including ischemic heart disease and heart rhythm disorders)	272	404
Hearing impairment	257	415
Orthopedic impairment	162	222
Cataracts	126	226
Chronic sinusitis	158	160
Diabetes	114	105
Visual impairment	71	112
Tinnitus	85	96

From National Center for Health Statistics (NCHS). (1994). Current estimates from the National Health Interview Survey, 1992. *Vital and Health Statistics*, Series 10, p. 189. Washington, DC: Government Printing Office.

Research Highlight

Physician Visits and Prescription Medications Increase for Elders

In 2001, the Centers for Disease Control and Prevention (CDC) issued a report on a nationwide study on primary health care usage by older Americans. This study revealed that between 1985 and 1999 physician visits for those 65 years of age and older increased by more than 20%, while visits by younger Americans stayed the same or, for some age groups, even declined. The increase was primarily for physicians specializing in internal medicine and cardiology and was largely attributed to the growing population of seniors. The following data are among the findings:

- About 33% of office visits by older adults were for acute problems.
- About 33% of office visits by older adults were for chronic problems.

- Preventative care comprised 16% of office visits.
- Diagnostic and screening services were provided at 75% of office visits.
- Therapeutic and counseling services (i.e., weight management, smoking cessation, and injury prevention) were provided at 33% of office visits.
- During the same time (1985 to 1999), physicians prescribed 33% more medications for seniors. In 1999, at two thirds of the office visits, one or more prescriptions were provided to clients. Drugs used to treat hypertension were the most frequently prescribed medications. Others also frequently prescribed were medications to treat arthritis, depression, asthma, and erectile dysfunction.

From Centers for Disease Control and Prevention (CDC). (2001). *Physician visits increase for older patients; doctors prescribe more medications for patients of all ages.* Retrieved 8/14/01 from http://www.cdc.gov/od/oc/media/pressrel/r010717.htm.

---

decreasing depression, nutritional deficits, and other related conditions associated with aging.

Nurses practicing in community settings frequently have an opportunity to work with older people and their families and to address these and related issues. This chapter describes tools for assessment of older adults, materials for health education, and resources for organizations that work with the elderly.

ASSESSMENT OF OLDER ADULTS

The Standards of Gerontological Nursing Practice require regular assessment in a comprehensive, accurate and systematic manner (American Nurses' Association [ANA], 1995). A comprehensive assessment should include gathering information on the individual's physical health, health history, functional ability, cognitive and mental state, and nutritional status. Consistent with use of the nursing process in other areas, interventions should be based on assessment findings and anticipated or potential threats to the health and well-being of the client.

GENERAL ASSESSMENT

A thorough health history is necessary to learn as much about the client as possible to discover issues and problems that might need attention and to assign priority. Most agencies have health history tools and assessment guides available for collecting this information. Minimal information should include the following (Luggen, 1996):

- Biographical data (name, age, date of birth, sex, race)
- Informant identification (self, relative, friend)
- Chief complaint (reason the client is seeking help)
- History of present illness (onset, location, and severity of symptoms; treatment or control methods; precipitating factors; associated symptoms)
- Past history (allergies, drug reactions, past illnesses, hospitalizations, current prescription and over-the-counter medications)
- Family history (diseases, particularly heart disease, diabetes, tuberculosis [TB], hypertension, arthritis, and cancer, in near relatives—parents, siblings, children)

- Psychosocial history (marital status; occupation; retirement history; current life situation; nutritional history; alcohol, smoking, or drug use; immunization history; education; leisure and exercise activities)
- Review of symptoms (history of concerns, symptoms or illnesses such as cardiovascular system [palpitations, murmur, hypertension], gastrointestinal system [nausea, abdominal pain, hemorrhoids], neurological problems [headache, syncope, seizures], and psychiatric problems [depression, memory loss, insomnia])
- Functional capacity (activities of daily living [ADL], such as bathing, toileting, feeding) and instrumental activities of daily living [IADL], such as driving, using the telephone, preparing meals)

Use of a comprehensive assessment tool that elicits essential information from clients regarding cognition, social support, financial status, and psychological health and physical health should be encouraged. The Comprehensive Older Person's Evaluation (COPE) tool (Appendix 12-A at the end of the chapter) is an example of one such tool. Use of a tool of this type can be valuable in ensuring that all factors that affect health are addressed.

COMMON HEALTH PROBLEMS

The process of aging results in several physical changes that contribute to development of chronic illnesses and conditions. Nurses who frequently care for older adults in community settings should assist in detection of unusual or abnormal findings during the assessment process. Table 12-2 presents some of the most common health problems encountered in older people, including etiology, symptoms, risk factors, identification, and clinical management.

NUTRITION

When assessing nutritional status in older people, the nurse must recognize physical changes and other factors that can influence dietary intake. Table 12-3 describes some factors and potential clinical manifestations. Nurses

who routinely work with older clients should assess for signs of nutritional deficiencies and develop interventions to minimize or eliminate them.

Several warning signs may indicate poor nutritional health. These include the presence of a disease or chronic condition (i.e., depression or diabetes) that changes the way the individual eats or makes it difficult to eat; missing, loose, or rotten teeth or dentures that do not fit well; economic hardship; reduced social contact; multiple medicines; involuntary weight loss or gain; needing assistance with IADL; and very old age (80+) (American Association of Retired Persons [AARP], 2001).

Interventions for nutritional deficits might include referral to a variety of providers or community resources that address the identified problem. For example, the nurse may obtain a referral for Meals on Wheels if the client is not able to cook or may obtain assistance for dental care or dentures for clients with missing teeth. Nutrition education is vitally important and the nurse might suggest the use of dietary supplements and tips on how to manage constipation.

PROMOTING FUNCTIONAL INDEPENDENCE

Functional independence refers to the extent to which the individual (in this case, the older adult) is able to complete normal and IADL without assistance from others. **Activities of daily living (ADL)** generally include bathing, dressing, eating, getting in and out of bed and chairs, walking, going outside, and toileting. The ability to perform necessary functions of life, such as taking transportation, preparing meals, shopping, and using the telephone, are examples of **instrumental activities of daily living (IADL)**. Managing money and accomplishing routine housework are additional examples.

In older adults, functional impairment can be caused by cognitive, physical, social, and/or psychological disorders. It is estimated that about

Text continued on p. 314

TABLE **12-2** Common Health Problems in Later Maturity

DISEASE/CONDITION	DEFINITION	RISK FACTORS	SIGNS/SYMPTOMS	MANAGEMENT/TREATMENT
CARDIOVASCULAR SYSTEM				
Coronary artery disease (CAD); angina	Progressive obstruction of blood flow through one or more coronary arteries caused by a build-up of plaque (cholesterol and lipids) on interior artery walls	Age (increases with age), gender, race, and genetic inheritance; elevated serum lipids, hypertension, smoking, obesity, diabetes, stress, sedentary lifestyle	Substantial chest pain that may radiate to the left arm, neck, jaw, or shoulder; tachycardia or bradycardia; apprehension; dyspnea; diaphoresis; nausea and vomiting; syncope; fatigue	Dependent on degree of damage and physical findings *Diagnosis:* history and physical, chest radiograph, ECG, serum enzyme levels, serum lipids, stress test, echocardiogram *Medication:* nitroglycerin (sublingual, patches, or ointment), beta-blocking agents, calcium channel blockers, antithrombotic therapy *Surgery:* coronary artery angioplasty or coronary artery bypass graft when indicated
Congestive heart failure (CHF)	Condition of altered cardiac function in which cardiac output is insufficient to meet demands of tissue metabolism	Age, hypertension, arteriosclerosis, CAD, other heart and lung conditions (arrhythmia, pneumonia, mitral stenosis, endocarditis)	Rales (crackles), difficulty breathing, tachypnea, confusion, insomnia, agitation, depression, nausea, anorexia, dyspnea, orthopnea, weight gain, bilateral ankle edema	*Medication:* digitalis, diuretics Other interventions: reduction in sodium intake, bed rest
Arrhythmias	Cardiac conduction irregularities characterized by chaotic electrical activity	Age, hypertension, CAD, valvular heart disease, CHF, diabetes, pulmonary embolus, hyperthyroidism	Irregular pulse, tachycardia, palpitations, light-headedness, fatigue, dyspnea, syncope, angina	Avoidance of risk (ethanol, caffeine, nicotine), management of underlying disease, prevention of complications (embolus) *Medication:* control ventricular rate (beta blockers, calcium channel blockers, cardiac glycosides), anticoagulants *Surgery:* surgical or invasive methods when appropriate (pacemaker implantation, implantable defibrillator)

Peripheral vascular disease (atherosclerotic occlusive disease)	Obstruction or narrowing of the arteries causing interruption of blood flow to extremities (most commonly to feet and legs)	Complication of atherosclerosis, smoking, hyperlipidemia, diabetes, hypertension, and physical stress	Intermittent claudication, diminished or absent pulses, affected limb is cold and pale	Smoking cessation, foot and limb care, exercise program, weight control, cholesterol management, management of diabetes; *Surgery:* bypass surgery, angioplasty, stent placement, amputate if necessary

RESPIRATORY SYSTEM

Chronic obstructive pulmonary disease (COPD)	Consists of chronic bronchitis (increased mucus production and recurrent cough), emphysema (destruction of interalveolar septa)	Cigarette smoking, passive smoking, aging, air pollution, occupational exposure, severe viral pneumonia early in life	*Chronic bronchitis:* cough, sputum production, frequent infections, dyspnea, cyanosis, wheezing, diminished breath sounds *Emphysema:* minimal cough, scant sputum, dyspnea, weight loss, occasional infections, barrel chest, use of accessory muscles of respiration, pursed-lip breathing, diminished breath sounds	Smoking cessation, aggressive treatment of infections, treat reversible bronchospasm, pulmonary rehabilitation, avoidance of cold weather *Medication:* anticholinergics, theophylline, corticosteroids, bronchodilators, expectorants; supplemental oxygen when necessary
Asthma	Reversible airway disease characterized by bronchial constriction, mucosal edema, and increased mucus production	Allergic factors (pollens, molds, dust mites, animal dander), smoke and other pollutants, viral infections, exercise, family history	Abnormal pulmonary function tests, wheezing, cough, prolonged expiration, hyperresonance, decreased breath sounds, nocturnal dyspnea, cyanosis, use of accessory respiratory muscles	*Medication:* steroids, beta-agonists, anticholingerics, theophylline; monitoring of peak expiratory flow (PEFR); identify and eliminate irritants
Pneumonia	Acute inflammation of the lungs caused by bacterial, viral, fungal, chemical, or mechanical agents; most commonly caused by viral or bacterial infection in adults	Age, viral infection, alcoholism, immunosuppression, smoking, COPD, diabetes, malnutrition, general anesthesia, malignancy, mechanical ventilation, altered LOC	Cough; fever; chest pain; chills; dark, thick, or bloody sputum; anorexia; anxiety; chest dull to percussion; crackles (rales); cyanosis; diminished breath sounds; dyspnea; pleuritic pain; rhonchi; tachypnea; tachycardia; weakness	*Medication:* antibiotic therapy; bed rest; in severe cases, oxygen therapy, mechanical ventilation, chest physiotherapy when necessary

continued

Data from Dambro, M. R. (1996). *Griffith's 5-minute clinical consult.* Baltimore: Williams & Wilkins; Eliopoulos, C. (1993). *Gerontological nursing* (3rd ed.). Philadelphia: J. B. Lippincott; Luggen, A. S. (1996). *Core curriculum for gerontological nursing.* St. Louis: Mosby; Murray, R., Zentner, J., & Pinnell, N. (1993). *Assessment and health promotion for the person in later maturity.* In R. B. Murray & J. P. Zentner (Eds.), *Nursing assessment and health promotion: Strategies through the life span* (5th ed., pp. 542–603). Upper Saddle River, NJ: Prentice Hall.

TABLE **12-2** Common Health Problems in Later Maturity—cont'd

DISEASE/CONDITION	DEFINITION	RISK FACTORS	SIGNS/SYMPTOMS	MANAGEMENT/TREATMENT
RESPIRATORY SYSTEM—cont'd				
Tuberculosis (TB)	Caused by infection with *Mycobacterium tuberculosis*; causative organism may invade any organ but usually develops in the lungs	Human immunodeficiency virus (HIV) infection, homelessness, institutionalization (i.e., correctional or other facility), chronic conditions such as diabetes, renal failure, malnutrition, close and prolonged exposure to an infected individual	Productive cough, hemoptysis, fever, night sweats, weight loss, pleuritic pain, fatigue	*Medication:* based on diagnostic testing; prophylaxis with isoniazid (INH) for positive purified protein derivative (PPD) skin test for 9 months; for active disease, three antiTB drugs for 6 to 12 months; careful monitoring of client and condition to ensure compliance with medication regimen
MUSCULOSKELETAL SYSTEM				
Osteoporosis	Progressive bone loss predisposing to atraumatic fractures, particularly of vertebra, upper femur, distal radius, humerus, and ribs; in women, may be from excessive and prolonged acceleration of bone resorption following menopausal loss of estrogen secretion	Gender (more common in women), age, family history, inadequate calcium and vitamin D intake, sedentary lifestyle, alcohol use, caffeine, smoking, steroid use, chemotherapy, radiation therapy	Acute or chronic back pain, kyphosis, scoliosis, atraumatic fractures, loss of height, absence of peripheral bone deformities	Weight reduction if appropriate; increase calcium intake to 1500 mg/day; avoid excess phosphate or protein intake; encourage ambulation and exercise; avoid exercise that increases compression and mechanical stress on spine *Medication:* hormone replacement therapy (estrogen/progesterone), synthetic calcitonins
Osteoarthritis	Degeneration of articular cartilage and hypertrophy of bone; leading cause of disability in elderly affecting between 33% and 90% of those over age 65; caused by biomechanical, biochemical, inflammatory, and immunological factors	Age, obesity, prolonged occupational or sports stress, injury	Slowly developing joint pain, pain following use of joint, stiffness (particularly in the morning), joint enlargement, decreased range of motion, possibly joint tenderness, local pain, and stiffness	Weight reduction, fitness program, heat, physical therapy, protection of joints *Medication:* nonsteroidal antiinflammatory agents, corticosteroids *Surgery:* may be indicated with advanced disease (joint replacement, debridement, osteotomy)

GENITOURINARY TRACT

Prostate conditions	Benign prostatic hyperplasia (BPH) is the benign growth of the prostate, which may result in bladder outlet obstruction; possibly arises from hormonal alterations associated with aging	Gender (male), age, family history	*Obstructive symptoms:* decrease in force of urine stream, hesitancy, postvoid dribbling, incomplete bladder emptying, overflow incontinence, urinary retention, inability to voluntarily stop stream *Irritative symptoms:* frequency, nocturia, urgency, urge incontinence *Other symptoms:* hematuria, distended bladder, enlarged prostate, renal failure from obstruction	*Medication:* alpha-adrenergic antagonist, hormonal agents *Surgery:* transurethral resection of prostate (TURP), open prostatectomy, other procedures

GASTROINTESTINAL TRACT

Periodontal disease (gingivitis)	Degeneration of tissues supporting the teeth; more than 80% of older adults have moderate periodontal disease and 50% of adults over age 65 have lost some teeth from tooth decay or periodontal disease	Malnutrition, aging, inadequate plaque removal, diabetes, poor dental hygiene, faulty dental restoration, irritation by faulty bridges or partial dentures)	Mouth odor, gum swelling, redness and bleeding, loose teeth, tooth loss	Removal of irritating factors (plaque, faulty dentures), promoting good oral hygiene, regular dental check-ups, smoking cessation *Medication:* antibiotic therapy sometimes indicated in severe cases
Diverticulitis (diverticular disease)	*Diverticulum of colon:* herniation of colon mucosa through the muscular layer; more common in sigmoid and distal colons *Diverticulitis:* an abscess or inflammation initiated by the rupture of a mucosal abscess; incidence increases with age; present in 40 to 50% of older population (aged 60 to 80 yr)	Low-fiber diet, defects in colon wall strength, age (>40 yr), low-residue diet, family history	*Diverticulosis:* 10 to 25% of individuals with diverticula have symptoms, pain, diarrhea, constipation, a palpable mass in the left iliac fossa; abdomen may be distended; no signs of peritoneal inflammation *Diverticulitis:* pain (acute, localized in left lower quadrant), fever, anorexia, nausea, vomiting, constipation or diarrhea, rebound tenderness, abdomen distended and tympanic, bowel sounds depressed	Nothing by mouth (NPO) status during acute diverticulitis; all clients with diverticula should increase dietary fiber intake *Medication:* oral treatment with antibiotics, analgesics *Surgery:* colon resection when indicated

continued

TABLE **12-2** Common Health Problems in Later Maturity—cont'd

DISEASE/CONDITION	DEFINITION	RISK FACTORS	SIGNS/SYMPTOMS	MANAGEMENT/TREATMENT
GASTROINTESTINAL TRACT—cont'd				
Constipation	Decrease in frequency from usual bowel elimination pattern or difficulty in defecating	More common with age, sedentary lifestyle, electrolyte abnormalities, concomitant illness, inadequate fluid intake, inadequate fiber or bulk, side effects of drugs, chronic abuse of laxatives; psychiatric, cultural, emotional, and environmental factors	Less frequency of bowel movements than the client perceives as normal (typically 3 to 5 times/wk), change in baseline defecating pattern, smaller stools than normal, impaction of stool, difficulty expelling feces from the rectum, painful evacuation, sensation of incomplete emptying of bowel, abdominal fullness	Encourage measures to improve bowel habits, routine time for toileting, avoid straining, respond to urge to defecate, daily physical exercise, increase fluid intake, increase dietary fiber *Medication:* bulk-forming agents (Metamucil, Citrucel), laxatives, stool softeners, lubricants (mineral oil), suppositories, cathartics, enemas
ENDOCRINE SYSTEM				
Diabetes	Noninsulin-dependent diabetes (NIDDM) (type II diabetes) accounts for 70 to 80% of all cases; hyperglycemia and glucose intolerance from defects in insulin secretion and peripheral insulin action; almost 50% of elderly may have glucose intolerance	Family history, obesity, age	Polyuria, polydipsia, and polyphagia (however, classical symptom triad may be absent in NIDDM); weight loss; constipation; numbness and tingling in peripheral extremities; diminished peripheral pulses; headache; weakness; fatigue; frequent infections; abnormal plasma glucose levels	Combination of diet management (increased complex carbohydrate intake; decreased fat intake; avoidance of alcohol); weight loss when appropriate; regular exercise; home monitoring of blood or urine glucose; careful instruction on self-monitoring for, and management of, complications *Medication:* oral hypoglycemic agents of insulin when necessary if conservative measures fail to control glucose levels
NEUROLOGICAL SYSTEM				
Alzheimer's disease	Degenerative organic mental disorder characterized by progressive brain	Family history, age, head trauma, low education level, Down syndrome	Progressive cognitive impairment lasting 3 to 20 years; three stages: early, middle, late	

	Cause	Signs and Symptoms	Interventions
	deterioration and dementia; usually occurs at age 65 years or older; cause unknown, although there is genetic predisposition (50% of all clients have a positive family history); other theories include excessive amount of an amyloid protein (beta-amyloid peptide), which is destructive to brain tissue; a virus; exposure to metals (particularly aluminum and mercury); an autoimmune disorder; and acceleration in aging	*Early (2 to 4 yr):* recent memory loss, forgets routine tasks, is distractible, forgets names or events, gets lost in familiar surroundings, has difficulty telling time and making decisions, is easily angered and aware of losses. *Middle (2 to 5 yr):* client has increased memory loss, may not recognize friends and family; wanders, confabulates; is preoccupied with thoughts; is immodest; experiences bowel and bladder incontinence; has decreased ability to understand and express language; has flat affect; has hallucinations and delusions; becomes suspicious *Late (1 to 3 yr):* inability to perform ADL, little response to stimuli, loss of body weight, seizures, loss of bodily functions	
Parkinson's disease	Neurodegenerative disorder of extra-pyramidal system; characterized by a combination of tremor at rest, rigidity, and bradykinesia; cause unknown, although probably the result of exposure to a toxic or infectious agent, or loss of dopamine neurons	Age; slightly more common in males	Rhythmic tremors of fingers, feet, lips, and head, with progressive rigidity of facial and trunk muscles; characteristic sign is shuffling gait while client is leaning forward at the trunk	Maintain activity to highest degree possible, use cane for walking, avoid tension and frustration, minimize emotional upsets; physical and occupational therapy may be indicated *Medication:* levodopa, dopamine agonists, monoamine oxidase (MAO) inhibitors, anticholinergics

continued

TABLE **12-2** Common Health Problems in Later Maturity—cont'd

DISEASE/CONDITION	DEFINITION	RISK FACTORS	SIGNS/SYMPTOMS	MANAGEMENT/TREATMENT
NEUROLOGICAL SYSTEM—cont'd				
Cerebrovascular accidents (CVAs)	Sudden onset of a focal neurological deficit resulting from infarction or hemorrhage within the brain. The second leading cause of death of people over 72 years of age.	Age, arteriosclerosis, hypertension, smoking, diabetes, family history	Symptoms depend on the site of CVA *Carotid (hemispheric):* hemianesthesia, aphasia, visual field defects, headache, seizure, amnesia, confusion *Vertebrobasilar (brainstem or cerebellar):* diplopia, vertigo, ataxia, facial paresis, dysphagia, dysarthria, impaired level of consciousness, behavioral changes	Maintain oxygenation; monitor cardiac rhythm; control hypertension; promote physical therapy, occupational therapy, and speech therapy when indicated *Medication:* antithrombotic measures (heparin, Coumadin, aspirin) *Surgery:* carotid endarterectomy when indicated
SENSORY DISORDERS				
Cataract	Clouding or opacity of lens; may be congenital, related to metabolic or systemic conditions, or traumatically induced; most commonly associated with aging ("senile" cataract) *Acute:* (closed-angle) (~10% of cases) *Chronic:* (open-angle) (~90% of cases)	Aging; exposure to ultraviolet B rays	Blurred vision, problems with visual acuity in bright light or at night, falls, or accidents; lens opacity on eye examination; pupil may appear cloudy or white	*Surgery:* removal of cataract if visual impairment produces symptoms that interfere with lifestyle or occupation or pose risk of injury; in most cases, the cataract is replaced by a plastic intraocular lens
Glaucoma	Damage to optic nerve and loss of visual field and visual acuity associated with high intraocular pressure	*Acute:* small cornea, Native Alaskan/Inuit ancestry, hyperopia, use of antidepressants or anticholinergics, cataract *Chronic:* positive family history, diabetes, African-American	*Acute:* severe eye pain, blurred vision, halos around lights, nausea and vomiting, elevated intraocular pressure *Chronic:* none until advanced, then gradual loss of peripheral vision, headaches, misty vision	*Acute:* medical emergency *Medication:* carbonic anhydrase inhibitors, hyperosmotic agents (e.g., mannitol) to lower pressure *Surgery:* peripheral iridotomy or iridotomy if glaucoma not managed through medication *Chronic:* *Medication:* used singly or in combination include topical beta-adrenergic blockers, carbonic anhydrase inhibitors, cholinergic agents *Surgery:* may be necessary if medical management is not successful

Hearing loss	Hearing loss may be complete or partial; may be classified as conductive or sensorineural. *Conductive:* cerumen impaction, perforation of tympanic membrane, serous otitis media, damage to ossicles, thickening of the tympanic membrane, growth of skin into middle ear. *Sensorineural:* noise induced (most common cause of hearing loss), acoustic tumor, Meniere's disease, heredity, congenital, viral, medication toxicity, or presbycusis (related to aging)	Eustacian tube obstruction, exposure to loud noise levels for extended periods; ototoxic medications; heredity; aging	Difficulty hearing (may be gradual or sudden); other symptoms include tinnitus, dizziness, pain, and blockage; otoscopy may reveal abnormalities; audiometry tests for pure tone and/or impedance (middle ear pressure) may indicate loss	*Conductive:* cerumen impaction—remove with suction and irrigation or use of a wire curet; serous otitis: decongestants; surgery if hearing loss persists; other conditions: tympanic membrane perforation, damaged ossicles, and thickening of eardrum may need surgical correction. *Sensorineural:* depending on etiology, client may require surgical correction (tympanoplasty, stapedectomy) or use of assistive devices (hearing aids, telephone enhancement aids)

MENTAL HEALTH

Depression	Clinical syndrome characterized by lowered mood, difficulty thinking, and somatic changes precipitated by feeling of loss (incidence higher in women) or guilt; between 10% and 65% of elderly may suffer from depression; it may be biochemical, genetic, or a deficiency in neurotransmitters, or situational (highest rate in persons with physical ailments)	Prior episode or diagnosis of depression, history of suicide attempt, lack of social support, stressful life events, gender, family history, substance abuse, alcoholism, chronic disease, chronic pain, retirement, age	Client reports depressive feelings, poor appetite, sleep disorder (insomnia or hypersomnia), fatigue, restlessness, irritability, withdrawal, lack of interest or lack of desire to seek pleasure, poor self-image, poor memory, inability to make decisions, suicidal thoughts. *Note:* in elderly, disorientation, memory loss, and distractibility may be signs of depression rather than dementia	Counseling or psychotherapy, often combined with antidepressants; in extreme cases, electroconvulsive therapy may be beneficial

TABLE **12-3** Factors That May Affect Nutrition in Later Maturity

FACTOR AND PROCESS	EFFECT	CLINICAL MANIFESTATION
INGESTION		
Loss of teeth; poor dentures; atrophy of jaws	Improper mastication; deletion of important foods from diet	Irritable bowel syndrome; constipation; malnutrition
Dietary habits	Overeating; eccentric diets	Obesity; malnutrition
Psychological losses and changes; changes in social environment; lack of socialization	Poor appetite	Anorexia; weight loss
Reduced income; difficulty with food preparation and ingestion	Excessive ingestion of carbohydrates	Obesity; malnutrition
Decreased fluid intake	Dry feces	Impacted stools
DIGESTION AND ABSORPTION		
Decreased secretion of hydrochloric acid and digestive enzymes	Interference with digestion	Dietary deficiencies
Hepatic and biliary insufficiency	Poor absorption of fats	Fat-soluble vitamin deficiency; flatulence
Atrophy of intestinal mucosa and musculature	Poor absorption; slower movement of food through intestine	Vitamin and mineral deficiencies; constipation
Decreased secretion of intestinal mucus	Decreased lubrication of intestine	Constipation
METABOLISM		
Impaired glucose metabolism and use	Diabetic-like response to glucose excesses	Hyperglycemia; hypoglycemia
Decrease in renal function	Inability to excrete excess alkali	Alkalosis
Impaired response to salt restriction	Salt depletion	Low-salt syndrome
Decline in basal metabolic rate	Lower caloric requirements, but same amount of food eaten	Obesity
Changes in iron and calcium (phosphorus, magnesium) metabolism	Iron deficiency; increased requirements for calcium	Anemia; demineralization of bone; osteoporosis
Changes in vitamin metabolism	Deficiency in vitamins K and C especially	Peripheral neuropathy, sensorimotor changes; easy bruising and bleeding tendencies

From Murray, R. B., Zentner, J. P., Pinnell, N. N., & Boland, M. H. (2001). Assessment and health promotion for the person in later adulthood. In R. B. Murray & J. P. Zentner (Eds.), *Nursing assessment and health promotion: Strategies through the life span* (7th ed.). Upper Saddle River, NJ: Prentice Hall.

20% of those over 70 years of age have difficulty performing at least one ADL (e.g., bathing, eating, dressing). Additionally, about 10% have difficulty performing at least one IADL (e.g., making meals, shopping, cleaning) (NCHS, 1999). The percentage of persons needing help with ADL increases significantly with age, rising from 15% for ages 65 to 69 years to 50% for those over age 85 years. Similarly, the percentage of persons needing help with IADL increases with age to approximately 55% by age 85 years.

Several objectives of *Healthy People 2010* address screening and referral of elderly clients for threats to functional independence (see the

Healthy People 2010 table earlier in the chapter). Areas specifically targeted include the following:
- Hearing deficits
- Vision deficits
- Cognitive impairment
- Depression
- Urinary incontinence

It is essential that all nurses working with older populations recognize potential threats and limitations to functional independence and associated health problems. Tools, health information, and teaching tips to prevent or manage threats to functional independence are described next.

HEARING DEFICITS

Some 33% of individuals aged 65 years and over, and more than half of those over age 85 years, have some degree of **hearing deficit** (USDHHS, 2000). As a result of embarrassment or frustration, hearing loss in the elderly can contribute to social isolation, depression, and exacerbation of coexisting psychiatric problems. The most common types of hearing loss and associated factors are the following:
- Presbycusis (most common in older adults): results from changes in the inner ear with aging and is manifested by slow decline in hearing ability
- Tinnitus: a symptom that results in auditory ringing or roaring; may be caused by cerumen, infection, aspirin, certain antibiotics, or a nerve disorder
- Conductive hearing loss: results from fluid in the middle ear, abnormal bone growth, or middle ear infection
- Sensorineural hearing loss: results form damage to parts of the inner ear or auditory nerve; may be from birth defects, head injuries, tumors, illnesses, certain prescription drugs, hypertension, or stroke (National Institute on Aging [NIA], 1999).

All older adults should be questioned about signs of hearing loss. If hearing loss is suspected or confirmed following questioning, the nurse should perform pure-tone testing using an audi-ometer (USDHHS/Office of Disease Prevention and Health Promotion [ODPHP], 1998).

Clients with evidence of hearing loss should be referred to a specialist because medical or surgical treatment may improve or restore hearing function. Hearing aids, when appropriate, are prescribed by specialists. Nurses in community settings, however, may be in a position to assist the client in exploring resources to help obtain a hearing aid and to instruct in its proper use and maintenance. See the Health Teaching box "Guidelines for Communicating with the Hearing-Impaired Person."

VISION DEFICITS

Vision loss in adults is common and the prevalence increases with age. It is estimated that more than 90% of older people require the use of corrective lenses and approximately 18% of all older people have significant visual deficits (NCHS, 1999). Cataracts, glaucoma, macular degeneration, and diabetic retinopathy often cause visual problems in the elderly. Loss of vision, in turn, may result in trauma from falls, automobile crashes, and other injuries and may significantly affect quality of life (USDHHS/ODPHP, 1998). Because most **vision deficits** can be successfully managed through medical or surgical treatment or use of corrective lenses, early detection and prompt treatment are very important.

A comprehensive eye examination, including screening for visual acuity and glaucoma, should be performed yearly for individuals aged 65 years and over. Use of a standard Snellen wall chart or a tumbling "E" chart at 20 feet is used for basic screening. The client should wear corrective lenses, if prescribed, during screening.

To determine the impact of visual impairment, the nurse should question the client regarding limitations to normal and IADL associated with poor vision. For example, the nurse might ask, "Does your vision make it difficult for you to feed yourself, read medication labels, groom yourself, handle money, or find your way around places outside of your home?" Determining whether the

health teaching

Guidelines for Communicating with the Hearing-Impaired Person

Do not start to speak to a hard-of-hearing person abruptly. Attract his or her attention first by facing the person and looking straight into the eyes. If necessary, touch the hand or shoulder lightly. Help him or her grasp what you are talking about right away by starting with a key word or phrase, for example, "Let's plan our weekend now" or "Speaking of teenagers...." If he or she does not understand you, do not repeat the same words. Substitute synonyms: "It's time to make plans for Saturday," and so on.

If the person to whom you are speaking has one good ear, always stand or sit on that side when you address him or her. Do not be afraid to ask a person with an obvious hearing loss whether he or she has a good ear and, if so, which one it is. The person will be grateful that you care enough to find out.

Facial expressions are important clues to meaning. Remember that an affectionate or amused tone of voice may be lost on a hard-of-hearing person.

In conversation with a person who is especially hard-of-hearing, do not be afraid occasionally to jot down key words on paper. If he or she is really having difficulty in understanding you, the person will be grateful for the courtesy.

Many hard-of-hearing persons, especially teenagers who hate to be different, are unduly sensitive about their disability and will pretend to understand you even when they do not. When you detect this situation, tactfully repeat your meaning in different words until it gets across.

Teach the family to avoid use of candles. Electric light gives the person a better chance to join the conversation because he or she can see the lips during conversation. Similarly, in choosing a restaurant or night club, remember that dim lighting may make lipreading difficult.

Teach family members that they do not have to exclude the hard-of-hearing person from all forms of entertainment involving speech or music. Concerts and operas may present problems, but movies, plays, ballets, and dances are often just as enjoyable to people with a hearing loss as to those with normal hearing. (Even profoundly deaf persons can usually feel rhythm and many are good and eager dancers.) For children, magic shows, pantomimes, and the circus are good choices.

When sending a telegram to someone who does not hear well, instruct the telegraph company to deliver your message, not telephone it.

The speech of a person who has been hard-of-hearing for years may be difficult to understand because natural pitch and inflection are the result of imitating the speech of others. To catch such a person's meaning more easily, watch the face while he or she talks.

Do not say such things as "Why don't you get a hearing aid?" or "Why don't you see a specialist?" to a person who is hard-of-hearing. Chances are he or she has already explored these possibilities and there is no need to emphasize the disability.

Use common sense and tact in determining which of these suggestions apply to the particular hard-of-hearing person you meet. Some persons with only a slight loss might feel embarrassed by any special attention you pay them. Others whose loss is greater are profoundly grateful for it.

From Murray, R., Zentner, J., & Pinnell, N. (1993). Assessment and health promotion for the person in later maturity. In R. B. Murray & J. P. Zentner (Eds.), *Nursing assessment and health promotion: Strategies through the life span* (5th ed., pp. 542-603). Upper Saddle River, NJ: Prentice Hall.

client is using visual assistance devices, such as glasses, contact lenses, magnifying lenses, or large print books, can be beneficial in recognizing the degree of adaptation. After a complete assessment, the nurse should refer clients with signi-

ficant changes in visual acuity or visual acuity of 20/40 or less with corrective lenses to an eye care specialist for further evaluation (USDHHS/ODPHP, 1998). In addition to identifying clients with visual difficulties and referring them for

health teaching

Guidelines for Helping the Blind Person

Talk to the blind person in a normal tone of voice. The fact that he or she cannot see is no indication that hearing is impaired.

Be natural when talking with a blind person.

Accept the normal things that a blind person might do such as consulting the watch for the correct time, dialing a telephone, or writing his or her name in longhand without calling attention to them.

When you offer assistance to a blind person, do so directly. Ask, "May I be of help?" Speak in a normal, friendly tone.

In guiding a blind person, permit him or her to take your arm. Never grab the blind person's arm, for he or she cannot anticipate your movements.

In walking with a blind person, proceed at a normal pace. You may hesitate slightly before stepping up or down.

Be explicit in giving verbal directions to a blind person. There is no need to avoid the use of the word "see" when talking with a blind person.

When assisting a blind person to a chair, simply place his or her hand on the back or arm of the chair. This is enough to give location.

When leaving the blind person abruptly after conversing with him or her in a crowd or where noise may obstruct hearing, quietly advise the person that you are leaving so that he or she will not be embarrassed by talking when no one is listening.

Never leave a blind person in an open area. Instead, lead him or her to the side of a room, to a chair, or some landmark from which he or she can obtain direction.

A half-open door is one of the most dangerous obstacles that blind people encounter.

When serving food to a blind person who is eating without a sighted companion, offer to read the menu, including the price of each item. As you place each item on the table, call attention to food placement by using the numbers of an imaginary clock. ("The green beans are at 2 o'clock.") If he or she wants you to cut up the food, he or she will tell you.

Be sure to tell a blind person who the other guests are so that he or she may know of their presence.

From Murray, R., Zentner, J., & Pinnell, N. (1993). Assessment and health promotion for the person in later maturity. In R. B. Murray & J. P. Zentner (Eds.), *Nursing assessment and health promotion: Strategies through the life span* (5th ed., pp. 542-603). Upper Saddle River, NJ: Prentice Hall.

follow-up treatment, the nurse may be able to help the client obtain needed treatment, visual aids (magnifying lenses, portable lights, large print books), or corrective lenses. See the Health Teaching box "Guidelines for Helping the Blind Person."

COGNITIVE IMPAIRMENT

Some degree of **cognitive impairment** is common among older individuals and often increases with age. An estimated 5% to 10% of individuals older than 65 years of age and almost 50% of those over 85 years of age experience some degree of mental impairment (USDHHS/ODPHP, 1998). Alzheimer's disease, vascular infarctions, and pharmaceuticals are frequently implicated as inducing cognitive changes.

Screening for cognitive function should include orientation, short-term memory, receptive and expressive language ability, attention, and visual-spatial ability. Use of a short screening instrument, such as the Mini Mental State Examination (Figure 12-1) may be helpful in eliciting important information quickly. If cognitive impairment is noted, consultation with family members and referral to a specialist may be indicated.

In regard to care of individuals with cognitive impairments, Alzheimer's disease is of particular concern for nurses who routinely work with the elderly. According to Selkoe (1992), Alzheimer's disease accounts for almost 56% of causes of dementia in older adults, followed by stroke (14.5%), multiple causes (12.2%), Parkinson's disease (7.7%), and other causes (9.9%).

Mini Mental Status Examination Sample Items

Orientation to Time

"What is the date?"

Registration

"Listen carefully,

I am going to say three words.

You say them back after I stop.

Ready? Here they are...

HOUSE (pause), CAR (pause), LAKE (pause).

Now repeat those words back to me."

[Repeat up to 5 times, but score only the first trial.]

Naming

"What is this?"

[Point to a pencil or pen.]

Reading

"Please read this and do what it says."

[Show examinee the words on the stimulus form.]

CLOSE YOUR EYES

Figure 12-1 Mini Mental State Examination sample items. (Reproduced by special permission of the Publisher, Psychological Assessment Resources, Inc., 16204 North Florida Avenue, Lutz, Florida 33549, from the Mini Mental State Examination, by Marshal Folstein and Susan Folstein, Copyright © 1975, 1998 by Mini Mental LLC, Inc. Published 2001 by Psychological Assessment Resources, Inc. Further reproduction is prohibited without permission of PAR, Inc. The Mini Mental State Examination can be purchased from PAR, Inc. by calling 800-331-8378 or 813-968-3003.)

Alzheimer's disease is a degenerative mental disorder characterized by progressive brain deterioration, resulting in impaired memory and in thought and behavioral changes. The Community Application box "Alzheimer's Disease" presents a review of the risk factors, manifestations, and clinical management. Box 12-2 lists current statistics and should be helpful to nurses who work with older people to understand the scope and significance of the problem.

COMMUNITY APPLICATION
Intervention Guidelines for Alzheimer's Disease

Direct goals toward helping the client experience the highest possible physical, emotional, intellectual, and social functions for as long as possible.

Client and caregiver education should focus on:

Manifestations of the disease
Stages and progression of the disease (what to expect)
Pharmacologic management (provide information on clinical drug trials)
Behavioral management
Provision of a consistent routine
Avoid chemical or physical restraints
Communication strategies
Simple commands and directions
Monitoring for acute illnesses and effects of medications

Caregiver and client counseling and referral should include:

Locating community resources
Legal/financial issues
Durable power of attorney
Conservatorship or guardianship
Establishment of trusts
Advance directives and living will
Financial assistance
Medicare
Medicaid
Long-term care insurance
Social Security Disability Insurance
Supplemental Security Income
Long-term care options (i.e., home care, respite care, nursing homes, Alzheimer's disease units)
Family and social support
Management of stress and lifestyle changes

Data from American Association of Retired Persons. (1993). *Coping & caring: Living with Alzheimer's disease.* Washington, DC: American Association of Retired Persons; Lukacs, K. (1996). Neurological/Alzheimer's disease. In A. S. Luggen (Ed.), *Core curriculum for gerontological nursing* (pp. 564-580). St. Louis: Mosby.

BOX 12-2 Alzheimer's Disease: Statistics

Approximately 4 million Americans have Alzheimer's disease and 14 million Americans will have it by the year 2050 unless a cure or prevention is found.
Alzheimer's disease is the fourth leading cause of death among adults.
One in 10 persons over age 65 and nearly half of those over 85 have Alzheimer's disease.
A person with Alzheimer's disease lives an average of 8 years after the onset of symptoms.
More than 70% of people with Alzheimer's disease live at home with care provided by family and friends.

Half of all nursing home patients have Alzheimer's disease or a related disorder that costs between $42,000 and $70,000 per person per year.
Alzheimer's disease is the third most expensive disease in the United States after heart disease and cancer.
The average lifetime cost of Alzheimer's disease per client is $174,000; neither Medicare nor private health insurance covers the long-term care most clients need.

Modified from Alzheimer's Disease Association. (2000). *Alzheimer's disease statistics.* Chicago, Alzheimer's Disease Association. Retrieved 8/14/01 from http://www.alz.org/hc/overview/stats.htm.

DEPRESSION

Depression in older adults causes distress and suffering and leads to mental and physical impairments and social isolation (USDHHS/ National Institute of Mental Health [NIMH], 1999). Although depression is common in older adults, it is often missed, untreated, or undertreated because as a person ages, the signs of depression are likely to be overlooked or ignored. Confusion or attention problems caused by depression can mimic Alzheimer's disease or other brain disorders. In addition, mood changes and other signs of depression can be caused by medications (NIA, 2000).

Depression is one of the most prevalent conditions among older adults and symptoms include feelings of despair, irritability, fatigue, and loneliness (Phillips, 2000). In addition, depression rates are highest among older adults who have a physical health problem. Indeed, between 8% and 20% of older adults in the community and up to 37% of older adults in health care institutions experience symptoms of depression (USDHHS/NIMH, 1999). To assess for depression, older adults should be evaluated for the following (NIA, 2000):

- Feelings of sadness and anxiety
- Tiredness and lack of energy
- Loss of interest in everyday activities
- Sleep problems
- Problems with eating and weight
- Crying
- Difficulty focusing, remembering, and making decisions
- Feelings of helplessness
- Irritability
- Thoughts of death or suicide

Counseling and antidepressants can assist in alleviating many of the symptoms of depression. Medications should be managed with care, however, because side effects, drug-drug interactions, comorbidities, and barriers to compliance may exist (USDHHS/NIMH, 1999).

Along with depression, older adults are at risk for suicide. In the United States, suicide rates increase dramatically with age. Indeed, older white men have a suicide rate more than six times that of the general population and individuals 65 years of age and older account for 20% of all suicides. Furthermore, the suicide rate for individuals 85 years of age and older is the highest in the country (USDHHS/NIMH, 1999).

Efforts to prevent depression in older adults should be encouraged. For example, grief counseling for widows and widowers and promoting participation in self-help groups can ameliorate depression and improve social adjustment.

Additionally, counseling and pharmacological treatment can be effective.

INCONTINENCE

Incontinence (the involuntary loss of urine) is a significant cause of disability and dependency in older adults. An estimated 10% to 15% of noninstitutionalized elderly persons experience urinary incontinence, which contributes to social isolation, embarrassment, feelings of loss of control, and low self-esteem (Lashley, 1995; NIA, 1996). Despite its prevalence, urinary incontinence is widely underdiagnosed and underreported. Reasons cited include lack of education about the condition on the part of health care providers and shame or embarrassment on the part of these individuals (USDHHS/Agency for Health Care Policy and Research [AHCPR], 1992).

The most common types of urinary incontinence are the following:

- Stress incontinence (most common): involuntary loss of urine associated with movements that put pressure on the bladder (e.g., exercise, coughing, sneezing, laughing, and lifting heavy objects)
- Urge incontinence: involuntary urine leakage before reaching a toilet; most often found in those with enlarged prostate, diabetes, infection, stroke, dementia, Parkinson's disease, multiple sclerosis, or those taking certain pharmaceuticals
- Overflow incontinence: involuntary urine leakage from an overdistended bladder; usually from urethral obstruction in older men and uterine prolapse in older women
- Functional incontinence: urine leakage that occurs in older adults who have a hard time getting to the toilet because of restricted mobility (NIA, 1999)

According to the Urinary Incontinence Guideline Panel, treatment can improve or cure most clients (USDHHS/AHCPR, 1992, p. xi). Following an intensive study, this panel recommended a vigorous information campaign targeting the public and health professionals about the problem, including effects, causes, and treatment options.

To comply with their recommendations, health care providers should routinely ask older clients about problems with bladder control using an open-ended question such as, "Do you have trouble with your bladder?" or "Do you have trouble holding your urine (water)?" If urinary incontinence is identified by questioning, detection of an odor, visualization of wetness, or client complaint, and if it represents a problem for the client or caregiver, further evaluation is needed.

A thorough health history should include questions regarding elimination patterns. Diagnosis is based on physical examination, measurement of postvoid residual volume, and urinalysis. Blood testing may be done to assess renal function and rule out diabetes. Treatment options are related to etiology and include a variety of behavior techniques, pharmacological therapy, surgery, or a combination of these.

HEALTH PROMOTION AND ILLNESS PREVENTION

Although health-promotion and illness-prevention interventions for older adults can be very beneficial in reducing death and disability and in improving quality of life, the health care system has not systematically encouraged or provided preventative health services for this population. Most older adults seek out medical care only in response to illness and are unlikely to see health care providers when they have no symptoms. They rely on health care professionals to recommend preventative tests and screenings. Because older clients may be unaware of activities that would improve their health and well-being, it is incumbent on providers in various community settings to seek opportunities to provide health teaching, perform screenings, and encourage other preventative services.

PREVENTATIVE SERVICES GUIDELINES

Healthy People 2010 encourages providers to improve access to primary care; to work to remove barriers to preventative care; and to provide clients with prescribed screening, counseling, and immunization services. The recommendations for screening and counseling for older adults from the U.S. Preventative Services Task Force are presented in Table 12-4.

Health care providers who routinely work with older clients should be familiar with these guidelines and should be prepared to perform the suggested assessments, laboratory tests, counseling, and immunizations as appropriate. Health professionals or specialists for referral should be determined in advance and mechanisms for timely, systematic, and streamlined care by specialists through interagency and interdisciplinary collaboration and communication should be strongly encouraged.

IMMUNIZATION RECOMMENDATIONS

Although primary prevention through immunization against a variety of illnesses is strongly encouraged (if not mandated) for children, immunization recommendations for older adults are often overlooked. As a result, deaths from vaccine-preventable diseases are quite common among older people. For example, approximately 90% of influenza deaths occur in individuals 65 years of age or older, particularly older adults with underlying health problems, such as pulmonary or cardiovascular disorders (USDHHS/ODPHP, 1998).

Improving the immunization status of Americans older than 65 years is addressed by several of the objectives of *Healthy People 2010* (see the *Healthy People 2010* box earlier in the chapter). The Immunization Practices Advisory Committee recommends that all older adults should have completed a primary series of diphtheria and tetanus toxoids (Centers for Disease Control and Prevention [CDC], 2000). In addition, a single dose of pneumococcal polysaccharide vaccine and annual vaccination against influenza should be strongly encouraged for all adults over age 65, particularly those with preexisting chronic health conditions. Table 12-5 summarizes **adult immunization** recommendations.

TABLE **12-4** Preventative Services Task Force Recommendations for Screenings, Service, and Referral for Older Adults

RISK FACTOR	PREVENTION TARGET CONDITION	PREVENTATIVE SERVICE AND/OR REFERRAL
Persons ages ≥50 years	Colorectal cancer	Fecal occult blood test; sigmoidoscopy
All perimenopausal and postmenopausal women	Osteoporosis	Hormone replacement counseling; nutritional counseling; exercise counseling
	Coronary heart disease	Obesity screening; blood pressure screening; cholesterol screening; nutritional screening; exercise counseling; smoking cessation counseling; aspirin therapy (if indicated)
Persons ≥60 years	Thyroid dysfunction	Thyroid function tests
Persons age ≥65 years	Influenza	Influenza vaccine
	Pneumococcal disease	Pneumococcal vaccine
	Tetanus	Check for last tetanus booster
	Visual problems including glaucoma	Snellen acuity test; referral for glaucoma screening
	Hearing impairment	Question regarding hearing
Persons >70 years with one or more of the following risk factors: psychoactive, antihypertensive or cardiac medication; impaired cognition, balance, or strength	Falls	Counsel regarding home safety; assess vision; counsel regarding polypharmacy; assess for cognitive/functional impairment

From U.S. Department of Health and Human Services/Office of Disease Prevention and Health Promotion (USDHHS/ODPHP). (1998). *Clinician's handbook of preventive services* (2nd ed.). McLean, VA: International Medical Publishing.

SAFETY CONCERNS FOR OLDER ADULTS

Several objectives from *Healthy People 2010* concerning older adults relate to safety. The document specifically addresses injuries from falls and poisoning caused by drug interactions and inadvertent overdosing. Additionally, encouraging health care providers to identify, treat, and refer victims of elder abuse is discussed as a component of the objectives to decrease violent and abusive behaviors.

FALLS

Falls are the second leading cause of death from injury for people aged 65 and older and, in 1997, more than 9000 elderly persons died as a result of falls (USDHHS, 2000). Falls and fall-related injuries are of special concern in older adults because of the severity of injuries combined with longer recovery periods and resultant threats to long-term health and functioning. In addition to the immediate pain and disability caused by the injury, falls are associated with loss of confidence in ability to function independently, restriction of

TABLE **12-5** Immunizations Recommended for Adults

VACCINATION	RECOMMENDED GROUP(S)
Tetanus/diphtheria	All adults should be screened and given boosters every 10 years
Influenza	Adults 50+; other adults in high-risk groups (e.g., those with chronic illnesses, health care providers)
Pneumococcal vaccine	Adults 65+: one dose; those who received pneumococcal vaccine before age 65 should be revaccinated if it has been more than 5 years since the first vaccine
Hepatitis B	Adults from high-risk groups (e.g., persons with occupational risk, hemodialysis patients, household contacts of those infected with hepatitis B virus [HBV], men who have sex with men)
Varicella	Any person without a reliable history of varicella disease or vaccination or who is seronegative for varicella
Measles/mumps/rubella	Anyone born after 1956 without written documentation of immunization on or after the first birthday should be given at least one dose; health care personnel born after 1956 who are at risk of exposure to clients with measles should have documentation of two doses of vaccine on or after their first birthday
Hepatitis A	Adults from high-risk groups (e.g., persons traveling to or working in countries with high or intermediate endemicity of infection; men who have sex with men; persons with chronic liver disease)

From Centers for Disease Control and Prevention (CDC). (2000). *Summary of adolescent/adult immunization recommendations.* Retrieved 8/14/01 from http://www.cdc.gov/nip/recs/adult-schedule.pdf.

physical and social activities, increased dependence, and increased need for long-term care.

Fall-related injuries contribute to 5.3% of all hospitalizations for those 65 years and older and falls account for nursing facility placement in 40% of the population seeking institutionalization (Meiner and Miceli, 2000). About one third of all elderly people have reported a fall during the previous 12 months.

Most falls occur in the home, although 30% to 40% occur in public places. Although most falls do not result in serious injury, between 5% and 15% of those who fall sustain fractures or other significant injuries. Fracture of the hip, femur, humerus, wrist, and ribs are the most common severe injuries from falls (Eliopoulos, 1997).

A number of risk factors for falling have been identified. Nurses working with older adults in any setting should be aware of risk factors for falls and should direct interventions accordingly. Intrinsic factors that contribute to falls include

(Meiner and Miceli, 2000; Stone and Chenitz, 1991):

- Age-related changes in vision, posture, and gait
- Emotional/mental state (agitated, depressed, rushed, distracted, confused, anxious)
- Weakness
- Fear of incontinence
- Denial of illness
- Pain
- Podiatric conditions (ingrown toenails, corns, bunions)
- Adjusting to a new environment (i.e., recent move, recent admission, transfer)
- Diagnosis of conditions that affect stability, mobility, and cognitive functions
- Alcohol
- Medications (e.g., sedatives/hypnotics, tricyclic antidepressants, antihypertensive agents, analgesics, and diuretics)

Extrinsic or environmental factors that may contribute to falls in elders include inappropriate lighting (i.e., dark, dim, glare, shadows); uneven, wet walking surfaces; inadequate handrails and poor step design on stairways; and furniture that is too low, too soft, or tips easily. In the bathroom, a slippery tub or shower and lack of rails for the tub or toilet often cause falls. Other factors include clothing that is too long or loose or shoes that are too large or have soles that are smooth and slippery (Meiner and Miceli, 2000; Stone and Chenitz, 1991). See the Health Teaching box "Guidelines for Prevention of Falls in the Home."

COMPLIANCE WITH MEDICATION

Another threat to the safety of older people is the use and misuse of medications. Elders consume approximately 35% of all prescription medications and, as a result, they are at risk for adverse drug reactions. Reactions are commonly from such factors as normal aging changes that affect absorption, metabolism, and excretion of drugs in the body; conditions that affect the body's response to drugs (i.e., bed rest, dehydration, stress); and the use of multiple drug regimens to treat concurrent health problems (Maurer, 2000a).

It is estimated that 25% to 30% of elderly persons are not compliant with their medication regimens (Maurer, 2000a). Nurses who work with older clients should be aware of factors that contribute to medication noncompliance, anticipate and recognize actual and potential problems, and be prepared to intervene. Box 12-3 provides a list of factors that can contribute to medication misuse. See the Community Application box "Barriers to Compliance."

Polypharmacy refers to the prescribing of multiple drugs for a client; it is a fairly common practice that affects many older people. Both prescription and nonprescription medications contribute to problems encountered in polypharmacy. To avoid problems associated with use of multiple medications, the nurse should perform the following:

- Help the client make and maintain a list of all prescription and over-the-counter medications, including purpose, dosage, frequencies, dates of use, and side effects.

- Simplify the medication regimen as much as possible.
- Ensure that the client brings all medications when seeing a practitioner.
- Evaluate potential medication interactions whenever a new medication is prescribed.
- Inform the client about possible side effects and symptoms of toxicity and explain what to do in the event of an occurrence.
- Use a medication box that can be filled weekly and distribute the medications based on the day (e.g., Sunday through Saturday) and time of day (morning, noon, evening, before bed).

ELDER ABUSE

Elder abuse refers to neglect, physical injury, or exploitation that results in harm to an older adult. As a result of widespread underreporting, the incidence of elder abuse is difficult to determine. One source estimates that 5% to 10% of older Americans are victims of abuse and neglect each year (Ballard, 2000). According to another source, more than one million cases of elder abuse occur each year in the United States (Maurer, 2000b). Elder abuse can take on several forms. The most common types of elder abuse are listed in Table 12-6.

It is estimated that only 8% to 25% of cases of elder abuse are reported. Clark (1999) cites the following reasons for failure to report abuse:
- Reluctance of older people to admit that their child or loved one might abuse them
- Love for abuser
- Dependence on the abuser
- Fear of further injury
- Inability to report the abuse

Further, health care providers may neglect to report elder abuse, often because of failure to recognize the problem, ignorance of their legal responsibilities to report suspected cases, and failure to adequately assess at-risk situations (Maurer, 2000b).

In most cases, the abuser is a caregiver, either a close family member or provider in a nursing home. Among family members, the spouse is most often the abuser (65% of cases), followed by

health teaching

Guidelines for Prevention of Falls in the Home

LIGHTS AND LIGHTING

1. Eyes tire quickly in improper lighting. Illuminate reading material or the object worked on. Illuminate steps, entranceways, and rooms before entering. Use 70- or 100-watt bulbs, not 60-watt bulbs.
2. Avoid glaring light caused by highly polished floors or large expanses of uncovered glass. Use sunglasses to avoid the glare of highway driving, but use light tints or photoray lenses.
3. Allow more time to adjust to changes in light levels. When going from a dark to a light room or vice versa, allow a minute or two for the eyes to accommodate to the change in light before proceeding.
4. Dirty glasses or outgrown prescription lenses inhibit vision. Keep glasses clean. Have regular eye examinations to identify changes and to get new glasses when needed. If possible, do not use bifocals when walking because you cannot see the ground clearly.
5. Ability to see up, down, and sideways decreases with age. Observe the lay of the land; learn to look ahead at the ground to spot and avoid hazards such as cracks in the side-walks. Use canes, walking sticks, and walkers that are prescribed.
6. At night, keep a nightlight on in your bedroom and bathroom. When getting out of bed at night, put the light on and wait a minute or two for the eyes to adjust before getting up. Have a telephone in the bedroom so you don't have to get out of bed to answer the phone. Before you go out in the evening or late afternoon, turn a light on for your return.

ACTIVITY

1. Get up from a chair slowly.
2. When getting out of bed, sit up, then wait a minute or two. Move to the side of the bed and wait another minute. Rise after you have sat for a few minutes.
3. If you are dizzy, sit down immediately. Sit on a step or a chair, or ease yourself to the sidewalk if you are outdoors.

4. Avoid tipping the head backward (extending the neck). Activities to avoid that extend the neck are washing windows, hanging clothes, and getting things from high shelves.
5. Use shelves at eye level. Avoid rapid turning of the head.
6. If weather is rainy and windy, avoid going out.
7. Use alcohol and tranquilizers with caution.
8. Exercise programs keep bodies limber. Consult your physician and then enroll in a senior exercise program.
9. Shoes and slippers should be flat and rubber-soled. Avoid clothing such as long robes and loose-fitting garments that may catch on furniture or door knobs.

AROUND THE HOUSE

1. Avoid scatter rugs and small bathroom mats that can slide. Repair loose, torn, wrinkled, or worn carpet.
2. Avoid slick, high polish on floors.
3. Put things in easy reach and avoid reaching to high shelves.
4. Use nonskid treads on stairs and nonskid mats in tub.
5. Install a grab rail in the bath, shower, and also by the toilet as needed.
6. Install handrails on both sides of the stairs. Paint stair edge in bright contrasting color.
7. Remove door thresholds.
8. Remove low-lying objects, such as coffee tables and extension cords.
9. Wipe up spills immediately.
10. Watch for pets underfoot and scattered pet food.
11. Check for even, nonglare lighting in every room, with easily accessible light switches.
12. Avoid floor coverings with complex patterns.
13. Avoid clutter in living areas.
14. Select furniture that provides stability and support, such as chairs with arms.
15. Check walking aids routinely, such as rubber tips on canes and screws on walkers.

From Chenitz, W. C., Kussman, H. L., & Stone, J. T. (1991). Preventing falls. In W. C. Chenitz, J. T. Stone, & S. A. Salisbury (Eds.), *Clinical gerontological nursing: A guide to advanced practice* (pp. 309-328). Philadelphia: W. B. Saunders.

BOX 12-3 Factors That Interfere with Medication Regimen Compliance in Elders

Physiologic changes associated with aging affecting absorption, metabolism, and excretion of drugs

Lack of knowledge or information about the reason for taking the medication and the prescribed regimen; stopping the medication when symptoms subside

Inaccessibility to pharmacy services

Problems with self-administration, such as failure to take the medication as prescribed, inability to open drug containers, forgetfulness, vision problems

Multiple prescriptions or related medications for the same condition from different providers

Lack of financial resources to purchase necessary medications (medications are not covered by Medicare)

Complexity of drug regimens and volume of drugs needed

Desire to avoid unpleasant side effects

Fear of drug dependency

Failure to discard discontinued or outdated medications

Sharing of prescription medications with spouse or others

Failure to report self-medication with over-the-counter drugs

Interactions between different medications

Data from Eliopoulos, C. (1993). *Gerontological nursing* (3rd ed., pp. 271-276). Philadelphia: J. B. Lippincott; Graves, M. (1988). Drug use and abuse. In M. O. Hogstel (Ed.), *Nursing care of the older adult* (2nd ed.). New York: John Wiley & Sons; Lashley, M. E. (1995). Elderly persons in the community. In C. M. Smith & F. A. Maurer (Eds.), *Community health nursing: Theory and practice.* (pp. 719-746). Philadelphia: W. B. Saunders.

TABLE **12-6** Types of Elder Abuse

TYPE OF ABUSE	EXAMPLE
Physical	Beating, slapping, rape and sexual molestation, murder
Confinement	Use of physical or chemical (sedatives) restraints, confinement to bed
Psychological or emotional	Verbal assault, isolation, exclusion, threats of abuse or abandonment, insults, humiliation, intimidation
Financial or material	Taking resources and possessions without consent; forcing or coercing elders to sign over properties and possessions
Neglect	Withholding food, adequate clothing, shelter, health care, or medications; deprivation of dentures or eyeglasses; failure to assist with ADL; abandonment; neglect may be passive or active
Abandonment	Desertion of elder by an individual who is the primary care taker or person who has assumed responsibility for providing care

Data from Ballard, D. (2000). Legal and ethical issues. In A. G. Lueckenotte (Ed.), *Gerontologic nursing* (2nd ed., pp. 34-62). St. Louis: Mosby; Pappas, A., & Hakala, K. L. D. (2001). Violence in the community. In M. Nies & M. McEwen (Eds.), *Community health nursing: Promoting the health of population* (pp. 596-623). Philadelphia: W. B. Saunders.

children (25% to 30% of cases). Risk factors common to victims of elder abuse include the following:

- The victim's dependency on the caregiver (physical, emotional, or financial)
- Confusion
- Incontinence
- Frailty
- Illness
- Mental disabilities

Characteristics of the abuser (Maurer, 2000b) include the following:

- A previous history of violence
- Being overwhelmed by the burden of providing care
- Feelings of frustration and resentment

Whenever working with older people in community or long-term settings, nurses should be aware of indicators of possible elder abuse and should direct interventions accordingly. Indicators

COMMUNITY APPLICATION
Barriers to Compliance and Interventions to Prevent and Treat Noncompliance in Elderly Clients

Barriers to Compliance	Nursing Intervention
Client-Related	
Impaired vision	Ask pharmacist to use large type on labels. Affix label on central axis. Use color-coding system.
Impaired hearing	Get client's attention before speaking. Speak clearly and slowly. Do not shout.
Impaired dexterity	Use nonchildproof medication container.
Memory loss	Write out medication schedule. Use compliance aids (medication boxes, medication calendars). Involve caregiver.
Social isolation	Suggest volunteer home visitor or telephone program.
Drug Therapy-Related	
Complex drug regimen	Work with physician and pharmacist to simplify schedule. Use compliance aids.
Cost of drugs	Suggest generic drugs. Discourage use of unnecessary nonprescription drugs. Suggest nondrug alternatives.
Health Professional-Related	
Inadequate knowledge about drug use	Provide specific detailed oral and written information about the drug regimen.
Diffidence of client toward health professionals	Ask about client's previous experience with health professionals. Allow time for questions and concerns.

From Hashizume, S. (1991). Home health care. In W. C. Chenitz, J. T. Stone, & S. A. Salisbury (Eds.), *Clinical gerontological nursing: A guide to advanced practice* (pp. 557-576). Philadelphia: W. B. Saunders.

may include (Campbell and Landenburger, 1996; Maurer, 2000b):

- Unexplained or repeated injury
- Discrepancies between injury and explanation
- Inappropriate use of medication (overuse or underuse)
- Fear of the caregiver
- Untreated wounds (decubitus ulcers)
- Evidence of poor care (an unclean or malnourished client)
- Withdrawal and passivity
- Failure to seek appropriate medical care
- Contractures resulting from immobility or restraints
- Unwillingness or inability of caregiver to meet the client's needs
- An unsafe home situation

In all states, nurses and other health care professionals have a legal responsibility to report suspected cases of elder abuse. Typically, the nurse would report possible cases to the adult protective services department of the area social services agency. According to Maurer (2000b), the state intervenes only in extreme cases.

Usually, interventions are directed at recognizing and reducing risks. Prevention activities for elder abuse are presented in the Community Application box "Elder Abuse Prevention." Referral to appropriate community agencies can assist in alleviating some of the stress of caregivers and thereby reduce the possibility of neglect and abuse. Respite care providers and adult day care centers can be used to allow the caregiver an opportunity to have

COMMUNITY APPLICATION
Elder Abuse Prevention

Each year hundreds of thousands of older persons are abused, neglected, and exploited by family members and others. Many victims are people who are older, frail, and vulnerable who depend on others to meet their most basic needs. According to adult protective services agencies, elder abuse increased 150% between 1986 and 1996. In response, the Administration on Aging recommended several prevention activities to address the problem of elder abuse. These include the following:

• Enhancing professional training through providing workshops for adult protective services personnel and other professional groups, by encouraging statewide conferences for all service providers with an interest in elder abuse, and developing training manuals, videos, and other materials for professional education

• Coordinating health service systems and service providers through creation of elder abuse hotlines for reporting, formation of statewide coalitions and task forces, and creation of local multidisciplinary teams and coalitions
• Providing technical assistance through development of policy manuals and protocols that outline the proper or preferred procedures for elder abuse protection, detection, and management.
• Enhancing efforts to develop public education campaigns including public service announcements, posters, flyers, and videos
• Supporting adult protective service agencies
• Providing crisis intervention and social and health services that older persons need

From Administration on Aging. (2000). *Elder abuse prevention.* Retrieved 8/14/01 from http://www.aoa.gov/factsheets/abuse.html.

time away from constant duty while providing supervision for the client. Meals on Wheels can assist in providing nutritious meals for individuals and senior citizens centers and state or local offices on aging can provide information and resources for older clients and their caregivers.

CARE ASSISTANCE FOR OLDER ADULTS

Only about 5% of older Americans reside in institutional settings (e.g., nursing homes) (Birchfield, 1996). The remainder live in their own homes, typically with their spouse or alone. If individuals have health problems or need assistance with normal or IADL, they may reside with someone who can assist them, usually a child, sibling, or other relative.

Whether the person lives at home or with someone else, many times assistance from an external organization or agency can be beneficial, even if not necessary. This **care assistance** might be temporary (e.g., home health care following hip replacement surgery) or more permanent (e.g., adult day care for a frail individual who lives with an adult child who is employed). Table 12-7 describes several types of community-based providers and agencies that assist in caring for older adults. Long-term care in a nursing home may ultimately be needed. See the Community Application box "Choosing a Nursing Home."

Referrals for assistance or services can be one of the most important interventions for nurses who work with older clients. The Resources box at the end of the chapter provides a collection of resources that can be used as a starting point for nurses in community settings. Each nurse, however, should assemble a list of local providers and services for quick referral for these individuals and their caregivers. For example, the nurse should have readily available the phone numbers for Meals on Wheels, a nearby respite care provider or adult day care center, and organizations that provide financial assistance to older people.

TABLE **12-7** Long- and Short-Term Care Providers and Facilities for Older Adults

SETTING/PROVIDER	CAREGIVERS	SERVICES
Home	Informal caregivers (spouses, children, neighbors)	Variable, depending on needs of the elder; assist with ADL, health care, meals
Home health agencies	Professional and paraprofessionals (nurses, therapists, aides)	Intermittent skilled nursing; various therapies; assistance with ADL, shopping, transportation, chores
Nursing homes (skilled nursing facilities and intermediate care facilities)	Professional and paraprofessionals (nurses, therapists, aides)	Skilled nursing, monitoring, various therapies, assistance with ADL, supervision as needed
Community-based services	Professional and volunteer staff	Preventative health care, on-site and delivered meals, legal and tax services, transportation, recreation
Adult day care	Professional, paraprofessional, and volunteer	Temporary care for elders who live at home with family or friends, but need supervision and assistance during the workday
Respite care	Professional, paraprofessional, and volunteer (friend/family)	Temporary care (few hours, day, week) for disabled or frail older person for the purpose of relieving the family or principal care provider
Housing services (retirement communities, assisted living board and care, halfway houses, congregate living)	Professional, paraprofessional	Services variable, based on individual need and functional ability; include room, meals, assistance with ADL, medication management, some protective oversight

Data from Evashwick, C. J. (1999). The continuum of long-term care. In S. J. Williams & P. R. Torrens (Eds.), *Introduction to health services* (5th ed., pp. 295-348). Albany, NY: Delmar Publishers; Richardson, H. (1995). Long-term care. In A. R. Kovner (Ed.), *Jonas's health care delivery in the United States* (5th ed., pp. 194-231). New York: Springer Publishing Co.

SUMMARY

The number and proportion of Americans over 65 years of age are growing at an astonishing rate. As a result, the United States needs many more health care professionals, particularly nurses, educationally prepared to work with older adults. In the case study, Frank provided nursing care in a senior health clinic and worked with clinic staff to address the many potential and actual health problems commonly found among elders. In addition, the client in this example was very typical of older adults seeking care in community settings.

Because most of the health care for elders is provided in community settings, nurses should be trained and equipped to manage care appropriately, focusing special attention on health promotion and illness prevention and recognizing the unique needs of this population. To help illustrate this important area of nursing, Box 12-4 creatively shows multiple roles and functions of the gerontological nurse.

KEY POINTS

- Because 22% of Americans will be older than 65 years by 2030, improving the health of and limiting disabilities in older adults are essential.
- Assessment of older adults should be comprehensive and include evaluation of physical health, health history, functional ability, cognitive and mental state, and nutritional status.

COMMUNITY APPLICATION
Choosing a Nursing Home

Approximately 1.5 million Americans reside in nursing homes, or about 5% of those 65 years of age or older. Choosing a nursing home is very difficult, and the Health Care Financing Administration (HCFA) presented the following 8-step process for this task:

Step 1: Talk to People You Trust—seek advice from family, friends, and health professionals (e.g., doctors, social workers, hospital discharge planners).

Step 2: Look at Options—various living arrangements offer different levels of care. Options include subsidized senior housing, assisted living arrangements, board and care homes, continuing care homes, and retirement communities.

Step 3: Gather Information—gather as much information about homes in the area as possible. Talk with healthcare professionals, ask friends, and look in the phone book. Also, speak with someone from the Long-term Care Ombudsman programs in the area and check Medicare's website. (See the Resources box at the end of the chapter for information on how to access this site from the book's website.)

Step 4: Evaluate Selection Factors—factors to consider include location, availability, staffing, acceptance of Medicare and Medicaid reimbursement, services and fees, religious and cultural preferences, and special needs.

Step 5: Paying for Care—paying for care is a major concern and several payment methods are possible. Medicare pays for some costs under certain circumstances; Medicaid pays most costs for people with limited income and assets. About half of nursing home residents pay costs from savings. Other possible sources are managed care plans, Medicare supplemental insurance, and long-term care insurance.

Step 6: Visit Nursing Homes—visit potential nursing homes, talk with staff and residents, and request a copy of the most recent inspection.

Step 7: Follow-up Visits—make several visits at different times of the day and on different days of the week. Critically examine the quality of life of the residents and the quality of care, nutrition, and safety.

Step 8: After Admission—ensure that you are treated with dignity and respect. Important issues include use of restraints, money management, privacy, respect of property, and guardianship and advance directives.

From U.S. Department of Health and Human Services/Health Care Financing Administration (USDHHS/HCFA). (2000). *Your guide to choosing a nursing home* (Publication No. HCFA-02174-B). Baltimore, MD: HCFA.

- Functional independence refers to the extent to which an individual is able to perform ADL and IADL without assistance from others.
- To promote functional independence, the nurse should identify and manage potential threats and limitations and associated health problems. Areas of assessment and intervention include hearing deficits, vision deficits, cognitive impairment, depression, and urinary incontinence.
- Health-promotion and illness-prevention guidelines adopted by the U.S. Preventative Services Task Force include recommendations on immunization, addressing safety concerns (falls and medication compliance), and assessment and intervention in elder abuse.
- Common health problems in older adults include cardiovascular conditions (CAD, CHF, peripheral vascular disease), respiratory diseases (chronic obstructive pulmonary disease, asthma), musculoskeletal problems (osteoporosis, arthritis), genitourinary conditions (prostate enlargement, incontinence), gastrointestinal problems, endocrine disorders (diabetes), neurological conditions (Alzheimer's disease, cerebrovascular accidents), sensory disorders (cataract, hearing impairment), and mental health problems (depression).
- Care assistance arrangements for older adults include nursing homes, home health agencies, adult day care providers, and respite care providers.

BOX 12-4 Functions of the Gerontological Nurse

Guide persons of all ages toward a healthy aging process
Eliminate ageism
Respect the rights of older adults and ensure that others do the same
Oversee and promote the quality of service delivery
Notice and reduce risks to health and well-being
Teach and support caregivers
Open channels for facing developmental tasks
Listen and support
Offer optimism and hope
Generate, support, implement, and participate in research
Implement restorative and rehabilitative measures
Coordinate services
Assess, plan, implement, and evaluate care in an individualized manner
Link services with needs
Nurture future gerontological nurses for advancement of the specialty
Understand the unique assets of each older individual
Recognize and encourage the appropriate management of ethical concerns
Support and comfort through the dying process
Educate to promote self-care and independence

From Eliopoulos, C. (1997). *Gerontological nursing* (4th ed.). Philadelphia: J. B. Lippincott.

Resources

General Aging

U.S. Department of Health and Human Services Administration on Aging
National Institute on Aging
Social Security Administration*

Social Issues

American Association of Retired Persons (AARP)†
Gray Panthers

Hearing Loss/Vision Impairment

National Institute of Deafness and other Communication Disorders
American Speech-Language-Hearing Association
Lions Club—Focus on Sight

Heart Disease and Stroke

American Heart Association
National Stroke Association
National Institute of Neurological Disorders and Stroke

Cancer

American Cancer Society
National Cancer Institute

Alzheimer's Disease

Alzheimer's Association

Parkinson's Disease

American Parkinson's Disease Association

Arthritis

Arthritis Foundation
National Institute of Arthritis and Musculoskeletal and Skin Disorders

Visit the book's website at
www.wbsaunders.com/SIMON/McEwen SIMON
for a direct link to the website for each organization listed.

*Local or regional offices available.
†Call for listings of state offices.

Learning Activities & Application to Practice

In Class

1. Discuss *Healthy People 2010* objectives that address older adults. What progress has been made in achieving the objectives? Outline strategies and interventions that nurses can implement to contribute to achieving the objectives.
2. Discuss recommendations of the Preventative Services Task Force for older adults (see Table 12-4). Are recommendations followed by primary care providers? Why or why not?

In Clinical

3. Visit providers of assistive care for elders (i.e., a local adult day care center, a nursing home or retirement center). What services are provided and who is the provider? What activities are

available? How are services funded? Share findings with the group.

4. Complete the COPE (Appendix 12-A) on one client being cared for in clinical practice. Use the questionnaire to develop a preventative plan of care for that client.

5. In a log or diary, record the chronic conditions identified in clinical practice. What percentage of elders encountered have more than one chronic condition? What are common combinations (e.g., chronic obstructive pulmonary disease and asthma, diabetes, peripheral vascular disease, CAD)? Share observations with members of the group.

6. Assess the home of an older client for threats to safety, particularly falls. Develop a plan or strategy to reduce identified threats.

REFERENCES

Administration on Aging. (2000). *Elder abuse prevention.* Retrieved 8/14/01 from http://www.aoa. gov/factsheets/abuse.html.

Alzheimer's Disease Association. (2000). *Alzheimer's disease statistics.* Chicago: Alzheimer's Disease Association. Retrieved 8/14/01 from http://www.alz.org/hc/overview/stats.htm.

American Association of Retired Persons (AARP). (2001). *Determine your nutrition health.* Retrieved 8/14/01 from http://www.aarp.org/contfacts/health/nutrihealth.html.

American Association of Retired Persons (AARP). (1993). *Coping & caring: Living with Alzheimer's disease.* Washington, DC: American Association of Retired Persons.

American Nurses' Association (ANA). (1995). *Scope and standards of gerontological nursing practice.* Washington, DC: American Nurses' Association.

Ballard, D. (2000). Legal and ethical issues. In A. G. Lueckenotte, (Ed.), *Gerontologic nursing* (2nd ed., pp. 34-62). St. Louis: Mosby.

Birchfield, P. C. (1996). Elder health. In M. Stanhope & J. Lancaster (Eds.), *Community health nursing: Promoting health of aggregates, families and individuals* (4th ed., pp. 581-600). St. Louis: Mosby.

Campbell, J., & Landenburger, K. (1996). Violence and human abuse. In M. Stanhope & J. Lancaster (Eds.), *Community health nursing: Promoting health of aggregates, families and individuals* (4th ed.). St. Louis: Mosby.

Centers for Disease Control and Prevention (CDC). (2000). *Summary of adolescent/adult immunization recommendations.* Retrieved 8/14/01 from http://www.cdc.gov/nip/recs/adult-schedule.pdf.

Centers for Disease Control and Prevention (CDC). (2001). *Physician visits increase for older patients; doctors prescribe more medications for patients of all ages.* Retrieved 8/14/01 from http://www.cdc.gov/od/oc/media/pressrel/r010717.htm.

Chenitz, W. C., Kussman, H. L., & Stone, J. T. (1991). Preventing falls. In W. C. Chenitz, J. T. Stone, & S. A. Salisbury (Eds.), *Clinical gerontological nursing: A guide to advanced practice* (pp. 309-328). Philadelphia: W. B. Saunders.

Clark, M. J. (1999). *Nursing in the community* (3rd ed.). Stamford, CT: Appleton & Lange.

Dambro, M. R. (1996). *Griffith's 5-minute clinical consult.* Baltimore: Williams & Williams.

Eliopoulos, C. (1997). *Gerontological nursing* (4th ed.). Philadelphia: J. B. Lippincott.

Evashwick, C. J. (1999). The continuum of long-term care. In S. J. Williams & P. R. Torrens (Eds.), *Introduction to health services* (5th ed., pp. 295-348). Albany, NY: Delmar Publishers.

Graves, M. (1988). Drug use and abuse. In M. O. Hogstel (Ed.), *Nursing care of the older adult* (2nd ed.). New York: John Wiley & Sons.

Hashizume, S. (1991). Home health care. In W. C. Chenitz, J. T. Stone, & S. A. Salisbury (Eds.), *Clinical gerontological nursing: A guide to advanced practice* (pp. 557-576). Philadelphia: W. B. Saunders.

Lashley, M. E. (1995). Elderly persons in the community. In C. M. Smith & F. A. Maurer (Eds.), *Community health nursing: Theory and practice* (pp. 719-746). Philadelphia: W. B. Saunders.

Luggen, A. S. (1996). Aging process. In A. S. Luggen (Ed.), *Core curriculum for gerontological nursing* (pp. 35-43). St. Louis: Mosby.

Lukacs, K. (1996). Neurological/Alzheimer's disease. In A. S. Luggen (Ed.), *Core curriculum for gerontological nursing* (pp. 564-580). St. Louis: Mosby.

Maurer, F. A. (2000a). Elderly persons in the community. In C. M. Smith & F. A. Maurer (Eds.), *Community health nursing: Theory and practice* (2nd ed., pp. 781-810). Philadelphia: W. B. Saunders.

Maurer, F. A. (2000b). Violence: A social and family problem. In C. M. Smith & F. A. Maurer (Eds.), *Community health nursing: Theory and practice* (2nd ed., pp. 571-606). Philadelphia: W. B. Saunders.

McEwen, M., & Davis, L. (2001). Senior health. In M. A. Nies & M. McEwen (Eds.), *Community health nursing: Promoting the health of populations* (3rd ed.). Philadelphia: W. B. Saunders.

Meiner, S. E., & Miceli, D. G. (2000). Safety. In A. G. Lueckenotte, (Ed.), *Gerontologic nursing* (2nd ed., pp. 232-255). St. Louis: Mosby.

Murray, R., Zentner, J., & Pinnell, N. (1993). Assessment and health promotion for the person in later maturity. In R. B. Murray and J. P. Zentner (Eds.), *Nursing assessment and health promotion: Strategies through the life span* (5th ed., pp. 542-603). Norwalk, CT: Appleton & Lange.

Murray, R., Zentner, J., & Pinnell, N. (2001). Assessment and health promotion for the person in later adulthood. In R. B. Murray & J. P. Zentner (Eds.), *Nursing assessment and health promotion: Strategies through the life span* (7th ed., pp. 745-834). Upper Saddle River, NJ: Prentice Hall.

National Center for Health Statistics (NCHS). (1994). Current estimates from the National Health Interview Survey, 1992. *Vital and Health Statistics,* Series 10, p. 189. Washington, DC: USDHHS, National Center for Health Statistics.

National Center for Health Statistics (NCHS). (1999). *Health, United States: 1999,* Hyattsville, MD: USDHHS, National Center for Health Statistics.

National Institute on Aging. (1999). *Hearing and older people.* Retrieved 8/14/01 from http://www.nia.nih.gov/health/agepages/hearing.htm.

National Institute on Aging. (2000). *Depression: A serious but treatable illness.* Retrieved 8/14/01 from http://www.nia.nih.gov/health/agepages/depresti.htm.

Pappas, A., & Hakala, K. L. D. (2001). Violence in the community. In M. Nies & M. McEwen (Eds.), *Community health nursing: Promoting the health of populations* (pp. 596-623). Philadelphia: W. B. Saunders.

Pearlman, R. A. (1987). Development of a functional assessment questionnaire for geriatric patients: The Comprehensive Older Person's Evaluation (COPE). *Journal of Chronic Diseases,* 40(suppl)1, 85S-98S.

Phillips, S. C. (2000). Preventing depression: A program for African American elders with chronic pain. *Family and Community Health, 22*(4), 57.

Richardson, H. (1995). Long-term care. In A. R. Kovner (Ed.), *Jonas's health care delivery in the United States* (5th ed., pp. 194-231). New York: Springer Publishing Co.

Selkoe, D. J. (1992). Aging brain, aging mind. *Scientific American, 267*(3), 134-142.

Stone, J. T., & Chenitz, W. C. (1991). The problem of falls. In W. C. Chenitz, J. T. Stone, & S. A. Salisbury (Eds.), *Clinical gerontological nursing: A guide to advanced practice* (pp. 291-308). Philadelphia: W. B. Saunders.

U.S. Department of Health and Human Services (USDHHS). (2000). *Healthy people 2010: Conference edition.* Washington, DC: Government Printing Office.

U.S. Department of Health and Human Services/ Health Care Financing Administration (USDHHS/ HCFA). (2000). *Your guide to choosing a nursing home* (Publication No. HCFA-02174-B). Baltimore, MD: HCFA.

U.S. Department of Health and Human Services/ Agency for Health Care Policy and Research (USDHHS/AHCPR). (1992). *Urinary incontinence in adults: Clinical practice guideline.* (AHCPR Pub. No. 92-0038). Rockville, MD: Agency for Health Care Policy and Research.

U.S. Department of Health and Human Services, National Institute of Mental Health. (1999). *Mental health: Report of the surgeon general.* Rockville, MD: USDHHS, SAMHSA, CMHS, NIH, NIMH.

U.S. Department of Health and Human Services/Office of Disease Prevention and Health Promotion (USDHHS/ ODPHP). (1998). *Clinician's handbook of preventive services* (2nd ed.). Washington, DC: Government Printing Office.

Appendix 12-A

Comprehensive Older Person's Evaluation (COPE)

PROVIDER NAME (PRINT): _____ DATE OF VISIT: _____

CHIEF COMPLAINT: _____

Today I will ask you about your overall health and function and will be using a questionnaire to help me obtain this information. The first few questions are to check your memory.

PRELIMINARY COGNITION QUESTIONNAIRE: RECORD IF ANSWER IS CORRECT WITH (+). IF ANSWER IS INCORRECT WITH (−). RECORD TOTAL NUMBER OF ERRORS.

(+, −)

A. What is the date today? _____

B. What day of the week is it? _____

C. What is the name of this place? _____

D. What is your telephone number? (RECORD ANSWER) _____ _____
IF SUBJECT DOES NOT HAVE PHONE, ASK: What is your street _____
address? _____

E. How old are you? (RECORD ANSWER) _____ _____

F. When were you born? (RECORD ANSWER FROM RECORDS IF PATIENT CANNOT _____
ANSWER) _____

G. Who is the President of the United States now? _____

H. Who was the President just before him? _____

I. What was your mother's maiden name? _____

J. Subtract 3 from 20 and keep subtracting from each new number you get, all the way down _____

(CORRECT: 17, 14, 11, 8, 5, 2)

TOTAL ERRORS_____

IF MORE THAN 4 ERRORS, ASK K. IF MORE THAN 6 ERRORS, COMPLETE QUESTIONNAIRE FROM INFORMANT.

K. Do you think you would benefit from a legal guardian, someone who would be responsible for your legal and financial matters?

4. Yes   2. Have functioning legal guardian (DESCRIBE: _____)

3. Have legal guardian   1. No

DEMOGRAPHIC SECTION

1. PATIENT'S RACE OR ETHNIC BACKGROUND (RECORD) _____

2. PATIENT'S GENDER (CIRCLE)   Male   Female

3. How far did you go in school?

6. 0–8 years   4. High school complete   2. Four year degree

5. High school incomplete   3. College or technical school   1. Post-graduate education

SOCIAL SUPPORT SECTION: Now there are a few questions about your family and friends.

4. Are you now married, widowed, separated, or divorced, or have you never been married?

1. Now Married   2. Widowed   3. Separated   4. Divorced   5. Never Married

Pearlman, R. A. (1987). Development of a functional assessment questionnaire for geriatric patients: The Comprehensive Older Person's Evaluation (COPE). *Journal of Chronic Diseases*, 40(suppl)1, 85S-98S.

5. Who lives with you? (CIRCLE ALL RESPONSES)
    1. Spouse   4. Live alone
    2. Other relative or friend (SPECIFY: _____)   5. Nursing home
    3. Group living situation (non-health)
6. Have you talked to any friends or relatives by phone during the last week?   1. Yes   2. No
7. Are you satisfied by seeing your relatives and friends as often as you want to, or are you somewhat dissatisfied about how little you see them?   1. Satisfied (SKIP TO #8)   2. Dissatisfied (ASK A)
    A. Do you feel you would like to be involved in a Senior Citizens Center for social events, or perhaps meals?   3. Yes   2. Am Involved (DESCRIBE: _____) 1. No
8. Is there someone who would take care of you for as long as you needed if you were sick or disabled?
    1. Yes   (SKIP TO C)   2. No   (ASK A)
    A. Is there someone who would take care of you for a short time?   1. Yes (SKIP TO C)   2. No (ASK B)
    B. Is there someone who could help you now and then?   1. Yes (ASK C)   2. No (ASK C)
    C. Whom would we call in case of an emergency? (RECORD NAME AND TELEPHONE) _____
_____

FINANCIAL SECTION: The next few questions are about your finances and any problems you might have.
9. Do you own, or are you buying, your own home?   1. Yes (SKIP TO #10)   2. No (ASK A)
    A. Do you feel you need assistance with housing?
    3. Yes (DESCRIBE: _____)
    2. Have subsidized or other housing assistance
    1. No
10. Are you covered by private medical insurance, Medicare, Medicaid, or some disability plan? (CIRCLE ALL THAT APPLY)
    1. Private insurance (SPECIFY BELOW AND SKIP TO #11) _____
    2. Medicare   3. Medicaid
    4. Disability (SPECIFY: _____)   (ASK A)
    5. None   6. Other (SPECIFY: _____)
    A. Do you feel you need additional assistance with your medical bills?   2. Yes   1. No
11. Which of these statements best describes your financial situation?
    3. My expenses are so heavy that I cannot meet my bills   (ASK A)
    2. My expenses make it difficult to meet my bills   (ASK A)
    1. My bills are no problem to me (SKIP TO #12)
    A. Do you feel you need financial assistance such as (CIRCLE ALL THAT APPLY)
    1. Food stamps   3. Assistance in paying your heating or electrical bills
    2. Social Security or disability payments   4. Other financial assistance? (DESCRIBE:_____)
PSYCHOLOGICAL HEALTH SECTION: The next few questions are about how you feel about your life in general. There are no right or wrong answers, only what best applies to you. *Please answer yes or no to each question.*
12. Is your daily life full of things that keep you interested?   1. Yes   2. No
13. Have you, at times, very much wanted to leave home?   2. Yes   1. No
14. Does it seem that no one understands you?   2. Yes   1. No
15. Are you happy most of the time?   1. Yes   2. No
16. Do you feel weak all over much of the time?   2. Yes   1. No
17. Is your sleep fitful and disturbed?   2. Yes   1. No
18. Taking everything into consideration, how would you describe your satisfaction with your life in general at the present time—good, fair, or poor?   1. Good   2. Fair   3. Poor
19. Do you feel you now need help with your mental health; for example, a counselor or psychiatrist?
    3. Yes   2. Have (SPECIFY: _____)   1. No
PHYSICAL HEALTH SECTION: The next questions are about your health.
20. During the past month (30 days), how many days were you so sick that you couldn't do your usual activities, such as working around the house or visiting with friends?   TOTAL NUMBER OF DAYS: _____
21. Relative to other people your age, how would you rate your overall health at the present time; excellent, good, fair, poor, or very poor?
    1. Excellent   (SKIP to #22)   3. Good (ASK A)   5. Poor (ASK A)
    2. Very Good   (SKIP TO #22)   4. Fair (ASK A)
    A. Do you feel you need additional medical services such as a doctor, nurse, visiting nurse, or physical therapy?   (CIRCLE ALL THAT APPLY)
    1. Doctor   2. Nurse   3. Visiting nurse   4. Physical therapy   5. None
22. Do you use an aid for walking, such as a wheelchair, walker, cane, or anything else? (CIRCLE AID USUALLY USED)   5. Wheelchair   4. Walker   3. Cane   2. Other (SPECIFY): _____   5. None

23. How much do your health troubles stand in the way of your doing things you want to do; not at all, a little, or a great deal?
    1. Not at all (SKIP TO #24)   2. A little (ASK A)   3. A great deal (ASK A)
    A. Do you think you need assistance to do your daily activities; for example, do you need a live-in aide or choreworker?
       1. Live-in aide   3. Have aide, choreworker or other assistance (DESCRIBE: _____)
       2. Choreworker   4. None needed

24. Have you had, or do you currently have, any of the following health problems? (IF YES, PLACE AN "X" IN APPROPRIATE BOX AND DESCRIBE [MEDICAL RECORD INFORMATION MAY BE USED TO HELP COMPLETE THIS SECTION.])

	HX	CURRENT	DESCRIBE
a. Arthritis or rheumatism?			
b. Lung or breathing problem?			
c. Hypertension?			
d. Heart trouble?			
e. Phlebitis or poor circulation problems in arms or legs?			
f. Diabetes or low blood sugar?			
g. Digestive ulcers?			
h. Other digestive problem?			
i. Cancer?			
j. Anemia?			
k. Effects of stroke?			
l. Other neurological problem? (SPECIFY): _____			
m. Thyroid or other glandular problem? (SPECIFY): _____			
n. Skin disorders such as pressure sores, leg ulcers, burns?			
o. Speech problem?			
p. Hearing problem?			
q. Vision or eye problem?			
r. Kidney or bladder problems, or incontinence?			
s. A problem of falls?			
t. Problem with eating or your weight? (SPECIFY): _____			
u. Problem with depression or your nerves? (SPECIFY): _____			
v. Problem with your behavior? (SPECIFY): _____			
w. Problem with your sexual activity?			
x. Problem with alcohol?			
y. Problem with pain?			
z. Other health problems? (SPECIFY): _____			

25. What medications are you currently taking, or have been taking, in the last month? (May I see your medication bottles?) (IF PATIENT CANNOT LIST, ASK CATEGORIES A–R AND NOTE DOSAGE AND SCHEDULE, OR OBTAIN INFORMATION FROM MEDICAL OR PHARMACY RECORDS AND VERIFY ACCURACY WITH THE PATIENT.)

	Rx (DOSAGE AND SCHEDULE)
a. Arthritis medication	
b. Pain medication	
c. Blood pressure medication	
d. Water pills or pills for fluid	
e. Medication for your heart	
f. Medication for your lungs	
g. Blood thinners	
h. Medication for your circulation	
i. Insulin or diabetes medication	
j. Seizure medication	
k. Thyroid pills	
l. Steroids	
m. Hormones	
n. Antibiotics	
o. Medicine for nerves or depression	
p. Prescription sleeping pills	
q. Other prescription drugs	
r. Other non-prescription drugs	

26. Many people have problems remembering to take their medications, especially ones they need to take on a regular basis. How often do you forget to take your medications? Would you say you forget often, sometimes, rarely, or never?   4. Often   3. Sometimes   2. Rarely   1. Never

ACTIVITIES OF DAILY LIVING: The next set of questions ask whether you would need help with any of the following activities of daily living.

27. I would like to know whether you can do these activities without any help at all, or if you need assistance to do them. Do you need help to: (IF YES, DESCRIBE, INCLUDING PATIENT NEEDS)

	Yes	No	DESCRIBE (INCLUDE NEEDS)
a. Use the telephone?			
b. Get to places out of walking distance? (Use transportation?)			
c. Shop for clothes and food?			
d. Do your housework?			
e. Handle your money?			
f. Feed yourself?			
g. Dress and undress yourself?			
h. Take care of your appearance?			
i. Get in and out of bed?			
j. Take a bath or shower?			
k. Prepare your meals?			
l. Have any problem getting to the bathroom on time?			

28. During the past six months, have you had any help with such things as shopping, housework, bathing, dressing, and getting around?

    2. Yes (SPECIFY: _____)

    1. No

Health Promotion and Illness Prevention for Families

objectives

Upon completion of this chapter, the reader will be able to:

1. Discuss the concept of family and explain the different types of families.

2. Describe characteristics common to all families and identify the purpose of the family.

3. Describe the stages of the family life cycle and give examples of tasks to be accomplished at each stage.

4. Perform a family assessment and develop a plan of care for a family including construction of a genogram, ecomap, and/or family health tree.

key terms

Blended family
Ecomap
Extended family
Family
Family assessment

Family crisis
Family health tree
Family roles
Genogram
Nuclear dyad

Nuclear family
Single-parent family
Stages of family
  development

See Glossary for definitions.

case study

Jessica Richardson is a registered nurse (RN) employed by a visiting nurse association (VNA) affiliated with a public health department in a large city. She specializes in caring for high-risk infants and their families. Most of the babies Jessica sees are low-birth-weight babies or they had complications following birth. In addition, several of the infants in her caseload have birth anomalies or genetic disorders.

On a recent Monday, Jessica admitted a new family into service. Jeffrey Smith was born 7 weeks prematurely and weighed just less than 3 pounds at birth. His mother, Sarah, is an unmarried 16-year-old high school junior, who lives with her mother, grandmother, and two siblings. Jeffrey spent almost 2 weeks in the neonatal intensive care unit (ICU) because of breathing problems before moving to the regular nursery. He was discharged at 6 weeks of age at 4.5 pounds. Because of his history of breathing difficulties and two episodes of apnea, Jeffrey needs to wear an apnea monitor 24 hours per day.

Jessica scheduled the initial home visit to occur within a few hours of the baby's discharge. She wanted to spend time with as many of the immediate family members as possible to do a thorough assessment of the family and the home environment. Jessica learned that Sarah and Jeffrey live with Sarah's mother Maggie (34 years of age), Maggie's mother Lucille (60 years of age), and Sarah's younger brother Pete (15 years of age) and sister Abby (13 years of age). Sarah's parents have been divorced for 10 years and the family moved to Lucille's home at that time so she could help care for the three grandchildren, then ages 3, 5, and 6 years.

Maggie is the primary breadwinner for the family. She is employed as a supervisor at a local paper mill and her income is adequate to meet the basic needs of the family. After the divorce, Mr. Smith relocated to another state. He is a construction worker, but is only periodically employed and rarely sends child support money. Lucille does not work outside the home because she is partially disabled as the result of a back injury. Pete and Sarah contribute to the family finances by working in fast food establishments, although Sarah has not worked since going into premature labor. Jeffrey's father is a high school student named Jimmy. Jimmy is no longer involved with Sarah and has shown minimal interest in the child; he provides no financial support.

For the initial meeting, Jessica interviewed Sarah and her mother and grandmother. Jessica was told that Lucille would be the primary caretaker of Jeffrey during the day while Sarah is completing her last 2 years of high school and while Maggie works. Sarah will provide most of his care during the evenings and on weekends.

The family lives in a three-bedroom, one-bath frame house. The sleeping arrangements have changed since the baby came home. Lucille has one bedroom alone and Maggie and Abby share another. Sarah and the baby have the third room and Pete sleeps on the couch. Jessica observed that the kitchen was clean and that there were ample supplies (e.g., diapers and bottles) for the infant. There is a baby bed in Sarah's room and Sarah acknowledged that Jeffrey will ride in a car seat at all times.

From her interview, Jessica learned that health care for the family is paid through insurance provided by Maggie's employer. Lucille receives Medicaid and Medicare because of her disability. They receive no other social services.

Sarah recovered from Jeffrey's birth without incident and stated that she has no current health problems. Maggie reported that she is in good health, although she smokes about two packages of cigarettes per day. She is also about 20 pounds overweight. In addition to her chronic back problem, Lucille is diabetic, and Jessica observed that she is about 50 pounds overweight. Maggie and Lucille explained that the other teenagers are all in good health, with no significant health problems. Jessica gained additional information about the extended family's health history.

Maggie reported that the family attends church weekly. Sarah is behind in school, but should be able to catch up and graduate. She hopes to go to beauty college after graduation and become a hair stylist. Pete is an adequate student, but Maggie expressed concern over some of his friends whom she knows smoke and drink and may be involved in drugs and gang activity. Abby is an excellent student and hopes to go to college to become a lawyer.

Jessica performed a complete physical assessment on Jeffrey. He had gained 1 ounce from the previous day and was breathing normally. The apnea monitor was attached and working properly. Her interventions for the first visit were directed toward teaching Sarah, Maggie, and Lucille how to care for Jeffrey. She focused on recognizing breathing problems and apnea and other health problems common to low-birth-weight and premature infants. She explained how to maintain the apnea monitor and what to do when the alarm sounds and she gave detailed instructions on emergency procedures and how to manage them, including when to call for assistance. She also provided the three women with teaching materials that supplemented what she taught.

The women asked questions and were able to repeat the instructions, indicating comprehension. Jessica made an appointment to return the following day for follow-up and additional teaching.

The **family** is the most basic social unit. Some forms of family can be found in all human societies. The family is the primary social group for each individual and contributes to his or her growth and experiences. The family impacts how the individual adapts and responds to changes and threats and directly influences health. The family has a major role in shaping the person.

Although the individual is usually the primary recipient of health care, many nurses, particularly those working in community settings, recognize the importance of providing interventions directed at the family level. For example, a nurse who works in a primary care pediatric clinic cares for several children from one family simultaneously, understanding that both acute and chronic illnesses can impact the entire family. Likewise, a home health nurse caring for an elderly diabetic man works with his spouse and extended family as she teaches the important points of managing diabetes. Finally, a hospice nurse cares for the entire family of a dying client, knowing that each member is affected by the illness and death of their loved one.

This chapter describes issues related to families and family health. It focuses on helping nurses who work in community settings understand the different types and stages of families and how to recognize both healthy and unhealthy family characteristics. Finally, the process of assessment and intervention for families is covered.

THE CONCEPT OF FAMILY

When most people think of a family, they think of a husband/breadwinner and wife/homemaker with one or more children living in the home. Sometimes, they include extended family members, in particular, grandparents, children living away (either single or married), and grandchildren. Others may consider sisters and brothers, aunts and uncles, cousins, godparents, and even very close friends to be family.

But what constitutes a family is not easily explained because family means different things to different people. Further, it has been pointed out that culture, not biology, determines family organization; therefore the meaning of family is different for people from different cultures (Murray et al., 2001). In addition, the concept of family is dynamic and evolving. In contemporary American society, conceptualizations of family have moved from a vision of the nuclear family and extended family to include a variety of households, such as unmarried adults living together with or without children, single parent households, divorced couples who combine households with children from previous marriages, and homosexual couples with or without children (Box 13-1) (Allender and Spradley, 2001a).

DEFINITIONS OF FAMILY

Many definitions for family can be found in the literature. According to Vaughn-Cole and colleagues (1998), traditional definitions of family are based on persistent myths. One of these myths is that the typical family is a nuclear family consisting of parents and children. Another myth relates to the ideal of the extended family of several generations working toward a common family goal. The authors pointed out that these are now the exception rather than the rule.

 13-1 Statistics of U.S. Families

Fewer than 20% of American families now have a working father, a full-time homemaker mother, and one or more children at home.
Approximately 25% of all families in the United States are headed by one adult, usually a woman.
The number of single households headed by men has increased to 3% of all families in 1998.
The proportion of children under 18 years who live with one parent increased from 12% in 1970 to 25% in 1990.
About 40% of all children will live part of their lives with a single parent.
Half of all marriages end in divorce and the median duration of marriages is approximately 7 years.

From Allender, J., & Spradley, B. (2001a). Theoretical bases for promoting family health. In J. A. Allender & B. W. Spradley (Eds.), *Community health nursing: Concepts and practice* (5th ed., pp. 427-445). Philadelphia: Lippincott.

Definitions for family are varied and numerous. The U.S. Census Bureau (1995) provided a relatively simple definition, calling the family "a group of two or more persons related by birth, marriage or adoption and residing together in a household." Other basic definitions for family include the following:

"A cluster of people whose relationship is stipulated by law in terms of marriage and descent, and whose precise membership varies according to the circumstances" (Farber, 1973, p. 2).

"A primary group of people living in a household in consistent proximity and intimate relationship" (Helvie, 1981, p. 64).

"An aggregate made up of a body of units, the individuals that represent the whole or the family" (Siegrist, 2001, p. 412).

More complete or complex definitions can also be found. For example, Allender and Spradley (2001a) stated that a "family consists of two or more individuals who share a residence or live near one another; possess some common emotional bond; engage in interrelated social positions, roles and task; and share a sense of affection and belonging" (p. 427).

A similar definition is proposed by Murray and others (2001) who explained that a family is "a small social system and primary reference group made up of two or more persons living together who are related by blood, marriage or adoption or who are living together by agreement over a period of time" (p. 158).

Finally, Craft and Willadsen (1992) wrote that the family is a "social context of two or more people characterized by mutual attachment, caring, long-term commitment, responsibility to provide individual growth, supportive relationships, health of members and of the unit, and maintenance of the organization and system during constant individual, family and societal change" (p. 519).

Stuart (1991) summarized the following conceptualizations of family:

- The family is a system or unit.
- Family members may or may not be related and may or may not live together.

- The unit may or may not contain children.
- Commitment and attachment exist among unit members and include future obligation.
- The unit caregiving functions consist of protection, nourishment, and socialization of unit members.

TYPES OF FAMILIES

Defining family is difficult because families can assume many different forms. Traditional families include the nuclear family, the nuclear-dyad (husband and wife with no children or with grown children), and single adult families where one adult lives alone. Other variations include multigenerational families, in which several generations or age groups live together in the same household; kin networks, in which several nuclear families live in the same household or near one another and share goods and services; blended families, in which single parents marry and raise children from one or both previous relationships; and single-parent families, in which one adult cares for a child or children as a result of a temporary relationship or a legal separation, divorce, or death of a spouse (Allender and Spradley, 2001a). Some types of both traditional and nontraditional families are described here and are summarized in Box 13-2.

Nuclear Family

The conjugal **nuclear family** is composed of a married husband and wife and children. The children may be either biological offspring or adopted. Several factors, such as the high rate of divorce, increased sexual freedom, decreased social stigma attached to illegitimacy, and alternative sexual lifestyles have contributed to changing the form of the nuclear family. As a result, the nuclear family is becoming less common. Indeed, only about 34% of American families consist of a married couple with children living at home.

Nuclear Dyad

A **nuclear dyad** (a married couple without children in the home) occurs by choice, because of infertility, or because children are grown and

BOX 13-2 Types of Families

Nuclear family: mother, father, and child(ren) living together, but apart from both sets of the father's and mother's parents

Nuclear dyad: husband and wife or other couple living alone without children

Single-parent family: mother or father living with either biological or adopted children; they may be tied emotionally, but not legally, to a partner

Extended family: nuclear family plus other relatives of one or both spouses; relatives may or may not live with the nuclear family and may include great-grandparents and great-great-grandparents

Stepfamily (blended family): one divorced or widowed adult with all or some of his or her children and a new spouse with all or some of his or her children;

may include the children born to this union so that parents, stepparents, children, and stepchildren or stepsiblings live together

Three generational family: any combination of the first, second, and third generation members living within a household

Single adult: never married, separated, divorced, or widowed individual living alone or with other single adults in a nonsexual relationship

Cohabitating couple: unmarried couple living together

Compound family: one man or woman with several spouses

Same-sex/homosexual family: gay or lesbian partners living together; may have children

From Cooley, M. (2000). A family perspective in community health nursing. In C. M. Smith & F. A. Maurer (Eds.), *Community health nursing: Theory and practice* (2nd ed., pp. 237-255). Philadelphia: W. B. Saunders; Murray, R. B., Zentner, P. P., Brockhaus, J. P. D., Brockhaus, R., & Sullivan, E. (2001). The family: Basic unit for the developing person. In R. B. Murray & J. P. Zentner (Eds.), *Health promotion strategies through the life span* (7th ed., pp. 157-212). Upper Saddle River, NJ: Prentice Hall.

away from home (Caudle, 1999). The nuclear dyad is the most common household arrangement, with almost half of all families (43%) being nuclear dyads.

Single-Parent Family

A **single-parent family** consists of an adult woman or man and children. Single-parent families result from divorce, out-of-wedlock pregnancies, absence or death of a spouse, or adoption by a single person. Most (86%) single-parent families are headed by women.

The number of single-parent families has risen sharply in the past few decades. Between 1970 and 1990, births to single women increased from 11% to 27% of all births and the proportion of single-parent households more than doubled (Caudle, 1999).

Extended Family

An **extended family** consists of the family kin network and includes grandparents, aunts, uncles, and cousins. Like the nuclear family, the extended family has been greatly affected by social changes. In the past, members of an extended family often lived in close proximity,

but because of increased mobility, families are more likely to live away from their extended kin network (Caudle, 1999).

Stepfamily or Blended Family

A stepfamily or **blended family** is composed of two adults, at least one of whom has remarried following divorce or death of a spouse. They can include children from either adult's previous marriage(s) and offspring from the new marriage.

Like single-parent families, blended families have increased rapidly in the United States over the last several decades. This is because approximately 50% of marriages end in divorce and two thirds of divorces involve children. Most divorced adults eventually remarry contributing to the formation of more than 250,000 stepfamilies each year (Caudle, 1999).

Cohabitating Family

A cohabitating family consists of a man and woman living together without being married. Cohabitation is becoming increasingly prevalent in the United States, and the number of unmarried couples increased from 2 million in 1985 to 4.2 million in 1998 (Caudle, 1999).

COMMUNITY APPLICATION
Grandparents Raising Grandchildren

Many older Americans approaching or in retirement suddenly find themselves raising their grandchildren. According to the Census Bureau, in 1997, 3.9 million children were living in homes maintained by their grandparents—a 76% increase since 1970. At some point, more than 10% of grandparents raise a grandchild for at least 6 months and typically grandparents are caregivers for much longer periods. The reasons for the increase in the number of grandparents caring for their grandchildren include death of parents, incarceration of parents, unemployment of parents, substance abuse by parents, teen pregnancy, family violence, and human immunodeficiency virus (HIV)/AIDS.

This phenomenon has important health consequences. Grandparents in the caregiving role are more prone to psychological and emotional strain and feelings of helplessness and isolation. Many grandparent caregivers face financial difficulties and grandparent caregivers are 60% more likely to live in poverty than are grandparents not raising grandchildren. Grandparent caregivers often neglect their own physical and emotional health because they give priority to the needs of their grandchildren.

In addition, the grandchildren in their care often have unmet physical, emotional, and developmental needs that may require special assistance. There may be legal issues because grandparents often must obtain legal authority to get their grandchildren medical care; enroll them in school; and enable them to receive immunizations, public assistance, and supportive services. Finally, grandparents may need respite services, affordable housing, and access to medical care.

From Administration on Aging (2000). *Grandparents raising grandchildren.* Retrieved 8/22/01 from http://www.aoa.gov/Factsheets/grandparents.html.

Homosexual Family

The homosexual family is a form of cohabitation in which a couple of the same sex lives together and shares a sexual relationship. Homosexual couples comprise about 2% of U.S. households. The homosexual family may include children (Caudle, 1999).

Communal Family

A communal family is made up of several adults and children living together, usually because of a common religious or ideological bond or financial necessity. Communal families typically resemble traditional extended families (Caudle, 1999).

Skip-Generation Family

A skip-generation family is one in which grandparents are raising their grandchildren. Skip-generation families typically occur because of working parents, drug or alcohol abuse, or child abandonment. Approximately 6% of U.S. children are being raised by grandparents (Caudle,

1999). See the Community Application box "Grandparents Raising Grandchildren." Box 13-3 gives statistics about all types of families.

CHARACTERISTICS OF FAMILIES

Although all families are unique, they all possess certain common qualities or characteristics. This is true regardless of whether they are nuclear families, nuclear dyads, foster families, homosexual families, or other family types (Allender and Spradley, 2001a). For example, each family can be thought of as a small social system in which each individual is a subsystem. The family system, as a whole, and each individual subsystem, interacts with other subsystems and the larger suprasystem in multiple ways.

Each family has a basic structure and function; these are dynamic and change with time and circumstances. Families are interdependent, meaning that family members rely on other members for assistance and to meet a variety of needs such as affection, love, loyalty, and financial commitment. Additionally, families set

BOX 13-3 The Changing Face of American Families

In 1970, 85% of children younger than 18 years were living with two parents; by 1998, that proportion declined to 59%.

Cohabiting, unmarried people increased from 523,000 in 1970 to 4.2 million in 1998.

About one third of cohabitating couple households include children.

In 1970, 12% of children lived with only one parent; by 1998, 32% of children were in single-parent homes.

Between 1980 and 1998, the birth rate for unmarried women 15 to 17 years increased from 21 to 32 per 1000.

In 1970, only 3% of children lived with their grandparents; by 1997, the figure was 6%.

About 45% of children in divorced families and 69% of children in never-married single-parent families live below or near the poverty level.

From U.S. Census Bureau. (1999). *Racial-ethnic and gender differences in returns to cohabitation and marriage: Evidence from the current population survey.* Washington, DC: U.S. Census Bureau; U.S. Department of Commerce. (1997). *Current population reports.* Series P23-193. Washington, DC: U.S. Department of Commerce.

and maintain boundaries (generation boundaries and family community boundaries), which result from shared experiences and expectations. Finally, all families create and maintain their own set of values, rules, and goals (Allender and Spradley, 2001a; Murray et al., 2001).

PURPOSES OF FAMILIES

Families exist to serve several purposes. For example, according to Murray and colleagues (2001), families provide physical safety and meet the economic needs of family members. The family helps members develop physically, emotionally, intellectually, and spiritually and creates a healthy environment for the family's well-being. The family should also help members develop a personal identity and a value system. This value system is generally built on spiritual and philosophic beliefs and the cultural and social system with which the family identifies.

Families also teach members social skills and how to communicate effectively. They teach gender roles and appropriate behaviors. Families provide security, support, encouragement, and motivation. Finally, families help members cope with crises and societal demands (Allender and Spradley, 2001a; Murray et al., 2001).

ROLES IN THE FAMILY

Roles are socially expected behavior patterns that are determined by a person's position or status. In families, roles are the assigned or assumed parts that members play during day-to-day

living; they are bestowed and defined by the family. In a given family, the specific roles to be played vary depending on the family's structure, needs, and patterns of functioning (Allender and Spradley, 2001a)

Within a family, each person occupies several roles by virtue of his or her position. For example, the adult woman in the house typically occupies the role of wife and mother. She may also be the cook, laundress, and housekeeper, as well as being a bread winner. The adult male in the house may be the primary bread winner. He may also be the disciplinarian and teacher.

Family roles may be well defined (formal) or less well defined (informal). Formal roles are expected sets of behaviors associated with family positions (i.e., husband, wife, mother, father, brother, sister, son, daughter). Informal roles are those behaviors not associated with a particular position, but which influence how and by whom emotional needs are met. Informal roles that may present within any family group include the encourager, the harmonizer, the follower, the martyr, the scapegoat, the go-between, and the blamer (Caudle, 1999). Children and adults take on multiple roles, both formal and informal.

Role conflict occurs when the demands of fulfilling several roles contradict or compete with each other. Role conflict can also occur when one individual's definition of a role does not correspond with someone else's definition of the same role (Caudle, 1999). For example, a husband may see his wife as the cook/housekeeper and

TABLE **13-1** Stages and Tasks of Middle-Class North American Family Life Cycle

STAGE	TASK
Launching: the single young adult leaves home	Coming to terms with the family of origin
	Development of intimate relationships with peers
	Establishment of self: career and finances
Marriage: the joining of families	Formation of identity as a couple
	Including spouse in realignment of relationships with extended families
	Parenthood: making decisions
Families with young children	Integration of children into family unit
	Adjusting tasks: childrearing, financial, and household
	Accommodation of new parenting and grandparenting roles
Families with adolescents	Development of increasing autonomy for adolescents
	Reexamine midlife marital and career issues
	Initial shift toward concern for the older generation
Families as launching centers	Establishment of independent identities for parents and grown children
	Renegotiation of marital relationship
	Readjust relationships to include in-laws and grandchildren
	Dealing with disabilities and death of older generation
Aging Families	Maintenance of couple and individual functioning while adapting to the aging process
	Support role of middle generation
	Support, yet allow, autonomy of older generation
	Preparation for own death and dealing with the loss of spouse and/or siblings and other peers

From Siegrist, B. C. (2001). Family health. In M. A. Nies & M. McEwen (Eds.), *Community health nursing: Promoting the health of populations* (3rd ed., pp. 409-456). Philadelphia: W. B. Saunders; Wright L. M., & Leahey M. (1994). *Nurses and families: A guide to family assessment and intervention* (2nd ed.). Philadelphia: F. A. Davis.

child care provider and the wife might expect her husband to help out around the house and take care of the children. Alternatively, a child might be responsible for caring for a younger sibling and need supervision himself.

DEVELOPMENTAL STAGES OF FAMILIES

Just as an individual grows through a series of developmental stages (i.e., infancy, toddlerhood, childhood), a normal family also evolves through a series of several stages. Indeed, the typical family goes through the following stages: beginning or establishment stage, early childbearing, families with young children, families with school-age children, families with adolescents, families as launching centers, middle-age families, and aging families (Box 13-4) (Siegrist, 2001).

Alterations in family development may occur that inhibit movement through these stages.

BOX 13-4 Stages of Family Development

Beginning family/establishment stage
Early childbearing family
Preschool children
School-age children
Teenage children
Launching family
Middle-age family
Aging family

From Siegrist, B. C. (2001). Family health. In M. A. Nies & M. McEwen (Eds.), *Community health nursing: Promoting the health of populations* (3rd ed., pp. 409-456). Philadelphia: W. B. Saunders.

Divorce and remarriage, for example, dramatically redefine the stages of family development. Likewise, having a late baby when other children are adolescents changes the family development cycle. Other alterations to the family life cycle occur with single parenting; infertility; and early, unexpected death. Table 13-1 provides a summary of tasks to be accomplished in each stage of the family's life cycle. Additionally, each **stage of family development**, as explained by McCarthy and Mandle (2000), is described briefly.

ESTABLISHMENT STAGE (BEGINNING FAMILY)

In the establishment stage, a couple goes through courtship and engagement. A commitment to a partner is made, usually through marriage. The new couple must develop and define their relationship and become free of parental domination. They establish their own home and life patterns and focus on the new lifestyle with the partner. At some point, the beginning family discusses parenting issues.

EARLY CHILDBEARING STAGE

In the early childbearing stage, the couple must resolve feelings and issues about pregnancy and parenthood. At a point, the woman becomes pregnant or the couple decides to adopt. This stage requires significant adjustment to changes in lifestyle and the couple must work through a number of related developmental tasks. When the infant arrives, they must adjust to caring for it. In addition, they need to renegotiate marital and extended family relationships.

FAMILIES WITH PRESCHOOL-AGE CHILDREN

In families with preschool-age children, the couple learns to adjust to family life, concentrating on adapting to the needs and interests of small children. They must learn to cope with energy depletion and lack of privacy as parents. Financial issues may be prevalent as the wife leaves the workforce or the family must pay for child care.

FAMILIES WITH SCHOOL-AGE CHILDREN

Families with school-age children need to adjust to growing children's activities. They should promote development of joint decision making by children and parents and encourage and support the children's education achievement.

FAMILIES WITH ADOLESCENTS

During the adolescent stage of family development, the family should strive to maintain open communication among family members. This is a good time to strengthen the family unit to support and encourage ethical and moral values. During this stage, it is important to balance freedom with responsibility as teenagers mature.

LAUNCHING FAMILIES

As the children become adults and leave home, the family must cope with different types of changes. They should be ready to release the young adults with appropriate rituals and assistance, while maintaining a supportive home base. During this stage, the husband and wife reestablish their relationship as couple.

MIDDLE-AGE FAMILIES

In the middle-age years, the family (possibly now a dyad) prepares for retirement. During this stage, a significant focus is on maintaining kin ties with both older and younger generations. In many cases, the middle-age family is called on to provide significant assistance to their own aging parents and to their own children who have been launched and begun their own families.

AGING FAMILIES

As the family ages, it is important to adjust to retirement. Other significant changes include loss of spouse, siblings, close friends, and possibly the loss of aging children. Often, the family must decide to close the family home or adapt it for elderly members (McCarthy and Mandle, 2000).

FAMILY HEALTH

Family health refers to the health status of a given family at a given point in time; it ranges along a continuum from wellness to illness (Allender and Spradley, 2001a). Family health is concerned with how well the family functions together as a unit and considers the health of each family member and how each member relates to other members. Family health also involves how well the family relates to and copes with the community outside the family. Because of the interactions between and among the family members and the interactions with the larger community, it is important for nurses who work in community settings to be aware of, and prepared to intervene in, issues that relate to family health.

HEALTHY PEOPLE 2010 AND FAMILY HEALTH

Although *Healthy People 2010* (U.S. Department of Health and Human Services [USDHHS], 2000) does not address families per se, a number of objectives related to families and family health can be found. In addition, other objectives can or should be addressed at the family level. The *Healthy People 2010* box lists several objectives related to family health.

CHARACTERISTICS OF HEALTHY FAMILIES

In healthy families, the family is the stable source for sustenance, nurturance, growth, and development of each member. There is mutual support as members share in problem solving and decision making. There is also recognition that the family is dynamic and that each member will become part of another family system at some point in time.

Healthy families maintain flexible boundaries that support and encourage exchange between the family and the larger society. There is a defined power structure, which results from clear role definitions and appropriate rules. In healthy families, power is shared among members, within parental roles and appropriate with age. Also, there is an open communication system in which there is honest, clear, and direct communication. Finally, the healthy family is

---

healthy people 2010

Objectives Related to Family Health

OBJECTIVE		BASELINE (1998)	TARGET
1.1:	Increase the proportion of persons with health insurance	86%	100%
1.6:	Reduce the proportion of families that experience difficulties or delays in obtaining health care or do not receive needed care for one or more family members	12%	7%
6.5:	Increase the proportion of adults with disabilities reporting sufficient emotional support	70%	79%
7.7:	Increase the proportion of health care organizations that provide client and family education	NA	NA
8.23:	Reduce the proportion of occupied housing units that are substandard	6.2%	3%
9.4:	Increase the proportion of pregnancies that are intended	51%	70%
9.12:	Reduce the proportion of married couples whose ability to conceive or maintain a pregnancy is impaired	13%	10%
11.1:	Increase the proportion of households with access to the Internet at home	26%	80%
15.34:	Reduce the rate of physical assault by current or former intimate partners	4.5 assaults per 1000	3.6 assaults per 1000
22.11:	Increase the proportion of children and adolescents who view television 2 or fewer hours per day	60%	75%
27.9:	Reduce the proportion of children who are regularly exposed to tobacco smoke at home	27%	10%

From U.S. Department of Health and Human Services (USDHHS). (2000). *Healthy people 2010: Conference edition.* Washington, DC: USDHHS.

adaptable, flexible, and resilient; this allows for coping with changing demands (Cooley, 2000).

The following specific characteristics or traits can be observed in healthy families:

- Members interact with each other repeatedly in many contexts (Figure 13-1).
- Members are encouraged to grow and develop as individuals and members of the family.
- Members are enhanced and fulfilled by maintaining contacts with a wide range of community groups and organizations.
- Members make efforts to master their lives by becoming members of groups, finding information and options, and making decisions.
- Members support and maintain a healthy environment and lifestyle.
- Members engage in flexible role relationships, share power, respond to change, support growth and autonomy of others, and engage in decision making that affects them.
- Members support mastery of developmental tasks leading to interdependence, progressive differentiation, and transformation to meet the requisites for survival of the system.
- Members provide nurturance and resources for growth and sustenance (Allender and Spradley, 2001b; Murray et al., 2001; Siegrist, 2001).

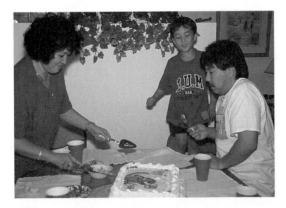

Figure 13-1. Family celebrations and traditions strengthen the role of the family. (From Potter, P. A., & Perry, A. G. [2001]. *Fundamentals of nursing* [5th ed.]. St. Louis: Mosby.)

CHARACTERISTICS OF UNHEALTHY FAMILIES

Just as there are characteristics common to healthy families, patterns can be identified among families that are not adaptive and might be termed unhealthy. Some of these characteristics include the following:

- Maladaptation: signs of strained or destructive family relationships
- Lack of understanding, communication, and helpfulness between members
- Each family member alternately acts as if the other did not exist or harasses others through arguments
- Lack of family decision making and lines of authority
- Parent's possessiveness of the children or the mate
- Children's derogatory remarks to the parents or vice versa
- Extreme closeness between husband and his mother or family, or between the wife and her mother or family
- Members not maintaining individuality, being too close or enmeshed, or too distant with each other
- Parents being domineering about performance of household tasks
- Few outside friends for parents or children
- Scapegoating or blaming each other for difficulties
- High level of anxiety or insecurity present in the home
- Lack of creativity and stability
- Pattern of immature or regressive behavior in parents or children
- Boundaries between generations not maintained (children carrying out parental roles because of parental inability or abandonment) (Murray et al., 2001)

When observing or assessing families, the nurse should watch for signs or indications that might show the family has unhealthy traits or characteristics. Table 13-2 lists some risk factors for unhealthy families based on life cycle stage.

TABLE **13-2** Family Stage-Specific Risk Factors and Related Health Problems

STAGE	RISK FACTORS	HEALTH PROBLEMS
Beginning childbearing family	Lack of knowledge about family planning Teenage marriage Lack of knowledge concerning sexual and marital roles and adjustments Underweight or overweight Lack of prenatal care Inadequate nutrition Poor food habits Smoking, alcohol, drug abuse Unmarried status First pregnancy before age 16 or after 35 History of hypertension and infections during pregnancy Rubella, syphilis, gonorrhea, and acquired immunodeficiency syndrome (AIDS) Genetic factors present Low socioeconomic and educational levels Lack of safety in the home	Premature baby Unsuccessful marriage Low-birth-weight infant Birth defects Birth injuries Accidents Sudden infant death syndrome Respiratory distress syndrome Sterility Pelvic inflammatory disease Fetal alcohol syndrome Mental retardation Child abuse Injuries
Family with school-age children	Home unstimulating Working parents with inappropriate use of resources for child care Poverty environment Abuse and/or neglect of children Generational pattern of using social agencies as a way of life Multiple, closely spaced children Low family self-esteem Children used as scapegoats for parental frustration Repeated infections, accidents, or hospitalizations Parents immature, dependent, and unable to handle responsibility Unrecognized or unattended health problems Strong beliefs about physical punishment Toxic substances unprotected in the home Poor nutrition (overeating and undereating)	Behavior disturbances Speech and vision problems Communicable diseases Dental caries School problems Learning disabilities Cancer Injuries Chronic diseases Homicide Violence
Family with adolescents	Racial and ethnic family origin Lifestyle and behavior patterns leading to chronic disease Lack of problem-solving skills Family values of aggressiveness and competition Socioeconomic factors contributing to peer relationships Family values rigid and inflexible Daredevil risk-taking attitudes Denial behavior Conflicts between parents and children Pressure to live up to family expectations	Violent deaths and injuries Alcohol and drug abuse Unwanted pregnancy Sexually transmitted diseases Suicide Depression

From McCarthy, N. C., & Mandle, C. L. (2000). Health promotion and the family. In C. L. Edelman & C. L. Mandle (Eds.), *Health promotion throughout the lifespan* (4th ed., pp. 144-170). St. Louis: Mosby.

continued

TABLE **13-2** Family Stage-Specific Risk Factors and Related Health Problems—cont'd

STAGE	RISK FACTORS	HEALTH PROBLEMS
Family with middle-age adults	Hypertension Smoking High cholesterol level Diabetes Overweight Physical inactivity Personality patterns related to stress Genetic predisposition Use of oral contraceptives Sex, race, and other hereditary factors Geographic area, age, occupational deficiencies Exposure to certain substances (sunlight, radiation, water or air pollution) Social class Residence	Cardiovascular disease Cancer Accidents Homicide Suicide Mental illness Depression
Family with older adults	Age Drug interactions Depression Metabolic disorders Chronic illness Retirement Loss of spouse Reduced income Poor nutrition Lack of exercise Past environments and lifestyle Lack of preparation for death	Periodontal disease and loss of teeth Mental confusion Reduced vision Hearing impairment Hypertension Acute illness Infectious disease Injuries (i.e., burns and falls) Depression Chronic disease Elder abuse Death without dignity

FAMILY CRISIS

Family crises are experienced in all families. Two basic types of family crises are the maturational crisis and the situational crisis. A maturational crisis is a normal transition point in which old patterns of communication and old roles must be exchanged for new patterns and roles. Every family experiences maturational crisis points whether or not a crisis is actually experienced. Examples of transitional periods in which maturational crises may occur are adolescence, marriage, and parenthood (Caudle, 1999).

A situational crisis can occur when the family experiences an event that is sudden, unexpected, and unpredictable. Such events threaten either biological, psychological, or social integrity leading to disorganization, tension, and severe anxiety. Examples of situational crises include illness, accidents, death, and natural disasters (Caudle, 1999).

A crisis state is associated with high stress and tension levels. The result of a crisis can be either resolution (resulting in a healthier, more positive state of being) or loss of well-being and a higher potential for recurrent crisis. Temporary relief can be gained from the use of defense mechanisms, environmental action, or both. During periods of crisis, families are more susceptible to change and are usually more open to help (Caudle, 1999).

Bergman (1993) identified the following key family characteristics that influence how people recover from and function during and after crises:

- Family cohesion: emotional bonding of family members and the degree of individual autonomy of each person in the family
- Family adaptation: the degree of flexibility evidenced by the ability to change roles, relationships, and power structures in response to stress
- Family social integration: the degree of social network with neighbors, friends, other family members, and religious or social organizations
- Degree of stress experienced by the family: includes combinations of stressors that may influence the family

If these characteristics are strong, in most cases the family can respond appropriately or positively to the crisis and adapt effectively. If the family characteristics are weak, the crisis may be more difficult to manage or resolve.

NURSING CARE OF FAMILIES

The concept of family nursing is not new. It has been taught in schools of nursing since Nightingale's time. Indeed, the National League for Nursing (NLN) has emphasized the importance of caring for the family in standard curricula guides for schools of nursing since 1917. Furthermore, many modern nurse theorists (i.e., Newman, King, Orem, Roy) extensively discuss the family and its importance to individuals and society (Siegrist, 2001).

FAMILY NURSING

Nurses working in community settings should be aware that the individual can best be understood within the social context of the family. Nurses approach family health care in two ways. The first is viewing the family as the context of care; the second is viewing the family as client. When families are treated as the context within which

individuals are assessed, the emphasis is primarily on the individual, keeping in mind that he or she is part of a larger system, the family (family as context). Conversely, when the nurse treats the family as a set of interacting parts and emphasizes assessment of the dynamics among these parts rather than the individual parts themselves (family members), the family as a whole rather than the individual members become the client (family as client) (Hitchcock, 1999).

In family nursing, care focuses on the individual family member, within the context of the family or the family unit, or in some cases, both. The nurse establishes a relationship with each family member within the unit and understands the influence of the unit on the individual and larger group or community (Siegrist, 2001). Birthing, parent-child relationships, adult day care, chronic illness, and home care are best addressed using nursing practice models emphasizing the family.

Friedman (1998) presented some reasons that nurses should work with families. This list included the following ideas:

- Within the family unit, any dysfunction that affects one or more family members will probably affect other family members and the family as a whole.
- The wellness of the family is highly dependent on the role of the family in every aspect of health care, from prevention to rehabilitation.
- The level of wellness of the whole family can be raised through care that reduces lifestyle and environmental risks by emphasizing health promotion, self-care, health education, and family counseling.
- Commonalities in risk factors and diseases shared by family members can lead to case finding within the family.
- A clear understanding of the functioning of the individual can be gained only when the individual is assessed within the larger context of the family.
- The family as a vital support system to the individual member needs to be incorporated into treatment plans.

FAMILY NURSING INTERVENTIONS

The nurse can provide several interventions to promote family health. For example, the nurse can act as a collaborator, helping the family to assess, improve, enhance, and evaluate their current health practices. The nurse can also assist the family in identifying high-risk behaviors and helping them make decisions about lifestyle choices. The nurse can provide information about health issues and give reinforcement for positive health practices. Finally, the nurse can act as a liaison for referral or collaboration between the family and community resources (Mandle, 2000). The Community Application box "Nursing Roles" lists other nursing roles and interventions for the family, based on the various family developmental stages.

FAMILY ASSESSMENT

A comprehensive **family assessment** should be the basis for promoting the health of a family. Several factors influence the assessment of the family: the nurse's perception of what constitutes a family, knowledge of theories, norms and standards, and ability to put the family at ease

(Mandle, 2000). When performing a comprehensive assessment of the family, Allender and Spradley (2001b) suggest that the nurse do the following:

1. Focus on the family as a total unit
2. Ask goal-directed questions
3. Collect data over time
4. Combine quantitative and qualitative data
5. Exercise professional judgment

In addition, Friedman (1998) lists 12 data-collection categories for family health assessment. These are shown in Box 13-5.

FAMILY HEALTH ASSESSMENT TOOLS

Completion of a family health assessment instrument may help the nurse identify the health status of individual members of the family and aspects of family composition, function, and process. A family health assessment may elicit information about the environment or community context and the family and enables the community health nurse to plan interventions appropriately (Siegrist, 2001).

The family assessment should be as comprehensive as possible. Many tools are available to assist the nurse in assessing the family. One

---

BOX 13-5 Data Collection Categories for a Comprehensive Family Assessment

1. Family demographics: family composition, socioeconomic status, education, ages, occupation, ethnicity, and religious affiliation of its members
2. Physical environment data: geography, climate, housing, space, social structures, food availability, and dietary patterns
3. Psychological and spiritual environment: relationships, mutual respect, and support; promotion of members' self-esteem, spiritual development, and goals
4. Family structure and roles: family organization, socialization processes, division of labor, authority and power patterns
5. Family function: Ability to carry out appropriate developmental tasks and provide for members' needs
6. Family values and beliefs: how to raise children, how to make and spend money, and emphasis on education, religion, work, health, and community involvement
7. Family communication patterns: frequency and quality of communication within a family and between the family and its environment
8. Family decision-making patterns: how decisions are made and implemented
9. Family problem-solving patterns: how the family handles its problems
10. Family coping patterns: how a family handles conflict and life changes; nature and quality of support systems and perception and responses to stressors
11. Family health behavior: family health history, current physical health status of members, use of health resources and health beliefs
12. Family social and cultural patterns: family discipline and limit-setting practices; promotion of members' initiative, creativity, and leadership; family goals; and development of meaningful relationships within and without the family

COMMUNITY APPLICATION
Possible Nursing Roles in Health Promotion and Disease Prevention Through Stages of Family Development

Stage	Possible Nursing Role
Couple	Counselor on sexual and role adjustment
	Teacher and counselor in family planning
	Teacher of parenting skills
	Coordinator for genetic counseling
Childbearing family	Monitor of prenatal care and referrer for problems of pregnancy
	Counselor on prenatal nutrition
	Counselor on prenatal maternal habits
	Supporter of amniocentesis
	Counselor on breastfeeding
	Coordinator with pediatric services
	Supervisor of immunizations
	Referrer to social services
	Assistant in adjustment to parental role
Family with preschool and school-age children	Monitor of early childhood development; referrer when indicated
	Teacher in first-aid and emergency measures
	Coordinator with pediatric services
	Counselor on nutrition and exercise
	Teacher in problem-solving issues regarding health habits
	Participant in community organizations for environmental control
	Teacher of dental care hygiene
	Counselor on environmental safety in the home
	Facilitator in interpersonal relationships
Family with adolescents	Teacher of risk factors on health
	Teacher in problem-solving issues regarding alcohol, smoking, diet, and exercise
	Facilitator of interpersonal skills with teenagers and parents
	Direct supporter, counselor, or referrer to mental health resources
	Counselor on family planning
	Referrer for sexually transmittable disease
Family with young or middle-age adults	Participant in community organizations on disease control
	Teacher in problem-solving issues regarding lifestyle and habits
	Participant in community organizations for environmental control
	Case finder in the home and community
	Screener for hypertension, Pap smear, breast examination, cancer signs, mental health, and dental care
	Counselor on menopausal transition
Family with older adults	Facilitator in interpersonal relationships among family members
	Referrer for work and social activity, nutritional programs, homemakers' services, and nursing home
	Monitor of exercise, nutrition, preventive services, and medications
	Supervisor of immunization
	Counselor on safety in the home
	Counselor on bereavement

From Mandle, C. L. (2000). Health promotion and the family. In C. L. Edelman & C. L. Mandle (Eds.), *Health promotion throughout the lifespan* (5th Ed., pp. 169-198). St. Louis: Mosby.

family assessment tool is provided in Appendix 13-A at the end of this chapter. An assessment tool of this type helps the nurse gather data on family characteristics, structure, and processes, and the environment (i.e., residence, neighborhood, and community). Not all information is appropriate for every family, however, and the assessment instrument should be modified and adapted as necessary to fit the individual family (Siegrist, 2001). Other tools for family assessment include the genogram, the family health tree, and the ecomap, described in the following sections.

GENOGRAM

A **genogram** is a tool that helps the nurse outline the family's structure. It is a way to diagram the family to view family patterns. The genogram may be developed during an early family interview and includes births, deaths, divorces, and remarriages. It might also identify other characteristics (race, social class), occupations, and places of family residence (Allender and Spradley, 2001b). Figure 13-2 shows commonly used genogram symbols and Figure 13-3 depicts a genogram that Jessica, the nurse from the opening case study, constructed from her assessment of the Smith family.

FAMILY HEALTH TREE

A **family health tree** is another tool that nurses in community-based practice may use. By expanding on the genogram, the family health tree provides a way to record pertinent data about a family's medical and health histories. Causes of death of deceased family members, when known, are important. Genetically linked diseases including heart disease, cancer, diabetes, hypertension, sickle cell anemia, allergies, asthma, and mental retardation are particularly important to assess. Environmental and occupational diseases, psychosocial problems (i.e., mental illness), obesity, and infectious disease should be noted.

From the health problems depicted in the family health tree, familial risk factors can be drawn. The family health tree can also be used to

plan or enhance positive familial influences on risk factors such as diet, exercise, coping with stress, or pressure to have a physical examination (Siegrist, 2001). Figure 13-4 is the family health tree Jessica developed for the Smith family.

ECOMAP

An **ecomap** is a tool that can be used to explain a family's linkages to their suprasystems or the larger environment. The ecomap visually illustrates the dynamic family-environment interactions and shows the connections between the family and the world. The ecomap depicts the important nurturing connections and conflicts, or areas of stress between family members. Figure 13-5 presents Jessica's ecomap of the Smith family. An ecomap can also demonstrate the flow or lack of resources; therefore it may help point to areas for conflict resolution or to where additional resources are needed (Siegrist, 2001).

An ecomap should be completed during an early family interview, noting persons, institutions, and agencies significant to the family. In constructing an ecomap, a central circle is drawn representing the family and smaller circles in the periphery represent people and systems (i.e., school, work, friends, church, health care) whose relationships with the family are significant (Allender and Spradley, 2001b).

APPLICATION OF THE NURSING PROCESS TO CARING FOR FAMILIES

When caring for families in community settings, typically one member of the family is identified as the client who is the primary recipient of nursing care. This client may have an identified health problem, a chronic illness that needs continued monitoring, or a significant potential problem. Often, however, a family has more than one member with actual or potential health problems. Because family members are interconnected, the health of each is a concern to the

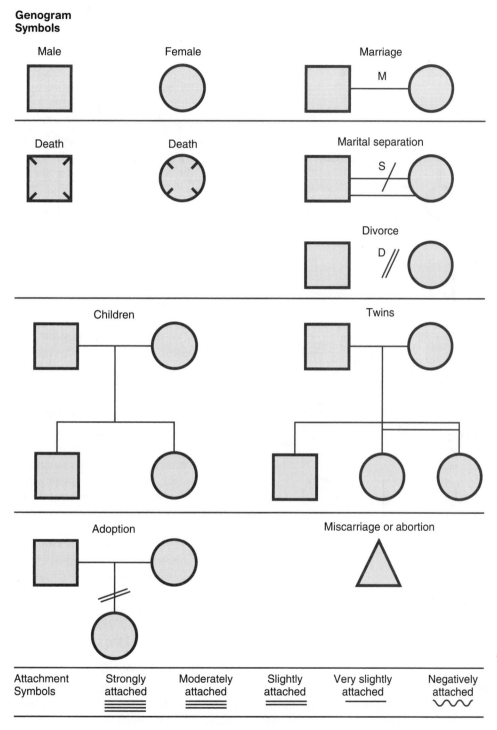

Figure 13-2. Genogram symbols.

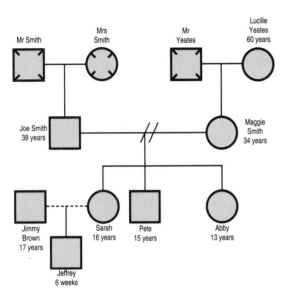

Figure 13-3. Genogram of the Smith family.

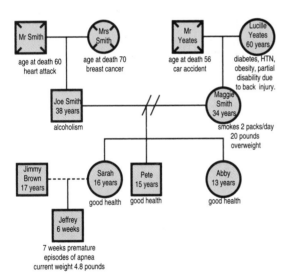

Figure 13-4. Family health tree of the Smith family.

nurse, and all family members may benefit from interventions (Cooley and Smith, 2000).

ASSESSMENT

Using tools or instruments such as those described earlier as a guide, the nurse should assess and reassess the family in their own envir-

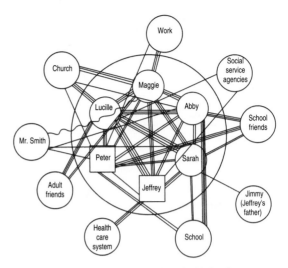

Figure 13-5. Ecomap of the Smith family.

onment and within the neighborhood. Data about the family should be collected from as many members of the family as possible. The nurse should assess verbal and nonverbal cues and environmental and behavioral information. When possible, the nurse should observe family dynamics, including communication patterns among family members, roles taken, and division of labor. Assessment should also include what is available to the family in terms of social support, schools, recreation, and religious activities.

Jessica, the nurse in the opening case study, performed a thorough assessment on the Smith family. She completed a family assessment instrument (much like the one in Appendix 13-A) by interviewing each of the adult family members and by observing the family's environment. In addition, she drew a genogram, ecomap, and family health tree (see Figures 13-3 to 13-5) illustrating her impression of relationships among family members and relationships between the family members and the larger society.

ANALYSIS AND DIAGNOSIS

Family assessments may provide massive amounts of data and are often complex and confusing. The information must be integrated and analyzed before decisions about the plan of care

BOX **13-6** Examples of Family Nursing Diagnoses

Altered family processes	Health-seeking behaviors
Altered parenting	Impaired home maintenance management
Anticipatory grieving	Impaired social interaction
Compromised family coping	Ineffective family coping
Decisional conflict	Knowledge deficit
Dysfunctional grieving	Parental role conflict
Family coping: potential for growth	

From North American Nursing Diagnosis Association (NANDA). (1999). *Nursing diagnoses: Definitions and classifications, 1999-2000.* Philadelphia: North American Nursing Diagnosis Association.

can be made. When analyzing data, the nurse might determine what style the family uses in day-to-day functioning (i.e., are they receptive, distant, resistant, disorganized, rigid, ordered, dependent?). The nurse would also identify family strengths and weaknesses and identify and prioritize health needs or areas of concern. For example, is the family dealing with normal growth and development issues? Is the family coping with illness or loss? Is the family dealing with external stressors? Does the family have adequate resources and support (Cooley and Smith, 2000)?

Following review and analysis, nursing diagnoses can be made for each individual family member and/or for the family as a whole. In addition to actual and potential health problems and developmental issues, nursing diagnoses may stem from problems in communication or roles and value conflicts. Examples of family nursing diagnoses are shown in Box 13-6.

In the chapter opening case study, Jessica identified several areas that needed intervention. First there was evidence of knowledge deficit on the part of Sarah, Lucille, and Maggie with regard to caring for a new infant with a chronic health problem. This is a priority issue.

Jessica also determined that several family processes were altered because the family had to adapt to the introduction of a new family member whose presence would affect each family member. There was also a potential for parental role conflict in Sarah because she wanted to help care for the infant, but needed to spend a great deal of time in school.

Maggie and Lucille both demonstrated health-seeking behaviors as they questioned Jessica about personal health issues—Maggie wanted to stop smoking and Lucille requested information on diet and exercise. Finally, Maggie shared with Jessica concerns over Pete's friend network and worried that he might become involved with drugs or gangs.

INTERVENTION

As explained, interventions are based on assessment and analysis. They are offered by the nurse to address actual and potential health problems of individuals within the family and the family as a whole.

In the case study, Jessica's primary interest is on helping the family adapt to the new infant and to meet his special needs. As mentioned, she taught the women how to care for the child, how to identify and manage potential problems, and emergency procedures. She also gave them information on social service programs they might be eligible for, including Women, Infants, and Children (WIC) and a community-sponsored day care program.

To address possible role conflicts with Sarah, Jessica talked at length with her about how she would help her grandmother care for the baby. Sarah recognized the importance of completing her education and knew that it was essential for her and Jeffrey's future. In confidence, Jessica also talked with Sarah about sexuality and contraception, explaining that it is common for teen mothers to become pregnant again. She left literature for Sarah on all of the issues they discussed.

For Maggie and Lucille's questions, Jessica stated that she would gather some literature from the health department on healthy lifestyles. She would also provide a referral for Maggie to attend a smoking cessation program. Finally, she suggested that Maggie make an appointment with Pete's school counselor to gather more information about drug and alcohol problems in the school and to see how Pete was doing in school. She also strongly encouraged Maggie to work to open communication patterns with Pete.

EVALUATION

Evaluation is the ongoing process of observing family progress toward meeting goals identified by the nurse and family. Evaluation is not merely a terminal phase, but should be ongoing within nursing care.

In the case study, Jessica continually evaluated responses to her health teaching. She encouraged questions and had the women verbally repeat her instructions. She also evaluated responses to her counseling and planned on following up to see if the family members complied with suggestions. For example, on a subsequent visit, she would ask Maggie if she had started her smoking cessation program and if she had met with Pete's counselor.

SUMMARY

Families are vital to promoting and preserving health. It is acknowledged that individuals can best be understood within the context of their family and the family can be essential in helping address individual health needs. Furthermore, the family itself may be healthy or unhealthy and may possess a number of risk factors that affect each member and the family as a whole. These health threats and risk factors are often best addressed at the family level. As a home health nurse working with high-risk infants, Jessica, the nurse from the opening case study, understood the impact of serious health problems and threats on the family and recognized

the necessity of caring for the entire family in many cases.

This chapter covers issues important to family health care. Through understanding the concept of family, recognizing the different types of families, and knowing the stages in a family's developmental life cycle, the nurse can more effectively assess, plan, implement, and evaluate family health. Nurses who work in community settings are frequently in a position to care for clients within the context of their family and to care for the family as a unit and should be prepared to intervene appropriately.

KEY POINTS

- Many definitions of family are found in the literature. In general, families are social units or systems comprised of two or more persons in a committed relationship. The family provides protection, nourishment, and socialization for family members.

- Several different types of families can be identified: the nuclear family, nuclear dyad, single-parent family, extended family, blended family, three-generational family, single adult, cohabitating couple, and homosexual family.

- Certain characteristics or traits are common to all families. For example, all families are social systems; families change; families are interdependent; families meet a variety of needs; and families create and maintain their own set of values, rules, and goals.

- Families exist to serve several purposes, including providing physical safety and meeting the economic needs of family members. They also help members develop physically, emotionally, intellectually, and spiritually and teach social skills and how to communicate.

- Each family member has both formal and informal roles within the family unit. Role conflict may occur when roles contradict or compete with each other, or when one person's role definition does not correspond with another's definition.

- Most families grow through a series of developmental stages: beginning family stage, early childbearing family stage, preschool children stage, school-age children stage, teenage children stage, launching family stage, middle-age family stage, and aging family stage.
- Family health refers to the health status of a given family at a point in time; it is concerned with how well the family functions together as a unit and how the family copes with the outside community.
- Healthy families share common characteristics including interaction with other family members, encouraging members to grow and develop, enhancing and fulfilling family members, maintaining a healthy environment, having flexible role relationships and shared power, and providing nurturance.
- Unhealthy families share common characteristics including lack of understanding, poor communication between members, lack of defined lines of authority, possessiveness of the children or mate, members not maintaining individuality, parents being domineering, few outside friends, high levels of anxiety or insecurity in the home, and immature or regressive behavior in parents or children.
- Family crises are experienced in all families and include maturational crises (related to normal developmental stages or transitions) and situational crises (related to sudden, unexpected and unpredictable events).
- Family nursing interventions should promote family health and include providing information, acting as a referral source, collaboration, and counseling.
- A family assessment should be thorough, covering such issues as demographics, the physical environment, the psychological environment, family roles, family function, family values, communication patterns, coping patterns, and family health behavior. Tools that nurses can use include a family assessment instrument, a genogram, a family health tree, and an ecomap.

- In family nursing, the nurse should apply each step of the nursing process to caring for an individual within the context of his/her family or caring for the family as a unit.

Resources

Family Health

Administration for Children and Families
Council on Family Health
Multicultural Family Institute
Office of Family Assistance
Family and Youth Services Bureau
National Clearinghouse on Families and Youth

Learning Activities & Application to Practice

In Class

1. Compose a definition of family. In groups of five or six, discuss criteria for a family.
2. Complete a genogram, family health tree, and/or ecomap for your own family. Identify potential areas for intervention at the individual and family level. Share with the rest of the class on a voluntary basis.

In Clinical

3. Identify a family from your clinical experience who is at risk for dysfunction. If the family is agreeable, complete a family health assessment and make nursing diagnoses and recommendations. Share findings with the clinical group.

REFERENCES

Allender, J., & Spradley, B. (2001a). Theoretical bases for promoting family health. In J. A. Allender & B. W. Spradley (Eds.), *Community health nursing: Concepts and practice* (5th ed., pp. 427-445). Philadelphia: Lippincott.

Allender, J., & Spradley, B. (2001b). Assessment of families. In J. A. Allender & B. W. Spradley (Eds.), *Community health nursing: Concepts and practice* (5th ed., pp. 446-469). Philadelphia: Lippincott.

Bergman, A. (1993). High-risk indicators for family involvement in social work in health care: A review of the literature. *Social Work, 38,* 282.

Caudle, P. (1999). Care of the family client. In M. J. Clark (Ed.), *Nursing in the community: Dimensions of community health nursing* (3rd ed., pp. 389-418). Stamford, CT: Appleton & Lange.

Cooley, M. (2000). A family perspective in community health nursing. In C. M. Smith & F. A. Maurer (Eds.), *Community health nursing: Theory and practice* (2nd ed., pp. 237-255). Philadelphia: W. B. Saunders.

Cooley, M., & Smith, C. M. (2000). The nursing process and families. In C. M. Smith & F. A. Maurer (Eds.), *Community health nursing: Theory and practice* (2nd ed., pp. 256-288). Philadelphia: W. B. Saunders.

Craft, M. J., & Willadsen, J. A. (1992). Interventions related to family. *Nursing Clinics of North America, 27,* 517-529.

Farber, B. (1973). *Family and kinship in modern society.* Glenview, IL: Scott Foresman.

Friedman, M. (1998). *Family nursing: Research, theory and practice* (4th ed.). Stamford, CT: Appleton & Lange.

Helvie, C. O. (1981). *Community health nursing: theory and process.* New York: Harper & Row.

Hitchcock, J. E. (1999). Frameworks for assessing families. In J. E. Hitchcock, P. E. Schubert, & S. A. Thomas (Eds.), *Community health nursing: Caring in action* (pp. 407-437). Albany, NY: Delmar.

Mandle, C. L. (2000). Health promotion and the family. In C. L. Edelman & C. L. Mandle (Eds.), *Health promotion throughout the lifespan* (5th ed., pp. 169-198). St. Louis: Mosby.

Murray, R. B. et al. (2001). The family: Basic unit for the developing person. In R. B. Murray & J. P. Zentner (Eds.), *Health promotion strategies through the life span* (7th ed., pp. 157-212). Upper Saddle River, NJ: Prentice Hall.

North American Nursing Diagnosis Association (NANDA). (1999). *Nursing diagnoses: Definitions and classifications, 1999-2000.* Philadelphia: North American Nursing Diagnosis Association.

Siegrist, B. C. (2001). Family health. In M. A. Nies & M. McEwen (Eds.), *Community health nursing: Promoting the health of populations* (3rd ed., pp. 409-456). Philadelphia: W. B. Saunders.

Stuart, M. (1991). An analysis of the concept of family. In Whall, A. & Fawcett, J. (Eds.), *Family theory development in nursing: State of the science and art.* Philadelphia: F. A. Davis.

U.S. Census Bureau. (1995). *Statistical abstracts of the United States.* (115th ed.). Washington, DC: U.S. Census Bureau.

U.S. Census Bureau. (1999). *Racial-ethnic and gender differences in returns to cohabitation and marriage: Evidence from the current population survey.* Washington, DC: U.S. Census Bureau.

U.S. Department of Commerce. (1997). *Current population reports.* Series P23-193. Washington, DC: U.S. Department of Commerce.

U.S. Department of Health and Human Services (USDHHS). (2000). *Healthy people 2010: Conference edition.* Washington, DC: U.S. Department of Health and Human Services.

Vaughn-Cole, B., Johnson, M. A., & Malone, J. A. (1998). *Family nursing practice.* Philadelphia: W. B. Saunders.

Wright, L. M., & Leahey M. (1994). *Nurses and families: A guide to family assessment and intervention* (2nd ed.). Philadelphia: F. A. Davis.

Family surname: _____
Household members (name, age, and relationship to head of household): _____
_____
_____
_____

Family composition: _____
_____

Genogram:

Family health tree (include health problems of individual members):

Ecomap (for social and health agencies include hours of service, distance and transportation, availability of interpreters, and criteria for receiving services such as age, sex, and income barriers):

Family characteristics	Source(s) of information	Date
Extended family Relatives living outside household		
Location of relatives		
Frequency and duration of contact		
Means of communication		
Family mobility Length of time living in residence		
Location of previous residence		
Frequency of geographic moves		
Country/area of origin		
Family structure Educational experiences		

Siegrist, B. C. (2001). Family health. In M. A. Nies & M. McEwen (Eds.), *Community health nursing: Promoting the health of populations* (3rd ed., pp. 409-456). Philadelphia: W. B. Saunders.

Family characteristics	Source(s) of information	Date
Employment history		
Financial resources		
Leisure time interests		
Division of labor		
Allocation of roles		
Distribution of authority and power		
Family cohesion Emotional bonding of family members		
Degree of individual autonomy		
Family adaptation Flexibility in role change		
Flexibility in power structures		
Family processes How members communicate		
How decisions are made		
How problems are solved		
How conflict is handled		
Family social integration Language(s) and/or dialect(s) spoken; where		
Literacy; ability to read or write in language(s)		
Degree of racial or cultural identity		
Degree of social network with neighbors, friends, and other family members		
Network with religious organizations		
Network with social organizations		
Degrees of stress experienced by the family Combinations of stressors: 1.		
2.		
3.		

Family characteristics	Source(s) of information	Date
Family health behavior Activities of daily living (how family spends typical day)		
Health history		
Health status (i.e., problems and priorities)		
Risk behaviors		
Self-care (health promotion and prevention)		

Health care resources
  Professionals and lay healers
  Working with family and agencies		

Family strengths		
Family priorities		
Family–nurse contract(s)		
Family cultural influences Values, attitudes, and beliefs about		
Spirituality		
Rituals (holidays and celebrations)		
Customs		
Dietary habits		
Child-rearing practices		
Health		
Folk diseases and folk medicine		
Cultural healers		
Care of ill family member		
Role of spiritual leader in care of ill family member		

Family characteristics	**Source(s) of information**	**Date**
Family–nurse contract(s)		

Family cultural influences
Values, attitudes, and beliefs about

Spirituality

Rituals (holidays and celebrations)

Customs

Dietary habits

Child-rearing practices

Health

Folk diseases and folk medicine

Cultural healers

Care of ill family member

Role of spiritual leader in care of ill family member

Family environment	**Source(s) of information**	**Date**
Family residence Adequacy of size		
Structurally safe		
Sanitation: water, sewage, and garbage		
Adequacy of sleeping arrangement		
Modes of transportation		

Resources
Grocery shopping

Pharmacy

Recreational (e.g., parks)

Educational

Religious

Emergency (i.e., fire and hospital)

Neighborhood interaction

Family environment	Source(s) of information	Date
Family community		
Industry and business		
Leadership		
Government		
Migration (i.e., in and out of community)		
Community memberships/interaction		
Social services		
Health services		
Primary care		
Institutions (e.g., hospital or nursing home)		

Nursing Care of Clients with Special Needs in Community Settings

Chapter 14

Vulnerable Groups

objectives

Upon completion of this chapter, the reader will be able to:

1. Describe the interaction of multiple risk factors that can lead to vulnerability and list several of these risk factors.

2. Discuss the concept of poverty and explain how poverty affects health.

3. Explain health threats common to homeless men, women, adolescents, and children and describe nursing interventions to address actual and potential health problems in this vulnerable group.

4. Explain health threats common to migrant workers and their families and describe nursing interventions to address actual and potential health problems in this vulnerable group.

5. Explain health threats common to disabled persons and describe nursing interventions to address actual and potential health problems in this vulnerable group.

6. Describe different types of disasters and explain the importance of preparedness and the role of the nurse.

key terms

American Red Cross (ARC)	Handicap	Poverty threshold
Disability	Homeless	Preparedness
Disaster	Impairment	Terrorism
Disempowerment	Marginalization	Vulnerability
Disenfranchisement	Migrant health centers (MHCS)	Vulnerable group
Federal Emergency Management Agency (FEMA)	Migrant workers	*See Glossary for definitions.*
	Poverty	

case study

Maria Chavez works as a registered nurse (RN) in the emergency department of a large hospital in an urban area. Like most Americans, Maria was stunned by the terrorist attacks on the World Trade Center and the Pentagon and, like most Americans, she wondered what she could do to combat such disasters. As a child in her native Honduras, she had been exposed to the devastation brought on by a hurricane, which had virtually destroyed the small town in which she lived, leaving her family homeless. Maria remembered the assistance provided to her family and other townspeople by the Red Cross and other relief organizations.

Because of her personal experience with disasters and the Red Cross, Maria suggested to a colleague that nurses from the hospital contact the local chapter of the Red Cross to learn what activities were being undertaken in their area and the opportunities for nurses to participate. Maria called the office and spoke to a volunteer about disaster planning. After learning about her background and interests, the volunteer suggested that Maria might want to become involved with the regional disaster planning group and told her whom to contact about the scheduled meetings.

Following the Red Cross volunteer's suggestion, Maria called the coordinator of the disaster cadre and talked with her at length about how nurses were trained in preparation for possible natural and man-made disasters. Because of the location of the city in the midwestern section of the country, Maria learned that much of the focus of the planning centered on such potential threats as tornadoes. The group also had plans in place for downed airliners and industrial accidents. Following the terrorists' attacks, however, there was a desire to enhance community preparedness for potential chemical and biological threats. There was a need, she learned, to help make members of the community less vulnerable to any terrorist incident.

After speaking with the disaster cadre coordinator, Maria was enthusiastic about learning more about the efforts being done and eager to become part of the group. She was given information on the next meeting and told the coordinator that she would attend.

Everyone is at risk for health problems or health threats related to some personal characteristic, a lifestyle habit, where they live, what they do, their education level, their family income, or a host of other factors. Men are at risk for heart disease, women are at risk for breast cancer, elders are at risk for problems related to aging, smokers are at risk for lung cancer, coal miners are at risk for black lung disease, and the list goes on. But some groups are at greater risk than others because of multiple risk factors; these are termed *vulnerable groups*.

Health issues related to some vulnerable groups (i.e., children, members of racial/ethnic minorities, elders, those with mental illnesses, pregnant teens) are described in other chapters. This chapter is concerned with describing health problems and health threats pertaining to certain particularly vulnerable groups. These are persons in extreme poverty, focusing on the homeless and migrant workers, disabled persons, and victims of disasters.

VULNERABLE GROUPS

As has been described previously, the interaction of many factors, both internal and external, can increase a person's risk of developing a health problem. These factors can include such things as a person's genetic makeup, lifestyle patterns, and the physical and social environments in which he or she lives and works. **Vulnerability** applies to a person or group that is more likely to develop a health-related problem or problems and to have more serious outcomes stemming from their exposure to multiple risks (Bushy, 2001).

Vulnerable groups are those people "who have an increased relative risk or susceptibility to adverse health outcomes" (Flaskerud and Winslow, 1998, p. 69). A vulnerable group is a subgroup of the population that is more likely to develop health problems as a result of exposure to risk(s) or to have worse outcomes from those health problems than the population as a whole (Sebastian, 2000).

Vulnerable groups share common risks or combinations of risk factors and their personal risk factors (i.e., personal habits, social environment, physical environment) make it more likely that they will develop a particular health problem or problems. It is the cumulative and interactive aspects of multiple risk factors that leave persons vulnerable (Bushy, 2001).

Healthy People 2010 (U.S. Department of Health and Human Services [USDHHS], 2000) recognizes that significant health disparities exist among different segments of the population. The objectives highlight the fact that differences occur based on combinations of factors such as age, gender, race/ethnicity, education, income, disability, location, and sexual orienta-

---

healthy people **2010**

Objectives Related to Vulnerable Groups

OBJECTIVE	BASELINE (1998)	TARGET
Poverty and Homelessness		
1.6: Reduce the proportion of families below poverty level that experience difficulties or delay in obtaining health care or do not receive needed care for one or more family members	17%	7%
8.23: Reduce the proportion of occupied housing units that are substandard	6.2%	3%
18.3: Reduce the proportion of homeless adults who have serious mental illness	25%	19%
19.12: Reduce iron deficiency among young children (lower income <130% of poverty threshold)	12%	5%
21.12: Increase the proportion of children and adolescents under age 19 years at or below 200% of the federal poverty level who received any preventive dental service during the past year	20%	57%
Rural and Migrant Health		
8.5: Increase the proportion of persons serviced by community water systems who receive a supply of drinking water that meets the regulations of the Safe Drinking Water Act	73%	95%
8.13: Reduce pesticide exposures that result in visits to a health care facility	27,156	13,500
20-1e: Reduce deaths from work-related injuries (agriculture, forestry, and fishing)	24.1 per 100,000	16.9 per 100,000
21.14: Increase the proportion of community-based health centers including migrant and homeless health centers that have an oral health component	34%	75%
Disabilities		
2.5: Increase the employment rate among adults with arthritis in the working-age population	67%	78%
6.5: Increase the proportion of adults with disabilities reporting sufficient emotional support	70%	79%
7.1: Increase high school completion of persons with disabilities	79%	90%
16.14a: Reduce the occurrence of developmental disabilities (mental retardation)	131 per 10,000	124 per 10,000

From U.S. Department of Health and Human Services (USDHHS). (2000). *Healthy people 2010: Conference edition.* Washington, DC: USDHHS.

tion, among others. Very often, vulnerable individuals and families belong to more than one of these at-risk groups. For example, a pregnant adolescent may be poor and Hispanic, or a rural elderly woman may be blind. The *Healthy People 2010* box gives examples of some of the objectives related to vulnerable groups.

Vulnerability is multidimensional and is exacerbated by the combined effects of limited resources, including physical and environmental resources (i.e., working and/or living in a hazardous environment); personal resources (i.e., poverty, limited social support); and biological, psychological, and social resources (i.e., presence of illness, genetic predisposition, family support). Contributing factors include disempowerment, disenfranchisement, and marginalization.

Vulnerability is a power issue because it involves a lack of control over critical resources needed to function effectively. **Disempowerment** is the loss of power or control over individual circumstances. Vulnerable groups often develop an external locus of control and they may believe that events are outside their control. An external locus of control makes it more difficult for people to initiate action or seek care for health problems. Health promotion and illness-prevention activities are not important or are ineffective (Sebastian, 2000).

Similarly, persons who are marginalized live on the margins, or edges, of society rather than in the mainstream (Zerwekh, 2001). Persons who are experiencing **marginalization** have limited control and power and often are overlooked by those in control.

Disenfranchisement refers to a feeling of separation from mainstream society in which the individual does not have an emotional connection with any group in particular or the larger social fabric in general. Vulnerable groups may be invisible to society and forgotten in health and social planning. Disenfranchisement, marginalization, and disempowerment suggest that vulnerable groups do not have the social supports necessary to effectively manage an emo-

tionally and physically healthy lifestyle. Indeed, many vulnerable individuals have limited support networks because they do not have well-established linkages with formal organizations in their communities, nor do they have other sources of support (i.e., family, friends, neighbors).

Social and economic factors predispose people to vulnerability. Poverty and social isolation are particularly associated with risk and vulnerability and being poor affects the health and well-being of individuals of all ages (Bushy, 2001). Vulnerability results from individual and family efforts to do what is necessary to manage. Social isolation is related to vulnerability (Sebastian, 2000).

Being at the extremes of age (very young or very old) can increase vulnerability. Additionally, disease processes (i.e., human immunodeficiency virus [HIV] infection, cancer) and physiological problems that result from injuries or congenital abnormalities or mental or physical disability can lead to vulnerability. Box 14-1 gives examples of vulnerable groups of special concern to nurses in community settings.

Vulnerable families are at risk because of an intensity or clustering of multiple stressors associated with life events. High-risk families include those who have a chronically ill or disabled family member or who have a family member who has a serious mental illness or

BOX **14-1 Particularly Vulnerable Groups**

Disabled persons
Homeless persons
Migrant workers
Persons in extreme poverty
Persons who are HIV positive
Persons with serious health problems
Pregnant adolescents
Refugees and recent immigrants
Severely mentally ill individuals
Substance abusers
Very young or very old individuals
Victims of disasters
Victims of violence

abuses alcohol or drugs. In addition, special or unexpected events can promote vulnerability in some families. This includes diagnosis of a fatal disease, sudden death, unemployment, and disasters. Finally, trauma-related events (i.e., accidents, domestic violence, sexual abuse) can predispose a family to subsequent health problems (Bushy, 2001).

PERSONS IN SEVERE POVERTY

A significantly large vulnerable group in the United States consists of those persons who are severely impoverished. Severe poverty affects health and well-being in a number of ways. People who are poor are more likely to live in hazardous environments that are overcrowded and have inadequate sanitation. Poverty is more likely to affect women, children, and the elderly, with over 80% of those in poverty being among these groups (Sebastian, 2000). Those who are poor frequently work at high-risk jobs, eat poorly, and have multiple stressors. Furthermore, poverty often reduces access to health care.

This section examines the health implications of poverty and focuses on two particularly vulnerable groups—the homeless and migrant workers. It provides information that helps nurses in community-based practice develop and implement effective interventions as they encounter persons from these vulnerable groups.

DEFINITION OF POVERTY

To be poor is to have few or no material possessions and to have inadequate access to family and community resources. Low socioeconomic status in American society is characterized by social and economic deprivation that combines poor income, no accumulated assets, no access to power, poor education, and a low-status occupation. People are indigent when they are impoverished and deprived of basic comforts (Zerwekh, 2001).

According to Sebastian (2000), **poverty** may be acute, such as cases occurring suddenly after a crisis (i.e., job loss or illness), or poverty may be

chronic and persist over many years. Poverty may also be described as absolute such as when food, shelter and clothing are lacking or relative, as when individuals or families subsist on less than average resources.

In most cases, in the United States, poverty is established by measuring and comparing family income with a predetermined index. Each year the Census Bureau provides a set of income thresholds that vary by family size and composition to determine who is poor. If a family's total income is less than the federally defined **poverty threshold**, then that family is considered poor. For example, in 2000, the poverty threshold for a family of four with two children was $17,463; the poverty threshold for a family of three with two children (single parent family) was $13,874 (U.S. Census Bureau, 2001). The poverty threshold is updated each year and affects eligibility to such programs as Medicaid, Head Start, subsidized housing, and food stamps (Zerwekh, 2001).

Characteristics of the Poor

According to the Census Bureau (2001), about 11.3% of the general population, or more than 31 million persons, lived in poverty in 2000; this was a slight decrease from previous years. Those who are extremely poor (less than half the official poverty threshold) are slightly less than half of the total, or 14.6 million Americans.

In terms of numbers, most impoverished Americans are white; however, a disproportionate number of racial and ethnic minority members are poor. For example, 21.2% of Hispanics and 22.1% of blacks are poor, compared with 7.5% of non-Hispanic whites. Children represent 40% of the poor population, with 16.9% of Americans under the age of 18 living in poverty. The majority of children under 6 who are poor live with single mothers because almost 25% of families with female heads live below the poverty level (U.S. Census Bureau, 2001).

Both urban and rural localities have significant poor populations as 16% of people in rural areas are poor and 19% of people in urban areas are poor. Finally, the states with the greatest percentage of people in poverty include New Mexico (19.3%), Louisiana (18.6%), Washington DC (17.3%), Montana (16.0%), Arkansas (15.8%), and West Virginia (15.8%) (U.S. Census Bureau, 2001).

Many of the poor are employed; however, only a small fraction have full-time jobs year round. Others have part-time employment, often in low-paying retail service industries or as migrant farmworkers or day laborers (Zerwekh, 2001).

Poverty and Health

Poverty directly affects health and well-being. Persons living in poverty and near-poverty have higher rates of chronic illness, higher infant morbidity and mortality, shorter life expectancy, more complex health problems, and more significant complications and physical limitations resulting from chronic diseases. These poor health outcomes are often secondary to barriers that impede access to health care, such as inability to pay for health care, lack of insurance, geographic location, language, maldistribution of providers, transportation difficulties, and negative attitudes of health care providers.

HOMELESSNESS

Poverty can lead to homelessness. Homelessness is a rather complex concept and not easily defined. Although it is easily agreed upon that persons living in bus stations, under bridges, or in shelters run by relief organizations (i.e., Salvation Army) are homeless, there is some disagreement in other cases. For example, is a woman and her children living temporarily in a shelter for abused women considered homeless? Is a teen runaway living in a friend's basement homeless? What about an autistic adult who is in a half-way house awaiting a permanent residence?

In general, a person is considered **homeless** if they lack a fixed, regular address and adequate sleeping arrangements. This includes people who have a primary night-time residence that is: a supervised publicly or privately operated shelter, an institution that provides a temporary residence (i.e., half-way house), or a public or private place not designated for sleeping (i.e., park benches). This definition addresses those persons who are literally homeless (living under bridges or in shelters), but does not include those who are living with relatives or in substandard housing (Bolla, 2000; Scholler-Jaquish, 2000).

The following types or stages of homelessness have been identified (Belcher, Scholler-Jaquish, and Drummond, 1991):

1. *Episodic homelessness* refers to individuals who live below or slightly above the poverty line and are socially stigmatized and vulnerable. Connection to a home is tenuous and may be episodic as persons move in and out of poverty.
2. *Temporary homelessness* refers to people who have recently become homeless. They still identify with the mainstream of their communities and view living on the streets or relying on shelters as an unacceptable lifestyle; most are attempting to regain a lost home, job, and social standing.
3. *Chronic homelessness* refers to people who have been homeless for a significant time and don't identify with most members of society. They accept their lives on the streets as normal and are more easily and clearly identifiable as homeless.

Homeless people are found in both rural and urban areas. Many sleep at night in shelters, streets, parks, alleys, shopping centers, libraries, and other places. They often seek shelter in public buildings, single-room occupancy hotels, all-night movie theaters, abandoned buildings, and vehicles (Bolla, 2000); therefore it is difficult to accurately estimate their numbers.

Since the 1980s, the number of homeless people has surpassed that of the Great Depression. Joining the traditional homeless, predominately composed of single males, are the new homeless. Today, the homeless include families with children, single women, adults who are unemployed and underemployed, immigrants, substance abusers, abandoned children, adolescent runaways, elders, persons who are mentally ill, and Vietnam-era veterans (Bolla, 2000; Droes and Hatton, 2001).

Factors that contribute to homelessness include unemployment, underemployment, poverty, a decrease in the number of affordable housing units, emergency demands on income, alcohol and drug addiction, and deinstitutionalization of chronically mentally ill persons. Other factors include a shift from goods production to services, which has changed the labor market and increased joblessness, lack of affordable health care, and domestic violence (Bolla, 2000; Droes and Hatton, 2001; Scholler-Jaquish, 2000).

Characteristics of Homelessness

In the first 70 years of the twentieth century, the homeless were largely men. Most were white and the vast majority had mental health problems, particularly alcoholism. At the beginning of the twenty-first century, the face of homelessness has changed. Although single men still make up the majority of the homeless, there are many single women and families with children. Box 14-2 shows characteristics that describe the homeless population.

BOX 14-2 Characteristics of the Homeless

43% are single men
37% are families (75% are headed by single women)
13% are single women
25% are children
  7% are unaccompanied minors (largely teenage runaways)
50% are black
31% are white
13% are Hispanic
  4% are Native American
  2% are Asian
45% are substance abusers
22% are veterans
22% are severely mentally ill
20% are employed

Source of data: Droes, N. S., & Hatton, D. C. (2001). Homeless populations. In M. A. Nies & M. McEwen (Eds.), *Community health nursing: Promoting the health of populations* (pp. 526-547). Philadelphia: W. B. Saunders; Scholler-Jaquish, A. (2000). *Homelessness in America.* In C. M. Smith & F. A. Maurer (Eds.), *Community health nursing: Theory and practice* (2nd ed., pp. 672-699). Philadelphia: W. B. Saunders.

Characteristics of the homeless and causes of homelessness vary, based on location. For example, approximately 60% of the urban homeless population is composed of members of racial and ethic minorities; rural homeless are mostly white. The large number of minorities among urban homeless are associated with poverty, unemployment, lack of low-income housing, and racial discrimination. Chronic homelessness for the white urban population is more likely to be related to substance abuse and mental illness (Scholler-Jaquish, 2000).

Homeless men make up the largest and most visible group of the homeless population. Most homeless men are mentally ill and/or substance abusers. Also, interestingly, between 20% and 40% of urban homeless are veterans (Scholler-Jaquish, 2000).

Homeless women are not as visible as are homeless men and they account for 14% to 25% of the homeless population. There are many types of homeless women including single women with a history of drug and alcohol abuse and "bag ladies" who are mostly white, over the age of 40, and mentally ill. These groups tend to seek refuge in public buildings or areas. The largest group of homeless women, however, consists of mothers with dependent children in their care. This group tends to be young and many have mental illnesses and/or substance abuse problems. Domestic abuse has been cited as the primary cause for homelessness for mothers and children and women with children are more likely to be found in shelters or welfare hotels than on the streets (Scholler-Jaquish, 2000).

As many as half a million teenagers leave home each year. Most are runaways, but others are "throwaways." Homeless teenagers have significant psychological issues and a high rate of drug abuse. Homeless youths tend to come from dysfunctional and single-parent homes and many report that their parents are substance abusers. There is often a history of family violence and physical and sexual abuse. Homeless youths typically live in neighborhoods among drug users and prostitutes and they often resort to such activities as prostitution and selling drugs. Because of this lifestyle, they frequently have serious and complex health problems (Scholler-Jaquish, 2000).

Homeless children make up almost 25% of the total homeless population. Most are preschoolers who live in overcrowded apartments or shelters. Many homeless children suffer from depression, anxiety, and learning disabilities (Scholler-Jaquish, 2000).

Health Problems of the Homeless

It is interesting to note that health problems are both a cause and effect of homelessness. Indeed, some health problems contribute to homelessness. Often these health problems lead to lack of employment and severance of support systems, resulting in a downward spiral toward homelessness. Examples of such problems are schizophrenia, dementia and personality disorders, substance abuse, and acquired immunodeficiency syndrome (AIDS) (Butts, 2001).

Other illnesses or health problems are the result of living on the streets or in shelters. These include skin problems, respiratory disorders, communicable diseases, malnutrition, physical assault, periodontal disease, and sexually transmitted diseases (STDs). Skin problems are often related to continual walking in inadequate or improper fitting shoes, lack of hygienic measures, and exposure to infections and parasites. Respiratory problems and communicable diseases are related to continued exposure to weather and crowded conditions in shelters. Malnutrition and poor dental health result from lack of regular, nutritious meals and lack of dental care. Physical assault is commonplace because sleeping in shelters and on the street leaves persons open to victimization (Butts, 2001).

Chronic health problems are exacerbated by homelessness. Successful management of such diseases as AIDS, diabetes, hypertension, renal disease, and liver disease is very difficult if not impossible and complications are common. Mental illnesses, in particular schizophrenia and depression, are seriously complicated by homelessness (Butts, 2001).

Health problems among the homeless vary, based on gender and age. For example, homeless men experience acute physical health problems, respiratory infections, trauma, and skin disorders at higher rates than do men in the general population. Chronic disorders, such as hypertension, musculoskeletal conditions, gastrointestinal problems, peripheral vascular disease, chronic obstructive pulmonary disease (COPD), neurological disorders (i.e., seizures), poor dental care, HIV/AIDS, and tuberculosis occur at higher rates than in the general population. Many health conditions are exacerbated by alcoholism, which occurs more frequently among homeless than nonhomeless men. Mental illness and drug abuse are also much more common (Droes and Hatton, 2001).

Homeless women have more physical health problems such as asthma, anemia, and ulcers compared with their nonhomeless counterparts. The incidence of STDs is about twice that of women in the general population. Pregnancy rates are higher and the outcomes of pregnancy are worse. Homeless women have more mental health-related problems, including anxiety, panic disorders, depression, substance abuse, eating disorders, self-mutilation, and suicidal behaviors. About 20% of homeless women are alcoholics, and 10 to 20% suffer from other drug problems (Droes and Hatton, 2001).

Among homeless adolescents, frequent health problems include pregnancy, STDs (including HIV/AIDS), alcohol and drug abuse, depression, and suicide (Droes and Hatton, 2001). Homeless children are more likely to be low birth weight and to experience immunization delays, upper respiratory tract and ear infections, asthma, skin disorders, and anemia. Homeless children are also more likely to lack personal and social skills, language skills, and gross and fine motor skills compared with poor, but housed preschoolers (Droes and Hatton, 2001). Table 14-1 summarizes health problems of the homeless.

TABLE **14-1** Physical Health Problems of the Homeless

Acute Physical Disorders	Upper respiratory conditions
	Trauma, including major and minor injuries
	Minor skin ailments
	Infestations (scabies and lice)
	Nutritional deficiencies
	Tuberculosis
Chronic Physical Disorders	Alcoholism
	Hypertension
	Gastrointestinal disorders
	Peripheral vascular disorders
	Dental problems
	Diabetes
	HIV/AIDS
	Neurological disorders
Problems Associated with Pregnancy	Lack of prenatal care
	Inadequate nutrition
	Obstetrical complications
Physical Illness in Children	Upper respiratory illnesses
	Minor skin ailments
	Ear disorders
	Gastrointestinal disorders
	Trauma
	Eye disorders
	Lice infestation

From Scholler-Jaquish, A. (2000). Homelessness in America. In C. M. Smith & F. A. Maurer (Eds.), Community health nursing: Theory and practice (2nd ed.). Philadelphia: W. B. Saunders.

Health Care for the Homeless

Health care for the homeless should address both the specific and general needs of this group. Primary prevention measures may include: working to improve living conditions in shelters, reducing exposure to communicable diseases, and enhancing efforts to improve hygiene to eliminate parasitic skin conditions (i.e., lice and scabies). Providing a good supply of socks and shoes, particularly athletic shoes, is important as are coats and other warm clothing in the winter. Flu shots should be offered in the fall, and if feasible, immunization against pneumonia and hepatitis B should be provided. Other primary prevention activities include provision of dental care in shelters and nutritional meals.

Secondary prevention efforts for the homeless can involve screening and referral for both acute and chronic health conditions including tuberculosis, HIV, hypertension, and diabetes. Tertiary prevention generally centers on management of chronic mental health problems (i.e., schizophrenia, depression, substance abuse) and physical problems (i.e., cirrhosis, diabetes, renal disorders, HIV/AIDS).

MIGRANT WORKERS

Migrant workers are individuals whose principal employment is in agriculture on a seasonal basis and who establish a temporary residence for such employment while traveling from location to location (Jones et al., 2001). In contrast, seasonal farmworkers live in one geographic location and work in the fields of that particular area.

Migrant farmworkers comprise a vulnerable population with regard to health risks because they have a low income and migratory status.

Additional variables, including cultural, linguistic, economic, and mobility factors, contribute to the nature and magnitude of health problems common among farmworkers (Henson, Chafey, and Butterfield, 2001). This population is vulnerable to isolation and neglect. Fear of deportation, poverty, and limited education intensify feelings of distrust of various segments of society; in many areas, nurses provide the only source for health care for migrant workers (Spencer and Morgan, 2001).

Demographics of Migrant Workers

The Office of Migrant Health estimates that in the United States 4.2 million persons are in migrant and seasonal farmwork (Jones et al., 2001). Most migrant farmworkers spend June to September doing seasonal harvesting, traveling from farm to farm to work. After harvest time, they are typically unemployed unless nonagricultural work can be found. Income for migrant workers is well below the poverty level and most earn about $5500 per year (Sandhaus, 2001).

Migrant farmworkers usually have their permanent residence in one of the border states (California, Texas, Arizona, Florida, New Mexico) or in Puerto Rico or Mexico. Migrant farmworkers move from place to place along predetermined routes called migrant streams. The eastern stream originates in Texas, Puerto Rico, and Florida and extends up the east coast to states east of the Mississippi River, reaching as far north as New York. This stream is ethnically diverse and includes Mexicans, blacks, whites, Haitians, and Jamaicans. The midwestern stream begins in Texas and reaches across the southwestern and midwestern states moving into Canada and covers areas both east and west of the Mississippi River. The western stream is the largest and originates in California and Arizona. This stream moves up the West Coast to all the western states. The midwestern and western streams are largely comprised of Mexicans, but groups of Native Americans and Southeast Asians are in certain areas (Sandhaus, 2001).

Characteristics of Migrant Workers

Most migrant farmworkers are multigenerational and their families have been farmworkers for several generations (Sandhaus, 2001). Farmwork provides the income that the family lives on for the entire year. Pay is hourly, at or below minimum wage, and only for the duration of the season (Spencer and Morgan, 2001).

Migrant farmworkers live in temporary housing for days or weeks. Housing is often substandard and crowded and typically consists of shacks and mobile homes. Sanitation and drinking water are variable and often not available in the fields. Some regions make an effort to provide schooling for the children.

Health Problems of Migrant Workers

Migrant workers face a wide a variety of risk factors including occupational risks associated with hazardous work and poor working conditions and socioeconomic risks from poverty and homelessness. Crowded living conditions, travel, and malnutrition are other risk factors and migrant workers are at risk for communicable diseases such as tuberculosis, hepatitis A, and hepatitis B (Sebastian, 2000). Box 14-3 and the Research Highlight give additional information about the health problems of migrant workers.

Work-Related Issues for Migrant Workers

Agriculture shares the highest rates of worker fatality for any U.S. industry and it accounted for 9% of all job-related fatalities in 1996. In that year, the rate of fatal injury for those employed in agriculture was 31 per 100,000 workers compared with a rate of 5 per 100,000 for all types of U.S. workers. Agricultural machinery is the most common cause of fatalities and nonfatal injuries of U.S. farmworkers; tractor-related accidents are the most frequent events associated with loss of life (Henson et al., 2001).

Work-related health conditions arise from physical demands of working 12- to 14-hour days. Injuries are not uncommon and result from working on ladders when harvesting fruit trees

BOX **14-3** Health Problems of Migrant Farmworkers

Migrant life expectancy is 49 years.

Migrant infant mortality is 125% higher than the national average.

The death rate from flu and pneumonia is 20% higher than the national average.

The rate of parasitic infection is 11 to 59 times higher than the general population.

The death rate from tuberculosis and other communicable diseases is 25 times higher than the general population.

Poor nutrition often results in infant deaths, anemia, dental problems, vision problems, and poor mental and physical development of children.

Data from Sandhaus, S. (2001). Migrant workers. In J. A. Allender & B. W. Spradley (Eds.), *Community health nursing: Concepts and practice* (5th ed., pp. 658-681). Philadelphia: Lippincott.

Research Highlight

Health Problems of Migrant Workers

In a recent study, the National Center for Farmworker Health sampled migrant and seasonal farmworkers to gather information on a number of issues. In the survey, the researchers assessed demographic patterns, socioeconomic conditions, lifestyle characteristics, and diseases and health conditions. The study showed that, compared with the general population, migrant farmworkers:

- Have different and more complex health problems
- Suffer more frequently from infectious diseases
- Have more clinic visits for diabetes, otitis media, pregnancy, hypertension, and contact dermatitis and eczema
- Have more young people and few older people
  Other findings included the following:
- More than 40% of all farmworkers have multiple and complex health problems

- Pregnancy is the most frequently present health condition for females 15 to 19 years of age.
- Dental disease is the most frequently present health condition for males 15 to 19 years of age.
- For those 30 to 44 years of age, two of the major problems for both males and females are diabetes and hypertension.
- Nearly half of all clinic visits for those 45 to 64 years of age are for diabetes, hypertension, or arthritis.
- The researchers concluded that the need for more services, care, and treatment for migrant farmworkers is urgent. Furthermore, there is a need to develop health policy and a research agenda that will address the unique needs of migrant farmworkers.

From National Center for Farmworker Health. (2001). *Profile of a population with complex health problems*. Retrieved 10/01/01 from http://www.ncfh.org/status.htm.

---

or using other equipment. Pesticide exposure is a particular concern. Associated health effects of exposure to pesticides include memory loss, difficulty with concentration, mood changes, abdominal pain, nausea, vomiting, diarrhea, headache, malaise, skin rashes, and eye irritation. Chronic exposure may lead to cancer, blindness, infertility, liver damage, polyneuropathy, and neurobehavioral problems (Jones et al., 2001).

Other major health care problems include women's health issues, high infant mortality,

malnutrition, diabetes, hypertension, respiratory illness, anemia, parasites, and delayed immunization. Mental and social problems include high rates of substance abuse and family violence. Occupational specific health problems include risk of motor vehicle accidents caused by high annual mileage, pesticide exposure, poor sanitation, farm accidents, skin diseases, and exposure to temperature extremes (Spencer and Morgan, 2001).

Dental problems are epidemic in migrant populations and many studies cite oral disease as the most frequent health problem among migrant workers. Despite this, dental care is a very low priority. Indeed, migrant families may seek to have teeth extracted when they become painful; little consideration is given to dental repair or restoration. Many migrant families do not even own a toothbrush and most have limited knowledge of dental care (Sandhaus, 2001).

Health Care for Migrant Workers

Migrant farmworkers experience limited access to health care. Financial, cultural, transportation, mobility, language, and occupational factors are frequently cited as the major barriers that limit access to health care. Access to dental, mental health, and pharmacy services are even more problematic (Jones et al., 2001).

The Migrant Health Act (1962) authorized federal aid for clinics serving migrant and agricultural workers and families (Bushy, 2000). The Migrant Health Act funds more than 100 **migrant health centers (MHCs)** in 40 states, but only 12% to 15% of eligible migrant workers use clinic services (Jones et al., 2001). The population served by the MHCs is limited to migratory and seasonal agricultural workers and their families. Services in an MHC are usually on a fee-for-service basis and a sliding fee schedule is used for those without insurance. In most areas, MHCs offer environmental health services (e.g., rodent control, field sanitation, sewage treatment), infectious and parasitic disease screening and control, and accident prevention programs (including prevention of excessive pesticide exposure) (Bushy, 2000).

Nursing care for migrant workers is typically broad based and general. Care is variable and services can include prenatal care, infant and childcare, home care for both acute and chronic illnesses, hospice care, school health, and mental health care (Henson et al., 2001). Goals identified by Sandhaus (2001) for working with migrant populations include the following:
- Reducing abuse of alcohol and other drugs
- Improving nutrition

- Improving mental health and preventing mental illness
- Reducing environmental health hazards
- Improving occupational safety and health
- Preventing unintentional injuries
- Reducing violence and abusive behavior
- Prevention and control of HIV infection and AIDS
- Immunizing against infectious diseases
- Improving maternal and infant health
- Improving oral health
- Reducing adolescent pregnancy
- Improving reproductive health
- Prevention, detection, and control of chronic diseases
- Improving access to health services

In caring for these very vulnerable populations, the nurse can work to evaluate and improve services. Nurses can help improve health care by using unique methods of health care delivery (i.e., mobile health vans, migrant ministries, and using vouchers to address gaps in health care). It is important that nurses network with other providers and use information tracking systems to ensure continuity of care. Finally, it can be helpful to use lay personnel from the ethnic groups served to enhance services and promote community outreach (Sandhaus, 2001).

PERSONS WITH DISABILITIES

Disability is a concept that is not well understood. Indeed, because disability has many different causes, it is often not recognized or acknowledged by nurses and other health care providers. Some disabled persons (i.e., blind persons, those with spinal cord injuries, and the severely mentally retarded) are easily identified, and others, such as persons with AIDS, serious asthma, schizophrenia, a severe heart condition, or a hearing difficulty, might not be recognized as being disabled.

The vulnerable groups described previously (i.e., the homeless and migrant farmworkers) are comprised of very small groups in specific locations and most health care providers rarely, if ever, encounter them. Disabled persons, on the other hand, are extremely common. Indeed, based on the most common definitions of disability, as many as 20% of the population could be considered disabled. However, the commonality of being disabled may lead to vulnerability. This section describes how nurses in community settings can be aware of the many factors that cause or contribute to disability and help direct in planning and providing care for this vulnerable group.

DEFINITIONS RELATED TO DISABILITY

A **disability** involves any restriction on or lack of ability to perform an activity in a normal manner or within the normal range, which results from a physical or psychological limitation. Other related, but different, terms are impairment and handicap. It is important, however, to distinguish among these concepts. An anatomical, mental, or psychological loss or another abnormality is an **impairment** and can lead to disability. A **handicap** is a disadvantage resulting from an impairment or disability (Treloar and Artinian, 2001). Table 14-2 presents an overview of terminology for impairment, disability, and handicap.

Limitations in functional activities (e.g., seeing, hearing, talking, walking, climbing, lifting items), activities of daily living (ADLs) (e.g., bathing, dressing, eating, toileting), and instrumental activities of daily living (IADLs) (e.g., shopping, banking, light housecleaning, preparing meals) determine disability. In short, disability is a measure of limitations in activity (Treloar and Artinian, 2001).

Disability indicates that an individual has some functional limitation from an alteration in anatomy (internal or external physical condition) or physiology. The Americans with Disabilities Act (ADA) defines disability as a physical or mental impairment that substantially limits one or more of the major life activities of an individual who has a record of such an impairment or is regarded as having such an impairment. Physical impairment is any physiological disorder or condition, cosmetic disfigurement, or anatomical loss affecting one or more of the body systems. Impairments include orthopedic abnormalities, visual and hearing difficulties,

TABLE **14-2** Terminology for Impairment, Disability, and Handicap

CHARACTERISTIC	IMPAIRMENT	DISABILITY	HANDICAP
Definition	Physical deviation from normal structure, function, physical organization, or development	Restricted ability to perform an activity in a normal or expected manner; what activity the person cannot perform	Disadvantage imposed by impairment or disability related to environment
Measurability	Objective and measurable	May be objective and measurable	Not objective or measurable; is an experience related to the responses of others
Illustrations	Spina bifida, spinal cord injury, amputation, and detached retina	Cannot walk unassisted; uses crutches and/or a manual or power wheelchair; blindness	Reflects physical and psychological characteristics of the person, culture, and specific circumstances
Level of analysis	Microlevel (e.g., body organ)	Individual level (e.g., person)	Macrolevel (e.g., societal)

From Treloar, L. L., & Artinian, B. (2001). Populations affected by disabilities. In M. A. Nies & M. McEwen (Eds.), *Community health nursing: Promoting the health of populations* (p. 498). Philadelphia: W. B. Saunders.

cerebral palsy, epilepsy, muscular dystrophy, multiple sclerosis, and HIV. Mental impairment is any serious or sustained mental or psychological disorder, such as mental retardation, emotional or mental illness, and specific learning disabilities (DeCoux and McDowell, 2001).

CHARACTERISTICS OF DISABLED PERSONS

Approximately 20.6% of the noninstitutionalized population (i.e., nearly 54 million people) has a disabling condition that interferes with life activities; more than half of these have a severe disability. Disability is age-related, rising from approximately 12% of the population under 20 years, to 36% of the population between 55 and 64, to over 70% of the population aged 80 and over (Treloar and Artinian, 2001).

CONDITIONS RELATED TO DISABILITY

As mentioned, there is a huge variety in the health problems and conditions associated with disability. These include AIDS-, alcohol-, or drug-related problems; arthritis or rheumatism; back or spine problems; blindness or other visual impairment; broken bones; cancer; cerebral palsy; deafness or serious trouble hearing; diabetes; epilepsy; head or spinal cord injury; heart trouble; high blood pressure; chronic renal disease; learning disability; lung or respiratory trouble (i.e., asthma, chronic bronchitis, COPD); mental retardation; missing limbs, hands, or fingers; paralysis; senility, dementia, or Alzheimer's disease; speech disorder; stiffness or deformity of the foot, leg, arm, or hand; stomach trouble; and stroke (McClellan, 2000).

The greatest numbers of disabilities are related to heart disease. Indeed, it is estimated that 14 million Americans have significant coronary artery heart disease and 500,000 have strokes each year; one third of these people become permanently disabled.

People with orthopedic disabilities represent 17% of the total number of Americans with disabilities. The two leading causes of disabilities include orthopedic impairment and arthritis, which inhibit a person's ability to work

and function independently. Asthma, diabetes, mental disorders, and learning disabilities are also frequent causes of limitation (Corasaniti, Hardinger, and Raimondi, 2000; Treloar and Artinian, 2001).

Many conditions are much more likely to be disabling than others. For example, although heart disease is the most common disabling condition, only around 31% of those with heart disease are considered disabled. Mental retardation, cerebral palsy, and paralysis of the extremities, which affect many fewer people, are nonetheless much more disabling to the individuals with those conditions. Table 14-3 lists those conditions most likely to be severely disabling.

MAJOR LEGISLATION RELATED TO DISABILITIES

As mentioned, the ADA (1990) defined a disability according to the limitations in a person's ability to carry out major life activities. Physical disabilities, sensory disabilities (e.g., being deaf or blind), intellectual disabilities, serious emotional disturbances, learning disabilities, significant chemical and environmental sensitivities, and health problems such as AIDS and asthma are examples of disabilities that may substantially limit at least one major life capacity (i.e., ability to breathe, walk, see, hear, speak, work, care for self, and learn) (Treloar and Artinian, 2001).

The Americans with Disabilities Act (ADA) (1990) (PL 101-336) took effect in 1992 and provided a mandate against discrimination toward people with disabilities in everyday activities. The ADA guarantees equal opportunities for people with disabilities related to employment, transportation, public accommodations, public services, and telecommunications (Treloar and Artinian, 2001).

The Education for All Handicapped Children act (1975) (PL 94-142), later renamed the Individuals with Disabilities Education Act (IDEA), was enacted in 1975 following other legislation and court cases ruling that children with disabilities should receive access to public education. IDEA

TABLE **14-3** Selected Chronic Conditions Causing 35% or More Limitations in Major or Outside Activity by Percentage With Limitation, United States 1990-1992

CHRONIC CONDITION	PERCENTAGE OF PERSONS WITH LIMITATIONS IN MAJOR OR OUTSIDE ACTIVITY
Mental retardation	87.5
Cerebral palsy	74.0
Multiple sclerosis	69.4
Paralysis of extremities (complete or partial)	65.5
Malignant neoplasms of stomach, intestines, colon, and rectum	62.1
Malignant neoplasm of the lung, bronchus, or other respiratory sites	60.6
Blindness—both eyes	60.3
Deformities or orthopedic impairments	54.4
Epilepsy	44.4
Cerebrovascular disease	35.9
Diabetes	35.9
Absence of lower extremities or parts of lower extremities	32.8
Ischemic heart disease	31.5

Data from Collins, J. D. (1997). Prevalence of selected chronic conditions: United States, 1990-1992. (USDHHS Publication No 97-1522). *Vital and Health Statistics*, Series 10(194). Washington, DC: USDHHS.

helps eligible children receive free, appropriate public education in the least restricted environment for their individual needs (Treloar and Artinian, 2001). This act has resulted in mainstreaming children with disabilities (many of which are extremely severe) into regular public schools. Additionally, the act mandates that the schools provide whatever health and custodial services the children need to function and to learn.

Nursing Care for People with Disabilities

Nurses who work with people with disabilities and their families provide nursing care in a variety of community-based sites. People affected by disabilities have many health care needs common to nondisabled people and other health care needs are unique because of the disability. For example, a middle-aged blind woman needs health education and preventative services to screen for breast and cervical cancer, diabetes, and heart disease like any other middle-aged woman. Because of her disability, however, how the nurse provides information is affected. If possible, the nurse should provide

teaching materials and instructions in Braille. In short, the nurse's role should be in response to the needs and resources of the client.

Guiding principles for providing nursing care for persons with disabilities were proposed by Treloar and Artinian (2001). They reported that nurses should recognize and understand that the client is an expert in his or her own health status. Nurses should listen and learn from the client and gather data from the perspective of the client and family. They should work to establish relationships that are responsive to the methods of the person and family for dealing with the disability. They should care for the client and family, not the disability. Finally, nurses should be well informed about the numerous community resources for disabled persons and should become a strong advocate.

VICTIMS OF DISASTERS

Disasters happen every day. They may be natural calamities, industrial accidents, terrorism, or war. Disasters can affect one family at a time and cause only a few thousand dollars in damage (i.e., a house fire), or they can kill thousands and have economic losses in the billions (i.e., the terrorist attacks on the World Trade Center and the Pentagon in September, 2001).

A **disaster** is any event that causes destruction and devastation that cannot be alleviated without assistance. The event need not cause injury or death. Disasters may be the result of natural or man-made occurrences. Natural disasters include climactic events such as hurricanes, tornadoes, floods, blizzards, typhoons, and droughts; topographical events such as earthquakes, avalanches, and volcanic eruptions; or communicable disease epidemics.

Man-made disasters include war, chemical and biological terrorism, civil disasters (riots and demonstrations), and accidents (transportation, structural collapse, explosion, and chemical and biological contamination). Fire can be either man-made (accidental or arson) or naturally occurring (lightning strike) (Beachley, 2000; Hassmiller, 2000).

Disasters can be destructive in terms of human life. It is estimated that approximately 3 million lives have been lost in the past 20 years as the result of earthquakes, volcanic eruptions, landslides, floods, tropical storms, droughts, and other natural disasters. Floods have been the most common type of natural disaster and account for more than one third of all disasters (Lundy and Butts, 2001).

Disasters are global and disproportionately affect persons from developing countries where poverty, urbanization, and overcrowding of cities have increased the danger of both natural and man-made disasters. Overcrowding promotes civil unrest and riots and warfare; rapid urbanization results in construction of substandard housing, which leaves persons particularly vulnerable. For example, the earthquake in Istanbul, Turkey, in 1999 resulted in thousands of deaths, many attributed to poor construction of housing (Lundy and Butts, 2001).

The use of terrorist tactics is not new, but terrorist bombings increased 400% between 1984 and 1994, and have climbed steadily since then.

Terrorism refers to the "unlawful use of force or violence against persons or property to intimidate or coerce a government or civilian population in the furtherance of political or social objectives" (Tait and Spradley, 2001, p. 403). Throughout the world, terrorism results in thousands of deaths and injuries and billions of dollars in property damage each year. In most cases, terrorists use explosives or incendiary devices against their targets, but there is growing concern over the potential for use of biologic organisms (i.e., anthrax, smallpox) or chemical agents (i.e., sarin gas, mustard gas) in a terrorist attack.

A major disaster can create a multiple casualty incident or a mass casualty incident. A multiple casualty incident is one in which between 2 and 100 persons are injured. Multiple casualties generally strain and, may in some cases overwhelm, the available emergency medical services and resources. A mass casualty incident is a situation with a large number of casualties (100 or greater) that significantly overwhelms available emergency services. When there are mass casualties (i.e., the September 11, 2001 terrorist attacks, the Oklahoma City federal building bombing, Hurricane Hugo), a community or region usually requires assistance of emergency personnel and resources from surrounding communities or states (Beachley, 2000). Table 14-4 lists recent multiple and mass casualty disasters.

IMPACT OF A DISASTER

How disasters affect individuals, families, and communities varies greatly depending on the disaster type, cause, location, magnitude, the extent of damage, duration, and amount of warning (Hassmiller, 2000). Victims of disasters include both direct and indirect victims. Direct victims are those people who experience the event and include the dead, injured, and the survivors. Indirect victims are the relatives and friends of direct victims and relief and aid workers (Tait and Spradley, 2001).

Disasters impact both individuals and communities. For example, individuals are affected when families have to leave their homes to escape the

TABLE **14-4** Major Disasters—United States, 1995 to 2001

DATE	TYPE OF DISASTER AND LOCATION	NUMBER OF DEATHS
April 19, 1995	Bombing of Murrah Federal Building	168
May, 1995	Floods in Texas, Louisiana, and Mississippi	27
July 11-27, 1995	Heat wave in Chicago, Illinois	465
July 17, 1996	Crash of TWA 800 (New York)	230
Sept, 1996	Hurricane Fran in South Carolina	37
March, 1997	Floods in South and Midwest	30+
Feb 21, 1998	Tornado in Florida	38
April, 1998	Tornado in Alabama	33
May, 1999	Tornado in Oklahoma	43
July, 1999	Heat wave in Midwest	21
Sept, 1999	Hurricane Floyd in Southeast United States	56
Jan 31, 2000	Crash of Alaska Air 261 (California)	88
June, 2001	Tropical Storm Allison in Southeast United States	41
Sept 11, 2001	Terrorist attacks, New York City, Washington DC, and Pennsylvania	Approximately 3000

From Federal Emergency Management Agency, Washington, DC, http://www.fema.gov.

effects of the disaster. The community is affected when it must provide temporary food, housing, and other services to those who are displaced.

Impact of a Disaster on Individuals

In individuals, responses to disaster can include fear, panic, disbelief, and anger. There is often reluctance to abandon property, disorientation, and difficulty in making decisions. Emotional responses include insomnia, headaches, apathy and depression, moodiness, irritability, anxiety about the future, domestic violence, frustration, feeling of powerlessness, and guilt. Physical disturbances include gastrointestinal upsets, diarrhea, and nausea (Hassmiller, 2000).

In general, individuals experience disasters in relation to how significantly they are directly affected. An individual's perception of a disaster may change over time as the person begins to acknowledge the full impact of the disaster. Beachley (2000) pointed out that psychological reactions fall into three categories: (1) mild to severe, (2) normal to pathological, and (3) immediate to delayed. A reaction may be severe, normal, or mild and yet abnormal. A few people are so overwhelmed by the disaster that they experience extreme psychological distress immediately. Others may appear unaffected initially, using denial as a defense mechanism to handle their thoughts and feelings.

If survivors do not recognize and deal effectively with emotional and psychological consequences, they may suffer long-term problems such as posttraumatic stress disorder. Most experts recommend that disaster victims and aid workers have critical stress debriefings and possible referral to a mental health care professional (Beachley, 2000).

Impact of a Disaster on the Community

During and immediately following a disaster, significant problems in a community can occur as public services personnel are being overworked. In some cases, important services such as telephone systems, television and radio broadcasting, electricity, transportation, and water and sanitation services may be disrupted. Resources such as food and medical supplies may be depleted. In cases such as floods, tornadoes, earthquakes, and terrorist attacks, public and private buildings may be destroyed or damaged (Beachley, 2000).

Beachley (2000) stated that there are four phases of a community's reaction to a disaster.

First, there is the heroic phase in which there is large-scale community support, with an emotional emphasis on helping people to survive and recover. The second phase is the honeymoon phase. Here there is a drawing together of people who simultaneously experienced the catastrophic event for support and sharing. This is followed by the disillusionment phase in which feelings of disappointment occur because of delays or failures when promises of aid are not fulfilled. Often, this is because people seek help to solve their own problems rather than community problems. Finally, there is the reconstruction phase. In this phase, there is reaffirmation of belief in the community when new buildings are constructed or other measures are taken to bring about closure (e.g., building of the memorial to the Oklahoma City bombing) (Beachley, 2000).

DISASTER MANAGEMENT

Historically, Americans have prepared for emergencies only in times of national threat, such as during World War II and in the early 1960s when there was concern over nuclear war with the Soviet Union. The occurrences of hurricanes and multiple earthquakes and terrorist attacks at Oklahoma City, the World Trade Center, and the Pentagon have created a concern across the nation for preparedness to meet both natural and man-made disasters (Beachley, 2000).

The federal, state, and local governments bear the primary responsibility for designing and implementing disaster relief. Local and national voluntary agencies, in particular the American Red Cross (ARC), also play a large part.

Disaster Services Provided by Governmental Agencies

Local governments are responsible for the safety and welfare of their citizens. Local disaster response organizations should include local area government agencies (i.e., fire departments, police departments, public health departments, emergency services, and the local branch of the ARC) (Beachley, 2000). Emergency operations plans should be based on the likelihood of a particular disaster and mock disaster exercises should be planned and conducted accordingly. For example, localities on the Gulf Coast should plan for hurricanes; certain locations on the West Coast should plan for earthquakes; midwestern and southern states should plan for tornadoes; and northern states should plan for blizzards.

State governments coordinate the state Emergency Operations Plan and establish emergency management agencies to manage the state's response to a disaster. If the disaster involves more than one local jurisdiction, the state may coordinate response services. When a disaster happens, the governor opens the Emergency Operations Center where some state agencies (i.e., state police, National Guard, and state health and social service agencies) work together to direct activities for disaster relief. If the state does not have the resources to respond and manage the disaster, the governor can request federal disaster relief assistance (Beachley, 2000).

The federal government enacts laws and provides funds to support state and local governments. The Public Disaster Act of 1974 (PL 93-288) provided consolidation of federal disaster relief activities and funding under a single agency. As a component of this Act, the **Federal Emergency Management Agency (FEMA)** was established in 1979. It is the federal agency that assesses and responds to disaster events in the United States; responsibilities include emergency planning, preparedness, mitigation, response, and recovery. Working closely with state and local governments, FEMA funds emergency programs and provides technical guidance and training in all phases of disaster management (Beachley, 2000; Tait and Spradley, 2001).

The Office of Emergency Planning/National Disaster Medical System (NDMS) within the Department of Health and Human Services is responsible for coordinating the health and medical response in a disaster event. The NDMS provides medical assistance to a disaster area; helps evaluate patients; and provides a national network of hospitals designated to accept patients in the event of a national emergency. The National

Guard provides transportation and assistance with evacuations and police services when local or area police resources are strained or overwhelmed by disaster needs (Beachley, 2000).

Disaster Services Provided by the American Red Cross

The **American Red Cross (ARC)** is a voluntary support agency founded in 1881 by Clara Barton. The ARC operates across the United States and has chapters in many localities throughout the country and throughout the world. The Disaster Relief Acts of 1970 and 1974 give the ARC the authority to act as the primary voluntary national disaster relief agency for the American people and to be ready for immediate action in every part of the United States (Beachley, 2000). As a result, the ARC provides disaster relief services to people 24 hours a day, 7 days a week. Each year, the ARC responds to more than 60,000 disasters including house or apartment fires (the majority of disaster responses), hurricanes, floods, earthquakes, and tornadoes among others (ARC, 2001).

Chapters of the ARC have been set up in more than 1300 communities to respond to needs of victims (ARC, 2001). The Red Cross chapters participate in drills and exercises that enable volunteers to respond efficiently and effectively. It has created five programs to meet human needs during a disaster (Table 14-5).

DISASTER PLANNING

The key to effective disaster management is pre-disaster planning and preparation. Planning requires the ability to forecast events, engineering to reduce risks, public education about potential hazards, a coordinated emergency response, and a systematic assessment of the effects of a disaster to better prepare for the future. Responsibility for addressing disaster planning is shared by the local, state, federal, and voluntary agencies. Beachley (2000) lists eight principles for disaster management:

1. Prevent the occurrence of the disaster whenever possible. Many disasters, particularly man-made ones, may be preventable through such activities as enforcement of building codes, proper land and water management, equipment maintenance, and safety education.

2. Minimize the number of casualties if the disaster cannot be prevented. Early warning systems can help alert the public to the possibility of immediate danger and help reduce the impact of predictable disasters. Additionally, information on an evacuation plan can be used to improve the chance of survival.

3. Prevent further casualties from occurring after the initial impact of the disaster. Identify and lessen any unsafe conditions that occur after a disaster; these often affect disaster workers (i.e., police and fire fighters).

TABLE **14-5** Programs Provided by the American Red Cross During Disasters

PROGRAM	EXAMPLES OF ACTIVITIES
Damage Assessment	Gather information about the physical damage resulting from a disaster
Mass Care	Provide food, shelter, and supplies (i.e., hygienic articles, toilet articles, cleaning supplies) to victims and disaster workers
Health Services	Provide health care to meet the emotional and medical needs of victims and disaster workers
Family Services	Emergency assistance to help families by providing food, clothing, shelter, medical needs, household furnishings, and occupational supplies and equipment
Disaster Welfare Inquiry Service	Gathers information about the disaster, including what and who are affected and individuals killed or injured; this information is disseminated to concerned relatives

From Beachley, M. (2000). Nursing in a disaster. In C. M. Smith & F. A. Maurer (Eds.), *Community health nursing: Theory and practice* (2nd ed., pp. 424-444). Philadelphia: W. B. Saunders.

4. Rescue the victims. Aid workers must locate and free trapped victims and then move them to a safe place.
5. Provide first aid to those injured.
6. Evacuate the injured to medical facilities. Aid workers must plan for transport vehicles and routes while considering current weather conditions, conditions of roads, and location of hospitals.
7. Provide medical care. All hospitals have disaster plans and hold disaster drills; how they are used during a disaster depends on the availability and location of medical care facilities and personnel.
8. Promote reconstruction of lives. Care should continue until recovery and both victims and disaster workers should receive psychological counseling and emotional support.

All communities should have a disaster plan. In addition, many organizations and groups (i.e., firefighters, police, emergency personnel, public health officials, hospitals) that would be called upon during a disaster must have their own plans to integrate with the community plan. Elements of a disaster plan include the following:

- Chain of authority (person or agency responsible for issuing warnings and for authority for delegation)
- Lines of communication
- Equipment and supplies
- Human resources (health professionals, disaster specialists, governmental officials, engineers)
- Team coordinators (persons assigned to coordinate aspects of a disaster)
- Modes of transportation
- Documentation
- Evacuation routes
- Rescue personnel and equipment
- Acute care (triage and first aid)
- Supportive care for victims and families
- Means for evaluation (Lundy and Butts, 2001; Tait and Spradley, 2001).

ROLE OF THE NURSE DURING DISASTERS

During a disaster, nurses and other emergency personnel are usually advised not to attempt to provide care until the situation has stabilized. Depending on the disaster, nurses may be involved in triage, in acute care/first aid for immediate treatment, or in shelters or other areas of support.

Triage

During a disaster, the first obligation of relief workers is to remove victims from danger. This job usually falls to firefighters and others trained in search and rescue and nurses are rarely involved.

After victims have been removed from danger, if there are multiple, severe casualties, disaster triage allows health care personnel to identify the most salvageable clients so that treatment can be initiated immediately. Prioritization of treatment may be very different in a mass casualty event. On a disaster site, a victim without a pulse or respirations most likely would be placed in a nonsalvageable category, allowing resource personnel to be used for those who have the best chance of survival.

Triage can determine where and how the victim is to be managed. In some circumstances, they might be treated onsite; in others they might be removed to a hospital via ambulance, helicopter, or other type of transport. Nurses may be involved in several areas. They may conduct the triage, monitoring those persons waiting for care, or working on the logistics of transfer.

Emergency Care/First Aid

Disaster nurses may provide care on-site at emergency treatment stations or they may work at local hospitals and clinics. At first aid stations, nurses are needed to provide direct nursing care, evaluate health care needs, and arrange for transport once victims are stabilized. They may also be involved in managing the procurement, distribution, and replenishing of supplies and providing on-the-job training and supervision of volunteer staff and assigning them to appropriate duties. In some cases, nurses may be called on to arrange for psychological and spiritual care of victims and in others they may be asked to care for bodies and notify families (Beachley, 2000; Tait and Spradley, 2001). They may also be involved in direct disaster counseling. See the Community Application box "Disaster Counseling."

Shelter Assistance

Shelters are managed by trained volunteers and the Red Cross. In widespread disasters, such as hurricanes, shelters are opened in several areas to house the local residents and victims who have traveled to escape more immediate danger. Each shelter has a team manager, a nurse, people to keep records, and numerous volunteers. Activities include keeping records; coordinating meals; providing snacks, cots, blankets, and other essentials; and providing health care (Lundy and Butts, 2001).

In shelters, nurses consult with the shelter manager on the health status of residents and workers and identify potential problems and needs. They may also monitor those who are particularly vulnerable for poor outcomes or health problems (i.e., pregnant women, elders, small children, ill or injured) and may refer clients for additional treatment or follow-up.

THE NURSE AND DISASTER PREPAREDNESS

Everyone should be encouraged to be prepared for a disaster. As health professionals, nurses in particular should be aware of potential dangers and prepare accordingly. In addition, nurses should know community resources that deal with disasters, and if interested, should join a local disaster action team or act as a liaison with local hospitals. Hassmiller (2000) suggests three levels of **preparedness** for nurses: (1) personal preparedness, (2) professional preparedness, and (3) community preparedness.

Personal preparedness addresses personal and family preparation and includes recognizing what would be the most likely type of disaster that will happen to the family (i.e., does the family live

---

COMMUNITY APPLICATION
Disaster Counseling

Disaster counseling involves both listening and guiding. Survivors typically benefit from talking about their disaster experiences and being assisted with problem solving and obtaining referrals to resources. These suggestions for disaster counselors are provided by the Center for Mental Health Services:

Establish Rapport: Survivors respond when workers offer caring eye contact and a calm presence. Rapport includes an attitude of interest and understanding and genuine concern. Conveying respect and being nonjudgmental are necessary for building rapport.

Active Listening: Workers listen when they take in information through their ears, eyes, and intuition to better understand the survivor's situation and needs. In active listening, the counselor should allow silence to give the survivor time to reflect and become aware of his or her feelings; attend nonverbally to the survivor by providing eye contact, head nodding, caring facial expressions, and occasional verbal acknowledgment; paraphrase to show understanding, interest, and empathy and to check for accuracy and clarification of

misunderstandings; acknowledge feelings that are shown in the survivor's tone of voice or nonverbal gestures that might suggest anger, sadness or fear; and allow expression of emotions through tears or angry venting and let the survivor know that it is all right to feel.

Dos and Don'ts
Do Say:
- These are normal reactions to a disaster.
- It is understandable that you feel this way.
- You are not going crazy.
- It wasn't your fault, you did the best you could.
- Things may never be the same, but they will get better and you will feel better.

Don't Say:
- It could have been worse.
- You can always get another pet/car/house.
- It's best if you just stay busy.
- I know just how you feel.
- You need to get on with your life.

From The Center for Mental Health Services. (2001). *Disaster counseling.* Retrieved 10/01/01 from http://www.mentalhealth.org/publications/allpubs/KEN-01-0096/default.asp.

in an area that might be hit by a hurricane? An earthquake? A blizzard?). The family should review disaster plans at the workplace or school and create a disaster plan for the home. The family should maintain emergency supplies in case of a disaster. This should include a 2-day supply of water (1 gallon per person per day); food that will not spoil; a change of clothing and blanket or sleeping bag for each person; a first aid kit that includes prescription medications, emergency tools, and supplies; and items needed for infants, elders, or disabled family members. See the Health Teaching box "Family Disaster Plan."

Professional preparedness refers to the need for nurses to be aware of and understand the dis-aster plans in the community. Items for nurses preparing to help in a disaster include a copy of their professional license, personal equipment (i.e., stethoscope), flashlight and extra batteries, weather-appropriate clothing, materials to keep records, and pocket-size reference books. In addition, all workers should be trained in first aid and CPR.

Community preparedness focuses on the community's ability to address a disaster. Some communities plan for disasters by having written disaster plans and participating in yearly disaster drills. Nurses can become a part of this process by becoming a member of the disaster team at work or in the community.

---

health teaching

Family Disaster Plan

A home disaster plan should be focused on the most likely or logical type of disaster that might happen. The plan should include an evacuation plan/escape route, emergency telephone numbers, being sure that insurance coverage is adequate, having a fire extinguisher and knowing where it is kept and how to use it, installing smoke detectors on each level of the home, and identifying safe spots in the home for various types of disasters. The disaster plan should also include assembling emergency supplies and a first aid kit. According to FEMA, the family disaster supplies kit should include the following:

Water: a minimum 3-day supply of water for each person in the household (1 gallon of water per person per day)

Food: a 3-day supply of nonperishable food. Foods should require no refrigeration, preparation or cooking, and little or no water. Include ready-to-eat canned meats, fruits and vegetables; canned juices; milk; soup; staples (e.g., sugar, salt, pepper); high-energy foods (e.g., peanut butter, jelly, crackers, granola bars); vitamins; foods for infants, elders, or persons on special diets; and comfort/stress foods (e.g., cookies, hard candy, cereals, instant coffee, tea bags)

First Aid Kit: sterile adhesive bandages in assorted sizes, sterile gauze pads, hypoallergenic adhesive tape, 2- and 3-inch sterile rolled bandages, scissors, tweezers, needle, moistened towelettes, antiseptic, thermometer, tongue blades, tube of petroleum jelly or other lubricant, assorted safety pins, cleansing agent/soap, latex gloves, sunscreen, and prescription and nonprescription drugs (pain reliever, antidiarrhea medication, antacid, syrup of Ipecac, laxative)

Tools and Supplies: paper cups, plates, and plastic utensils; battery-operated radio and extra batteries; flashlight and extra batteries; cash or traveler's checks; a credit card; extra car keys; extra eye glasses; nonelectric can opener; fire extinguisher; pliers; tape; compass; candles and matches in a waterproof container; aluminum foil; plastic storage containers; signal flare; paper and pencil; needles and thread; wrench to turn off household gas and water; whistle; plastic sheeting; regional map; toilet paper; soap and liquid detergent; feminine supplies; plastic garbage bags; disinfectant; chlorine bleach

Clothing and Bedding: sturdy shoes or work boots, rain gear, blankets or sleeping bags, hat and gloves, thermal underwear, sunglasses

Special Items: for family members with special needs (i.e., infants, elders); include formula, diapers, medications, extra eyeglasses

Important Family Documents (kept in a portable, waterproof container): wills, insurance policies, stocks and bonds, passports, Social Security cards, immunization records, bank account numbers, credit card account numbers, and an inventory of valuable household goods, important telephone numbers, and family records (birth, marriage, and death certificates)

From Federal Emergency Management Agency (FEMA). (2001). *Your family disaster plan*. Jessup, MD: FEMA.

SUMMARY

This chapter has presented a great deal of information on vulnerability and vulnerable groups. Some of the groups described (i.e., those with disabilities) are large and have both general and specific health problems. Others, such as the homeless and migrant workers, are relatively small and have more easily defined and identified health risks and health problems. Nurses who work in community settings should be aware of the risks and needs of these groups and recognize how multiple risks factors can interact to increase health problems and to make them more difficult to manage.

The final section addressed how nurses can be used during disasters to intervene in the problems that can suddenly leave individuals, families, groups, and even entire communities vulnerable. In many cases, nurses, like Maria from the chapter-opening case study, have recognized the need to be prepared for such situations and to encourage preparedness in their own families, professional groups, and communities. The Resources box at the end of the chapter presents a number of resources that may be used by nurses who work with impoverished people, the homeless, migrant workers, those who are disabled, and victims of disasters.

KEY POINTS

- Vulnerable groups are those people who have an increased risk or susceptibility to adverse health outcomes; risk factors tend to be cumulative and interactive.
- Vulnerability is exacerbated by the combined effects of limited resources. Contributing factors include disempowerment, disenfranchisement, and marginalization.
- Poverty is established by comparing family income with the federally defined poverty threshold. The poverty threshold for a family of four with two children was $17,463 in 2000.

- About 11.3% of Americans have incomes below the poverty threshold. The majority of the poor are white, but members of racial and ethnic minority groups are overrepresented among the poor. Families headed by single mothers are likely to live in poverty.
- Persons in poverty have poorer health than those not impoverished. Health problems include higher rates of chronic illness, higher infant morbidity and mortality, shorter life expectancy, more complex health problems, and more significant complications from chronic diseases.
- Persons are considered homeless if they sleep in a supervised shelter, an institution that provides a temporary residence, or in a public or private place not designated for sleeping.
- Factors that contribute to homelessness include unemployment, underemployment, poverty, a decrease in the number of affordable housing units, emergency demands on income, alcohol and drug addiction, domestic violence, and deinstitutionalization of chronically mentally ill persons.
- The largest group of homeless is comprised of single men; however, the number of families with children and single women are growing.
- Health problems are a cause and an effect of homelessness. Health problems that can contribute to a person becoming homeless include schizophrenia and other severe mental disorders, substance abuse, and AIDS. Health problems that result from living on the streets or in shelters include skin problems, respiratory disorders, communicable diseases, malnutrition, physical assault, periodontal disease, and STDs.
- Migrant farmworkers are individuals whose principal employment is in agriculture on a seasonal basis and who establish a temporary residence for employment while traveling from location to location.
- Migrant farmworkers are at risk for a number of health problems related to hazardous work and poor working and living conditions and socioeconomic risks of poverty.

- Health care for migrant farmworkers is often provided in MHCs, which are supported by the Migrant Health Act (1962).
- Almost one in five Americans has some type of disability that limits their ability to perform an activity in a normal manner. Limitations in functional activities, ADL, and IADL determine disability.
- Disability is age related; about 12% of the population under 20 years has a disability and over 70% of those over age 80 have a disability. The most common causes of disability are heart disease and orthopedic problems including arthritis. Other common causes of disability are asthma, hearing or visual impairment, cerebral palsy, and head or spinal cord injury.
- The ADA (1990) prohibits discrimination toward people with disabilities in everyday activities and affects such areas as employment, transportation, public accommodations, public services, and telecommunications.
- Disasters are daily occurrences and include natural disasters (e.g., hurricanes, floods, earthquakes) and man-made disasters (e.g., war, terrorism, major accidents). Mass casualty disasters refer to those in which more than 100 persons are injured.
- In individuals, disasters cause fear, panic, disbelief, and anger. Emotional responses include insomnia, headaches, apathy and depression, frustration, and guilt. Physical disturbances include gastrointestinal problems, diarrhea, and nausea.
- Governmental agencies are largely responsible for management of disasters. Local groups lead by fire departments, police departments, public health departments, and emergency services usually manage small-scale disasters. In larger disasters that affect more than one community, state governments may be involved to coordinate response services. The FEMA group is responsible for assessment of and response to major disaster events in the United States.

- The ARC is the primary voluntary agency that provides disaster relief in the United States. The Red Cross has more than 1300 local chapters throughout the United States that respond to disasters.
- Predisaster planning and preparedness are key to effective disaster management. Planning includes attempting to forecast events, engineering to reduce risks, public education about potential hazards, and developing a coordinated emergency response plan.
- During disasters, nurses generally help in triage, provide emergency first aid, or work in shelters.

Resources

Nurses Caring for Vulnerable Groups

Impoverished/Homeless

National Coalition for the Homeless
National Health Care for the Homeless Council
U.S. Department of Veterans Affairs
Health Care for the Homeless

Migrant Workers

Farmworker Health Program
National Center for Farmworker Health
Health Resources and Services Administration
Bureau of Primary Health Care Migrant Health Program

Disabled Persons

Administration on Developmental Disabilities
American Spinal Injury Association
Brain Injury Association of America
Christopher Reeve Paralysis Foundation
Disability Rights Education and Defense Fund
Disability Resources on the Internet
National Council on Disability

Victims of Disasters

American Red Cross
Federal Emergency Management Agency (FEMA)
Office of Emergency Preparedness/National Disaster Medical System

Visit the book's website at
www.wbsaunders.com/SIMON/McEwen   SiMON
for a direct link to the website for each organization listed.

Learning Activities & Application to Practice

In Class

1. In groups of four to six, work with classmates to draft personal, professional, and community preparedness plans.

In Clinical

2. If feasible, spend at least one clinical day working in a setting that provides health care for one of the vulnerable groups described (i.e., the homeless, migrant workers). What health problems were observed that are related to risk factors?

3. At a local hospital, find out as much as you can about their plan for disaster. Look for the elements of the disaster plan described in the chapter. Share findings with the clinical group.

REFERENCES

American Red Cross (2001). *Red Cross facts.* Retrieved 10/01/01 from http://www.redcross.org/services/disaster/aboutdis/facts.html.

Beachley, M. (2000). Nursing in a disaster. In C. M. Smith & F. A. Maurer (Eds.), *Community health nursing: Theory and practice* (2nd ed., pp. 424-444). Philadelphia: W. B. Saunders.

Belcher, J. R., Scholler-Jaquish, A., & Drummond, M. (1991). Three stages of homelessness: A conceptual model for social workers in health care. *Health and Social Work, 16*(2), 87-93.

Bolla, C. D. (2000). Poverty and homelessness. In M. Stanhope & J. Lancaster (Eds.), *Community & public health nursing* (5th ed., pp. 666-683). St. Louis: Mosby.

Bushy, A. (2000). Rural health. In C. M. Smith & F. A. Maurer (Eds.), *Community health nursing: Theory and practice* (2nd ed., pp. 870-898). Philadelphia: W. B. Saunders.

Bushy, A. (2001). Vulnerability: An overview. In K. S. Lundy & S. Janes (Eds.), *Community health nursing: Caring for the public's health* (pp. 576-591). Boston: Jones and Bartlett Publishers.

Butts, J. B. (2001). Urban and homeless populations. In K. S. Lundy & S. Janes (Eds.), *Community health nursing: Caring for the public's health* (pp. 594-617). Boston: Jones and Bartlett Publishers.

The Center for Mental Health Services. (2001). *Disaster counseling.* Retrieved 10/01/01 from http://www.mentalhealth.org/publications/allpubs/KEN-01-0096/default.asp.

Collins, J. D. (1997). Prevalence of selected chronic conditions: United States, 1990-1992. (USDHHS Publication No. 97-1522). *Vital and Health Statistics, Series 10*(194). Washington, DC: USDHHS.

Corasaniti, R. P., Hardinger, M. E., & Raimondi, D. S. (2000). Rehabilitation clients in the community. In C. M. Smith & F. A. Maurer (Eds.), *Community health nursing: Theory and practice* (2nd ed., pp. 733-754). Philadelphia: W. B. Saunders.

DeCoux, V. M., & McDowell, L. G. (2001). Disabilities and health. In K. S. Lundy & S. Janes (Eds.), *Community health nursing: Caring for the public's health* (pp. 660-681). Boston: Jones and Bartlett Publishers.

Droes, N. S., & Hatton, D. C. (2001). Homeless populations. In M. A. Nies & M. McEwen (Eds.), *Community health nursing: Promoting the health of populations* (pp. 526-547). Philadelphia: W. B. Saunders.

Federal Emergency Management Agency (FEMA). (2001). *Your family disaster plan.* Jessup, MD: FEMA.

Flaskerud, J. H., & Winslow, B. J. (1998). Conceptualizing vulnerable populations health-related research. *Nursing Research, 47*(2), 69.

Hassmiller, S. B. (2000). Disaster management. In M. Stanhope & J. Lancaster (Eds.), *Community & public health nursing* (5th ed., pp. 400-415). St. Louis: Mosby.

Henson, D., Chafey, K., & Butterfield, P. G. (2001). Rural and migrant health. In M. A. Nies & M. McEwen (Eds.), *Community health nursing: Promoting the health of populations* (pp. 548-582). Philadelphia: W. B. Saunders.

Jones, K. D. et al. (2001). Migrant health issues. In M. Stanhope & J. Lancaster (Eds.), *Community & public health nursing* (5th ed., pp. 701-713). St. Louis: Mosby.

Lundy, K. S., & Butts, J. B. (2001). The role of the community health nurse in disasters. In K. S. Lundy & S. Janes (Eds.), *Community health nursing: Caring for the public's health* (pp. 546-573). Boston: Jones and Bartlett Publishers.

McClellan, M. A. (2000). The physically compromised. In M. Stanhope & J. Lancaster (Eds.), *Community & public health nursing* (5th ed., pp. 613-635). St. Louis: Mosby.

National Center for Farmworker Health. (2001). *Profile of a population with complex health problems.* Retrieved 10/01/01 from http://www.ncfh.org/status.htm.

Sandhaus, S. (2001). Migrant workers. In J. A. Allender & B. W. Spradley (Eds.), *Community health nursing: Concepts and practice* (5th ed., pp. 658-681). Philadelphia: Lippincott.

Scholler-Jaquish, A. (2000). Homelessness in America. In C. M. Smith & F. A. Maurer (Eds.), *Community health nursing: Theory and practice* (2nd ed., pp. 672-699). Philadelphia: W. B. Saunders.

Sebastian, J. G. (2000). Vulnerability and vulnerable populations: An overview. In M. Stanhope & J. Lancaster (Eds.), *Community & public health nursing* (5th ed., pp. 638-665). St. Louis: Mosby.

Spencer, G. A., & Morgan, L. L. (2001). Rural populations. In K. S. Lundy & S. Janes (Eds.), *Community health nursing: Caring for the public's health* (pp. 618-635). Boston: Jones and Bartlett Publishers.

Tait, C., & Spradley, B. (2001). Communities in crisis: Disasters, group violence and terrorism. In J. A. Allender & B. W. Spradley (Eds.), *Community health nursing: Concepts and practice* (5th ed., pp. 391-407). Philadelphia: Lippincott.

Treloar, L. L., & Artinian, B. (2001). Populations affected by disabilities. In M. A. Nies & M. McEwen (Eds.), *Community health nursing: Promoting the health of populations* (pp. 496-525). Philadelphia: W. B. Saunders.

U.S. Census Bureau. (2001). *Poverty in the United States: 2000.* Washington, DC: Government Printing Office.

U.S. Department of Health and Human Services (USDHHS). (2000). *Healthy people 2010: Conference edition.* Washington, DC: USDHHS.

Zerwekh, J. V. (2001). Clients living in poverty. In J. A. Allender & B. W. Spradley (Eds.), *Community health nursing: Concepts and practice* (5th ed., pp. 641-557). Philadelphia: Lippincott.

Mental Health Issues

objectives

Upon completion of this chapter, the reader will be able to:

1. Explain the concept of mental health and discuss the importance of mental health promotion.

2. Describe some of the most common types of mental illnesses encountered in community settings including depression, anxiety disorders, eating disorders, and attention deficit hyperactivity disorder.

3. Discuss the different types of substance abuse and explain risk factors and treatment.

4. Discuss the problem of suicide and recognize risk factors.

5. Describe different types of treatment for mental disorders, including use of psychotherapeutic medications, psychotherapy, and behavior therapy.

key terms

12-step programs	Bulimia nervosa	Posttraumatic stress disorder (PTSD)
Agoraphobia	Depression	Psychotherapeutic medications
Anorexia nervosa	Mental health	Psychotherapy
Anxiety disorders	Mental illness	Substance abuse
Attention deficit hyperactivity disorder (ADHD)	Obsessive-compulsive disorder (OCD)	Suicide
Behavioral therapy	Panic disorder	
	Phobia	*See Glossary for definitions.*

case study

Kay Morton is a registered nurse (RN) working in a public-sponsored primary care clinic for indigent and homeless people in a large southwestern city. The clinic is housed in a center that provides comprehensive care for the poor. The center provides two meals per day; counseling; and assistance with job training and employment, housing, child care, and a number of other services. In addition to administrative and support personnel, the center employs five social workers, two psychologists, two RNs, and a physician's assistant.

Residents from an area medical school provide psychiatric and medical care and other local physicians volunteer their services periodically. In addition to primary medical care, other related services offered at the center include drug and alcohol counseling and 12-step programs, psychological counseling, and psychiatric care.

Recently, Kay saw Jeannie Smith for follow-up psychiatric care. Jeannie is 22 years old and a participant in the center's intensive case management program. Jeannie has three children (ages 6, 5, and 2 years) and has been receiving public assistance for more than 6 years. During that time, her children have been in foster care on several occasions. She admits to using crack cocaine, marijuana, and several other street drugs in addition to alcohol. She was diagnosed with bipolar disorder 2 years ago and is currently on medication. Since beginning the program, Jeannie has been clean, has passed a high school equivalency examination, is enrolled in a local community college, and works part time as a cashier. She and her children live in a subsidized apartment and the center assists her with child care.

At the center, Jeannie was first seen by her caseworker for her weekly visit. Following that, she went to the clinic. Kay admitted her and following routine clinic procedures, questioned her about compliance with her medication regimen; any observed side effects and use of illicit drugs; and asked if she had any other problems, questions, or concerns.

Jeannie replied that she had been taking her medications as prescribed and had noticed no side effects. Also, she had not been using any substances prohibited in the program. She reported that her children have been well, her job is satisfactory, and school is fairly difficult, but she is managing. Kay took Jeannie's vital signs and weighed her. The weight and vital signs were all consistent with previous readings. Following agency protocols and a physician's order, Kay collected a urine specimen from Jeannie to be sent for drug screening.

Following the interview with Kay, the psychiatric resident talked with Jeannie for about 20 minutes. To ensure that Jeannie's lithium levels were in therapeutic range, the physician asked Kay to obtain a sample of blood. Kay drew a small sample of blood from Jeannie's right arm, using careful sterile technique and attention to universal precautions. She reviewed the purpose of the test with Jeannie and explained that the results would be back in a day or two. Jeannie verbalized understanding and left to keep her appointment with her psychologist.

"Mental health is a state of successful performance of mental function, resulting in productive activities, fulfilling relationships with other "people, and the ability to adapt to change and to cope with adversity" (U.S. Department of Health and Human Services [USDHHS], 2000, p. 18-3). Mental health refers not only to the absence of mental disorders, but also to the ability of an individual to negotiate daily challenges and social interactions of life without experiencing cognitive, emotional, or behavioral dysfunction. Mental health and mental disorders can be affected by numerous factors such as biologic and genetic vulnerabilities, acute or chronic physical dysfunction, environmental conditions, and stressors.

Consider the following statistics (USDHHS, 1995; 2000):
- Mental disorders affect an estimated 40 million Americans (22% of the population) each year.
- About 20% of children and adolescents (9 to 17 years of age) have a diagnosable mental disorder (e.g., depression, autism, and attention deficit disorder [ADD]) during a given year.
- Schizophrenia affects about 1% of the adult population at any one time.
- Depression and associated affective/mood disorders affect about 5% of the population of the United States at any one time.
- Suicide, a potential outcome of mental illness and mental disorders, is the eighth leading cause of death in the United States.

- Only about 25% of persons with a mental disorder obtain help for their illness in the health care system.
- Mental disorders cost an estimated $69 billion in 1996 in direct costs and an additional $75 billion in lost productivity and disability insurance payments because of illness or premature death.
- Persons hospitalized with major depression account for more bed days than any impairment except cardiovascular disorders.
- Individuals with job-related stress and depression miss an average of 16 work days annually.

The use and abuse of illicit drugs and alcohol is strongly related to mental disorders and is both a cause and an effect of mental disorders. Use of drugs and alcohol is directly associated with violence, suicide, birth defects (including mental retardation), accidental injury, and long-term health problems (e.g., liver disease, heart disease, some forms of cancer, and acquired immunodeficiency syndrome [AIDS]). The impact of drug and alcohol abuse in the United States is evident in the following statements (USDHHS, 1995; 2000):

- Substance abuse is the cause of 120,000 deaths each year (100,000 attributed to alcohol and 20,000 attributed to drug use and associated AIDS).
- Alcohol and drug problems cost U.S. citizens some $276 billion per year, or more than $1000 for each citizen.
- Alcohol is implicated in nearly half of all deaths caused by motor vehicle crashes.
- Between 24% and 40% of all general hospital patients are there because of complications related to alcoholism.

- About 25% of adolescents are at high risk for alcohol and other drug problems.
- Alcohol use during pregnancy is the leading preventable cause of birth defects.
- Alcohol and drug abuse may be both a cause and an effect of homelessness.

Table 15-1 gives an overview of the prevalence rates for the major groups of mental disorders. Early identification, appropriate treatment, and rehabilitation can significantly reduce the duration and level of disability associated with mental disorders and decrease the possibility of relapse. Interventions to promote mental health and decrease mental disorders include focusing on decreasing stressors and/or increasing the capacity of the individual to cope with stress. Other interventions include the use of pharmacological agents and psychosocial interventions such as strengthening interpersonal, psychological, and physical resources through counseling, support groups, and training.

Two focus areas of *Healthy People 2010* (USDHHS, 2000) address the related issues of mental health and problems associated with substance abuse. Mental Health and Mental Disorders (Focus Area #18) and Substance Abuse (Focus Area #26) contain a number of objectives concerning mental health and related issues. The *Healthy People 2010* box lists selected objectives from these focus areas.

Over the last 50 years, psychiatry and mental health services have changed dramatically. Until the mid-1900s, treatment of the mentally ill was largely carried out in long-term psychiatric hospitals. The development of psychotropic drugs in the 1950s led to dramatic breakthroughs in the

TABLE **15-1** One-Year Prevalence Rates for Mental Disorders

Substance abuse	2.0%
Anxiety disorders (e.g., phobias, general anxiety disorder, obsessive compulsive disorder, posttraumatic stress disorder)	13.0%
Mood disorders (e.g., manic depressive episode, dysthymia, schizophrenia, anorexia)	10.3%
Any disorder	20.9%

From U.S. Department of Health and Human Services (USDHHS). (1999). *Mental health: Report of the surgeon general.* Rockville, MD: USDHHS.

treatment of mental illness and enabled thousands of clients to be treated on an outpatient basis (Richardson and Shiu-Thornton, 1999). The process of deinstitutionalization began in the early 1960s in response to legislation intended to move mental health care into the community. The Mental Retardation Facilities and Community Mental Health Centers Construction Act of 1964 (PL 88-164) was written to improve inpatient, outpatient, emergency, and day treatment, and consultation and education services for persons with mental disorders. As a result of these developments, between 1955 and 1980, the census of state and county mental hospitals declined from 559,000 to 138,000 (Sharfstein, Stoline, and Koran, 1999).

In 1955, 75% of patient care for mental illnesses took place in state hospitals. Today, 75% of client care for mental disorders occurs in community-based settings (Sharfstein et al., 1999). Ambulatory, or outpatient, care for mental disorders can be provided in many settings and by a variety of professionals, parapro-fessionals, and volunteers. Persons with mental problems may seek assistance from physicians and other professional clinicians (e.g., psychologists, counselors) in private practice, hospital outpatient departments, mental health centers or clinics, alcohol and drug units or outpatient clinics, emergency departments, family or social service agencies, crisis centers, volunteer services such as self-help programs (e.g., Alcoholics Anonymous [AA], Narcotics Anonymous [NA]), and clergy or religious counselors.

The number of health professional visits that a client needs varies greatly, depending on the mental health problem, diagnosis, or disorder. Therapeutic mental health services include individual, family, and group psychotherapy; hypnosis; psychodrama; expressive therapies (e.g., art therapy); milieu therapy; medications; electroconvulsive therapy; and psychosurgery (Sharfstein et al., 1999).

This chapter discusses some of the most common mental disorders encountered by nurses in community-based practice. The correlating and

---

healthy people **2010**

Objectives Related to Mental Health

OBJECTIVE		BASELINE (1998)	TARGET
18.1:	Reduce the suicide rate	10.8 suicides per 100,000	6 suicides per 100,000
18.5:	Reduce the relapse rates for persons with eating disorders including anorexia nervosa and bulimia nervosa	NA	NA
18.9a:	Increases the proportion of adults aged 18 to 54 years with serious mental disorders who receive treatment	47%	55%
26.1a:	Reduce deaths caused by alcohol-related motor vehicle crashes	6.1 per 100,000	4 per 100,000
26.2:	Reduce cirrhosis deaths	9.4 per 100,000	3 per 100,000
26.3:	Reduce drug-induced deaths	5.1 per 100,000	1 per 100,000
26.6:	Reduce the proportion of adolescents who report that they rode, during the previous 30 days, with a driver who had been drinking alcohol	37%	30%
26.9c:	Increase proportion of high school seniors never using alcoholic beverages	19%	29%
26.11b:	Reduce the proportion of college students engaging in binge drinking during the past 2 weeks	39%	20%

From U.S. Department of Health and Human Services (USDHHS). (2000). *Healthy people 2010: Conference edition.* Washington, DC: USDHHS.

contributing health problems and risks posed by the use of alcohol and illicit drugs are also described. Nursing roles and interventions are included throughout.

MENTAL HEALTH AND MENTAL ILLNESS

As discussed, mental health is more than absence of mental illness. There are varying degrees of mental health and not one characteristic is indicative of good mental health, nor can lack of one characteristic indicate a mental illness. In general, **mental health** is determined by how a person feels about himself or herself, how a person feels about others, and how a person meets the demands of everyday life (National Mental Health Association, 1996). Mental health refers to the ability to adapt to distress by mobilizing internal and external resources to minimize tension. Mentally healthy individuals are independent, have high self-esteem, and are able to form meaningful interpersonal relationships (Antai-Otong, 1995).

In contrast, **mental illness** refers to maladaptive responses to distress and an inability to mobilize resources. The mentally ill person is often dependent, has low self-esteem, and has difficulty forming interpersonal relationships (Antai-Otong, 1995). In the *Diagnostic and Statistical Manual of Mental Disorders IV* (DSM-IV), (American Psychiatric Association [APA], 2000) the APA has classified mental illnesses and outlined diagnostic criteria for some 300 mental disorders. Some of the most common disorders are discussed here. These include depression, anxiety disorders, ADD, eating disorders, and substance abuse. In addition, suicide, a consequence of mental illness, is also described. Assessment and treatment of mental disorders concludes the chapter.

DEPRESSION

Depression affects almost 19 million Americans (9.5% of the adult population) each year. It is estimated about 25% of all women and 12% of all men will suffer at least one episode or occurrence of depression during their lifetime and approximately 3% to 5% of teenagers experience clinical depression each year. Most people (almost two thirds) with a depressive illness do not seek treatment, although most, even those with the most severe disorders, can be helped (National Institute of Mental Health [NIMH], 2000b). Estimates of the cost of depression in the United States range from $30 to $44 billion. In addition to direct costs, factors to be considered include the value of lost workdays and impact on productivity (Greensberg, Stiglin, Finkelstein, and Berndt, 1993).

The most prevalent types of depression are major depression, dysthymia, and bipolar disorder. Major depression is diagnosed when an individual experiences symptoms that interfere with the ability to work, sleep, eat, and enjoy once pleasurable activities for a period of at least 2 weeks (APA, 2000). These symptoms may include depressed mood, diminished interest in most activities, significant weight loss or weight gain, and diminished ability to think or concentrate (Box 15-1).

Dysthymia is chronic, mild depression that lasts a minimum of 2 years. In dysthymic disorder, the individual experiences depressive symptoms that are not disabling, but keep him or her from functioning or from feeling good. As with major depression, persons with dysthymia may have poor appetite or may overeat; they often have insomnia or hypersomnia, and experience low energy or fatigue. In dysthymia, the symptoms cause significant distress or impairment in social, occupational, or other areas of functioning, and some people with dysthymia also experience major depressive episodes (APA, 2000).

Bipolar disorder (manic-depressive illness) produces cycles of depression and mania. During a manic episode, the individual will experience a period of abnormally and persistently elevated expansive or irritable mood that lasts for a week or longer. During this period, the individual often

BOX 15-1 Diagnostic Criteria for Major Depressive Episode

A. Five (or more) of the following symptoms have been present during the same 2-week period and represent a change from previous functioning; at least one of the symptoms is either (1) depressed mood or (2) loss of interest or pleasure.

Note: Do not include symptoms that are clearly due to a general medical condition or mood-incongruent delusions or hallucinations.

1. Depressed mood most of the day, nearly every day, as indicated by either subjective report (e.g., feels sad or empty) or observation made by others (e.g., appears tearful). *Note:* In children and adolescents, can be irritable mood.
2. Markedly diminished interest or pleasure in all, or almost all, activities most of the day, nearly every day (as indicated by either subjective account or observation made by others).
3. Significant weight loss when not dieting or weight gain (e.g., a change of more than 5% of body weight in a month) or decrease or increase in appetite nearly every day. *Note:* In children, consider failure to make expected weight gains.
4. Insomnia or hypersomnia nearly every day.
5. Psychomotor agitation or retardation nearly every day (observable by others, not merely subjective feelings of restlessness or being slowed down).
6. Fatigue or loss of energy nearly every day.

7. Feelings of worthlessness or excessive or inappropriate guilt (which may be delusional) nearly every day (not merely self-reproach or guilt about being sick).
8. Diminished ability to think or concentrate, or indecisiveness, nearly every day (either by subjective account or as observed by others).
9. Recurrent thoughts of death (not just fear of dying), recurrent suicidal ideation without a specific plan, or a suicide attempt or a specific plan for committing suicide.

B. The symptoms do not meet criteria for a Mixed Episode.
C. The symptoms cause clinically significant distress or impairment in social, occupational, or other important areas of functioning.
D. The symptoms are not due to the direct physiological effects of a substance (e.g., a drug of abuse, a medication) or a general medical condition (e.g., hypothyroidism).
E. The symptoms are not better accounted for by Bereavement (i.e., after the loss of a loved one); the symptoms persist for longer than 2 months or are characterized by marked functional impairment, morbid preoccupation with worthlessness, suicidal ideation, psychotic symptoms, or psychomotor retardation.

Reprinted with permission from the *Diagnostic and statistical manual of mental disorders* (4th ed., Text Revision). Copyright 2000, American Psychiatric Association.

experiences inflated self-esteem or grandiosity. He or she may have a decreased need for sleep and may be more talkative than usual. They may also experience racing thoughts, have difficulty concentrating, and are easily distractible. Lastly, during a manic episode, the individual may pursue pleasurable activities (e.g., drug abuse, spending sprees, irresponsible sexual activity) that have a high potential for painful consequences. Bipolar disorder is diagnosed if the mood disturbance is severe enough to impair occupational functioning or necessitates hospitalization to prevent harm to self or others (APA, 2000).

RISK FACTORS AND SYMPTOMS

Nurses working in community-based settings should be aware of risk factors for developing depression and of symptoms that might indicate a depressive episode. They can then work to reduce risk factors and teach others to be aware of these symptoms. Health education should also include information on when and how to obtain treatment. Symptoms of depression and mania are included in Box 15-2. The following are risk factors for depression (USDHHS/Office of Disease Prevention and Health Promotion [ODPHP], 1998):

- Prior episode(s) of depression
- Family history of depressive disorder
- Prior suicide attempt(s)
- Female gender
- Postpartum period
- Medical comorbidity
- Lack of social support
- Stressful life events

15-2 Symptoms of Depression and Mania

DEPRESSION

Persistent sad or empty mood

Feelings of hopelessness, pessimism

Feelings of guilt, worthlessness, helplessness

Loss of interest or pleasure in ordinary activities, including sex

Decreased energy, fatigue, being slowed down

Difficulty concentrating, remembering, making decisions

Insomnia, early-morning waking, or oversleeping

Appetite and/or weight loss or overeating and weight gain

Thoughts of death or suicide; suicide attempts

Restlessness, irritability

Persistent physical symptoms that do not respond to treatment (e.g., headaches, digestive disorders, chronic pain)

MANIA

Abnormal or excessive elation

Unusual irritability

Decreased need for sleep

Grandiose notions

Increased talking

Racing thoughts

Increased sexual desire

Markedly increased energy

Poor judgment

Inappropriate social behavior

From National Institute of Mental Health. (2000b). *Depression.* (NIH Publication No. 00-3561). Rockville, MD: National Institute of Mental Health.

- Personal history of sexual abuse
- Current substance abuse

The accompanying Health Teaching box presents risk factors specifically for depression in women.

The highest rates of depressive disorders are found among those 25 to 44 years of age, with rates apparently increasing among those born after 1945. This trend may be the result of psychosocial factors (e.g., single parenting, changing roles, stress). Married people and those in ongoing intimate relationships have a lower rate of clinical depression than do those living alone. Overall, however, unhappily married people have the highest rates, whereas happily married men have the lowest. About 32% of clinically depressed individuals have some form of substance abuse or dependence.

DEPRESSION IN CHILDREN AND ADOLESCENTS

According to the USDHHS/ODPHP (1998), approximately 2% to 4% of prepubertal children and almost twice that number of adolescents have major depressive disorders. A family history of depression is a major risk factor for childhood depression. Other associated factors that may

increase the risk of depression in children and adolescents include a history of verbal, physical, or sexual abuse; frequent separation from or loss of a loved one; poverty; mental retardation; ADD; hyperactivity; and chronic illness. Complications of depression in children and adolescents include poor school performance, poor peer relations, alcohol and drug abuse, promiscuity, teenage pregnancy, other psychiatric illnesses, and suicide (USDHHS/ODPHP, 1998). It should be noted that suicide is the third leading cause of death among persons 15 to 25 years and that the rate of suicide among young males is five times that among young females.

Health care providers should recognize the symptoms of depression and refer for treatment as appropriate. Box 15-3 summarizes characteristics of depression that may be seen in all age groups.

TREATMENT

Treatment for depression includes pharmacological therapy, electroconvulsive therapy, psychotherapy, behavior therapy, or a combination of these (NIMH, 2000b). Antidepressant medication has been shown to effectively treat depression and is the first-line of treatment if the depression

---

health teaching

Risk Factors for Depression in Women

DEVELOPMENTAL ROLES

Adolescence: Female high school students have higher rates of depression, anxiety disorders, eating disorders, and adjustment disorders than male students; contributing factors may include changes in roles and expectations and physical, intellectual, and hormonal changes.

Adulthood: Multidimensional stresses (e.g., responsibilities at home and work, single parenthood, caring for children and aging parents); lack of an intimate, confiding relationship; and marital disputes increase depression.

REPRODUCTIVE LIFE CYCLE

Menstruation and premenstrual syndrome: Depressed feelings, irritability, and other behavioral and emotional changes may occur; these symptoms usually begin after ovulation and worsen until menstruation begins. Premenstrual syndrome is probably attributable to the variations in estrogen and other hormones.

Pregnancy: Pregnancy (if desired) seldom contributes to depression. Having an abortion does not appear to lead to a higher incidence of depression. Women with infertility problems may be subject to extreme anxiety or sadness.

Postpartum depression: Many women experience sadness ranging from transient "blues" to major depression to severe, incapacitating psychotic depression. Many women who experience

depressive illness after childbirth have had prior depressive episodes (although they may have not been diagnosed).

Maternal depression: Maternal depression may negatively affect a child's behavioral, psychological, and social development.

Menopause: In general, menopause is not associated with an increased risk of depression.

VICTIMIZATION

Women molested as children are more likely to have clinical depression at some time in their lives than are those with no history of abuse. There may be a higher incidence of depression among women who were raped as adults and women who experience physical abuse and/or sexual harassment; this may be the result of fostering low self-esteem, helplessness, self-blame, and social isolation.

POVERTY

Low economic status contributes to isolation, uncertainty, frequent negative events, and poor access to resources.

DEPRESSION IN LATER ADULTHOOD

Depression in elderly women may be most often related to widowhood; this is usually temporary and often subsides within a year.

Data from National Institute of Mental Health. (1994b). *Helpful facts about depressive illness.* (NIH Publication No. 94-3875). Rockville, MD: National Institute of Mental Health.

---

is severe, if the person has psychotic features, if the person is melancholic or has atypical symptoms, if the client prefers medication, and/or if psychotherapy by a trained, competent psychotherapist is not available (Frank, Karp, and Rush, 1993). Treatment for all mental disorders is addressed in greater detail later in this chapter.

ANXIETY DISORDERS

Anxiety disorders are a group of mental illnesses characterized by feelings of severe anxiety, resulting symptoms, and efforts (sometime extreme) to avoid those symptoms. Anxiety disorders are the most common of all of the mental disorders, affecting as many as 13% of the general population at any time. Anxiety disorders may be attributed to genetic makeup and life experiences of the individual. Some of the more commonly encountered anxiety disorders are generalized anxiety disorder (GAD), panic disorder (sometimes accompanied by agoraphobia), phobias, obsessive-compulsive disorder (OCD), and posttraumatic stress disorder

BOX **15-3** Characteristics of Depression Across the Life Span

CHILDHOOD

Infants and Preschoolers

Insidious onset
Apathy, fatigue, withdrawal
Poor appetite, weight loss
Agitation, sleeplessness
Rarely, spontaneous disclosure of feeling sad

Prepubertal Children

Possible disclosure of sadness, suicidal thoughts
Irritability, self-criticism, weepiness
Decreased initiative and responsiveness to stimulation, apathy
Fatigue, sleep disturbance
Enuresis, encopresis
Weight loss, anorexia
Somatic complaints
Poor school performance
Social withdrawal, increased aggressiveness

ADOLESCENCE

Feelings of sadness less frequent than in other age groups
Unhappy, restlessness, boredom, irritability
Intense, labile affects
Low self-esteem, hopelessness, worthlessness
Associated anxiety
Feelings of loneliness and being unloved
Pessimism about the future
Loss of interest in friends and activities, apathy
Low frustration tolerance
Poor school performance
Argumentativeness
Increased conflict with peers
Acting-out behavior (e.g., running away, stealing, physical violence)
Sexual activity
Substance abuse
Complaints of headaches, abdominal pain
Hypersomnia

EARLY AND MIDDLE ADULTHOOD

Depressed mood
Anhedonia
Feelings of worthlessness, hopelessness, guilt
Reduced energy, fatigue
Sleep disturbance, especially early morning awakening and multiple nighttime awakenings
Decreased sexual interest and activity
Psychomotor retardation
Anxiety
Decreased appetite and weight loss or increased appetite and weight gain

LATER ADULTHOOD

Unlikely to complain of depressed mood or present with tearful affect
Feelings of helplessness
Pessimism about the future
Ruminating about problems
Critical and envious of others
Loss of self-esteem
Guilt feelings
Longer and more severe depressions than in middle adulthood
Perceived cognitive deficits
Somatic complaints
Constipation
Social withdrawal
Loss of motivation
Change of appetite

CORE SYMPTOMS ACROSS AGE GROUPS

Suicidal ideation
Diminished concentration
Sleep disturbance

From Tommasini, N. R. (1995). The client with a mood disorder (depression). In D. Antai-Otong (Ed.), *Psychiatric nursing: Biological and behavioral concepts* (pp. 157-190). Philadelphia: W. B. Saunders.

(PTSD) (USDHHS/Public Health Service [PHS], 1999). These are discussed briefly here.

GENERALIZED ANXIETY DISORDER

Generalized anxiety disorder is characterized by chronic, unrealistic, and exaggerated worry and tension about one or more life circumstances lasting 6 months or longer without anything seeming to provoke it (USDHHS/PHS, 1999). Approximately half of cases of GAD begin in childhood or adolescence and it is more common in women than in men.

Symptoms of GAD include trembling, twitching muscle tension, headaches, irritability, sweating or hot flashes, dyspnea, nausea, and feeling a lump in the throat. It typically fluctuates with periods of increasing symptoms that are usually associated with life stressors or impending difficulties.

PANIC DISORDER

Some 2% to 4% of the population will suffer from panic disorder during their lifetime; women experience approximately double the rate of men (USDHHS/PHS, 1999). Panic disorder can occur at any age, but it most often begins in young adulthood (average age, 17 to 30 years). **Panic disorder** typically develops in three stages, with clients potentially stopping at any stage or progressing through all three. Individuals often have their first attack or cluster of attacks after a variety of life stresses. The initial attack may occur suddenly and unexpectedly while the client is performing everyday tasks. Typically, he or she experiences tachycardia; dyspnea; dizziness; chest pain; nausea; numbness or tingling of the hands and feet; trembling or shaking; sweating; choking; or a feeling that he or she is going to die, go crazy, or do something uncontrolled. This can be extremely frightening. A diagnosis of panic disorder is made when attacks occur with some degree of frequency or regularity.

During the second stage, the anxiety attacks become increasingly frequent and severe and the individual develops anticipatory anxiety (fear of having a panic attack). During this phase, events and circumstances associated with the attack may be selectively avoided, leading to phobic behaviors (e.g., if a woman has an attack while driving, she may become anxious the next time she needs to drive and she may begin to avoid driving and then refuse to drive altogether). In this phase, the client's life may become progressively constricted.

As the avoidance behavior intensifies, the third stage may develop, in which the client begins to withdraw further to avoid being in places or situations from which escape may be difficult or embarrassing or help may be unavailable in the event of a panic attack (e.g., church, elevators, movie theaters) (Katon, 1994). The fear of being in these situations or places can lead to **agoraphobia** (literally, fear of the marketplace or open places). Agoraphobics frequently progress to the point where they cannot leave their homes without experiencing anxiety. Agoraphobia is the most common phobia leading to the use of health services, particularly when accompanied by panic attacks. About one third of all people who experience panic attacks eventually develop agoraphobia.

Panic disorder is often accompanied by other conditions. If not treated, approximately 50% to 65% of clients with panic disorder will develop a major depression at some time in their lives (USDHHS/PHS, 1999). Alcoholism is also common. Cognitive-behavioral therapy and medication can help 70% to 90% of people with panic disorder. Box 15-4 contains diagnostic criteria for panic disorder with and without agoraphobia.

PHOBIAS

A **phobia** is an irrational fear of something (an object or situation) and as many as 8% of Americans are affected by phobias at any given time. Adults with phobias realize their fears are irrational, but facing the feared object or situation might bring on severe anxiety or a panic attack. Phobias may begin in childhood, but usually first appear in adolescence or adulthood.

Social phobia, or social anxiety disorder, is a persistent and intense fear of, and compelling desire to avoid, something that would expose the individual to a situation that might be humiliating and embarrassing. Its tendency is familial and may be accompanied by depression or alcoholism. Social phobia often begins in childhood or early adolescence. Individuals suffering from social phobia think that others are very competent in public, but that they are not. Small mistakes are exaggerated. The most common social phobia is a fear of public speaking. Other examples include being unable to urinate in a public bathroom and not being able to answer questions in social situations. Most people with social phobias can be

BOX 15-4 Diagnostic Criteria for Panic Disorder with and without Agoraphobia

DIAGNOSTIC CRITERIA FOR PANIC DISORDER WITHOUT AGORAPHOBIA	**DIAGNOSTIC CRITERIA FOR PANIC DISORDER WITH AGORAPHOBIA**
A. Both 1 and 2. 　1. Recurrent unexpected Panic Attacks 　2. At least one of the attacks has been followed by 1 month (or more) of one (or more) of the following: 　　a. Persistent concern about having additional attacks 　　b. Worry about the implications of the attack or its consequences (e.g., losing control, having a heart attack, "going crazy") 　　c. A significant change in behavior related to the attacks B. Absence of Agoraphobia. C. The Panic Attacks are not due to the direct physiological effects of a substance (e.g., a drug of abuse, a medication) or a general medical condition (e.g., hyperthyroidism). D. The Panic Attacks are not better accounted for by another mental disorder, such as Social Phobia (e.g., occurring on exposure to feared social situations), Specific Phobia (e.g., on exposure to a specific phobic situation), Obsessive-Compulsive Disorder (e.g., on exposure to dirt in someone with an obsession about contamination), Posttraumatic Stress Disorder (e.g., in response to stimuli associated with a severe stressor), or Separation Anxiety Disorder (e.g., in response to being away from home or close relatives).	A. Both 1 and 2. 　1. Recurrent unexpected Panic Attacks 　2. At least one of the attacks has been followed by 1 month (or more) of one (or more) of the following: 　　a. Persistent concern about having additional attacks 　　b. Worry about the implications of the attack or its consequences (e.g., losing control, having a heart attack, "going crazy") 　　c. A significant change in behavior related to the attacks B. The presence of Agoraphobia. C. The Panic Attacks are not caused by the direct physiological effects of a substance (e.g., a drug of abuse, a medication) or a general medical condition (e.g., hyperthyroidism). D. The Panic Attacks are not better accounted for by another mental disorder, such as Social Phobia (e.g., occurring on exposure to feared social situations), Specific Phobia (e.g., on exposure to a specific phobic situation), Obsessive-Compulsive Disorder (e.g., on exposure to dirt in someone with an obsession about contamination), Posttraumatic Stress Disorder (e.g., in response to stimuli associated with a severe stressor), or Separation Anxiety Disorder (e.g., in response to being away from home or close relatives.)

Reprinted with permission from the *Diagnostic and statistical manual of mental disorders* (4th ed., Text Revision). Copyright 2000, American Psychiatric Association.

treated with cognitive-behavior therapy and medication.

Simple phobias (excluding panic attack or social phobia) involve a persistent fear of, and compelling desire to avoid, certain objects or situations. Common objects of phobias are spiders, snakes, dogs, cats, and situations such as flying, heights, and closed-in spaces. The person often recognizes that the fear is excessive or unreasonable, but nonetheless avoids the situation or endures it with intense anxiety. Systematic desensitization and normal exposure are the most effective treatments for simple phobias. Medication produces minimal benefit (Katon, 1994).

OBSESSIVE-COMPULSIVE DISORDER

Obsessive-compulsive disorder (OCD) is characterized by anxious thoughts and rituals that the individual has difficulty controlling. The person with OCD is overcome with the urge to engage in some ritual to avoid a persistent frightening thought, idea, image, or event—the obsession. Compulsions are the rituals or behaviors that are repeatedly performed to prevent, neutralize, or dispel the dreaded obsession. When the individual tries to resist the compulsion, anxiety increases. Common compulsions include hand washing, counting, checking, or touching (Robinson, 1996).

Obsessive-compulsive disease is diagnosed only when the compulsive activities consume at least an hour a day and interfere with daily life. Most individuals recognize that what they are doing is senseless, but are unable to control the compulsion. About 2% of Americans are afflicted with OCD, which often appears in the teenage years or early adulthood. Depression or other anxiety disorders often accompany OCD. Clomipramine (Anafranil) and fluoxetine (Prozac) have been effective in treating OCD. Behavioral therapy may also help.

POSTTRAUMATIC STRESS DISORDER

Posttraumatic stress disorder (PTSD) is a debilitating condition that follows a terrifying event. Individuals with PTSD have recurring, persistent, frightening thoughts and memories of their ordeal. Traumatic incidents that trigger PTSD may have threatened that individual's life or the life of someone else. Incidents include "shell shock" or "battle fatigue" common to war veterans, violent attack (e.g., kidnapping, rape, mugging), serious accidents, natural disasters (e.g., earthquake, tornado), or witnessing mass destruction or injury, such as an airplane crash. Sometimes the individual is unable to recall an important aspect of the traumatic event (Katon, 1994). Interestingly, about 30% of Vietnam veterans experience PTSD at some point after the war (NIMH, 2001a).

People with PTSD repeatedly relive the trauma in the form of nightmares and/or disturbing recollections, flashbacks, or hallucinations during the day. As a result, they often have sleep disturbances, depression, and feelings of detachment or emotional numbness, and/or are easily startled. They may avoid places or situations that bring back memories (e.g., a woman raped in an elevator may refuse to ride in elevators) and anniversaries of the event are often very difficult. It occurs at all ages and may be accompanied by depression, substance abuse, and/or anxiety. It usually begins within 3 months of the trauma and the course of the disorder varies. Some individuals recover within 6 months;

the condition becomes chronic in others. Infrequently, the illness does not manifest until years after the traumatic event.

Posttraumatic stress disorder is treated with antidepressants and antianxiety medications and psychotherapy. Support from family and friends can be very beneficial.

EATING DISORDERS

Eating disorders are becoming increasingly prevalent in the United States. Indeed, the most common eating disorders, anorexia nervosa and bulimia nervosa, affect about 3 million U.S. residents. Currently, it is estimated that anorexia affects 0.5% to 3.7% of girls and women during their lifetime (NIMH, 2001b). Additionally, as many as 2% to 8% of adolescent and college-aged women have some symptoms of bulimia (Decker and Freeman, 1996).

Eating disorders almost exclusively affect females; males account for only 5% to 10% of bulimia and anorexia cases. Most clients diagnosed with eating disorders are white. This, however, may be because of socioeconomic factors rather than race because females in middle and upper socioeconomic groups are most frequently affected. Anorexia and bulimia are often triggered by developmental milestones (e.g., puberty, first sexual contact) or another crisis (e.g., death of a loved one, ridicule over weight, starting college).

BULIMIA NERVOSA

"The essential features of bulimia are binge eating and inappropriate compensatory methods to prevent weight gain" (APA, 2000, p. 545). A binge is defined as eating an abnormal amount of food at a discrete time (usually less than 2 hours) (APA, 2000). For example, a bulimic might eat an entire pie, half a cake, or a half gallon of ice cream at one sitting. Snacking throughout the day is not considered bingeing.

To lose or maintain weight, the bulimic practices purging, which usually involves self-induced vomiting caused by gagging, using an emetic, or simply mentally willing the action. Laxatives, diuretics, fasting, and excessive exercise may also be employed to control weight.

Bulimia nervosa typically begins in adolescence or during the early 20s and usually in conjunction with a diet. Members of certain professions that emphasize weight and/or appearance (e.g., dancers, flight attendants, athletes, actors, models) are at high risk (Decker and Freeman, 1996).

A number of health problems may result from bulimia. Electrolyte imbalance can result in fatigue, seizures, muscle cramps, arrhythmias, and decreased bone density. Vomiting can damage the esophagus, stomach, teeth, and gums.

ANOREXIA NERVOSA

The person suffering from **anorexia nervosa** becomes obsessed with a fear of fat and with losing weight. Anorexia nervosa often develops with a fairly gradual decrease in caloric intake. However, the decrease in caloric intake continues until the anorexic is consuming almost nothing. Anorexia usually begins in early adolescence (12 to 14 years is the most common age group) and may be limited to a single episode of dramatic weight loss within a few months followed by recovery or the illness may last for many years.

As stated earlier, anorexia nervosa almost exclusively affects white adolescent girls. Other characteristics of girls who develop anorexia are that they are well-behaved and eager to please; are perfectionists; may have a poor self-image; are dependent on others' opinions, introverted, and insecure; are overly compliant and deferential to others' wishes; and are emotionally reserved (Decker and Freeman, 1996).

In response to the severely decreased caloric intake, the body tries to compensate by slowing down body processes. Menstruation ceases; blood pressure, pulse, and respiration rates slow; and thyroid activity diminishes. Electrolyte imbalance can become very severe. Other symptoms include mild anemia, joint swelling, and reduced muscle mass. Anorexia nervosa can be

life threatening and has a mortality rate of 5% to 18%. In 1990, 70 deaths in the United States were attributed to anorexia.

TREATMENT

Treatment for eating disorders includes nutrition counseling, psychotherapy, and behavior modification and may take a year or more. Hospitalization may be required for clients with serious complications. Self-help groups and support groups can be very beneficial for both the client and the family. Many bulimics appear to respond to antidepressants. Anorexia nervosa, however, does not appear as responsive to medication.

Nurses who frequently work with adolescent girls and young women in community settings such as schools and clinics should be aware of the risk factors, signs, and symptoms of anorexia and bulimia and be prepared to intervene.

ATTENTION DEFICIT HYPERACTIVITY DISORDER

One of the most common conditions encountered by nurses who work with children in community settings is ADD or **attention deficit hyperactivity disorder (ADHD)**. (Here the disorder is referred to as ADHD.) In the United States, ADHD affects 3% to 5% of all children (about 2 million) (NIMH, 2000a). Behaviors that might indicate ADHD usually appear before age 7 years and are often accompanied by related problems, such as learning disability, anxiety, and depression. The three major characteristics of ADHD are inattention, hyperactivity, and impulsivity. Box 15-5 presents the diagnostic criteria for ADHD.

The cause of ADHD is not known, but it is important to note that it is not caused by minor head injuries, birth complications, food allergies, too much sugar, poor home life, poor schools, or too much television. Maternal substance use and abuse (e.g., alcohol, cigarettes, cocaine) may affect the brain of the developing baby and produce symptoms of ADHD later in life. This, however, accounts for only a small percentage of those affected (NIMH, 1994a).

BOX 15-5 Diagnostic Criteria for Attention Deficit/Hyperactivity Disorder

A. Either (1) or (2):

1. Six (or more) of the following symptoms of inattention have persisted for at least 6 months to a degree that is maladaptive and inconsistent with developmental level

INATTENTION

a. Often fails to give close attention to details or makes careless mistakes in schoolwork, work, or other activities

b. Often has difficulty sustaining attention in tasks or play activities

c. Often does not seem to listen when spoken to directly

d. Often does not follow through on instructions and fails to finish schoolwork, chores, or duties in the workplace (not because of oppositional behavior or failure to understand instructions)

e. Often has difficulty organizing tasks and activities

f. Often avoids, dislikes, or is reluctant to engage in tasks that require sustained mental effort (such as schoolwork or homework)

g. Often loses things necessary for tasks or activities (e.g., toys, school assignments, pencils, books, or tools)

h. Is often easily distracted by extraneous stimuli

i. Is often forgetful in daily activities

2. Six (or more) of the following symptoms of hyperactivity-impulsivity have persisted for at least 6 months to a degree that is maladaptive and inconsistent with developmental level

HYPERACTIVITY

a. Often fidgets with hands or feet or squirms in seat

b. Often leaves seat in classroom or in other situations in which remaining seated is expected

c. Often runs about or climbs excessively in situations in which it is inappropriate (in adolescents or adults, may be limited to subjective feelings of restlessness)

d. Often has difficulty playing or engaging in leisure activities quietly

e. Is often "on the go" or often acts as if "driven by a motor"

f. Often talks excessively

IMPULSIVITY

g. Often blurts out answers before questions have been completed

h. Often has difficulty awaiting turn

i. Often interrupts or intrudes on others (e.g., butts into conversations or games)

B. Some hyperactive-impulsive or inattentive symptoms that caused impairment were present before age 7 years

C. Some impairment from the symptoms is present in two or more settings (e.g., at school [or work] and at home)

D. There must be clear evidence of clinically significant impairment in social, academic, or occupational functioning

E. The symptoms do not occur exclusively during the course of a Pervasive Developmental Disorder, Schizophrenia, or other psychotic disorder and are not better accounted for by another mental disorder (e.g., Mood Disorder, Anxiety Disorder, Dissociative Disorder, or a Personality Disorder)

Code based on type:

314.01: Attention-Deficit/Hyperactivity Disorder, Combined Type: if both Criteria A1 and A2 are met for the past 6 months

314.00: Attention-Deficit/Hyperactivity Disorder, Predominantly Inattentive Type: if Criterion A1 is met, but Criterion A2 is not met for the past 6 months

314.01: Attention-Deficit/Hyperactivity Disorder, Predominantly Hyperactive-Impulsive type: if Criterion A2 is met, but Criterion A1 is not met for the past 6 months

Coding note: For individuals (especially adolescents and adults) who currently have symptoms that no longer meet full criteria, "In Partial Remission" should be specified.

Reprinted with permission from the *Diagnostic and statistical manual of mental disorders* (4th ed., Text Revision). Copyright 2000, American Psychiatric Association.

Attention disorders run in families, as children diagnosed with ADHD usually have at least one close relative who also has ADHD, and at least one third of all fathers who had ADHD as children have children with symptoms. Additionally, in the majority of sets of identical twins in which one has the disorder, the other does also (NIMH, 2000a). Although parents may notice symptoms and signs, it is often teachers who recognize the behaviors consistent with attention deficit disorders and suggest referral for assessment and treatment.

Experts caution that diagnosis of attention disorders should be made following a comprehensive physical, psychological, social, and behavioral evaluation and not based solely on anecdotal reports from parents. The evaluation should rule out other possible reasons for the behavior (e.g., emotional problems, poor vision or hearing, physical problems) and should include input from teachers, parents, and others who know the child well. Intelligence and achievement testing may also be performed to rule out or identify a learning disability.

Symptoms of ADHD are typically managed through a combination of behavior therapy, emotional counseling, and practical support. Use of medication is becoming increasingly commonplace in the management of ADHD. It is very important, however, that children with attention disorders and their families understand that medication does not cure the disorder; it just temporarily controls symptoms.

Curiously, stimulants are the medications that have been shown to be successful in treating attention disorders in both children and adults. The most commonly used medications are methylphenidate (Ritalin) and amphetamines (Dexedrine, Dextrostat, or Adderall). About 90% of children with ADHD show improvement when taking one of these drugs. These medications are short acting (lasting 2 to 4 hours) and therefore may need to be taken several times each day. Recently, sustained-release preparations, which require fewer doses, have been made available for some of the medications (NIMH, 2000c).

Effective doses vary among children and drug regimens for treatment of ADHD vary among physicians. Some physicians recommend keeping children on medication only during school and have the child stop taking the medication on weekends and during summer vacation. Others prescribe medication every day, assuming that this regimen is more beneficial in helping establish positive behavioral patterns and work habits.

Medications used to treat ADHD have some potential adverse effects. Appetite suppression is fairly common and may contribute to growth retardation. Periodic assessment of height and weight is therefore important. Sleeping difficulties are also possible. There is concern that long-term use of pemoline (Cylert) may affect the liver. Therefore liver function must be assessed periodically in clients taking this medication (NIMH, 2000c).

SUBSTANCE ABUSE

Substance abuse refers to patterns of use of alcohol and/or other drugs that result in health consequences or impairment in social, psychological, and occupational functioning. A diagnosis of substance abuse may be made if an individual brings about hazardous situations from substance abuse (i.e., driving an automobile while impaired) or if the individual experiences substance-related legal problems. Substance dependence occurs when the individual develops a tolerance for the substance and needs increased amounts to achieve the desired effect. In substance dependence, there may be problems associated with withdrawal of the substance, a need to take the substance more often and in larger amounts, and an unsuccessful desire to cut down or control substance use. The person who is substance dependent may spend an inordinate amount of time in activities to obtain the substance or to recover from it and may neglect or abandon social, occupational, or recreational activities because of the substance (APA, 2000).

The toll caused by alcohol and other drugs on society is staggering. The economic costs of alcohol alone are massive. Alcohol and drug use is involved in several of the leading causes of morbidity and mortality in the United States, including accidental injury, suicide, homicide, liver disease, certain types of cancer, and AIDS (USDHHS, 2000). A number of legal and illegal substances used by many Americans, including alcohol, cigarettes, marijuana, heroin, and many others, are harmful.

BOX **15-6** Fast Facts About Alcohol Use and Abuse

Alcohol abuse costs U.S. residents almost $167 billion annually, the majority being in productivity losses associated with illness and death.

During the past decade, alcohol consumption in the United States has declined, most notably because of a decrease in consumption of distilled liquor; in contrast, beer consumption has remained stable and wine consumption has increased slightly.

By eighth grade, almost 70% of adolescents state that they have tried alcohol at least once; the average age of first use is 14 years.

Abuse varies markedly based on cultural and ethnic groups; white, Native American, and Hispanic high

school seniors reportedly drink the most (45% to 48% of boys drink heavily); by comparison, only 19% of Asian-Americans and 24% of black high school seniors drink heavily.

Alcohol consumption is highest between 18 and 34 years of age when about 62% of individuals report using alcohol during the last month.

Binge drinking and heavy alcohol use peak at 21 years of age.

About 41% of all fatal traffic accidents involve alcohol.

Drinking also contributes to a large percentage of deaths from falls, fires or burns, homicides, suicides, and drownings.

Data from Robert Wood Johnson Foundation. (1993). *Substance abuse: The nation's number one health problem.* Waltham, MA: Institute for Health Policy, Brandeis University; U.S. Department of Health and Human Services (USDHHS). (2000). *Healthy people 2010: Conference edition.* Washington, DC: USDHHS; U.S. Department of Health and Human Services/Substance Abuse and Mental Health Services Administration (USDHHS/SAMHSA). (1999). *Findings from the 1999 national household survey on drug abuse.* Washington, DC: USDHHS.

ALCOHOL ABUSE

Alcoholism is the largest drug problem in the United States today. Indeed, about 10% of the adult population has a chronic, heavy intake of alcohol and shows symptoms of alcoholism. Box 15-6 lists some facts about alcohol abuse.

ILLICIT DRUG USE

Illicit drugs used in the United States include opioids (e.g., heroin, morphine), cocaine (e.g., crack), amphetamines, hallucinogens (e.g., lysergic acid diethylamide [LSD], phencyclidine [PCP]), marijuana, and inhalants (e.g., airplane model glue, spray paint, nail polish remover, gasoline). Box 15-7 lists a few relevant statistics on the use and abuse of illicit drugs.

RISK FACTORS FOR SUBSTANCE ABUSE

Several risk factors have been identified that can contribute to the likelihood that an individual might abuse alcohol and/or other drugs. Box 15-8 lists these by developmental stage. The Research Highlight box discusses the relationship between stress and substance abuse. Nurses who work in community settings such as clinics, physicians' offices, schools, and work sites should be knowledgeable about risk factors that

contribute to substance abuse and when to intervene to reduce them, whenever possible.

SIGNS AND SYMPTOMS OF SUBSTANCE ABUSE

Nurses should also be aware of the signs and symptoms that might indicate use and/or abuse of alcohol and other drugs. To help nurses recognize these symptoms of substance use and withdrawal and identify appropriate treatment, Table 15-2 describes each.

TREATMENT FOR SUBSTANCE ABUSE

An estimated 18 million people who use alcohol and other drugs are in need of treatment and less than one fourth will get it. Unlike health care for other conditions, most of the funding for drug and alcohol treatment facilities comes from federal block grants and state and local government funds. Private insurance, Medicaid, and other public insurance programs contribute less than a third of the total funding for treatment.

Substance abuse treatment is effective for many people and most people need some kind of treatment to recover from substance abuse (Plumlee, 1995). The key to effective treatment is

15-7 Fast Facts About the Use and Abuse of Illicit Drugs

Drug abuse costs U.S. residents about $110 billion annually; in contrast to alcohol abuse, much of the costs of illicit drug use are from costs related to crime, property destruction, and public attempts to control their use.

The use of illicit drugs has declined over the last several decades. In the late 1970s, almost 40% of high school seniors reported using drugs compared with 14% in 1992; marijuana use among those 18 to 25 years of age peaked at 35% in 1979 and fell to 13% in 1991; likewise, cocaine use peaked in 1979 at 13% and dropped to 2% in 1991.

Drug use among adolescents doubled between 1992 and 1997 from 5.3% to 11.4%; marijuana is the major illicit drug used by this group.

Males are more than three times as likely as females to be heavy drinkers and more than twice as likely to use marijuana weekly; males and females are equally likely to use cocaine.

At least half of all people arrested for major crimes (homicide, theft, assault) were using illicit drugs at the time of their arrest.

Deaths from illicit drugs are often from a combination of two or more illicit drugs or drugs combined with alcohol; heroin or cocaine is involved in two thirds of drug deaths; almost 40% of illicit drug deaths are among adults between 30 and 39 years (perhaps indicating chronic problems because of drug abuse); blacks are more than twice as likely to die from the direct effects of illicit drugs as are whites.

About one third of new AIDS cases occur among injecting drug users or people having sexual contact with them.

Among convicted inmates, 84% of women reported they had used illicit drugs at some time and 40% reported daily use; for those arrested for prostitution, 85% tested positive for illicit drugs and 65% of women arrested for homicide tested positive for illicit drugs.

In contrast, men most likely to be under the influence were arrested for drug sales or possession (80%) or larceny or theft (65%).

Data from Robert Wood Johnson Foundation. (1993). *Substance abuse: The nation's number one health problem.* Waltham, MA: Institute for Health Policy, Brandeis University; U.S. Department of Health and Human Services (USDHHS). (2000). *Healthy people 2010: Conference edition.* Washington, DC: USDHHS; U.S. Department of Health and Human Services/Substance Abuse and Mental Health Services Administration (USDHHS/SAMHSA). (1999). *Findings from the 1999 national household survey on drug abuse.* Washington, DC: USDHHS.

Research Highlight

Stress and Substance Abuse

Many clinicians and addiction medicine specialists suggest that stress is the primary cause of relapse to drug abuse, including smoking. It is hypothesized that stress leads to an increase in the brain levels of a peptide known as corticotrophin releasing factor (CRF). An increase in CRF levels triggers biological responses that promote relapse. Also people subject to chronic stress or those with symptoms of PTSD often have hormonal responses that are not properly regulated and do not return to normal when the stress is over. This may make these individuals more prone to stress-related illnesses and may prompt relapse to drug use. Among the research findings on stress and drug use relapse are the following:

- Studies report that individuals exposed to stress are more likely to abuse alcohol and other drugs or undergo relapse.

- High stress was found to predict continued drug use among opiate addicts.
- Acute stress can improve memory, whereas chronic stress can impair memory and may impair cognitive function.
- Among drug-free cocaine abusers in treatment, exposure to personal stress led to consistent and significant increases in cocaine craving.
- A study of smokers who had completed a smoking cessation program showed that there is a strong relationship between stress coping resources and the ability to sustain abstinence.
- A risk factor for substance abuse is PTSD.

From National Institute on Drug Abuse (2001). *Stress and substance abuse: A special report.* Retrieved 8/20/01 from http://www.nida.nih.gov/stressanddrugabuse.html.

BOX **15-8** Risk Factors for Alcohol and Other Drug Abuse by Stage of Life

CHILDHOOD

Fetal exposure to alcohol and other drugs (AOD)
Parents who are substance abusers
Physical, sexual, or psychological abuse
Economic disadvantage
Delinquency
Mental health problems such as depression and
   suicidal ideation
Disability

ADOLESCENCE

Parental use of AOD
Low self-esteem
Depression
Psychological distress
Poor relationship with parents
Low sense of social responsibility
Lack of religious commitment
Low academic performance and motivation
Peer use of AOD
Participation in deviant, aggressive behavior

YOUNG ADULTHOOD

Exposure to drug users in social and work environments
Marital and work instability
Unemployment
Divorce
Psychological or psychiatric difficulties

MIDDLE ADULTHOOD

Bereavement, especially as a result of loss of spouse
   or significant other
Adverse work conditions or unemployment
Changes in health status or appearance
Socioeconomic stressors
Environmental changes or relocation
Divorce, separation, or remarriage
Difficulties with children or changes in child-rearing
   responsibilities

OLDER ADULTHOOD

Retirement or role status change
Loss of loved ones
Changes in health status and mobility
Increased sensitivity to effects of alcohol and other
   drugs
Housing relocations
Affective changes (e.g., anxiety and depression)
History of previous misuse or abuse of AOD
Solitude or social contexts that foster use of AOD
Negative self-concept

From U.S. Office of Substance Abuse Prevention. (1992). *Nurse training course: Alcohol and other drug abuse prevention.* Rockville, MD: National Training System, U.S. Public Health Service.

to match the client's needs with the intervention strategy most appropriate for him or her. The vast majority of clients in alcohol and/or drug treatment programs are outpatients. Alcohol and drug treatment services are provided by family practitioners, internists, psychiatrists, and other medical specialists and in emergency rooms. Self-help groups are an important part of recovery for many. The most common models of treatment consist of education and participation in twelve-step programs (Plumlee, 1995).

Education

Intense and ongoing education about the disease of alcoholism or other drug addiction to break

the abuser's denial may be helpful, including the following:
- Initiation of the Twelve Steps of AA
- Required reading of literature from AA or NA (as appropriate)
- Attendance at AA or NA meetings
- Skill building to maintain abstinence

Twelve-Step Programs

Participation in **twelve-step programs** (e.g., NA and AA) gives social support and structure that assists in the recovery process. Nurses who are in a position to identify those in need of these services should be knowledgeable about these programs and ready to supply information and

TABLE **15-2** Signs of Intoxication, Indications of Withdrawal, and Treatment Modalities for Selected Psychoactive Substances

SUBSTANCE	SIGNS OF INTOXICATION	INDICATIONS OF WITHDRAWAL	TREATMENT MODALITIES
Alcohol	Decreased alertness, impaired judgment, slurred speech, nausea, double vision, vertigo, staggering, unpredictable emotional changes, stupor, unconsciousness, increased reaction time	Anxiety, insomnia, tremors, delirium, convulsions	Detoxification, psychotherapy, group therapy, family therapy, self-help groups (AA, Al-Anon), pharmacological therapy, residential programs, referral for vocational rehabilitation and social services as needed
Sedatives, hypnotics, anxiolytics	Slurred speech, slow and shallow respiration, cold and clammy skin, nystagmus, weak and rapid pulse, drowsiness, blurred vision, unconsciousness, disorientation, depression, poor judgment, motor impairment	Anxiety, insomnia, tremors, delirium, convulsions (may occur up to 2 weeks after stopping use of anxiolytics)	Detoxification, psychotherapy, and group therapy (for underlying psychiatric disorders)
Opioids	Sedation, hypertension, respiratory depression, impaired intellectual function, constipation, pupillary constriction, watery eyes, increased pulse and blood pressure	Restlessness, irritability, tremors, loss of appetite, panic, chills, sweating, cramps, watery eyes, runny nose, nausea, vomiting, muscle spasms, impaired coordination, depressed reflexes, dilated pupils, yawning	Pharmacological therapy (methadone, opioid antagonists), therapeutic communities (Synanon, Odyssey House, Phoenix House), group therapy, assistance with social skills, vocational training and job placement, family therapy, self-help groups (NA, Chemical Dependency Anonymous), psychotherapy
Cocaine	Irritability; anxiety; slow and weak pulse; slow and shallow breathing; sweating; dilated pupils; increased blood pressure; insomnia; seizures; disinhibition; impulsivity; compulsive actions; hypersexuality; hypervigilance; hyperactivity	*Early crash:* agitation, depression, anorexia, high level of craving, suicidal ideation *Middle crash:* fatigue, depression, no craving, insomnia *Late crash:* exhaustion, hypersomnolence, hyperphagia, no craving *Early withdrawal:* normal sleep and mood, low craving, low anxiety	Hospitalization, self-help groups, contingency contracting (client agreement to urinary monitoring and acceptance of aversive contingencies for positive results), pharmacological therapy (tricyclic antidepressants)

continued

Adapted from Clark, M. J. (1999). Substance abuse. In M. J. Clark (Ed.), *Nursing in the Community* (3rd ed., pp. 859–886). Stamford, CT: Appleton & Lange.

TABLE **15-2** Signs of Intoxication, Indications of Withdrawal, and Treatment Modalities for Selected Psychoactive Substances—cont'd

SUBSTANCE	SIGNS OF INTOXICATION	INDICATIONS OF WITHDRAWAL	TREATMENT MODALITIES
Amphetamines	Sweating, dilated pupils, increased blood pressure, agitation, fever, irritability, headache, chills, insomnia, agitation, tremors, seizures, wakefulness, hyperactivity, confusion, paranoia	*Middle and late withdrawal:* anhedonia, anxiety anergy, high level of craving exacerbated by conditioned cues *Extinction:* normal hedonic response and mood, episodic craving triggered by conditioned cues	No established treatment guidelines; may be similar to treatment for cocaine abuse
Hallucinogens	Dilated pupils, mood swings, elevated blood pressure, paranoia, bizarre behavior, nausea and vomiting, tremors, panic, flushing, fever, sweating, agitation, aggression, nystagmus (with PCP)	Fatigue, hunger, long period of sleep, disorientation, severe depression Slight irritability, restlessness, insomnia, reduced energy level, depression	Detoxification, psychotherapy (for underlying psychiatric disorders), group therapy, residential programs
Cannabis (marijuana, hashish)	Reddened eyes; increased pulse, respiration, and blood pressure; laughter; confusion; panic; drowsiness	Insomnia, hyperactivity, decreased appetite	Same as for hallucinogens; self-help groups
Inhalants	Giddiness, drowsiness, increased vital signs, headache, nausea, fainting, stupor, fatigue, slurred speech, disorientation, delirium	None reported	Psychosocial interventions, psychotherapy (for underlying psychiatric disorder), sociodrama, vocational rehabilitation, family therapy, social support services
Nicotine	Headache; loss of appetite; nausea; increased pulse, blood pressure, and muscle tone	Nervousness, increased appetite, sleep disturbances, anxiety, irritability	Aversive conditioning, desensitization, substitution, hypnotherapy, group therapy, relaxation training, supportive therapy, abrupt abstinence

BOX **15-9** The Twelve Steps of Alcoholics Anonymous

Admitted we were powerless over alcohol—that our lives had become unmanageable

Came to believe that a Power greater than ourselves could restore us to sanity

Made a decision to turn our will and our lives over to the care of God as we understood Him

Made a searching and fearless moral inventory of ourselves

Admitted to God, to ourselves, and to another human being the exact nature of our wrongs

Were entirely ready to have God remove all these defects of character

Humbly asked Him to remove our shortcomings

Made a list of all persons we had harmed and became willing to make amends to them all

Made direct amends to such people wherever possible, except when to do so would injure them or others

Continued to take personal inventory and, when we were wrong, promptly admitted it

Sought through prayer and meditation to improve our conscious contact with God as we understood Him, praying only for knowledge of His will for us and the power to carry that out

Having had a spiritual awakening as the result of these steps, we tried to carry this message to alcoholics and to practice these principles in all our affairs

The Twelve Steps are reprinted with permission of Alcoholics Anonymous World Services, Inc. Permission to reprint this material does not mean that AA has reviewed or approved the contents of this publication, nor that AA agrees with the views expressed herein. AA is a program of recovery from alcoholism—use of the Twelve Steps in connection with programs and activities that are patterned after AA, but address other problems, does not imply otherwise.

referral. To this end, Box 15-9 presents the Twelve Steps of AA. Further information can be obtained by contacting local programs or national offices (see the Resources box at the end of the chapter).

SUICIDE

Suicide is the most serious potential outcome of mental disorders and is the eighth leading cause of death in the United States. Each year, more than 30,000 U.S residents take their own lives. Depression, schizophrenia, panic disorder, and alcohol and other drug abuse have been implicated in both attempted and completed suicides (USDHHS, 2000). Box 15-10 lists some statistics regarding suicide of which the nurse in community-based practice should be aware.

Risk factors for adolescent suicide include a strong family history of psychiatric disorders (e.g., depression or suicidal behavior), previous suicide attempts, serious medical illness, family violence, alcohol and other drug abuse, and accessibility to firearms (USDHHS/ODPHP, 1998). To combat the high rates of suicide among adolescents and young adults, the National Center for Injury Prevention and Control outlined general recommendations, which are listed in the Community Application box "Examples of Suicide Prevention Programs."

IDENTIFICATION OF MENTAL DISORDERS

Whether the nurse is working in a physician's office, a clinic, home health, a school, occupational health, or another setting, recognition of signs and symptoms that might indicate a mental disorder is an important component of practice. For example, a student might come to the school nurse's office concerned about a friend who induces vomiting in the bathroom after lunch each day; an occupational health nurse might observe signs consistent with alcohol abuse in an employee; or a client might visit a clinic for a routine visit, but mention that for the last several weeks she has been unable to sleep, has lost several pounds, and is no longer interested in her normal activities. In each of these situations, the nurse should continue to assess for other signs and symptoms that might indicate a mental disorder and be prepared to intervene should concerns be supported.

Often, the assessment process includes direct questioning or observation. At other times, a standardized assessment tool or questionnaire

BOX 15-10 Suicide Facts

COMPLETED SUICIDES (UNITED STATES, 1997)

Suicide is the eighth leading cause of death in the United States, accounting for 1.3% of all deaths (in contrast, 31% of deaths are from heart disease, 23% are from cancer, and 7% are from cerebrovascular disease—the three leading causes).

More men than women die by suicide.

The gender ratio is more than 4:1.

More than 72% of all suicides are committed by white men.

Nearly 80% of all firearm suicides are committed by white men.

The highest suicide rates are for persons older than 85 years (rate 65/100,000).

Suicide is the third leading cause of death among young people 15 to 24 years of age (following unintentional injuries and homicide) in this age group.

The total number of deaths in 1997 was 34,489.

The gender ratio was 5:1 (men:women).

RISK FACTORS (FREQUENTLY OCCUR IN COMBINATION)

One or more diagnosable mental or substance abuse disorder(s)

Impulsivity

Adverse life events

Family history of mental or substance abuse disorder

Family history of suicide

Family violence, including emotional, physical, or sexual abuse

Prior suicide attempt

Firearm in the home

Incarceration

Exposure to the suicidal behavior of others (e.g., family members, peers, and/or the media in news or fiction stories)

ATTEMPTED SUICIDES

There are an estimated 8 to 25 attempted suicides to one completion; the ratio is higher in women and youth and lower in men and the elderly.

More women than men report a history of attempted suicide (gender ratio 2:1).

The strongest risk factors for attempted suicide in adults are depression, alcohol abuse, cocaine use, and separation or divorce.

The strongest risk factors for attempted suicide in youth are depression, alcohol or other drug use disorder, and aggressive or disruptive behaviors.

The majority of suicide attempts are expressions of extreme distress that need to be addressed and not just a harmless bid for attention.

PREVENTION

Because suicide is a highly complex behavior, preventative interventions must also be complex and intensive to have lasting effects.

Recognition of mental and substance abuse disorders and appropriate treatment are the most promising ways to prevent suicide in older persons.

Limiting young people's access to firearms and other forms of responsible firearm ownership, especially in conjunction with the prevention of mental and addictive disorders, may be beneficial for prevention of firearm suicides.

School-based, information-only prevention programs focusing on suicide may actually increase distress in the young people who are most vulnerable.

School and community prevention programs designed to address suicide as part of a broader focus on mental health (e.g., incorporating coping skills in response to stress, substance abuse, aggressive behaviors) are most likely to be successful.

Adapted from National Institute of Mental Health (NIMH). (1999). *Suicide facts*. Retrieved 8/20/01 from http://www.nimh.nih.gov/research/suifact.htm.

might be employed. Figures 15-1 through 15-3 contain examples of instruments that are available to elicit information about symptoms of anxiety or depression or conditions such as alcohol abuse. However, whenever using these or other screening tools, the nurse should be prepared in advance to intervene based on assessment data. Very frequently, this involves referral to other health professionals for further assessment, testing, counseling, and treatment.

For example, the nurse who suspects that a student has an eating disorder can talk with his or her parents and teachers, the school counselor and principal, and others to determine the best course of action to follow up on assessment findings and associated concerns. If a client describes signs and symptoms consistent with depression, the nurse should chart the reported information and explain to the client's physician the comments that were voiced. When an em-

COMMUNITY APPLICATION

Examples of Suicide Prevention Programs and General Recommendations for Prevention of Suicide Among Adolescents and Young Adults

Suicide Prevention Programs

School gatekeeper training: School staff are taught to identify and refer students at risk for suicide.

Community gatekeeper training: Community members (e.g., clergy, police, recreation staff) and clinical health care providers who see adolescent clients are trained to identify and refer persons who are at risk for suicide.

General suicide education: Students are taught about suicide, including warning signs and how to seek help for themselves or others.

Screening programs: Questionnaires or other screening instruments are used to identify high-risk adolescents and young adults and provide further assessment and treatment.

Peer support programs: Peer relationships and competency in social skills among high-risk adolescents and young adults are encouraged.

Crisis centers and hotlines: Trained volunteers and paid staff provide telephone counseling and other services for suicidal persons.

Restriction of access to lethal means: Activities and programs that restrict access to handguns, drugs, and other common means of suicide are encouraged.

Intervention after a suicide: Focus on friends and relatives of persons who have committed suicide to help prevent or contain suicide clusters and help adolescents and young adults cope effectively with feelings of loss that follow the sudden death or suicide of a peer.

Suicide Prevention Recommendations

Ensure that suicide prevention programs are linked as closely as possible with professional mental health resources in the community.

Avoid reliance on one prevention strategy: Use of more than one of the types of programs detailed above is recommended.

Expand suicide prevention efforts for young adults.

Incorporate evaluation efforts into suicide prevention programs.

From Centers for Disease Control and Prevention (CDC). (1994). Programs for the prevention of suicide among adolescents and young adults, *MMWR Morbidity and Mortality Weekly Report, 43*(RR-6), 3-8.

ployee is suspected of alcohol abuse, the occupational nurse should follow company policy on how, when, and under what circumstances the employee and his or her supervisor should be informed of the concerns. The employee should be given information on available treatment options and support groups.

TREATMENT OF MENTAL DISORDERS

The goals of treatment for mental illness are to reduce symptoms, improve personal and social functioning, develop and strengthen coping skills, and promote behaviors to improve the individual's life. Basic approaches to the treatment of mental disorders include pharmacotherapy, psychotherapy, and/or behavior therapy (USDHHS/PHS, 1999).

PSYCHOTHERAPEUTIC MEDICATIONS

Psychotherapeutic medications do not cure mental illness; they act by controlling symptoms (NIMH, 1995). As with medications for physical health problems, the appropriateness of psychotherapeutic medications and their prescribed regimen depends on the diagnosis, side effects, and client response. Table 15-3 lists some of the most commonly used psychotherapeutic medications. Indications and adverse effects and nursing implications for the different types of medications are briefly discussed.

Antipsychotic Medications

Antipsychotic medications are used to reduce symptoms of schizophrenia. Most antipsychotic medications are neuroleptics. Neuroleptics are quite effective, but may produce some side effects. The most common are drowsiness, tachy-

During the Past Week	Rarely or None of the Time (Less than 1 Day)	Some or a Little of the Time (1-2 Days)	Occasionally or a Moderate Amount of the Time (3-4 Days)	Most or All of the Time (5-7 Days)
1. I was bothered by things that don't usually bother me.	0	1	2	3
2. I did not feel like eating; my appetite was poor.	0	1	2	3
3. I felt that I could not shake off the blues even with the help of my family or friends.	0	1	2	3
4. I felt that I was just as good as other people.	3	2	1	0
5. I had trouble keeping my mind on what I was doing.	0	1	2	3
6. I felt depressed.	0	1	2	3
7. I felt everything I did was an effort.	0	1	2	3
8. I felt hopeful about the future.	3	2	1	0
9. I thought my life had been a failure.	0	1	2	3
10. I felt fearful.	0	1	2	3
11. My sleep was restless.	0	1	2	3
12. I was happy.	3	2	1	0
13. I talked less than usual.	0	1	2	3
14. I felt lonely.	0	1	2	3
15. People were unfriendly.	0	1	2	3
16. I enjoyed life.	3	2	1	0
17. I had crying spells.	0	1	2	3
18. I felt sad.	0	1	2	3
19. I felt that people disliked me.	0	1	2	3
20. I could not get "going."	0	1	2	3

Figure 15-1. Center for Epidemiologic Studies depression scale. Interpretation: A total score of 22 or higher is indicative of depression when the scale is used in primary care. (From Radloff, L. S. [1977]. The CES-D scale: A self-report depression scale for research in the general population. *Applied Psychologic Measurement, 1,* 385-401. Copyright 1977, West Publishing Company/Applied Psychological Measurement, Inc. Reproduced by permission.)

Rank	Life Event	Mean Value	Rank	Life Event	Mean Value
1	Death of spouse	100	23	Son or daughter leaving home	29
2	Divorce	73	24	Trouble with in-laws	29
3	Marital separation	65	25	Outstanding personal achievement	28
4	Jail term	63			
5	Death of close family member	63	26	Wife begins or stops work	26
6	Personal injury or illness	53	27	Begin or end school	26
7	Marriage	50	28	Change in living conditions	25
8	Fired at work	47	29	Change in personal habits	24
9	Marital reconciliation	45	30	Trouble with boss	23
10	Retirement	45	31	Change in work hours or conditions	20
11	Change in health of family member	44			
12	Pregnancy	40	32	Change in residence	20
13	Sex difficulties	39	33	Change in schools	20
14	Gain of new family member	39	34	Change in recreation	19
15	Business readjustment	39	35	Change in church activities	19
16	Change in financial state	38	36	Change in social activities	18
17	Death of close friend	37	37	Mortgage or loan less than $10,000	17
18	Change to different line of work	36			
19	Change in number of arguments with spouse	35	38	Change in sleeping habits	16
			39	Change in number of family get-togethers	15
20	Mortgage over $10,000	31			
21	Foreclosure on mortgage or loan	30	40	Change in eating habits	15
22	Change in responsibilities at work	29	41	Vacation	13
			42	Christmas	12
			43	Minor violations of the law	11

Life Crisis Categories and LCU Scores*

No life crisis	0-149
Mild life crisis	150-199
Moderate life crisis	200-299
Major life crisis	300 or more

Figure 15-2. Social readjustment rating scale. (Reprinted by permission of the publisher from Holmes, T. H., & Rahe, R. H. [1967]. The social readjustment rating scale. *Journal of Psychosomatic Research, 11,* 213-217. Copyright 1967 by Elsevier Science Inc.)

cardia, orthostatic hypotension, weight gain, photosensitivity, and menstrual irregularities. Often, side effects diminish after a few weeks.

More serious adverse effects of neuroleptics include "extrapyramidal reactions" (movement disorders resulting from the effect of the drug on the extrapyramidal motor system) (Lehne and Scott, 1996). Acute dystonia (characterized by spasms or cramping of the muscles of the tongue, face, neck, or back), parkinsonism (including bradykinesia, masklike face, drooling, tremor, rigidity, shuffling gait), and akathisia (restlessness characterized by constant pacing and squirming) are extrapyramidal reactions sometimes seen early in treatment with antipsychotic drugs (Lehne and Scott, 1996; Pennebaker and Riley, 1995). These adverse effects tend to decrease with time or can be managed with other medications (e.g., antiparkinsonian agents).

The most serious extrapyramidal adverse effect of use of antipsychotic agents, however, is tardive dyskinesia. Tardive dyskinesia develops in 20% to 40% of clients during long-term therapy and produces involuntary movement of the tongue and face. Eating difficulty and weight loss may result. Tardive dyskinesia is permanent, although some symptoms decline after the dosage is reduced or the drug is withdrawn (Lehne and Scott, 1996).

> "Have you ever felt you ought to **C**ut down on drinking?"
> "Have people **A**nnoyed you by criticizing your drinking?"
> "Have you ever felt bad or **G**uilty about your drinking?"
> "Have you ever had a drink first thing in the morning to steady your nerves or get rid of a hangover (**E**ye-opener)?"
> One "yes" response should raise suspicions of alcohol abuse. More than one "yes" response should be considered a strong indication that alcohol abuse exists.

Figure 15-3. The CAGE questionnaire. (From Ewing, J. A. [1984]. Detecting alcoholism: The CAGE questionnaire. *Journal of the American Medical Association, 252* (14), 1905-1907. Copyright 1984, American Medical Association.)

Clozapine (Clozaril) and risperidone (Risperdal) are termed *atypical neuroleptics.* These are relatively new medications that have been shown to be more effective than traditional antipsychotic medications for some people with schizophrenia. These medications have less risk of extrapyramidal side effects, including tardive dyskinesia, than other antipsychotics. Other complications or adverse effects are possible, however. Clozapine, the most commonly used atypical neuroleptic, is known to cause agranulocytosis in 1% to 2% of clients. Because this condition is potentially fatal, persons on Clozapine must have weekly white blood cell counts performed to assess for signs of agranulocytosis. Treatment is stopped if the white blood cell count is below 3000 or the granulocyte count is under 1500. Risperidone, the newest atypical neuroleptic, was introduced in 1994 and has fewer side effects and no reported cases of agranulocytosis (Lehne and Scott, 1996).

Antimanic Medications

Lithium is the most frequently used medication for treatment of bipolar disorders. Response to treatment with lithium varies somewhat between individual clients. In addition, the range between an effective dose and a toxic dose is small, so serum lithium levels must be monitored closely. It is recommended that levels be checked routinely at the beginning of treatment and every few months thereafter to determine the optimal maintenance dosage (NIMH, 1995).

Side effects are often worse during the initial stage of lithium therapy and include drowsiness, weakness, nausea, vomiting, fatigue, hand tremors, increased thirst, and weight gain. Long-term lithium use may affect thyroid function; therefore thyroid function tests should also be performed periodically.

Anticonvulsants

Occasionally, anticonvulsants, such as Valproate and Carbamazepine, are used to treat mania. The most common side effects of anticonvulsants include drowsiness, dizziness, confusion, visual disturbances, memory impairment, and nausea. Periodic blood tests are needed to monitor white blood cell counts and for anemia (NIMH 2001c).

Antidepressants

Antidepressants are used most often for serious depression, but they can also be helpful for mild depression and anxiety. The choice of medications is usually based on the individual client's symptoms. Most medications take 1 to 3 weeks before improvement is seen. If little or no change occurs in symptoms after 5 to 6 weeks, a different medication should be tried. Treatment is usually continued for a minimum of several months and may last up to a year or more.

Tricyclic antidepressants are commonly used for treatment of major depression. Side effects vary somewhat between medications and the reaction of the individual to the medication. Potential side effects include drowsiness, blurred vision, dry mouth, constipation, weight gain, orthostatic hypotension, dysuria, fatigue, and weakness. Often, side effects diminish or disappear during the course of treatment. Tricyclics may interfere with other medications and substances, including thyroid hormone, antihy-

TABLE **15-3** Psychotherapeutic Medications

GENERIC NAME	TRADE NAME	GENERIC NAME	TRADE NAME
Antipsychotic Medications		**Antidepressant Medications—cont'd**	
Chlorpromazine	Thorazine	Imipramine	Tofranil
Chlorprothixene	Taractan	Isocarboxazid (MAOI)	Marplan
Clozapine	Clozaril		(discontinued
Fluphenazine	Permitil		in 1994)
—	Prolixin	Maprotiline	Ludiomil
Haloperidol	Haldol	Nefazodone	Serzone
Loxapine	Daxolin	Nortriptyline	Aventyl
Mesoridazine	Serentil	—	Pamelor
Molindone	Lidone	Parozetine (SSRI)	Paxil
Perphenazine	Trilafon	Phenelzine (MAOI)	Nardil
Pimozide (for Tourette's	Orap	Protriptyline	Vivactil
syndrome)		Sertraline (SSRI)	Zoloft
Risperidone	Risperdal	Tranylcypromine (MAOI)	Parnate
Thioridazine	Mellaril	Trazodone	Desyrel
Thiothixene	Navane	Trimipramine	Surmontil
Trifluoperazine	Stelazine	Venlafaxine	Effexor
Trifluopromazine	Vesprin	**Antianxiety Medications (All of These Medications,**	
Antimanic Medications		**Except Buspirone, are Benzodiazepines)**	
Carbamazepine	Tegretol	Alprazolam	Xanax
Divalproex sodium	Depakote	Buspirone	BuSpar
Lithium carbonate	Eskalith	Chlordiazepoxide	Librax
—	Lithane	—	Libritabs
Lithium citrate	Cibalith-S	—	Librium
Antidepressant Medications		Clorazepate	Azene
		Diazepam	Valium
Amitriptyline	Elavil	Halazepam	Paxipam
Amoxapine	Asendin	Lorazepam	Ativan
Bupropion	Wellbutrin	Oxazepam	Serax
Desipramine	Norpramin	Prazepam	Centrax
—	Pertofrane	**Stimulants (Given for Attention**	
Doxepin	Adapin	**Deficit/Hyperactivity Disorder)**	
—	Sinequan		
Clomipramine	Anafranil	Destroamphetamine	Dexedrine
Fluvoxamine (SSRI)	Luvox	Methylphenidate	Ritalin
Fluoxetine (SSRI)	Prozac	Pemoline	Cylert

From National Institute of Health (NIH). (1995). *Medications*. (NIH Publication No. 95-3929). Rockville, MD: National Institute of Mental Health.

pertensives, oral contraceptives, sleeping medications, antipsychotic medications, diuretics, antihistamines, aspirin, vitamin C, alcohol, and tobacco.

An overdose of tricyclic antidepressant medications may produce tachycardia, dilated pupils, and flushed face. In extreme cases, overdose may cause agitation, which may progress to confusion, loss of consciousness, seizures, arrhythmias, cardiorespiratory collapse, and death (NIMH, 1995).

Monoamine oxidase inhibitors (MAOIs) are more often used for atypical depression in which symptoms like anxiety, panic attacks, and phobias are present. The MAOIs may cause a serious reaction with certain foods (e.g., aged cheeses, foods containing monosodium glutamate), beverages (e.g., red wines), and medications (e.g., antihistamines, decongestants, local anesthetics, amphetamines, insulin, some narcotics, and antiparkinsonian medications). Reactions may produce hypertension, headache, nausea, vomiting, tachycardia, confusion, psychotic symptoms, seizures, stroke, and coma (NIMH, 1995). Persons taking MAOIs should be given a list of restricted foods, beverages, and medications and encouraged to strictly comply with the restrictions.

Selective serotonin reuptake inhibitors (SSRIs) are the newest class of antidepressants available in the United States and have a more rapid onset of action than do other antidepressants. Improvement is usually seen in 1 to 3 weeks after initiation of therapy (Pennebaker and Riley, 1995). Gastrointestinal problems, headache, insomnia, anxiety, and agitation are the most common side effects of SSRIs. Ejaculatory delay in men and skin rashes, which may be severe, have also been noted (Lehne and Scott, 1996). In addition, SSRIs may decrease appetite.

Serious complications have resulted when SSRIs are used in conjunction with other medications. In particular, fluoxetine (Prozac) should not be combined with MAOIs and should only be used with caution with tricyclic antidepressants (Lehne and Scott, 1996). Finally, although apparently rare, suicidal thoughts and overtly violent behaviors have been traced to Prozac.

Antianxiety Medications

Benzodiazepines are medications used to treat most anxiety disorders. They have been shown to be safe and effective and have low addictive potential. The most commonly used benzodiazepines are alprazolam (Xanax), diazepam (Valium), clonazepam (Klonopin), and lorazepam (Ativan). Antianxiety medications usually act rapidly. Dosage varies greatly, depending on the symptoms and the individual's body chemistry. Common side effects include drowsiness, loss of coordination, fatigue, and mental slowing or confusion. Combination of benzodiazepines and alcohol can produce serious interactions and potentially life-threatening complications and clients should be warned accordingly.

Stimulants

Stimulants are primarily used to treat symptoms of ADHD and narcolepsy. The most common side effects are decreased appetite and difficulty in falling asleep. Some children report gastrointestinal problems, headache, and depression. Growth retardation has been documented in some children and careful, ongoing assessment of growth patterns is recommended while children are taking stimulants.

PSYCHOTHERAPY

"Psychotherapies rely primarily on structured conversation aimed at changing a patient's attitudes, feelings, beliefs, defenses, personality, and behavior. The therapist's procedures vary across schools of psychotherapy and with the nature of the patient's problem" (Sharfstein et al., 1999, p. 249). **Psychotherapy** is often used in conjunction with medication to treat many mental disorders. Various types of psychotherapy include the following (NIMH, 1994b):

- *Individual or interpersonal therapy* focuses on the client's current life and relationships within the family, social, and work environments.
- *Family therapy* involves discussions and problem-solving sessions with every member of a family—sometimes with the entire group, sometimes with individuals.
- *Couple therapy* is used to develop the relationship and minimize problems through understanding how individual conflicts are expressed in the couple's interactions.
- *Group therapy* involves a small group of people with similar problems who, with the guidance of a therapist, discuss individual issues and help each other with problems.
- *Play therapy* is a technique used for establishing communication and resolving problems with young children.

- *Cognitive therapy* works to identify and correct distorted thought patterns that can lead to troublesome feelings and behaviors; is often combined with behavioral therapy.

Short-term psychotherapy is often used when situational stresses (e.g., death in the family, divorce, physical illness) produce problems. In these cases, therapy may only last a few weeks or months, with the goal of helping the individual resolve the problem as quickly as possible. Long-term therapy may last for several months to several years and emphasize underlying problems that started in childhood (NIMH, 1994b).

BEHAVIORAL THERAPY

Behavioral therapy uses learning principles to change thought patterns and behaviors systematically. Behavior therapy is used to encourage the individual to learn specific skills to obtain rewards and satisfaction. Stress management, biofeedback, and relaxation training are examples of behavior therapy (NIMH, 1994b).

SUMMARY

As discussed throughout this chapter, mental disorders are very common and are most often identified and treated in community settings. Therefore all nurses who work in the community should be knowledgeable about risk factors and signs and symptoms that might indicate a mental disorder and be prepared to intervene. In the opening case study, Kay, who works in a clinic for indigent persons, understood the types of mental health problems commonly observed in community settings. As a result, she was prepared to effectively address the needs of her clients.

This chapter describes some of the more common mental disorders, including assessment of risk factors and symptoms, overview of diagnostic criteria, and basic treatment regimens. For more information on any of the topics covered, nurses should consult the Resources box at the end of the chapter. Brochures and teaching materials are available free of charge from many organizations listed and a supply of appropriate materials can be made available for all who come in contact with the health care provider. For example, a school nurse can display brochures on eating disorders, depression in teenagers, and prevention of alcohol and drug abuse in adolescents in or near the school clinic. Likewise, a variety of educational materials describing threats to mental health and mental disorders should be easily accessible in work site settings and primary care clinics. These measures can help demystify mental illness and assist those who need treatment to seek care. In addition to these resources, the nurse in community-based practice is strongly encouraged to develop a list of area individuals, groups, agencies, and organizations that provide services for persons with mental disorders and their families.

KEY POINTS

- Mental health refers to the absence of mental disorders and the ability of an individual to negotiate the daily challenges and social interactions of life without experiencing cognitive, emotional, or behavioral dysfunction.
- Approximately 75% of client care for mental disorders occurs in community-based settings. Providers include physicians, psychologists, counselors, clergy, and laypersons. Settings for care include outpatient departments, mental health centers and clinics, alcohol and drug units, emergency departments, family or social service agencies, crisis centers, and volunteer services (self-help programs).
- Depression affects almost 19 million people in the United States each year. Nurses in community-based practice should be aware of risk factors and symptoms of depression and routinely assess those in high-risk groups. Treatment for depression includes pharmacological therapy, electroconvulsive therapy, behavior therapy, and/or psychotherapy.
- Anxiety disorders are the most common mental disorder, affecting up to 13% of the general population. The most common anxiety disorders are GAD (chronic, unrealistic, and exaggerated worry), panic disorder (sometimes

accompanied by agoraphobia), phobias, OCD, and PTSD. Anxiety disorders are treated with antidepressants, antianxiety medications, behavior therapy, and psychotherapy.

- Eating disorders are becoming increasingly prevalent in the United States. Bulimia is characterized by binge eating and purging (self-induced vomiting, use of laxatives, diuretics, fasting, and excessive exercise). Individuals with anorexia nervosa are obsessed with a fear of fat and with losing weight. Anorexia and bulimia usually develop during adolescence. Nurses who work with adolescents and young adults should be aware of the signs and symptoms of eating disorders and screen those considered to be at risk. Treatment includes counseling, psychotherapy, and behavior modification.

- Attention deficit hyperactivity disorder affects 3% to 5% of all children and is characterized by inattention, hyperactivity, and impulsivity. A diagnosis of ADD or ADHD should be made following a comprehensive physical, psychological, social, and behavioral evaluation to rule out other possible reasons for the behavior. It is usually managed through a combination of behavior therapy, emotional counseling, practical support, and medication.

- A number of legal and illegal substances used by Americans are potentially harmful. Alcoholism is the greatest drug problem in the United States today. Illicit drugs used include opioids (e.g., heroin, morphine), cocaine, amphetamines, hallucinogens, marijuana, and inhalants. Nurses in community-based settings should be aware of risk factors of substance abuse, signs of intoxication and withdrawal, and treatment of the most common psychoactive substances and refer accordingly.

- Suicide is the most serious potential outcome of mental disorders and is the eighth leading cause of death in the United States. Risk factors for suicide include a family history of psychiatric disorders, previous suicide attempts, serious medical illness, family violence, alcohol and other drug abuse, and accessibility to firearms.

- Treatment of mental disorders includes use of psychotherapeutic medications (e.g., antipsychotics, antimanics, anticonvulsant medications, antidepressants, antianxiety medications, stimulants), psychotherapy, and behavior therapy.

Resources

Mental Health and Mental Disorders

Mental Health/Mental Illness

American Academy of Child and Adolescent Psychiatry
American Psychiatric Association
American Psychological Association
American Psychiatric Nurses Association
Center for Mental Health Services
National Alliance for the Mentally Ill
National Institute of Mental Health
National Mental Health Association
Substance Abuse and Mental Health Services Administration (SAMHSA)

Depression

Depression and Related Affective Disorders Association
National Depressive and Manic Depressive Association
National Foundation for Depressive Illness, Inc. (NAFDI)

Suicide

Suicide Crisis Center
National Adolescent Suicide Hotline
  800-621-4000; 800-SUICIDE

Anxiety Disorders

Anxiety Disorders Association of America
National Anxiety Foundation
Panic Disorder Information Line
  800-64-PANIC (800-647-2642)

Attention Deficit/Hyperactivity Disorder

Attention Deficit Information Network (AD-IN)
Children and Adults with Attention Deficit Disorders (CHADD)
Federation of Families for Children's Mental Health
National Center for Learning Disabilities

Eating Disorders

National Eating Disorders Association
Harvard Eating Disorders Center
National Association of Anorexia Nervosa and
Associated Disorders

Alcohol and Drug Abuse

Al-Anon/Alateen
Alcoholics Anonymous World Services
Center for Substance Abuse Treatment (CSAT)
Center for Substance Abuse Prevention (CSA)
Narcotics Anonymous World Services
National Institute on Alcohol Abuse and
Alcoholism
National Institute on Drug Abuse
Substance Abuse and Mental Health Services
Administration
National Drug and Alcohol Treatment Hotline
800-662-HELP
Cocaine Hotline
800-COCAINE (800-262-2463)

Visit the book's website at
www.wbsaunders.com/SIMON/McEwen
for a direct link to the website for each
organization listed.

Learning Activities & Application to Practice

In Class

1. In groups of four to six, discuss one of the commonly encountered mental health problems described in this chapter (e.g., depression, anxiety disorders, eating disorders, substance abuse). Share if you have encountered the problem in practice and if so describe how the problem was identified and treated. In the group, devise primary, secondary, and tertiary prevention strategies to address the mental health problem and share ideas with the class.

2. Discuss the *Healthy People 2010* objectives related to "Alcohol and Other Drugs" and "Mental Health and Mental Disorders." Examine differences related to age, race/ethnic group, and gender (e.g., suicide is most common among white males; alcohol-related motor vehicle deaths for American Indians are 400% higher than for the population as a whole). Identify factors that contribute to differences and outline strategies to address these factors.

In Clinical

3. Identify, investigate, and visit area organizations and providers that care for persons with mental disorders or work to improve mental health. During the visit learn what services are available, how services are accessed, what interventions are provided, and what the responsibilities of nurses are. Share findings with the clinical group.

4. Identify the most common mental disorder encountered in the community-based setting in which you are assigned (e.g., if you are in elementary school—ADD; if in a high school—eating disorders or substance abuse; if working with women or elders—depression). Compile or develop materials that could be used for health education in that setting. Develop a forum to share the materials with other health professionals at the setting or with members of the group or community (e.g., a seminar for parents of children diagnosed with ADD/ADHD).

REFERENCES

American Psychiatric Association. (2000). *Diagnostic and statistical manual of mental disorders* (4th ed., Text Revision). Washington, DC: American Psychiatric Association.

Antai-Otong, D. (1995). Foundations of psychiatric nursing practice. In D. Antai-Otong (Ed.), *Psychiatric nursing: Biological and behavioral concepts* (pp. 65-78). Philadelphia: W. B. Saunders.

Centers for Disease Control and Prevention (CDC). (1994). Programs for the prevention of suicide among adolescents and young adults, *MMWR Morbidity and Mortality Weekly Report, 43*(RR-6), 3-8.

Decker, W. A., & Freeman, M. (1996). The journey challenged by eating disorders. In V. B. Carson & E. N. Arnold (Eds.), *Mental health nursing: The nurse-patient journey* (pp. 909-926). Philadelphia: W. B. Saunders.

Ewing, J. A. (1984). Detecting alcoholism: The CAGE questionnaire. *Journal of the American Medical Association, 252*(14), 1905-1907.

Frank, E., Karp, J. F., & Rush, A. J. (1993). Efficacy of treatments for major depression. *Psychopharmacology Bulletin, 29*(4), 457-475.

Greensberg, P. E., Stiglin, L. E., Finkelstein, S. N., & Berndt, E. R. (1993). The economic burden of depression in 1990. *Journal of Clinical Psychiatry, 54*(11), 405-418.

Holmes, T. H., & Rahe, R. H. (1967). The social readjustment rating scale. *Journal of Psychosomatic Research,* 11, 213-217.

Katon, W. (1994). *Panic disorder in the medical setting* (NIH Publication No. 94-3482). Washington, DC: National Institutes of Mental Health.

Lehne, R. A., & Scott, D. (1996). Psychopharmacology. In V. B. Carson & E. N. Arnold (Eds.), *Mental health nursing: The nurse-patient journey* (pp. 523-570.) Philadelphia: W. B. Saunders.

National Institute of Mental Health (NIMH). (1994a). *Attention deficit hyperactivity disorder.* (NIH Publication No. 94-3572). Rockville, MD: National Institute of Mental Health.

National Institute of Mental Health (NIMH). (1994b). *Helpful facts about depressive illnesses.* (NIH Publication No. 94-3875). Rockville, MD: National Institute of Mental Health.

National Institute of Mental Health (NIMH). (1995). *Medications.* (NIH Publication No. 95-3929). Rockville, MD: National Institute of Mental Health.

National Institute of Mental Health (NIMH). (1999). *Suicide facts.* Rockville, MD: National Institute of Mental Health.

National Institute of Mental Health (NIMH). (2000a). *Attention deficit hyperactivity disorder—questions and answers.* Retrieved 8/20/01 from http://www.nimh.nih.gov/publicat/adhdqa.cfm.

National Institute of Mental Health (NIMH). (2000b). *Depression.* (NIH Publication No. 00-3561). Rockville, MD: National Institute of Mental Health.

National Institute of Mental Health (NIMH). (2000c). *Treatment of children with mental disorders.* (NIH Publication No. 00-4702). Rockville, MD: National Institute of Mental Health.

National Institute of Mental Health (NIMH). (2001a). *Eating disorders.* (NIH Publication No. 01-4901). Rockville, MD: National Institute of Mental Health.

National Institute of Mental Health (NIMH). (2001b). *Mental disorders in America.* Retrieved 8/20/01 from http://www.nimh.nih.gov/publicat/numbers.cfm.

National Institute of Mental Health (NIMH). (2001c). *Bipolar disorders.* (NIH Publication No. 01-3679). Rockville, MD: National Institute of Mental Health.

National Mental Health Association. (1996). *Mental health and you.* Alexandria, VA: National Mental Health Association.

Pennebaker, D. F., & Riley, J. (1995). Psychopharmacological therapy. In D. Antai-Otong (Ed.), *Psychiatric nursing: Biological and behavioral concepts* (pp. 543-576). Philadelphia: W. B. Saunders.

Plumlee, A. A. (1995). The client with addictive behaviors. In D. Antai-Otong (Ed.), *Psychiatric nursing: Biological and behavioral concepts* (pp. 357-386). Philadelphia: W. B. Saunders.

Radloff, L. S. (1977). The CES-D scale: A self-report depression scale for research in the general population. *Applied Psychological Measurement,* 1, 385-401.

Richardson, M., & Shiu-Thornton, S. (1999). Mental health services. In S. J. Williams & P. R. Torrens (Eds.), *Introduction to health services* (5th ed., pp. 349-380). Albany, NY: Delmar Publishers.

Robert Wood Johnson Foundation. (1993). *Substance abuse: The nation's number one health problem.* Waltham, MA: Institute for Health Policy, Brandeis University.

Robinson, L. (1996). The journey threatened by stress and anxiety disorders. In V. B. Carson & E. N. Arnold (Eds.), *Mental health nursing: The nurse-patient journey* (pp. 691-724). Philadelphia: W. B. Saunders.

Sharfstein, S. S., Stoline, A. M., & Koran, L. (1999). Mental health services. In A. R. Kovner & S. Jonas (Eds.), *Jonas & Kovner's health care delivery in the United States* (6th ed., pp. 243-278). New York: Springer Publishing Co.

Tommasini, N. R. (1995). The client with a mood disorder (depression). In D. Antai-Otong (Ed.), *Psychiatric nursing: Biological and behavioral concepts* (pp. 157-190). Philadelphia: W. B. Saunders.

U.S. Department of Health and Human Services (USDHHS). (1995). *Healthy people 2000: Midcourse review and 1995 revisions.* Washington, DC: Government Printing Office.

U.S. Department of Health and Human Services (USDHHS). (2000). *Healthy people 2010: Conference edition.* Washington, DC: USDHHS.

U.S. Department of Health and Human Services/Office of Disease Prevention and Health Promotion (USDHHS/ODPHP). (1998). *Clinician's handbook of preventive services* (2nd ed.). Washington, DC: Government Printing Office.

U.S. Department of Health and Human Services/Public Health Service (USDHHS/PHS). (1999). *Mental health: A report of the surgeon general.* Rockville, MD: USDHHS.

U.S. Department of Health and Human Services/ Substance Abuse and Mental Health Services Administration (USDHHS/SAMHSA). (1999). *Findings from the 1999 national household survey on drug abuse.* Washington, DC: USDHHS.

Communicable Disease: Prevention and Intervention

objectives

Upon completion of this chapter, the reader will be able to:

1. Discuss the changes in incidence and prevalence of communicable disease patterns in the United States over the past century and describe the impact of immunization on those patterns.

2. Describe the various ways that communicable disease may be transmitted.

3. Explain the process of reporting communicable diseases.

4. Describe the process of immunization and explain the pediatric immunization schedule including contraindications, precautions, and reporting of adverse events.

5. Discuss the incidence and prevalence of sexually transmitted diseases and present prevention strategies.

6. Identify potential emerging infectious diseases and discuss their prevention.

7. Discuss health issues related to international travel, focusing on prevention of communicable diseases.

key terms

Active immunity	Indirect transmission	Vaccine Adverse Event Reporting System (VAERS)
Direct transmission	Passive immunity	
Emerging infectious diseases	Reportable diseases	Vaccine-preventable disease
Immunity	Sexually transmitted diseases (STDs)	*See Glossary for definitions.*
Immunization schedule		

case study

Mark Mitchell works as a nurse for the public health department in a midsized city. Mark's primary responsibility is investigation and follow-up of suspected cases of reportable diseases. One recent Monday, Mark received a call from a local pediatrician who reported a possible case of measles in a 3-year-old boy named Grant. To gather information about the case, Mark reviewed the child's presenting symptoms with the physician. The symptoms were a fever of over 101°F for 2 days, a mild cough, runny nose, conjunctivitis, and a red rash, which his mother reported began on his face and had progressed to his trunk. Upon prompting from Mark, the pediatrician looked inside the child's mouth and discovered small red spots with bluish-white centers on the buccal mucosa (Koplik's spots). Additionally, the pediatrician stated that according to her records, Grant's immunization status was incomplete because he had received only his initial diphtheria/pertussis/tetanus (DPT), Haemophilis influenzae b (HIB), and polio vaccinations at her office. The mother denied that the child had received shots at any other clinic. The pediatrician concluded that although Grant was quite ill, he did not need to be hospitalized, but would be treated with cough medication, antipyretics, and decongestants as an outpatient.

Mark was aware that during the past 6 weeks, 10 cases of measles had been confirmed in the county and about 20 others were suspect. Because of the presence of the disease in the area, Mark determined that with Grant's symptoms, and his incomplete immunization status, it was probable that Grant was ill with measles. Mark instructed the pediatrician to obtain a sample of blood to send to the state laboratory for confirmation of the diagnosis. According to department protocols, Mark obtained the boy's name and address and made a visit to the boy's home later that day.

Grant was the youngest of three (Joseph, 6, and Brittany, 9). While in the home, Mark questioned Grant's parents regarding the immunization status of their other two children and reviewed their immunization records. Both children's records were complete and included two injections of measles/mumps/rubella (MMR) vaccine, as required by the state for all children in school. Both of Grant's parents were born before 1957 and reported they had been ill with measles as children.

Next, Mark gathered as much information as the parents could provide pertaining to other children that Grant had been around the previous 2 weeks. He discovered that Grant had spent a few hours at a baby sitter's house on two separate days and in the church's nursery for about 3 hours the previous Sunday. Mark called the nursery director at their church. She stated there had been about 10 children in Grant's class on Sunday and she knew of none that were sick. She agreed to call all of the parents and explain that their children had possibly been exposed to measles. Further, she would instruct them to call their pediatricians to check their children's immunization status.

The baby sitter was then called. She reported that one of the children she keeps on a sporadic basis had been very ill with a fever about 10 days previously, but she did not know what was wrong with her. Mark obtained that child's name and her parent's telephone number and address and continued the process of communicable disease surveillance.

Caring for individuals with communicable diseases was one of the earliest functions of nurses. Later, prevention of the spread of communicable diseases through advocating cleanliness and use of immunizations and medications became an integral part of nursing practice. Indeed, the first intervention learned by virtually every nursing student relates to the spread of communicable diseases: "Wash your hands!" The importance of frequent and thorough handwashing is repeatedly stressed and cannot be overstated for prevention of the spread of communicable diseases.

Around 1900, communicable diseases accounted for 4 of the top 10 causes of death for Americans. At that time, pneumonia and influenza were designated collectively as the leading cause of death, followed closely by tuberculosis (TB). Diarrhea and enteritis were collectively the third major cause of death and diphtheria was tenth. A similar list for 2000 contains only one notation of communicable diseases. Pneumonia and influenza was the sixth leading cause of death that year, accounting for about 3.9% of all deaths (National Center for Health Statistics [NCHS], 2000). Acquired immunodeficiency syndrome and human immunodeficiency virus (AIDS and HIV) infection is also one of the leading causes of death in certain age groups. With these exceptions, communicable disease as a cause of mortality has largely been managed. In terms of morbidity, however, although there has been much improvement, many Americans are sickened each year by a variety of communicable diseases ranging from mild (colds or stomach flu) to serious and life threatening (influenza or TB). In addition, the possibility of emerging infectious diseases is a continuing threat.

This chapter presents an overview of contemporary health problems and issues that relate to communicable disease prevention, transmission, and management. *Healthy People 2010* (U.S. Department of Health and Human Services [USDHHS], 2000) lists three priority areas that specifically target the prevention and management of communicable diseases. These are HIV

Infection (Area 13), Immunization and Infectious Diseases (Area 14), and Sexually Transmitted Diseases (STDs) (Area 25). Examples of goals from these priority areas are shown in the *Healthy People 2010* box.

COMMUNICABLE DISEASE TRANSMISSION

Communicable diseases may be transmitted either directly, through physical contact between infected individuals, or indirectly, through a source other than another human. **Direct transmission** can be through physical contact including biting, kissing, and touching (e.g., for influenza, colds, strep throat) or sexual contact (e.g., for HIV, STDs, hepatitis B [HBV]). **Indirect transmissions** can be vehicleborne through *fomites* (objects that absorb and transmit infectious material such as toys, telephones, money) or substances (food, water,

healthy people **2010**

Objectives Related to Epidemiology

OBJECTIVE		BASELINE (1998)	TARGET
13.1:	Reduce AIDS among adolescents and adults	19.5 per 100,000	1 per 100,000
13.2:	Reduce the number of new AIDS cases among adolescent and adult men who have sex with men	17,847	13,385
13.6:	Increase the proportion of sexually active persons who use condoms	23%	50%
14.1d:	Reduce or eliminate indigenous cases of HBV in people aged 2 to 18	945	9
14.1g:	Reduce or eliminate indigenous cases of pertussis in children under age 7	3417	2000
14.9:	Reduce new cases of hepatitis C	2.4 per 100,000	1 per 100,000
14.22d:	Achieve and maintain effective vaccination coverage levels for two doses of MMR vaccine	92%	90%
14.29a:	Increase the proportion of adults who are vaccinated annually against influenza	63%	90%
25.1b:	Reduce the proportion of females aged 15 to 24 attending STD clinics with *Chlamydia trachomatis* infections	12.2%	3.0%
25.2:	Reduce new cases of gonorrhea	123 per 100,000	19 per 100,000
25.6:	Reduce the proportion of females who have ever required treatment for PID	8%	5%

From U.S. Department of Health and Human Services (USDHHS). (2000) *Healthy people 2010: Conference edition.* Washington, DC: Public Health Service.
AIDS, Acquired immunodeficiency syndrome; *MMR,* measles, mumps, rubella; *PID,* pelvic inflammatory disease; *STD,* sexually transmitted disease.

TABLE **16-1** Types of Transmission

DIRECT TRANSMISSION	INDIRECT TRANSMISSION
PHYSICAL CONTACT	**VEHICLEBORNE**
Biting	Fomites (toys)
Touching	Substances (food, blood)
Spitting	
	VECTORBORNE
SEXUAL CONTACT	Mechanical
Fecal-oral	Biological
Anal intercourse	
Oral-genital	**AIRBORNE**
	Dust and droplets
AIRBORNE	Droplet nuclei
Dust and droplets	
Droplet nuclei	

From Dash, D. (1993). Communicable disease. In J. Swanson & S. Albrecht (Eds.), *Community health nursing: Promoting the health of aggregates*. Philadelphia: W. B. Saunders. Data from Mausner, J. S., & Kramer, S. (1985). *Epidemiology: An introductory text*. Philadelphia: W. B. Saunders.

blood). Communicable disease may also be transmitted indirectly through *vectors* such as animals (e.g., rabies, anthrax, toxoplasmosis) or arthropods (e.g., malaria, Lyme disease, Rocky Mountain spotted fever). Airborne transmission through dust and droplet and droplet nuclei may be either direct (spray from body fluids such as sneezing or coughing—in colds, influenza) or indirect (contaminated dusts or droplet nuclei—in legionellosis, TB) (Table 16-1). Figure 16-1 illustrates communicable disease transmission.

Efforts to prevent spread of communicable diseases must incorporate primary prevention strategies designed to stop transmission. Encouraging frequent handwashing, use of tissues to cover the mouth and nose when coughing or sneezing, mosquito control, rabies inoculation for all pets, and promoting sexual abstinence or appropriate use of condoms are examples of primary prevention interventions that attempt to stop the spread of communicable diseases.

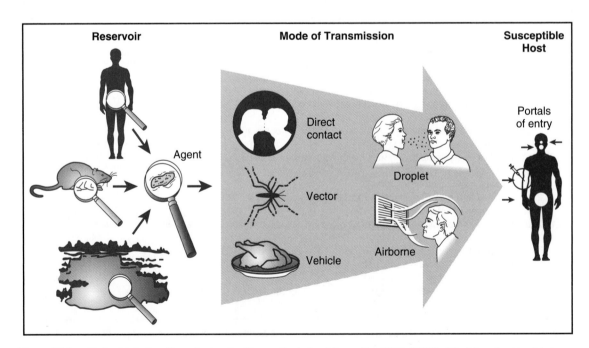

Figure 16-1. Chain of infection. (From Centers for Disease Control and Prevention (CDC). [1992]. *Principles of epidemiology* [2nd ed.]. Atlanta, GA: Centers for Disease Control and Prevention.)

REPORTABLE COMMUNICABLE DISEASES

Each state has an established reporting system to monitor communicable diseases. Typically, state laws or regulations empower the state board or department of health to establish and modify reporting requirements. The individual states are then required to report selected data to the Centers for Disease Control and Prevention (CDC). The CDC monitors communicable disease and provides aggregate reports and interpretation of trends. In response to findings, it issues recommendations through weekly updates and periodic publications.

According to the CDC (1992), state regulations usually specify:

- The disease and conditions that must be reported
- Who is responsible for reporting
- What information is required on each case of disease reported
- How, to whom, and how quickly the information is to be reported
- Control measures to be taken for specified diseases

REPORTABLE DISEASES

Reportable diseases and those that require notification of authorities vary slightly from state to state. Box 16-1 provides a list of diseases and conditions that are required to be reported nationally and other diseases about which authorities must be notified according to individual state regulations.

WHO IS RESPONSIBLE FOR REPORTING

Although there may be differences based on state regulations, most states require reporting of known or suspected cases of reportable diseases by physicians, dentists, nurses, and other health professionals (medical examiners, laboratory directors, chiropractors, veterinarians) and administrators of hospitals, clinics, nursing homes, schools, and nurseries (CDC, 1992). Typically, organizations (e.g., clinics, doctor's offices, hospi-

tals) designate one individual who is responsible for this activity and who has been trained in the process.

WHAT INFORMATION IS REQUIRED

Data to be collected vary based on the disease. Usually, case reports include the name, age, sex, race or ethnicity, date of birth, address, and telephone number of the patient. Case reports then describe the disease, including its date of onset, the attending physician, and the method of diagnosis. Some diseases (e.g., chicken pox or influenza during an outbreak) may only be reported by number of cases.

HOW, WHEN, AND TO WHOM TO REPORT

Individual state regulations dictate the process for reporting. Some diseases, such as those that are rare, potentially very infectious, or involved in unusual outbreaks, are to be reported immediately by telephone. These typically include plague, rabies, measles, and poliomyelitis. Others are usually reported on a weekly basis either by telephone or by written report. Examples of illness reported weekly include AIDS and other STDs, TB, Lyme disease, and mumps.

Most frequently, the health professional identifying a reportable disease reports to the local health department. The local health department in turn reports to the state health department, which then reports to the CDC.

STEPS TAKEN TO CONTROL SPREAD

States may have specific instructions to follow when certain diseases are identified. These instructions can include sending out surveillance teams to investigate and confirm reported cases; instruction on collecting of specimens; and specified control techniques such as environmental sanitation, immunization, quarantine, and education on prevention of transmission (CDC, 1992). Nurses working in public health departments, hospital infection control departments, ambulatory settings, schools, and industry should be aware of the most frequently

BOX 16-1 National Notifiable Diseases, United States, 1999

AIDS	Lyme disease
Anthrax	Malaria
Botulism	Measles
Brucellosis	Meningococcal disease
Chancroid	Mumps
Chlamydia trachomatis (genital infections)	Pertussis
Cholera	Plague
Coccidioidomycosis (regional)	Poliomyelitis (paralytic)
Cryptosporidiosis	Psittacosis
Cyclosporiasis	Rabies (animal)
Diphtheria	Rabies (human)
Ehrlichiosis	Rocky Mountain spotted fever
Encephalitis (California serogroup)	Rubella
Encephalitis (human monocytic)	Rubella (congenital syndrome)
Encephalitis (Eastern equine)	Salmonellosis
Encephalitis (Western equine)	Shigellosis
Encephalitis (St. Louis)	Streptococcal disease (invasive group A)
Escherichia coli (0157:H7)	Streptococcus pneumoniae (drug-resistant invasive disease)
Gonorrhea	
Haemophilus influenzae (invasive disease)	Streptococcal TSS
Hansen's disease	Syphilis
Hantavirus pulmonary syndrome	Syphilis (congenital)
Hemolytic uremic syndrome, postdiarrheal	Tetanus
Hepatitis A	Toxic shock syndrome
Hepatitis B	Trichinosis
Hepatitis C (non-A/non-B)	Tuberculosis
HIV infection (adult)	Typhoid fever
HIV infection (pediatric)	Varicella deaths
Legionellosis	Yellow fever

Data from Centers for Disease Control and Prevention (CDC). (2001c). Summary of notifiable diseases, United States—1999. *MMWR Morbidity and Mortality Weekly Report, 48*(53), 1-104.

encountered communicable diseases in their settings and learn the appropriate measures to take when a reportable disease is suspected or confirmed.

IDENTIFYING COMMUNICABLE DISEASES

Table 16-2 presents information on identification of some of the most common communicable diseases. Included are incubation period, mode of transmission, symptoms, and treatment. Familiarity with these illnesses allows nurses to assist in identification, prevention, and treatment.

INCIDENCE OF SELECTED REPORTABLE DISEASES

Control of communicable diseases requires careful monitoring of trends and disease patterns. Table 16-3 lists several reportable diseases and the number of cases for selected years dating from 1950. This table graphically illustrates the effectiveness of immunization efforts in the reduction of **vaccine-preventable diseases** and trends in some communicable diseases that are interesting (fluctuation of gonorrhea, relative stability of hepatitis A), concerning (recent rise in pertussis), and encouraging (1 case of diphtheria in 1999). This table also allows insight into recent

Text continued on p. 443

TABLE 16-2 Identifying Selected Communicable Infectious Diseases

DISEASE (CAUSATIVE AGENT)	SYMPTOMS	MODE OF TRANSMISSION	COMPLICATIONS AND COMMUNITY HEALTH CONCERNS	SPECIFIC TREATMENT (IF ANY)
RESPIRATORY ROUTE				
Chicken pox (varicella-zoster virus)	Incubation period, 12 to 21 days. Low-grade fever, listlessness. Lesions within 2 to 4 days. Rash has three phases: raised spots, fluid-filled vesicles, and scabs. Rash itches and is found over entire body, including mucous membranes such as mouth.	Very contagious (person-to-person direct contact or contact with airborne droplet). Vesicles are contagious, scabs are not. Communicable 2 days before to 6 days after vesicles appear. Primarily affects children.	Grandparents and older adults should avoid caring for children because they may develop shingles.	Immunosuppressed persons should be treated with γ-globulin. Vaccine is available.
Diphtheria (Corynebacterium diphtheria)	Flulike symptoms with sore throat, fever, and involvement of adenoids and larynx with potential respiratory distress. Characterized by formation of yellow-white membranes on tonsils and pharyngeal walls.	Person-to-person direct contact or contact with airborne droplet. Usually affects children under 15 years, but may affect adults.	Asymptomatic carrier state possible; should be treated with antibiotics.	Antitoxin immediately on diagnosis and antibiotics (e.g., penicillin and/or erythromycin). Isolate until three negative throat cultures.
Pertussis or whooping cough (Haemophilus pertussis bacteria)	Incubation period, 7 to 10 days. Characteristic cough is nonproductive with quick expiratory phase followed by inspiratory "whoop." Pneumonia and ear infections may be present. Small scleral and conjunctival hemorrhages can occur because of severe coughing. Convulsions may occur.	Person-to-person contact or droplet spread. Very contagious. Affects females more than males. Infants younger than 1 year are severely affected.	Incidence has increased in recent years because of lower immunization rates and concern about side effects of vaccine. Severity of illness and risk of death far surpass the risks from vaccination.	Antibiotics. Hospitalization with oxygen support and nasotracheal suctioning may be necessary.

continued

From Matocha, L. K. (1995). Communicable disease. In C. M. Smith & F. A. Maurer (Eds.), *Community health nursing: Theory and practice.* Philadelphia: W. B. Saunders. Compiled by L. K. Matocha & F. A. Maurer.

TABLE **16-2** Identifying Selected Communicable Infectious Diseases—cont'd

DISEASE (CAUSATIVE AGENT)	SYMPTOMS	MODE OF TRANSMISSION	COMPLICATIONS AND COMMUNITY HEALTH CONCERNS	SPECIFIC TREATMENT (IF ANY)
RESPIRATORY ROUTE—cont'd				
German measles/ rubella (rubella virus)	Incubation period, 14 to 21 days. Mild in adults and young children, with a macular rash on scalp, body, and limbs lasting 1 to 3 days. Severe in early fetal development and can result in congenital malformations and death; late fetal infection carries risk of birth defects Conditions associated with fetal infections include low birth weight, deafness, cataracts, glaucoma, heart disease, and mental retardation.	Person-to-person direct contact or droplet spread. Communicable 4 days before to 4 days after rash appears. Highly contagious. Common in children 5 to 10 years of age.	Women of childbearing years should be immunized before pregnancy. Vaccine is live, so it must not be given to pregnant women. Reinfections can occur, but are rare.	None
Measles/rubeola (rubeola virus)	Incubation period, 7 to 21 days. Rash, usually starting on the face and spreading to body, lasting 6 days. Koplik's spots in mouth that are bluish white and very fine. Coldlike symptoms and cough. Lasts 4 to 5 days.	Person-to-person direct contact with saliva or droplets. Common disease of childhood. More common in poorly immunized populations and in adolescents.	Complications are pneumonia and encephalitis. No congenital malformations, but can cause spontaneous abortion and prematurity. Children who are HIV positive and asymptomatic should be considered for the vaccine because the illness could be fatal. Persons allergic to eggs may have severe reactions to vaccine.	None
Mumps (mumps virus)	Incubation period, 14 to 26 days. Low-grade fever, headache, earache, pain, and swelling of parotid glands (unilateral or bilateral). Swelling lasts about a week. Early fetal infections can	Person-to-person direct contact with saliva or droplets. More commonly a childhood disease. Communicable 6 days before to 9 days after swelling.	Infrequent complications are encephalitis and meningitis. Orchitis occurs in males who have reached puberty, but sterility is rare. Potential for spontaneous abortion if woman is	None

Disease	Symptoms	Transmission	Treatment/Prevention
		result in spontaneous abortion.	infected in early pregnancy. Persons allergic to eggs may have severe reaction to vaccine.
Tuberculosis (*Mycobacterium tuberculosis*)	Low-grade fever, listlessness, night sweats, respiratory congestion, cough, hemoptysis. Sites other than the lungs may be infected; if so, symptoms are specific to the site. (Other sites include meninges, joints, bladder, and lymphatic system.)	Inhalation from droplet containing bacteria. Risk factors include poverty, poor health, and age. Very young and very old are most susceptible.	Infection with the bacteria produces disease in approximately 10% of cases in the United States. Mantoux test is used to screen for infection and disease. Incidence is on the rise from increased incidence in HIV patients and rise of drug-resistant strains of TB.	Multiple drug therapy with 3 to 6 drugs for 6 to 12 months for persons with the disease. Persons infected are treated prophylactically with one medication for for up to 6 months. Drug-resistant individuals may need a variety and mix of drugs over time to ensure appropriate treatment.
Influenza (influenza type A or B virus, or potentially a third [type C] virus)	Respiratory symptoms such as runny nose or cough. May be accompanied by headache and fever. Sometimes may be accompanied by gastrointestinal symptoms such as nausea and vomiting.	Inhalation from droplet spread. Very contagious.	Rapid antigenic variation makes it difficult for the host to develop immune response. Influenza causes more pandemics than any other organism. Complications include pneumonia, croup, Reye's syndrome, toxic shock syndrome, myocarditis, and myocardial infarction.	Antiviral drugs (e.g., amatadine, rimantadine, zanamivir, oseltamivir) can treat and help prevent influenza in exposed individuals. Yearly vaccination recommended for susceptible individuals (i.e., elderly and chronically ill persons). Vaccine must be reconfigured each year to meet the specific characteristics of the current strain.

continued

TABLE **16-2** Identifying Selected Communicable Infectious Diseases—cont'd

DISEASE (CAUSATIVE AGENT)	SYMPTOMS	MODE OF TRANSMISSION	COMPLICATIONS AND COMMUNITY HEALTH CONCERNS	SPECIFIC TREATMENT (IF ANY)
INTEGUMENTARY ROUTE				
Pediculosis (parasitic lice)	Incubation period, 2 weeks. Lice and eggs may be present in scalp hair or pubic hair or on the body. Itching and other signs of skin irritation, such as a rash or swollen glands, may be present.	Direct contact or indirect transfer of adult lice, nits, or eggs via body contact, or contact with personal items that are infected with the parasites.	Nuisance disease; not easily transmitted from person to person.	Hair and pubic lice are treated with medicated shampoos such as Kwell in several applications. Nits (eggs) should be removed from scalp hair with a fine-toothed comb. Body lice are eliminated by dusting clothes with 15 malathion powder and washing all affected garments in very hot water.
Impetigo (group A streptococcal or staphylococcal bacteria)	Incubation period, 4 to 10 days. Skin blisters usually found in the corners of the mouth or near edge of nose. Blisters break and form yellow crusts that resolve with little or no scarring; blisters may be itchy, and scratching may occur. Fever, malaise, and headache may be present.	Direct contact with lesions or secretions. Very contagious. Scratching spreads the disease to other areas of the body or other persons. Communicable as long as lesions persist.	Most common in hot, humid climates. Very contagious and problematic in children. Infected children should be kept from school until completely healed.	Penicillin and/or erythromycin and topical antibiotics to treat skin eruptions.
Rabies (rabies virus)	Three phases: prodromal, neurological, and coma. Prodromal: wound heals and symptoms of minor infection are present lasting 2 to 10 days; these include fever, headache, chills, sore throat, and pain at site of bite.	Transmitted through bites from an infected animal.	Treatment is difficult and fatality rate is high. Prevention is the main community health thrust. Domestic animals should be immunized and populations educated to avoid wild (e.g., fox, raccoon) or unknown animals.	Rabies vaccine. Hospitalization with isolation.

	Neurological: lasts up to 7 days and includes hallucinations, stiffness, disorientation, and seizures. Coma: death may occur if treatment is not given.			
Scabies (parasitic mite)	Incubation period, 2 to 6 weeks; reinfections in 1 to 4 days. Skin rash, scratching may occur. Burrows on skin look like gray-white tracts; lesion may be evident around wrists and belt line.	Direct contact. Transmitted by mites that burrow under skin and lay eggs. Clothing and other personal items may hold mites or eggs. Communicable as long as eggs or mites are alive.	Concerns similar to those for pediculosis.	Hot bath, vigorous body scrub followed by application of 5% solution of benzyl benzoate or Kwell. Application should be repeated in approximately 1 week. Bedding and clothing must be thoroughly cleaned.

GASTROINTESTINAL ROUTE

Candidiasis (Candida fungus)	Depend on site of infection. Gastrointestinal infection produces diarrhea and may be accompanied by cramping. Vaginal infections have vaginal symptoms.	Highly infectious. Found on skin and under finger and toenails and may be passed to gastrointestinal tract by hand-to-mouth transmission. Vaginal infection common in females, easily transferred to males during sexual contact.	Infants can be infected during vaginal delivery.	Multiple oral and topical drugs depending on site of infection, including nystatin, clotrimazole, and amphotericin B.
Salmonellosis (several types of Salmonella bacteria)	Incubation period, 6 to 72 hours. Sudden onset of acute gastroenteritis with abdominal cramps, diarrhea, nausea, and sometimes vomiting and dehydration. Headache and fever are present. Stools are loose for days after acute episode.	Direct via person-to-person oral-fecal contact or indirectly by ingestion of food contaminated with feces containing Salmonella. Communicable during entire period of infection, which may be as long as 1 year or more.	Infections most frequent from July to November with warm weather. Uncooked eggs and meats are major harborers of bacteria. Carriers continue to excrete organisms in stool for more than 1 year after symptoms disappear. Drug-resistant strains becoming more common.	Antibiotics for severe symptoms. Carriers treated with ampicillin.

continued

TABLE **16-2** Identifying Selected Communicable Infectious Diseases—cont'd

DISEASE (CAUSATIVE AGENT)	SYMPTOMS	MODE OF TRANSMISSION	COMPLICATIONS AND COMMUNITY HEALTH CONCERNS	SPECIFIC TREATMENT (IF ANY)
GASTROINTESTINAL ROUTE—cont'd				
Polio (strains of poliovirus)	Incubation period, 7 to 14 days or longer. Muscle weakness progressing to paralysis. May affect any muscle group, including limbs and respiratory muscles. Pain may accompany muscle weakness. There is little or no loss of sensation despite paralysis.	Direct contact of virus with mouth.	Humans are the only natural host and reservoir of the virus. Localized outbreaks in the United States are usually in unvaccinated or undervaccinated communities.	None
Shigellosis (variety of bacterial agents)	Incubation period, 1 to 7 days. Diarrhea, fever, and nausea. Can progress to toxemia, vomiting, and tenesmus. Blood, mucus, and pus may be found in stool.	Person-to-person by fecal-oral route, or, more rarely, from contaminated water. Communicable as long as organism is present, which may be a month or more. Infants and young children are more often infected because of poor hygiene.	Most contagious condition caused by bacteria. Seasonal; more common in warm weather.	Antibiotics for severe symptoms
Intestinal parasites (roundworms and pinworms)	Abdominal pain; bloody stools or diarrhea may be present. Occasional nausea and vomiting.	Transmitted via ingestion of eggs of the worms, either directly via hand and fingernails or through food and water containing eggs.	Diagnosis of pinworms made by application of cellophane tape to anal area early in the morning to confirm eggs.	Treat with mebendazole until stools are clear of parasites.
Toxoplasmosis (protozoa)	Most persons have no symptoms or only mild symptoms, including enlarged lymph nodes, fever, night sweats, sore throat, or rash. Immunosuppressed persons, including HIV-positive individuals, may develop toxoplasmic encephalitis; hemiparesis, seizures, visual complications, mental disorientation, and listlessness.	Contact with the protozoa via uncooked or undercooked meat or via airborne contact from the feces of cats.	Health education related to proper preparation of meats and care of cat litter is important. Toxoplasmosis screening should be done on pregnant women.	Immunosuppressed individuals are treated with a variety of drugs for up to 4 to 6 weeks after symptoms resolve; infected pregnant women are also treated.

	Symptoms	Transmission	Comments	Prevention/Treatment
	Fetal infection may result in spontaneous abortion, stillbirth, or varied complications after birth, e.g., blindness, encephalitis, hydrocephalus, and anemia.			
Hepatitis A (hepatitis A virus)	Incubation period, 15 to 30 days. Rapid onset of flulike symptoms, nausea and vomiting, abdominal cramps, jaundice; may also be asymptomatic. Long period of recovery (1 to 3 months).	Person-to-person by oral-fecal route. Very contagious and spreads rapidly. Also may be spread indirectly if virus is present in milk, undercooked shellfish, or contaminated water.	Common in daycare centers, homosexuals, and illicit IV drug users.	Immune serum globulin can be administered if exposed individuals are identified. Vaccine is recommended for those in high-risk areas
SERUM ROUTE				
Hepatitis B (hepatitis B virus)	Incubation period, 1 to 6 months. General flulike symptoms or no symptoms. Liver deterioration, if present, is noted by markedly enlarged liver, dark urine, light stool, jaundiced eyes and skin, skin eruptions. Symptoms last 4 to 6 weeks.	Exposure to infected blood (e.g., through sexual activity and IV drug paraphernalia). In health care workers, exposure to infected blood is often via accidental needle puncture.	Complications include chronic hepatitis, cirrhosis, liver cancer, and death. Persons who need frequent blood transfusions are at increased risk. Health care workers are at increased risk to exposure. Chronic carriers can transmit disease to others; drug users are at risk for carrier status.	Vaccination for at-risk populations is recommended.
Human immunodeficiency virus (HIV)	Incubation period, potentially 10 years or more. Flulike symptoms may or may not be noted immediately after infection. Symptoms of immune compromise including opportunistic infections and cancers that allow for the diagnosis of AIDS (i.e., Kaposi's sarcoma, *Pneumocystis carinii* pneumonia, toxoplasmosis, candidiasis, cryptococcus, cytomegalovirus, herpes simplex, and others).	Exchange of secretions and semen during sexual intercourse; parenteral exposure of blood and blood products from mother to fetus; breast milk.	Testing for HIV infection is confidential. Persons testing positive for HIV infection may be asymptomatic for years, which is problematic because they may unknowingly engage in behavior that puts others at risk. Health teaching about safe sexual and personal habits is a concerted community health effort to control spread.	Treatment depends on specific presenting opportunistic illness or disease. Zidovudine (formerly called azidothymidine [AZT]), didanosine (DDI), and (dideoxycytidine (DDC) appear to slow the the spread of the virus. AZT is particularly toxic and cannot be tolerated by many.

continued

TABLE **16-2** Identifying Selected Communicable Infectious Diseases—cont'd

DISEASE (CAUSATIVE AGENT)	SYMPTOMS	MODE OF TRANSMISSION	COMPLICATIONS AND COMMUNITY HEALTH CONCERNS	SPECIFIC TREATMENT (IF ANY)
SERUM ROUTE—cont'd				
Human immunodeficiency virus (HIV)—cont'd	Eventual outcome is death.		HIV screening requires retesting at intervals after possible infection because the virus is not immediately detectable. There is a window period of approximately 1 to 12 weeks after infection when test results may be negative. People must be encouraged to retest as needed to ensure accurate testing results.	Research continues in an attempt to find an effective treatment; at present none exists. Efforts at vaccine development continue.
Herpes (herpes simplex virus, HSV 1, oral; HSV 2, genital)	Incubation period, 2 weeks. Lesions at site of infection are fluid filled and rupture and ulcers form scabs. Lesions may or may not be painful. Virus stays dormant in body, and successive eruptions occur commonly as a result of stress or other illnesses. HSV 2 symptoms may include fever and other flulike symptoms. In women, vaginal discharge, painful intercourse, and painful urination may be present.	Direct contact with oral and genital secretions. HSV 1 and HSV 2 viruses have recently been found in genital and oral sites previously thought to be exclusive to one or the other.	Complications include increased risk of cervical cancer. Infants exposed through the birth canal may experience blindness, brain damage, or death. Recurrence in infected individuals places new sexual partners at risk. Protection of sexual partner during infectious periods should be stressed; condom use is important.	Incurable; acyclovir is given to treat existing cases and suppress recurrent episodes.
Cytomegalovirus (CMV)	Incubation period varies. If symptomatic, resembles mononucleosis; adults are mostly asymptomatic. Virus remains in body for life. Fetal infections can result in congenital anomalies, e.g., mental retardation, deafness, jaundice, chorioretinitis, hydrocephaly, and epilepsy.	Transmitted through blood transfusions, organ transplants, breast milk, from children's urine and respiratory tract, and through sexual contact with semen and vaginal secretions.	Immunosuppressed individuals are at risk for frequent infectious episodes.	Gancyclovir is used to treat retinal CMV, but is not successful against gastrointestinal, respiratory, and systemic CMV. Vaccine development is experimental and minimally useful to date.

Disease	Symptoms	Transmission	Complications	Treatment
Venereal warts (papillomavirus)	Symptoms in newborns may not be immediately evident at birth but are usually present during the first 6 months. Condylomata warts, which may or may not be painful. Infants may develop respiratory symptoms.	Close contact with warts; may also be sexually transmitted. Passed to infants during passage through the birth canal.	Most serious complication is the link between the disease and malignancies of the cervix and genital tract.	Cryotherapy, laser therapy, or podophyllin in tincture of benzoin compound to remove or destroy warts.
Gonorrhea (Neisseria gonorrhoeae)	Incubation period, 2 to 30 days. Frequently asymptomatic, especially in men. Symptoms: women—pain, heavy purulent vaginal discharge, pain in the genital and pelvic area; men—discharge from penis, pain on urination, urinary frequency.	Primarily sexual contact. Can be transmitted to mucous membranes other than genitalia.	Complications include arthritis, blood, meningeal and heart infections, and sterility. In women, pelvic inflammatory disease; in men, narrowing of the urethra and swelling of the testicles. Children born during an active case may contract ophthalmia neonatorum, leading to blindness. Incidence is alarmingly high and most prevalent in young adults 15 to 35 years old.	One-time dose of ceftriaxone, cefixime, ciprofloxacin, or ofloxacin. Antibiotics appropriate to treat for Chlamydia and trichomoniasis are often prescribed simultaneously. Test of cure in 4 to 7 days after treatment ends to ensure treatment effectiveness is especially important, because drug-resistant strains are becoming more frequent.
Chlamydia (Chlamydia bacteria)	Incubation period, 1 to 3 weeks. Symptoms consist of other infections such as nongonococcal urethritis, pelvic inflammatory disease, inflammation of cervix, and conjunctivitis. In infants, as a result of vaginal delivery, eye infections and pneumonia.	Primarily sexual contact, but infections can occur in other areas of the body if contact is made with the bacteria.	Complications in women include pelvic inflammatory disease and cervical dysplasia; in men, prostatitis and epididymitis occur. Frequently occurs with other STDs. This is the most frequently occurring STD.	Doxycycline, axithromycin, tetracycline, or erythromycin. Test of cure in 4 to 7 days after treatment is completed.

continued

TABLE **16-2** Identifying Selected Communicable Infectious Diseases—cont'd

DISEASE (CAUSATIVE AGENT)	SYMPTOMS	MODE OF TRANSMISSION	COMPLICATIONS AND COMMUNITY HEALTH CONCERNS	SPECIFIC TREATMENT (IF ANY)
SERUM ROUTE—cont'd				
Syphilis (*Treponema pallidum*)	Incubation period, first stage, 10 to 90 days. Disease has three stages if left untreated. First stage: canker sore at site of infection (genital, rectum, lips); sore is usually painless. Second stage: occurs 3 to 6 weeks later; generalized flulike symptoms and may have body rash, sores, inflamed eyes. Third stage: starts when disease becomes dormant, which may last years. Symptoms may recur, including blindness, deafness, brain damage, paralysis, heart disease, and death.	Sexual contact	Incidence is increasing, especially among young adults. Complications of untreated syphilis include blindness, deafness, brain damage, paralysis, heart disease, and death.	Large-dose intramuscular penicillin; if individual is allergic to penicillin, oral tetracycline or doxycycline is given. Patients must be rescreened at 3, 6, and 12 months because some infections are resistant to treatment. Drug-related strains are becoming problematic.
Pelvic inflammatory disease (gonorrhea, *Chlamydia*, *Trichomonas* bacteria, and other organisms)	Abnormal vaginal discharge, severe abdominal/pelvic pain and tenderness, painful intercourse, irregular vaginal bleeding, chills, fever, and nausea and vomiting. Can be fatal.	Infections caused by STD that spread to the upper genital tract of women.	Most common complication is sterility. Others include chronic abdominal pain; chronic infection of fallopian tubes, uterus, and ovaries; ectopic pregnancies.	Oral antibiotics, outpatient care; if no substantial improvement within 72 hours, hospitalization is necessary. Antibiotics should be specific for the particular organism causing the infection.
Trichomoniasis (protozoa *Trichomonas vaginalis*)	Incubation period, 1 to 6 weeks. Men usually asymptomatic, but can have slight, clear penile discharge and itch on urination. Women have thin yellow-green–gray vaginal discharge with odor and burning, redness, itching of genitalia; may have frequency of urination.	Sexual contact with exchange of body fluids.	Sexual partners must be treated at the same time, even though men are commonly asymptomatic.	Metronidazole (flagyl, Protostat, or Metryl) given orally for 7 to 10 days. Vinegar douche may alleviate vaginal symptoms.

TABLE **16-3** Selected Reportable Diseases by Year

DISEASE	NUMBER OF CASES						
	1950	1960	1970	1980	1990	1994	1999
AIDS	N/A	N/A	N/A	N/A	41,595	78,279	45,104
Diphtheria	5796	918	435	3	4	2	1
Gonorrhea	286,746	258,933	600,072	1,004,029	690,169	418,068	360,076
Hepatitis A	2820	41,666	56,797	29,078	31,441	29,796	17,047
Hepatitis B	Non-Specific	Non-Specific	8310	19,015	21,102	12,517	7694
Measles	319,124	441,703	47,351	13,506	27,786	963	100
Mumps	N/A	N/A	104,953	8576	5292	1537	387
Pertussis	120,718	14,809	4249	1730	4570	4617	7288
Poliomyelitis	33,300	3190	33	9	6	—	—
Rubella	N/A	N/A	56,552	3904	1125	227	267
Syphilis	217,558	122,538	91,382	68,832	134,255	81,696	35,628
Tuberculosis	121,742	55,494	37,137	27,749	25,701	24,361	17,531
Varicella	N/A	N/A	N/A	190,894	173,099	151,219	46,016

From Centers for Disease Control and Prevention (CDC). (2001c). Summary of notifiable diseases, United States —1999. *MMWR Morbidity and Mortality Weekly Report*, 48(53), 1-104.

TABLE **16-4** Comparison of Maximum and Current Morbidity from Vaccine-Preventable Diseases

DISEASE	MAXIMUM CASES (*N* [YEAR])	1999 CASES (*N*)	CHANGE (%)
Diphtheria	206,939 (1921)	1	–99.9
Measles	894,134 (1941)	100	–99.9
Mumps	152,209 (1968)	387	–99.7
Pertussis	265,269 (1934)	7288	–97.3
Polio (paralytic)	21,269 (1952)	0	–100.0
Rubella	57,686 (1969)	267	–99.5
Tetanus	601 (1948)	40	–93.3

From Centers for Disease Control and Prevention (CDC). (1995a). *Epidemiology & prevention of vaccine-preventable diseases.* Atlanta, GA: Centers for Disease Control and Prevention; Centers for Disease Control and Prevention (CDC). (2001c). Summary of notifiable diseases, United States —1999. *MMWR Morbidity and Mortality Weekly Report*, 48(53), 1-104.

changes in the immunization schedules (e.g., the addition of a booster for MMR following the outbreak of measles in 1989 to 1990 and the addition of immunization against chicken pox).

VACCINE-PREVENTABLE DISEASES

Vaccination against communicable diseases has very dramatically affected morbidity and mortality from infectious diseases, as Table 16-3 shows. The worldwide eradication of small pox in 1980 is an example of the success that is pos-

sible through the use of global efforts to control disease through immunization. Efforts to eradicate other diseases, such as measles and polio, have been less successful to date, primarily because of failure to appropriately immunize all those who are susceptible. Table 16-4 further illustrates the impact of routine vaccinations.

The routine pediatric immunization schedule has become very complex in recent years. Recommendations have been modified a number of times since the early 1980s with the addition of new vaccines, changes in the ages for administration, requirements for informed consent, and reporting of serious side effects. Nurses who primarily work with children in schools, clinics, and doctor's offices, and who administer immunizations, must be aware of a number of components of immunization delivery. In addition to a basic understanding of the principles behind immunization, nurses should know the pediatric immunization schedule and standards, contraindications and precautions, requirements for parent education and consent, and the process for reporting adverse vaccine events. Each is discussed here.

IMMUNITY

- **Immunity** refers to protection from infectious disease. There are two basic mechanisms for acquiring immunity—active and passive.
- **Passive immunity** is protection produced by an animal or human and transferred to another human. Passive immunity often provides effective protection, but this protection usually wanes in a few weeks or months.
- **Active immunity** is protection that is produced by the person's own immune system. This type of immunity is generally long lasting (CDC, 1995a, p. 12).

Examples of passive immunity include transplacental transfer of immunity from a mother to her infant and injection of constituents of blood products from human donors (e.g., homologous pooled human antibody, immune globulin). Active immunity occurs following the stimulation of the body's immune system to produce antibodies and cellular immunity, often after a person has had a disease. Active immunity can also be achieved through administration of a vaccine that produces an immunological memory similar to that of the natural disease (CDC, 1995a).

Vaccines are classified as live attenuated and inactivated. Live attenuated vaccines are produced by modifying a disease-producing virus or bacterium in the laboratory. The altered vaccines allow production of an immune response as the organism replicates in the vaccinated person. Although the organisms in live attenuated vaccines replicate, they usually do not cause the disease; or if they do, the case is usually much milder than the natural disease (CDC, 1995a). Live attenuated vaccines must be handled and stored carefully because they may be destroyed by heat and light. Examples of live attenuated vaccines include those for MMR, oral polio, varicella, and TB (bacille Calmette-Gurin vaccine [BCG]).

Inactivated vaccines are produced by growing the organism in a culture media, then inactivating it with heat or chemicals. The organisms in inactivated vaccines do not replicate and the vaccine's effectiveness depends on the body's immune system to develop protection following a second or third dose. Influenza, pertussis, HBV, tetanus, and HIB are examples of diseases that a person can be inoculated against with inactivated vaccines (CDC, 1995a).

IMMUNIZATION SCHEDULE

The recommended **immunization schedule** for routine pediatric vaccinations has undergone several major changes over the last decade. Changes include the addition of vaccination for HIB in the early 1980s, the addition of an MMR booster in 1990, the inclusion of vaccination against HBV in 1992, additions of vaccination against varicella in 1997, addition of vaccination against hepatitis A in high-risk areas, addition of a series to protect against pneumococcal disease in 2000, and HBV vaccination for adolescents. Other changes have occurred following approval of new vaccines, such as that for acellular DPT and a combined DPT and HIB vaccine. The current recommended schedule for pediatric immunization is presented in Figure 16-2.

IMMUNIZATION STANDARDS

The Standards for Pediatric Immunization Practices were published in 1993 "to eliminate barriers and obstacles...that impede efficient vaccine delivery and to encourage providers to take advantage of all health care visits as opportunities to provide vaccination" (CDC, 1993, p. 1). These standards, with numerous programs at each local, state, and federal level of the public health system, have been quite successful in improving the rates

Recommended Childhood Immunization Schedule United States, 2002

Age Vaccine	Birth	1 mo	2 mos	4 mos	6 mos	12 mos	15 mos	18 mos	24 mos	4-6 yrs	11-12 yrs	13-18 yrs
		Range of recommended ages				Catch-up vaccination				Preadolescent assessment		
Hepatitis B[1]	Hep B #1	only if mother HBsAg(-)									Hep B series	
			Hep B #2			Hep B #3						
Diphtheria, Tetanus, Pertussis[2]			DTaP	DTaP	DTaP		DTaP			DTaP	Td	
Haemophilus influenzae type b[3]			Hib	Hib	Hib	Hib						
Inactivated Polio[4]			IPV	IPV		IPV				IPV		
Measles, Mumps, Rubella[5]						MMR #1				MMR #2	MMR #2	
Varicella[6]						Varicella				Varicella		
Pneumococcal[7]			PCV	PCV	PCV	PCV			PCV	PPV		
Hepatitis A[8]											Hepatitis A series	
Influenza[9]					Influenza (yearly)							

Vaccines below this line are for selected populations

This schedule indicates the recommended ages for routine administration of currently licensed childhood vaccines, as of December 1, 2001, for children through age 18 years. Any dose not given at the recommended age should be given at any subsequent visit when indicated and feasible. ▆▆▆▆ Indicates age groups that warrant special effort to administer those vaccines not previously given. Additional vaccines may be licensed and recommended during the year. Licensed combination vaccines may be used whenever any components of the combination are indicated and the vaccine's other components are not contraindicated. Providers should consult the manufacturers' package inserts for detailed recommendations.

Approved by the Advisory Committee on Immunization Practices (www.cdc.gov/nip/acip), the American Academy of Pediatrics (www.apa.org), and the American Academy of Family Physicians (www.aafp.org).

1. **Hepatitis B vaccine (Hep B).** All infants should receive the first dose of hepatitis B vaccine soon after birth and before hospital discharge; the first dose may also be given by age 2 months if the infant's mother is HBsAg-negative. Only monovalent hepatitis B vaccine can be used for the birth dose. Monovalent or combination vaccine containing Hep B may be used to complete the series; four doses of vaccine may be administered if combination vaccine is used. The second dose should be given at least 4 weeks after the first dose, except for Hib-containing vaccine which cannot be administered before age 6 weeks. The third dose should be given at least 16 weeks after the first dose and at least 8 weeks after the second dose. The last dose in the vaccination series (third or fourth dose) should not be administered before age 6 months.

   Infants born to HBsAg-positive mothers should receive hepatitis B vaccine and 0.5 mL hepatitis B immune globulin (HBIG) within 12 hours of birth at separate sites. The second dose is recommended at age 1-2 months and the vaccination series should be completed (third or fourth dose) at age 6 months.

   Infants born to mothers whose HBsAg status is unknown should receive the first dose of the hepatitis B vaccine series within 12 hours of birth. Maternal blood should be drawn at the time of delivery to determine the mother's HBsAg status; if the HBsAg test is positive, the infant should receive HBIG as soon as possible (no later than age 1 week).

2. **Diphtheria and tetanus toxoids and acellular pertussis vaccine (DTaP).** The fourth dose of DTaP may be administered as early as age 12 months, provided 6 months have elapsed since the third dose and the child is unlikely to return at age 15-18 months. **Tetanus and diphtheria toxoids (Td)** is recommended at age 11-12 years if at least 5 years have elapsed since the last dose of tetanus and diphtheria toxoid-containing vaccine. Subsequent routine Td boosters are recommended every 10 years.

3. **Haemophilus influenzae type b (Hib) conjugate vaccine.** Three Hib conjugate vaccines are licensed for infant use. If PRP-OMP (PedvaxHIB® or ComVax® [Merck]) is administered at ages 2 and 4 months, a dose at age 6 months is not required. DTaP/Hib combination products should not be used for primary immunization in infants at ages 2, 4 or 6 months, but can be used as boosters following any Hib vaccine.

4. **Inactivated polio vaccine (IPV).** An all-IPV schedule is recommended for routine childhood polio vaccination in the United States. All children should receive four doses of IPV at ages 2 months, 4 months, 6-18 months, and 4-6 years.

5. **Measles, mumps, and rubella vaccine (MMR).** The second dose of MMR is recommended routinely at age 4-6 years but may be administered during any visit, provided at least 4 weeks have elapsed since the first dose and that both doses are administered beginning at or after age 12 months. Those who have not previously received the second dose should complete the schedule by the 11-12 year old visit.

6. **Varicella vaccine.** Varicella vaccine is recommended at any visit at or after age 12 months for susceptible children, i.e. those who lack a reliable history of chickenpox. Susceptible persons aged >13 years should receive two doses, given at least 4 weeks apart.

7. **Pneumococcal vaccine.** The heptavalent **pneumococcal conjugate vaccine (PCV)** is recommended for all children age 2-23 months. It is also recommended for certain children age 24-59 months. **Pneumococcal polysaccharide vaccine (PPV)** is recommended in addition to PCV for certain high-risk groups. See MMWR. 2000;49(RR-9):1-35.

8. **Hepatitis A vaccine.** Hepatitis A vaccine is recommended for use in selected states and regions, and for certain high-risk groups; consult your local public health authority. See MMWR. 1999;48(RR-12):1-37.

9. **Influenza vaccine.** Influenza vaccine is recommended annually for children age > 6 months with certain risk factors (including but not limited to asthma, cardiac disease, sickle cell disease, HIV, diabetes; see MMWR. 2001;50(RR-4):1-44), and can be administered to all others wishing to obtain immunity. Children aged ≥ 12 years should receive vaccine in a dosage appropriate for their age (0.25 mL if age 6-35 months or 0.5 mL if age ≥ 3 years). Children aged ≤ 8 years who are receiving influenza vaccine for the first time should receive two doses separated by at least 4 weeks.

For additional information about vaccines, vaccine supply, and contraindications for immunization, please visit the National Immunization Program Web site at www.cdc.gov/nip or call the National Immunization Hotline at (800) 232-2522 (English) or (800) 232-0233 (Spanish).

Figure 16-2. Recommended childhood immunization schedule United States, January to December 2001. (From American Academy of Pediatrics. [2001]. *Recommended childhood immunization schedule United States, January-December 2001.* Chicago, IL: The Academy.)

BOX 16-2 Standards for Pediatric Immunization Practices

1. Immunization services are readily available.
2. There are no barriers or unnecessary prerequisites to the receipt of vaccines.
3. Immunization services are available free or for a minimal fee.
4. Providers utilize all clinical encounters to screen and, when indicated, vaccinate children.
5. Providers educate parents and guardians about immunization in general terms.
6. Providers question parents or guardians about contraindications and, before vaccinating a child, inform them in specific terms about the risks and benefits of the vaccinations their child is to receive.
7. Providers follow only true contraindications.
8. Providers administer simultaneously all vaccine doses for which a child is eligible at the time of each visit.
9. Providers use accurate and complete recording procedures.
10. Providers coschedule immunization appointments in conjunction with appointments for other child health services.
11. Providers report adverse events following vaccination promptly, accurately, and completely.
12. Providers operate a tracking system.
13. Providers adhere to appropriate procedures for vaccine management.
14. Providers conduct semiannual audits to assess immunization coverage levels and to review immunization records in the patient populations they serve.
15. Providers maintain up-to-date, easily retrievable medical protocols at all locations where vaccines are administered.
16. Providers practice patient-oriented and community-based approaches.
17. Vaccines are administered by properly trained persons.
18. Providers receive ongoing education and training regarding current immunization recommendations.

From Centers for Disease Control and Prevention (CDC). (1993). Standards for pediatric immunization practices. *MMWR Morbidity and Mortality Weekly Report, 42*(RR-5), 3.

of complete immunization for U.S. children (CDC, 1994b). The standards are outlined in Box 16-2.

CONTRAINDICATIONS

Standards 6 and 7 of the Standards for Pediatric Immunizations relate to contraindications and precautions to vaccine administration. Although adverse reactions to vaccines are uncommon, they do occur and may be severe. Reactions can occur because of allergies to vaccine components (e.g., eggs, egg proteins, antibiotics, preservatives, and adjuvants). Therefore patient allergies should be considered before administration of specific vaccines (Bond, Labat, and Langthorn, 2001).

Mild illness with or without low-grade fever is not a contraindication for vaccination. However, vaccination should be postponed in cases of moderate or severe febrile illness to avoid confusion between a vaccine side effect and an unknown underlying cause (Bond, Labat, and Langthorn, 2001).

Pregnancy is not a contraindication for immunization using inactivated vaccines, antitoxins, or immune globulins. However, pregnant women should avoid live vaccines (i.e., MMR, varicella, and yellow fever) unless the risk of infection is very high (CDC, 2000a). Likewise, immunocompromised patients should not receive live vaccines, although MMR can be administered to asymptomatic HIV-infected people and varicella can be given to people with humoral immunodeficiency and some asymptomatic HIV-infected people, as determined by their physician (CDC, 2000a).

PARENTAL EDUCATION AND CONSENT

Standards 5 and 6 of the standards for pediatric immunization practices refer to parental education and providing information on the risks of vaccination. In October 1994, the CDC instituted a requirement that all health care providers administering any vaccine for DPT, MMR, or polio provide parents with Vaccine Information Statements (VIS). The VIS were written to simplify explanations on the benefits and risks associated with MMR, polio, DPT, and tetanus/diphtheria vaccines. Since that time, all providers are required to provide a copy of the relevant VIS each time a patient is vaccinated (CDC, 1995a). The VIS have been translated into Chinese, French, Spanish, and Vietnamese and can be obtained from the CDC and the state health departments. Information can also be found on the CDC's website (see the book's website at **www.wbsaunders.com/SIMON/McEwen** $\widehat{\text{SIMON}}$ to access this site).

DOCUMENTATION

Legal documentation of vaccinations is important for both the individual and the provider for future administration and follow-up of hypersensitivity reactions. Both individual and provider immunizations should be maintained and the health care provider is responsible for maintaining accurate records. These records should include the patient name; dates immunized; vaccine type; vaccine manufacturer; vaccine lot number; date of the VIS; and the name, title, and address of the person administering the vaccine (Bond, Labat, and Langthorn, 2001).

REPORTING ADVERSE VACCINE EVENTS

Standards 11 and 12 of the Pediatric Immunization Practices Standards relate to tracking and reporting adverse events following immunization. The **Vaccine Adverse Event Reporting System (VAERS)** was developed to comply with the National Childhood Vaccine Injury Act of 1986 to "provide a single system for the collection and analysis of reports on all adverse events associated with the administration of any U.S. licensed vaccine in all groups" (Chen et al., 1994, p. 542). Examples of reportable adverse events appear in Table 16-5. The VAERS is operated by the CDC and Food and Drug Administration; additional information can be obtained by calling a 24-hour toll-free telephone number (1-800-822-7967).

ADULT IMMUNIZATION

In general, people are aware of pediatric immunizations, but most adults, and many health care providers, are unaware of recommended immunizations for adults. For example, the CDC reports that fewer than 28% of persons in high-risk categories have received pneumococcal polysaccharide vaccine (CDC, 1995). Appropriately vaccinating adults should be a priority for all health care providers.

Vaccination recommendations for adults were presented in Chapter 12, but there also have been recent calls for routine vaccination of adolescents and young adults. Indeed, many adolescents and young adults suffer needlessly from vaccine-preventable diseases such as HBV, varicella, influenza, and meningitis. To address this problem, in 1996 a routine health care visit was recommended for adolescents 11 to 12 years of age to ensure that this group would receive HBV, varicella vaccine (if no history of the disease), a second dose of MMR vaccine, and a booster dose of tetanus and diphtheria vaccine if it had been more than 5 years since their last booster (Bond, Labat, and Langthorn, 2001). Also, many colleges and universities are now requiring some minimal level of proof of immunization before enrollment for new students. In 1999, the CDC recommended that vaccination against meningococcal disease be provided to freshmen and other undergraduate students who request the vaccine, although routine vaccination is not recommended (CDC, 2000b).

SEXUALLY TRANSMITTED DISEASES

The number and type of different **sexually transmitted diseases (STDs)** has increased dramatically over the last several decades. Because of this, STDs have been termed a "hidden epidemic of tremendous health and economic consequence in the United States" (USDHHS, 2000, p. 25.3). Indeed, of the top 10 infections reported to the CDC in 1998, five were STDs (chlamydia,

TABLE **16-5** Vaccine Injury Table

VACCINE	ILLNESS, DISABILITY, INJURY, OR CONDITION*	TIME FOR FIRST SYMPTOM OR MANIFESTATION OF ONSET OR OF SIGNIFICANT AGGRAVATION AFTER VACCINE ADMINISTRATION
DTP; P; DT; Td; or tetanus toxoid; or in any combination with polio; or any other vaccine containing whole cell pertussis bacteria, or partial cell pertussis bacteria, or specific pertussis antigen(s)	Anaphylaxis or anaphylactic shock	24 hours
	Encephalopathy (or encephalitis)	3 days
	Shock-collapse or hypotonic or hyporesponsive collapse	3 days
		3 days
	Residual seizure disorder[†]	
MMR, or any vaccine containing any of the foregoing as a component	Anaphylaxis or anaphylactic shock	24 hours
	Encephalopathy (or encephalitis)	15 days (for mumps, rubella, measles, or any vaccine containing any of the foregoing as a component)
		3 days (for DT, Td, or tetanus toxoid)
	Residual seizure disorder[†]	Same as for encephalopathy
Polio vaccines (other than inactivated polio vaccine)	Paralytic polio	
	In a nonimmunodeficient recipient	30 days
	In an immunodeficient recipient	6 months
	In a vaccine-associated community case	Not applicable
Inactivated polio vaccine	Anaphylaxis or anaphylactic shock	24 hours

From Centers for Disease Control and Prevention (CDC). (1995a). *Epidemiology & prevention of vaccine-preventable diseases.* Atlanta, GA: Centers for Disease Control and Prevention.
*Any acute complication or sequela (including death) of an illness, disability, injury, or condition that arose within the time prescribed is also subject to the presumption of causation.
[†]Defined as follows: Patient did not suffer a seizure or convulsion unaccompanied by fever or accompanied by a fever of less than 102°F before the first seizure or convulsion after the administration of the vaccine involved and in the case of measles, mumps, or rubella vaccine or any combination of such vaccines, the first seizure or convulsion occurred within 15 days after administration of the vaccine and two or more seizures or convulsions occurred within 1 year after the administration of the vaccine, which were unaccompanied by fever or accompanied by a fever of less than 102°F; and in the case of any other vaccine, the first seizure or convulsion occurred within 3 days after the administration of the vaccine and two or more seizures or convulsions occurred within 1 year after the administration of the vaccine, which were unaccompanied by a fever or accompanied by a fever of less than 102°F.

gonorrhea, AIDS, syphilis, and HBV), and it is estimated that more than 15 million cases of STDs occur each year in the United States (USDHHS, 2000). It is of particular concern that 86% of STDs occur in people aged 15 to 29 years (USDHHS/Office of Disease Prevention, Health Promotion [ODPHP], 1998). People considered at risk for STDs and HIV infection include the following:

- Those who are contacts of, or have a previous history of, documented STD and HIV infection
- Pregnant women

- Individuals who are or were recently sexually active (especially those with multiple sexual partners)
- Individuals living in areas with high prevalence of HIV and STDS
- Homosexual and bisexual men
- Drug and alcohol abusers
- Those involved in the exchange of sex for drugs or money (USDHHS/ODPHP, 1998)

Until as recently as the early 1980s, the only STDs (called venereal diseases at the time) commonly recognized by the public were syphilis and gonorrhea. By the end of the 1990s, more than a dozen STDs were recognized. Table 16-6 lists some of the most common STDs in the United States and gives their incubation periods, symptoms, possible complications, and treatment information. The next two sections describe primary and secondary prevention of STDs.

PRIMARY PREVENTION OF SEXUALLY TRANSMITTED DISEASES

Primary prevention of STDs is based on changing the sexual behaviors that place individuals at risk. Education and counseling on abstinence, high-risk behaviors, and safer sex strategies (e.g., the use of condoms and other barriers and spermicides) is essential in primary prevention of STDs. It is the responsibility of the health care provider to counsel and educate those at risk to change their behaviors (see the Health Teaching box "Basics of Sexually Transmitted Disease and Human Immunodeficiency Virus Counseling"). When counseling clients at risk for STDs, it is also important to use language and terminology that the client understands and to reassure them that treatment will be provided regardless of ability to pay, citizenship or immigration status, language spoken, or lifestyle.

Sexual intimacy in a mutually monogamous relationship between partners known to be disease free and sexual abstinence are the only certain ways to prevent infection. To reduce the possibility of exposure, safer sex counseling should include correct use of latex condoms for each sexual encounter, avoidance of sex with high-risk partners, avoiding anal intercourse, and avoiding the use of substances that impair judgment (e.g., alcohol, cocaine, marijuana). See the Health Teaching box "Guidelines for Condom Use."

SECONDARY PREVENTION AND SEXUALLY TRANSMITTED DISEASES

Early diagnosis and prompt, appropriate treatment are essential in stopping the spread of STDs. Treatment must include instruction on medication compliance and referral for treatment of all sex partners. In most cases, partners of clients with STDs should be examined. Resources for referral should be identified in advance and information should be made available where STDs are most likely to be detected (e.g., drug treatment and HIV treatment centers).

TRENDS IN INCIDENCE AND PREVALENCE OF SELECTED COMMUNICABLE DISEASES

Nurses who work in community-based settings should continually watch for changes in rates of communicable diseases. It is particularly important to monitor trends in area populations and communities. Several diseases are discussed here because of their importance to nurses in community-based practice.

ACQUIRED IMMUNODEFICIENCY SYNDROME AND HUMAN IMMUNODEFICIENCY VIRUS

It is well known that HIV is transmitted primarily by sexual contact involving the exchange of body fluids (e.g., vaginal secretions and semen) with an infected individual. It is also transmitted by the following means: blood transfusion or exposure to blood, blood products, or tissues of an infected person; by perinatal transmission from an infected mother to fetus during pregnancy, delivery, or when breastfeeding; and by sharing needles or syringes with an infected person. The infection of HIV is widespread and an estimated 47 million adults and children have AIDS worldwide. In the United States, between 650,000 and 900,000 people are HIV positive and in recent years incidence rates have stabilized at about 40,000 cases per year (USDHHS, 2000).

At the inception of the epidemic, HIV and AIDS was largely found in white men who had sex with men; however, this has changed dramatically over the last decade. Indeed, the proportion of cases among whites has decreased from 60% to 41% and the proportion of cases has increased correspondingly among minorities (blacks from 25% to 41% and Hispanics from

TABLE **16-6** Sexually Transmitted Diseases

DISEASE	INCUBATION PERIOD	SYMPTOMS	TREATMENT	POSSIBLE COMPLICATIONS
Chlamydia	7 to 14 days+	Often there are no symptoms; females have slight vaginal discharge, itching and burning of the vagina; males may have a penile discharge, burning during urination, and burning and itching at the urethral opening.	Antibiotics—not penicillin	Women—pelvic inflammatory disease (PID), ectopic pregnancy, and infertility. Men—prostatitis, epididymitis.
Gonorrhea	2 to 7 days (can be longer)	Males usually have burning on urination and purulent discharge from the urethra (5 to 20% have no symptoms); females may have a genital discharge, but most have no symptoms.	Antibiotics—some strains have become resistant to penicillin in recent years.	Women—PID, infertility. Men—narrowing of urethra, sterility. Newborns—eye, nose, lung, and/or rectal infections.
Herpes simplex	2 to 12 days	Painful blisters or sores on the genitals, rectum, or mouth that break, crust over, and heal in 2 to 4 weeks. The sores may reappear throughout life.	No cure at this time. Medication (acyclovir) may be given to shorten the outbreak; medications may be given to prevent bacterial infection in the open sores and to control pain.	Women—possible increased risk of cervical cancer. Newborns—blindness, brain damage, and/or death to baby passing through birth canal of mother with active lesions; cesarean section is indicated if mother has active lesions at the time of delivery.
HIV	Unknown, 1 to 3 months to 10 years	No symptoms for years; eventually, fever, weight loss, fatigue, swollen glands, and diarrhea; opportunistic infections and conditions follow.	No medical cure. AZT and other medications are being used with success.	Multiple opportunistic infections; death.
Human papillomavirus	1 to 20 months (average is 4 months)	Sometimes there are no symptoms. Typically, there are pink or dirty gray warts appearing on the moist areas of the genitals and anus.	Removal of the warts through freezing, laser therapy, surgical removal, or application of a topical medication.	Blockage of vaginal, rectal, or throat openings; cervical dysplasia; cervical cancer (possibly).

Disease	Incubation	Symptoms	Treatment	Complications
Syphilis	10 days to 3 months	Primary stage: painless chancre (sore) at site of entry; swollen glands. Secondary stage: 1 week to 6 months after chancre—may include rash, patchy hair loss, sore throat, and swollen glands.	Antibiotics	If untreated—blindness, deafness, brain damage, heart disease, death. Newborns—damage to skin, eyes, teeth, and/or liver.
Chancroid	3 to 5 days to 14 days	Single or multiple painful, necrotizing ulcers at the site of infection; swelling and pain in the regional lymph nodes. May be asymptomatic in women.	Antibiotics	Increases risk of HIV transmission; fluctuant lymphadenopathy.
Hepatitis B	45 to 180 days; average: 60 to 90 days	Variable. Fatigue, weakness, anorexia, abdominal pain, muscle or joint pain, nausea and vomiting, jaundice, and dark urine.	No cure. Treatment is palliative.	Chronic hepatitis; cirrhosis; liver cancer.
Trichomoniasis	4 to 20 days; average: 7 days	Many women and most men have no symptoms. Women may have a white or greenish-yellow odorous discharge, vaginal itching and soreness and/or painful urination. Males may have a slight itching of the penis, painful urination and/or clear penile discharge.	Oral medication (Flagyl)	None identified.
Scabies	2 to 6 weeks in initial infection; 1 to 4 days after reexposure	Small raised, red bumps or blisters on the skin with severe itching. Generally affects webs of the fingers, elbows, underarms, external genitalia.	Over-the-counter (OTC) and prescription medications Laundering all bedding, clothing, and towels in hot water.	Secondary bacterial infection.
Pediculosis pubis	3 to 14 days	Intense itching, blue or gray spots and insects or nits in the pubic area	OTC (NIX, RID) or prescription (lindane, Kwell) medications	None identified.

Adapted from Benenson, A. S. (1990). *Control of communicable diseases in man.* Washington, DC: American Public Health Association; Texas Department of Health. (1992). *Educator's guide to sexually transmitted diseases* (3rd ed.). Austin, TX: Texas Department of Health.

health teaching

Basics of Sexually Transmitted Disease and Human Immunodeficiency Virus Counseling

Determine client's risk for STDs and tailor counseling to the behaviors, circumstances, and special needs of the person being served. Risk reduction messages should be personalized and realistic, culturally appropriate and sensitive to issues of sexual identity, developmentally appropriate, and linguistically specific.

Provide educational materials about STD transmission and prevention that are appropriate for the client's culture and educational level.

Advise all clients that any unprotected sexual behavior poses a risk for STDs and HIV infection; caution patient to avoid sexual contact with persons who may be infected with HIV and to not make decisions about sexual activity while under the influence of alcohol or other drugs that cloud judgment and permit risk-taking behavior.

Provide educational material and information that explain that STDs and HIV infection are best prevented by abstinence; limiting sexual relationships to those between mutually monogamous partners known to be HIV negative; avoiding sex with high-risk partners; avoiding anal intercourse; and using latex condoms if having sex with anyone other than a single, mutually monogamous partner know to be HIV-negative.

Provide educational materials and information explaining that infection can be transmitted even if males withdraw before ejaculation and that infection can be transmitted during all forms of sexual intercourse including oral sex.

Provide educational information indicating that the risk of HIV infection is increased during coinfection with other STDs (i.e., syphilis, genital herpes, and gonorrhea).

Instruct all sexually active individuals about the effective use and limitations of condoms.

Use client-centered counseling by establishing a trusting, caring relationship, listening carefully to identify any specific barriers to preventing STDs and HIV infection, and providing counseling that is culturally appropriate and sensitive to issues of sexual orientation.

From U.S. Department of Health and Human Services (USDHHS). (1998). *Clinician's handbook of preventive services* (2nd ed.). Washington, DC: Government Printing Office.

health teaching

Guidelines for Condom Use

Use only latex (rubber) condoms.

Use only condoms that are not in damaged packages and are not brittle, sticky, discolored, or past expiration date.

Use only reservoir-tip condoms or leave one-half inch space at the tip of the condom to collect semen.

Use only water-based lubricants. Lubricants made with petroleum jelly, mineral oil, cold cream, or vegetable oils may damage the condom.

Spermicides containing nonoxinol-9 inside the condom or inside the vagina may increase protection against STDs and HIV. However, if spermicides cause local irritation, they may increase the risk of HIV transmission.

The condom should be placed on an erect penis and unrolled slowly and completely to the base before the penis comes in contact with a body opening.

If a condom breaks, it should be replaced immediately.

After ejaculation, withdraw the penis while it is still erect. Hold the condom carefully against the base of the penis so that it remains in place.

Dispose of condoms properly. Never reuse condoms.

Remember that other contraceptives (birth control pills, Depo-Provera, and intrauterine devices) cannot protect against STDs and HIV.

Condom failure rates are 10% to 15%, either as a result of product failure (breakage) or incorrect or inconsistent use.

Adapted from American College Health Association (1990). *Safer sex* [brochure]. Baltimore, MD: American College Health Association; U.S. Department of Health and Human Services (USDHHS). (1998). *Clinician's handbook of preventive services* (2nd ed.). Washington, DC: Government Printing Office.

COMMUNITY APPLICATION
Tuberculosis in the United States

Beginning in 1993, there has been a steady downward trend in the number of cases of TB in the United States. In 2000, there were a total of 16,377 cases, which was an all-time low. The decline has been promoted by strengthening of TB control activities such as screening and treatment. Despite this drop, rates remain high in some areas.

The CDC has reported that the states with the highest TB rates are Alaska, Hawaii, California, New York, Georgia, Arkansas, Louisiana, Florida, Texas, and South Carolina, respectively. In addition, there is a growing global TB epidemic, which could reverse the declines made in the United States. This highlights the need for all communities to remain diligent in fighting this health problem. Defense systems must be maintained to address the threat of TB, and health care providers must remain diligent, particularly in high-risk areas, to work to identify and treat or refer suspected cases of TB.

From Centers for Disease Control and Prevention (CDC). (2001a). *CDC issues report on the top ten states with the highest rates of TB*. Washington, DC: Author. Retrieved 07/11/01 from http://www.cdc.gov/od/oc/media/pressrel/r010613.htm.

14% to 18%). Over the same period the proportion of cases transmitted through homosexual contact decreased from 64% to 45% and increased through intravenous (IV) drug use and heterosexual transmission. The prevalence among women has also risen and women now account for 20% of all cases (USDHHS, 2000). Fortunately, however, because of widespread testing of pregnant women and treatment with zidovudine (formerly called azidothymidine [AZT]), perinatal transmission rates have declined substantially.

Treatment for HIV and AIDS has become relatively effective over the last decade changing AIDS from a death sentence to a chronic disease for those who have access to care. Management of HIV and AIDS, however, is highly complex, very expensive, and changes frequently. In addition, side effects can be significant and debilitating. Drugs used to treat HIV infection include antiemetics, antimicrobials, antifungals, antivirals, protease inhibitors, antimycobacterials, and antiretrovirals, among others.

Prevention efforts should be targeted at creating awareness of risk and reduction of risk behaviors in high-risk populations and preventing transmission of HIV infection by people who are infected. Periodic testing of those in high-risk groups (e.g., those practicing unprotected sex, IV

drug users) should be encouraged and referrals for treatment should be planned in advance.

TUBERCULOSIS

After decades of decreasing incidence of TB in the United States, the number of reported cases increased slowly, but steadily, from the mid-1980s, before dropping off somewhat in the late 1990s. The rise in cases is attributed, in part, to opportunistic infections in those who are HIV positive. Additionally, many new cases are identified in immigrants and those in other high-risk groups. This trend is cause for concern, in particular because of the emergence of multiple-drug resistant strains (USDHHS/ODPHP, 1998). See the Community Application box "Tuberculosis in the United States."

Persons at risk for TB include the medically underserved (particularly those of black, Hispanic, Asian, Native American, and Alaskan Native heritage); foreign-born individuals from high-prevalence areas (Asia, Africa, and Latin America); those in close contact with infectious TB cases; individuals with medical conditions known to increase the risk of TB (e.g., HIV, diabetes, chronic renal failure, conditions requiring prolonged corticosteroid therapy); alcoholics and IV drug users; residents of high-risk environments (long-term care facilities, correctional institutions, and mental institutions), and health care workers who serve high-risk clients (USDHHS/ODPHP, 1998). Guidelines for TB screening are as follows:

- Screening for TB should be performed on children and adults from high-risk groups.
- The Mantoux text (intradermal injection of 0.1 ml of purified protein derivative in the long axis of the forearm) should be performed whenever possible.
- The Mantoux test should be read 48 to 72 hours after placement by palpating the margin of induration and measuring and recording the diameter. Treatment is indicated if induration is greater than 5 mm to greater than 15 mm depending on exposure, age, risk factors, and presence of symptoms.
- It should be recognized that absence of a reaction does not exclude a diagnosis of TB infection, particularly when the individual has symptoms of active disease. Induration of less than 5 mm may occur early in the course of TB infection or in individuals with altered immune function (e.g., clients with AIDS).
- Vaccination with BCG may cause false-positive Mantoux reactions, but this decreases with time and rarely causes an induration of 15 mm or greater.
- Live vaccines such as MMR and oral polio vaccine may interfere with response to the Mantoux test. Tuberculosis testing may be administered either concurrently with these vaccines or 4 to 6 weeks afterward.

Additional testing after positive Mantoux results consists of chest radiograph and sputum smear and culture to determine if there is active disease. If the results of these tests are negative, the client is usually placed on a preventative medication regimen, typically oral isoniazid (INH) 300 mg daily for 6 to 12 months (CDC, 1994c). For clients with active TB, as evidenced by radiographs and sputum cultures, therapy consists of administration of multiple drugs over a period of several months depending on symptoms, exposure, preexisting conditions, and sputum cultures.

HEPATITIS B

The reported incidence of HBV decreased 63% between 1990 and 1999 (CDC, 2001c). This decline is largely attributed to a reduction in the number of cases among homosexual men and IV drug users. These decreases are thought to result from an increase in AIDS awareness and subsequent behavioral changes (e.g., safer sex and needle-using practices) (CDC, 1994a).

The availability of the HBV vaccine and recommended use for at-risk populations has also contributed to the decreased incidence. Identification of these individuals and recommendation of immunization are important interventions for nurses who work in ambulatory settings. Those identified as at risk for contracting HBV include the following:

- Persons with occupational risk
- Clients and staff of institutions for the developmentally disabled
- Hemodialysis patients
- Sexually active homosexual men
- Users of illicit injectable drugs
- Recipients of certain blood products
- Household and sexual contacts of HBV carriers
- Adoptees from countries of high HBV endemicity
- Other contacts of HBV carriers
- Populations with high endemicity of HBV infection in the United States (Alaskan natives, Pacific Islanders, and refugees from HBV-endemic areas)
- Sexually active heterosexual persons (particularly those requiring treatment for STDs, prostitutes, and those with a history of multiple partners)
- International travelers residing for more than 6 months in areas with high endemicity (CDC, 1990)

Routine testing of pregnant women for HBV and treatment for the infants of those who tested positive with immune globulin and vaccine was instituted in the early 1990s. As described earlier, efforts to further reduce the incidence of HBV include initiation of routine immunization of all infants in 1992 and the more recent recommendation to immunize adolescents.

EMERGING INFECTIONS

Emerging infectious diseases are those diseases whose incidence in humans has increased within the past two decades or threatens to increase in the near future. They can be new or previously unrecognized infectious diseases, reemerging diseases, or infectious diseases that have developed resistance to previously effective antimicrobial drugs. Factors identified as contributing to concern over emerging infectious diseases include social and environmental changes, explosive population growth, expanding poverty, urban migration, international travel, changes in the way food is processed and distributed, and technology (CDC, 1998).

Box 16-3 lists several emerging infections of which nurses who work in community-based settings should be aware. Other potentially important emerging infections that have been the subject of concern are *Escherichia coli* 0157:H7, group A streptococcal disease, Hantavirus pulmonary syndrome, and drug-resistant pneumococcus (CDC, 1994a). All health care providers should monitor current concerns or trends in communicable diseases in their community to assist in identification of suspect cases and to provide education, prevention, and early treatment where indicated. See the Health Teaching box "Facts About Anthrax," a disease that has recently been used as a method of bioterrorism.

To address concerns about emerging infections, the CDC has developed a set of goals and objectives (CDC, 1998). These include objectives to strengthen infectious disease surveillance and response; to improve methods for gathering and evaluating surveillance data; to ensure the use of surveillance data to improve public health practice and medical treatment; and to strengthen global capacity to monitor and respond to emerging

---

BOX **16-3** Emerging Infections

NEW VARIANT CREUTZFELDT-JAKOB DISEASE

New variant Creutzfeldt-Jakob disease (nvCJD) first appeared in the United Kingdom in the early 1990s and cases have been identified in a number of countries in northern Europe and elsewhere around the world. It is thought that nvCJD is caused by a newly recognized type of transmissible agent called a *prion*. New variant Creutzfeldt-Jakob disease is possibly transmitted by ingestion of beef from animals afflicted with bovine spongiform encephalopathy (mad cow disease).

VIRULENT STRAIN OF INFLUENZA (HONG KONG INFLUENZA)

In 1997, an avian strain of influenza that had never before infected humans began to kill previously healthy persons in Hong Kong.

FOODBORNE OUTBREAKS

The United States has had several multistate foodborne outbreaks including outbreaks caused by *Cyclospora* parasites on fresh raspberries; hepatitis A on frozen strawberries; and *Escherichia coli* 0157:H7 bacteria in apple cider, lettuce, alfalfa sprouts, and ground beef.

TUBERCULOSIS (STRAIN W)

Tuberculosis strain W is multidrug resistant and appears more frequently in persons with HIV infection; strain W has become endemic in New York.

VANCOMYCIN-RESISTANT ENTEROCOCCI (VRE) AND *STAPHYLOCOCCUS AUREUS*

From 1989 through 1993, the percentage of nosocomial enterococci resistant to vancomycin reported from hospitals participating in the National Nosocomial Infections Surveillance System increased from 0.3% to 7.9%. During this period, numerous VRE outbreaks (occurring primarily among immunocompromised patients) were reported. Also, cases of vancomycin-resistant *Staphylococcus aureus* have recently been reported in the United States and Japan.

From Centers for Disease Control and Prevention (CDC). (1998). Preventing emerging infectious disease: A strategy for the 21st century overview of the updated CDC plan. *MMWR Morbid Mortal Weekly Report, 47*(RR15), 1-14.

health teaching

Facts About Anthrax

The terrorist attacks in the fall of 2001 made the world aware of the threat of anthrax. The following information can be shared with clients in community settings.

Anthrax is an acute infectious disease caused by the spore-forming bacterium *Bacillus anthracis.* Anthrax most commonly occurs in hoofed mammals (i.e., cattle, sheep), but can also infect humans.

Symptoms of anthrax vary depending on how the disease was contracted, but usually occur within 7 days after exposure. The forms of human anthrax are inhalation anthrax, cutaneous anthrax, and intestinal anthrax.

Initial symptoms of inhalation anthrax infection may resemble a common cold or the flu. After several days, the symptoms may progress to severe breathing problems and shock. Inhalation anthrax is often fatal.

The intestinal disease form of anthrax may follow the consumption of contaminated food and is characterized by an acute inflammation of the intestinal tract. Initial signs of nausea, loss of appetite, vomiting, and fever are followed by abdominal pain, vomiting of blood, and severe diarrhea.

Direct person-to-person spread of anthrax is extremely unlikely. Therefore there is no need to immunize or treat contacts of persons ill with anthrax unless they were also exposed to the same source of infection.

In persons exposed to anthrax, infection can be prevented with antibiotic treatment. Early antibiotic treatment of anthrax is essential—delay lessens chances for survival. Anthrax is usually susceptible to penicillin, doxycycline, and fluorquinolones.

An anthrax vaccine can also prevent infection. Vaccination against anthrax is not recommended for the general public, however, and is not available.

From Centers for Disease Control and Prevention (CDC). (2001b). *Facts about anthrax.* Washington, DC: CDC. Retrieved 07/11/01 from http://www.bt.cdc.gov/Agent/Anthrax/AnthraxGen.asp.

infectious diseases. The areas targeted for preventing emerging infectious diseases are the following:

- *Antimicrobial resistance:* The emergence of drug resistance in bacteria, parasites, viruses, and fungi is concerning and many drug choices for treatment of common infections are becoming increasingly limited.
- *Foodborne and waterborne diseases:* Changes in the ways that food is processed and distributed are causing more multistate outbreaks of foodborne infections; a new group of waterborne pathogens has emerged that is unaffected by routine disinfection methods.
- *Vectorborne and zoonotic diseases:* Many emerging or reemerging diseases are acquired from animals or transmitted by arthropods; environmental changes can affect the incidence of these diseases by altering the habitats of disease vectors.

- *Disease transmitted through blood transfusions or blood products:* Improvements in blood donor screening, serologic testing, and transfusion practice have helped make the U.S. blood supply relatively safe, but continued vigilance is needed.
- *Chronic diseases caused by infectious agents:* Several chronic diseases and some forms of cancer, heart disease, and ulcers might be caused or intensified by infectious agents.
- *Vaccine development and use:* Although many childhood diseases have been virtually eliminated, additional vaccines are needed to prevent diseases that are a burden in the United States or internationally (e.g., HIV, hepatitis C, malaria).
- *Diseases of persons with impaired host defenses:* Opportunistic infections are rising because of the number of persons whose defenses are

impaired by illness, medical treatment, or as a result of age.

- *Diseases of pregnant women and newborns:* Some asymptomatic infections in pregnant women can increase the infant's risk of prematurity, low birth weight, long-term disability, or death; effective and accessible prenatal care is essential to prevention of infection in pregnant women and babies.
- *Diseases of travelers, immigrants, and refugees:* Persons who cross international boundaries are at increased risk for contracting infectious diseases and can also disseminate diseases to new places (CDC, 1998).

INTERNATIONAL TRAVEL

International travel may greatly increase exposure to a number of communicable diseases. Jong and McMullen (1995) state that international travelers should seek medical advice 4 to 6 weeks in advance of departure to allow "adequate time for immunizations to be scheduled, for advice and prescriptions to be given, and for specific information to be obtained when needed" (p. 3). Destinations obviously dictate travel precautions with regard to health. Of particular concern are enteric diseases, malaria, rabies and other vectorborne diseases, STDs and HIV, and other illnesses. Individual research into specific risks and careful planning of primary and secondary prevention is vitally important.

Before leaving the United States, a traveler's health history should be completed by the traveler and carried in a safe place throughout the trip. This document should contain immunization records, list of current medications, list of medical problems, known drug allergies, blood type, name and telephone number of the regular doctor, and name and telephone number of the closest relative or friend in the United States.

The traveler should also prepare a medical kit to take that anticipates needed supplies and medications. To be included are any prescription and nonprescription medications (i.e., aspirin, acetaminophen or ibuprofen, antibiotic ointment, antifungal powder or cream, decongestant tablets, diarrhea prevention medications, and hydrocortisone cream). General health and first aid supplies include antiseptic solution, Band-Aids, extra eyeglasses, insect repellent (if applicable), sanitary supplies, sunscreen, and premoistened towelettes. Women may want to take sanitary supplies and antifungal vaginal cream or suppositories.

Immunizations and prophylactic pharmacological treatment recommendations are based on location of travel. Vaccines may be taken to protect against cholera, hepatitis A, HBV, Japanese encephalitis, typhoid, meningococcal disease, and yellow fever. Additionally, recommendations for taking prophylactic medication for malaria should be followed. Specific information can be obtained from the local health department and from the CDC's website (see the book's website at **www.wbsaunders.com/SIMON/McEwen** SiMoN to access this site). See the Health Teaching box "Pretravel Medical Recommendations."

SUMMARY

Primary and secondary prevention of communicable diseases is one of the most important functions of nurses who work in community-based settings. This chapter discusses several aspects of communicable disease control, including identification and reporting of suspected cases, prevention through immunization, and education and counseling efforts to reduce transmission of STDs. Encouraging monitoring of selected diseases and emerging infections and disease prevention during international travel concludes the discussion.

In the opening case study, Mark was a public health nurse responsible for investigating cases of reportable communicable diseases and because of this he had a direct, defined role in communicable disease control. However, it is important to remember that all nurses need to be aware of communicable diseases in their area of

health teaching

Pretravel Medical Recommendations

1. Consult personal physician, local Public Health Department, or travel clinic about recommendations for immunizations and malaria chemoprophylaxis after selection of the travel itinerary, but preferably 4 to 6 weeks in advance of departure.
2. Prepare a traveler's health history and medical kit.
3. Carry a telephone credit card that can be used for international telephone calls or make sure that the friends or relatives listed in the health history would accept an international collect call in case of an emergency.
4. Make sure to have the telephone number of your personal physician, including office and after-hours numbers, and a fax number if available. A business card attached to the traveler's health history is a handy way to carry this information.
5. Check medical insurance policy or health plan for coverage of illness or accidents occurring outside the United States.
6. Specifically inquire if the regular insurance policy or health plan covers emergency medical evacuation by an air ambulance.
7. Arrange for additional medical insurance coverage or for a line of credit as necessary for a medical emergency situation.

From Jong E. C. (1995). The travel medical kit and emergency medical care abroad. In E. C. Jong & R. McMullen (Eds.), *The travel & tropical medicine manual* (2nd ed.). Philadelphia: W. B. Saunders.

practice and to know how and when to report them.

In addition to the Reference list at the end of the chapter, the Resources box at the end of the chapter lists resources for further information on the major topics. Each of these agencies and organizations provides literature for health care providers and many offer educational materials for clients.

KEY POINTS

- Although improvement in morbidity and mortality from communicable diseases has been dramatic, particularly vaccine-preventable diseases (e.g., measles, diphtheria, polio), a number of threats and risks still exist for all people from communicable illnesses (HIV, TB, influenza).
- Communicable diseases may be transmitted directly (kissing, touching, sexual contact) or indirectly (through fomites, substances, or vectors). Airborne transmission may be either direct or indirect.
- The CDC and the individual state legislatures have identified Reportable Communicable Diseases. Guidelines for reporting include who is responsible for reporting; what information is required; how, when, and to whom to report; and steps taken to control spread.
- Many communicable diseases are preventable through immunization. The recommended immunization schedule for infants and children is complex and has changed several times in recent years. Providers should be aware of contraindications and precautions for vaccines, parent education materials, consent requirements, and reporting of adverse vaccine events.
- The number and incidence of STDs have increased dramatically over the last several decades. The most common STDs include chlamydia, gonorrhea, herpes, HIV, human papillomavirus, syphilis, and scabies.
- Nurses working in community-based settings should watch for changes in rates of communicable diseases. Diseases that should be closely monitored include TB, HIV and AIDS, and emerging infections.
- Often, nurses in community settings are asked to advise clients on issues related to international travel. Information that might be needed includes pretravel recommendations and immunization requirements and recommendations.

Resources

Communicable Disease Prevention

American Academy of Pediatrics
Centers for Disease Control and Prevention
National Center for Infectious Diseases
National Immunization Program
National Institute of Allergy and Infectious
    Diseases
Centers for Disease Control—Travelers' Health
National Center for HIV, STD and TB
    prevention
World Health Organization

Visit the book's website at
www.wbsaunders.com/SIMON/McEwen
for a direct link to the website for each
organization listed.

Learning Activities & Application to Practice

In Class

1. Discuss modes of communicable disease transmission. Identify and outline primary prevention strategies to reduce or eliminate each type of transmission.
2. Visit the local public health department to discuss surveillance and control of communicable diseases. Find out about local and regional trends in communicable diseases. Learn about the process of reporting.
3. Discuss the current pediatric immunization schedule and the Standards for Pediatric Immunization Practices with classmates. Become aware of recent changes and contraindications and precautions.

In Clinical

4. In a log or diary, compile a list of communicable illnesses encountered in the clinical setting. When possible, participate in the process of reporting of communicable diseases.
5. Participate in a pediatric immunization clinic or work with nurses who routinely immunize children. If possible, help screen children for possible contraindications. Also provide the required parent education.

REFERENCES

American College Health Association (1990). *Safer sex* [brochure]. Baltimore, MD: American College Health Association.

Benenson, A. S. (1990). *Control of communicable diseases in man* (15th ed.). Washington, DC: American Public Health Association.

Bond, M., Labat, V., & Langthorn, D. C. (2001). Communicable disease and public health. In M. Nies & M. McEwen (Eds.), *Community health nursing: Promoting the health of populations* (3rd ed.). Philadelphia: W. B. Saunders.

Centers for Disease Control and Prevention (CDC). (1990). Protection against viral hepatitis: Recommendations of the Advisory Committee on Immunization Practices. *MMWR Morbidity and Mortality Weekly Report, 39,* 5-22.

Centers for Disease Control and Prevention (CDC). (1992). *Principles of epidemiology* (2nd ed.). Atlanta, GA: Centers for Disease Control and Prevention.

Centers for Disease Control and Prevention (CDC). (1993). Standards for pediatric immunization practices. *MMWR Morbidity and Mortality Weekly Report, 42*(RR-5), 1-19.

Centers for Disease Control and Prevention (CDC). (1994a). Addressing emerging infectious disease threats: A prevention strategy for the United States. *MMWR Morbidity and Mortality Weekly Report, 43*(RR-5), 1-23.

Centers for Disease Control and Prevention (CDC). (1994b). General recommendations on immunization. *MMWR Morbidity and Mortality Weekly Report, 43*(RR-1), 1-48.

Centers for Disease Control and Prevention (CDC). (1994c). Vaccine coverage of 2-year-old children, United States. *MMWR Morbidity and Mortality Weekly Report, 43*(39), 705-709.

Centers for Disease Control and Prevention (CDC). (1995). *Epidemiology and prevention of vaccine-preventable diseases.* Atlanta, GA: Centers for Disease Control and Prevention.

Centers for Disease Control and Prevention (CDC). (1998). Preventing emerging infectious disease: A strategy for the 21st century overview of the updated CDC plan. *MMWR Morbidity and Mortality Weekly Report, 47*(RR15), 1-14.

Centers for Disease Control and Prevention (CDC). (2000a). *Epidemiology and prevention of vaccine-preventable diseases (pink book)* (6th ed.). Atlanta, GA: Public Health Foundation.

Centers for Disease Control and Prevention (CDC). (2000b). Meningococcal disease and college students, recommendations of the Advisory Committee on Immunization Practices (ACIP). *MMWR Morbidity and Mortality Weekly Report 49*(RR-07), 11-20.

Centers for Disease Control and Prevention (CDC). (2001a). *CDC issues report on the top ten states with the highest rates of TB.* Washington, DC: Author. Retrieved 7/11/01 from http://www.cdc.gov/od/oc/media/pressrel/r010613.htm.

Centers for Disease Control and Prevention (CDC). (2001b). *Facts about anthrax.* Washington, DC: CDC. Retrieved 7/11/01 from http://www.bt.cdc.gov/Agent/Anthrax/AnthraxGen.asp.

Centers for Disease Control and Prevention (CDC). (2001c). Summary of notifiable diseases, United States—1999. *MMWR Morbidity and Mortality Weekly Report, 48*(53), 1-104.

Chen, R. T., Rastogi, S. C., Mullen, J. R., et al. (1994). The vaccine adverse event reporting system (VAERS). *Vaccine, 12*(6), 542-550.

Dash, D. (1993). Communicable disease. In J. Swanson & S. Albrecht (Eds.), *Community health nursing: Promoting the health of aggregates.* Philadelphia: W. B. Saunders.

Jong, E. C. (1995). The travel medical kit and emergency medical care abroad. In E. C. Jong & R. McMullen (Eds.), *The travel and tropical medicine manual* (2nd ed.). Philadelphia: W. B. Saunders.

Jong, E. C., & McMullen, R. (1995). Sexually transmitted disease and foreign travel. In E. C. Jong & R. McMullen (Eds.), *The travel and tropical medicine manual* (2nd ed.). Philadelphia: W. B. Saunders.

Matocha, L. K. (1995). Communicable diseases. In C. M. Smith & F. A. Maurer (Eds.), *Community health nursing: Theory and practice.* Philadelphia: W. B. Saunders.

Mausner, J. S., & Kramer, S. (1985). *Epidemiology: An introductory text.* Philadelphia: W. B. Saunders.

National Center for Health Statistics (NCHS). (2000). Deaths: Final data for 1998. *National Vital Statistics Reports, 48*(11), 1-106, Washington, DC: National Center for Health Statistics.

Texas Department of Health. (1992). *Educator's guide to sexually transmitted diseases* (3rd ed.). Austin, TX: Texas Department of Health.

U.S. Department of Health and Human Services (USDHHS). (2000). *Healthy people 2010: Conference edition.* Washington, DC: Government Printing Office.

U.S. Department of Health and Human Services/Office of Disease Prevention, Health Promotion (USDHHS/ODPHP). (1998). *Clinician's handbook of preventive services* (2nd ed.). Washington, DC: Government Printing Office.

Glossary

The number in parentheses after each term represents the chapter in which that term is found.

A

Active immunity (16): protection against a communicable disease that is produced by the person's own immune system. Active immunity occurs following the stimulation of the body's immune system to produce antibodies and cellular immunity, often after a person has had a disease. Active immunity can also be achieved through administration of a vaccine that produces an immunological memory similar to that of the natural disease.

Activities of daily living (ADL) (12): normal activities of living that generally include bathing, dressing, eating, getting in and out of bed and chairs, walking, going outside, and toileting.

Adult immunization (12): recommendations of the Immunization Practices Advisory Committee that all older adults should have completed a primary series of diphtheria and tetanus toxoids, a single dose of pneumococcal polysaccharide vaccine, and annual vaccination against influenza.

Advocate (2): someone who acts on behalf of, or intercedes for, the client. Advocates ensure that clients receive necessary care and services.

Agent (6): a factor, such as a microorganism, chemical substance, or form of radiation, whose presence, excessive presence, or (in deficiency diseases) relative absence is essential for the occurrence of a disease.

Agoraphobia (15): literally, fear of the marketplace or open places. About one third of all people who experience panic attacks eventually develop agoraphobia. Persons with agoraphobia frequently progress to the point where they cannot leave their homes without experiencing anxiety.

Alzheimer's disease (12): a degenerative mental disorder characterized by progressive brain deterioration, resulting in impaired memory and changes in thought patterns and behaviors. Approximately 4 million Americans have Alzheimer's disease, and it is a leading cause of death among adults.

Ambulatory care (3): personal health care or health services (e.g., outpatient surgery and chemotherapy, diagnostic tests, and procedures) provided to noninstitutionalized patients. Ambulatory care includes care, procedures, and services provided in settings such as home, work, church, and school.

American Red Cross (ARC) (14): a voluntary support agency founded in 1881 by Clara Barton. The ARC has more than 1300 local chapters throughout the United States and provides disaster relief services to people around the clock.

Ambulatory nursing practice (3): refers to provision of comprehensive nursing care for individuals or families in community-based settings. Ambulatory nursing care is largely focused on health promotion, primary prevention, screening for early identification of disease, and assisting in treatment regimens for both acute and chronic illnesses (e.g., colds, influenza, ear infection, hypertension, diabetes).

Ambulatory oncology nursing practice (3): is nursing care provided in oncology clinics, physician's offices, and 23-hour and 24-hour clinics and day hospitals. Ambulatory oncology nursing practice includes patient counseling, health care maintenance, primary care, patient education, therapeutic care, normative care, nonclient-centered care, and telephone triage.

Ambulatory surgery (3): refers to the process in which patients have surgery, recover, and are discharged home the same day. Nurses who work in outpatient surgical centers may provide preoperative care, intraoperative care, or postanesthesia care.

Anemia screening (9): recommended routine screening of hemoglobin or hematocrit levels during infancy (6-9 months) and early childhood to detect iron deficiency anemia. Screening for adolescent females is also recommended.

Anorexia nervosa (15): eating disorder that occurs when a person becomes obsessed with a fear of fat and with losing weight. Anorexia nervosa usually begins in early adolescence and often develops with a fairly gradual decrease in caloric intake. However, the decrease in caloric intake continues until the anorexic is consuming almost nothing.

Anxiety disorders (15): a group of mental disorders characterized by feelings of severe anxiety, resulting symptoms, and efforts to avoid those symptoms. Anxiety disorders are the most common of all of the mental disorders, affecting as many as 13% of the general population at any time. Some of the more commonly encountered anxiety disorders are generalized anxiety disorder (GAD), panic disorder, phobias, obsessive-compulsive disorder, and posttraumatic stress disorder (PTSD).

Assisted reproduction technology (11): therapies that have been developed to treat infertility. Some of the available options include in vitro fertilization, gamete intrafallopian transfer (GIFT), zygote intrafallopian transfer, donor ovum transfer, donor embryo, and therapeutic donor insemination.

Atmospheric quality (7): the purity of the air available for breathing purposes. Atmospheric quality is threatened by air pollutants such as ozone, carbon monoxide, nitrogen dioxide, particulates, sulfur dioxide, and lead, which can cause lung damage, inflammatory responses, and respiratory symptoms.

Attention deficit hyperactivity disorder (15): affects 3% to 5% of all children and is characterized by inattention, hyperactivity, and impulsivity.

B

Behavioral therapy (15): use of learning principles to change thought patterns and behaviors systematically. Behavior therapy is used to encourage the individual to learn specific skills to obtain rewards and satisfaction. Stress management, biofeedback, and relaxation training are examples of behavior therapy.

Blended family (13): a family that is comprised of one divorced or widowed adult with all or some of his or her children and a new spouse with all or some of his or her children; may include the children born to this union so that parents, stepparents, children, and stepchildren or stepsiblings live together.

Bottle mouth syndrome (9): destruction of teeth in older infants and toddlers who are allowed to fall asleep with a bottle of formula or milk or another sweetened fluid in their mouth.

Breast cancer (11): the most common cancer among women in the United States (excluding skin cancer) and the second leading cause of cancer deaths in women. In the United States a woman's average lifetime risk for developing breast cancer is approximately one in eight.

Breastfeeding (11): the recommended sole form of infant feeding for the first 5 to 6 months. Benefits and advantages of breastfeeding include that it is more economical and convenient and provides a number of health benefits to both mother and infant.

Bulimia nervosa (15): eating disorder characterized by binge eating and "purging" (self-induced vomiting, use of laxatives, diuretics, fasting, and excessive exercise) to prevent weight gain.

C

Capitation (5): in managed care, capitation describes a negotiated, prepaid fixed fee for each covered individual or family. For the capitation fee, the managed care organization agrees to provide the services for which the contract calls, for a specified time period.

Carbon monoxide (7): a colorless, odorless gas that results from burning of fossil fuels. More than 200 deaths each year are caused by accidental carbon monoxide poisoning.

Care assistance (12): professional or institutional residential facilities that provide services for about 5% of older Americans. Care assistance arrangements for older adults include nursing homes, home health agencies, adult day care providers, and respite care providers. Care assistance is temporary in some cases and permanent in others.

Carrier (6): a person or animal without apparent disease who harbors a specific infectious agent and is capable of transmitting the agent to others.

Case management (4): the process of identifying needs for and arranging, coordinating, monitoring, and evaluating quality, cost-effective, primary, secondary, and tertiary prevention services to achieve designated health outcomes. In case management one professional is responsible for assessing needs, targeting services to meet the needs, and monitoring and evaluating client status to ensure that needs are met adequately.

Child abuse (9): any physical or mental injury, sexual abuse or exploitation, negligent treatment or maltreatment of a child by a person who is responsible for the child's welfare.

Child safety (9): includes efforts to protect children from injury. Potential threats targeted by childhood safety measures include motor vehicle accidents, bicycle accidents, violence, poisoning, drowning, burns, sports-related accidents, asphyxiation, and falls.

Chlorofluorocarbons (CFCs) (7): gases that are found in refrigerants, aerosols, and some solvent cleaning agents and are theorized to contribute to stratospheric ozone depletion.

Cognitive impairment (12): mental impairment that is common among older individuals and often increases with age. An estimated 5% to 10% of individuals older than 65 years of age and almost 50% of those over 85 years of age experience some degree of cognitive impairment. Alzheimer's disease, vascular infarctions, and pharmaceuticals are frequently implicated as inducing cognitive changes.

Cohort (6): a well-defined group of people who have had a common experience or exposure, who are then followed up for the incidence of new diseases or events, as in a cohort or prospective study.

Coinsurance (5): a predetermined amount or percentage of the cost of covered services that the beneficiary will pay. The coinsurance may be an agreed-on percentage of the fee or the balance of the total for fixed price services.

Collaborator (2): someone who participates in the process of making decisions regarding health care management with individuals from various professions. Collaborators work with the client and the family or caregivers to jointly determine the course of care.

Common source outbreak (point source) (6): an outbreak that results from a group of persons being exposed to a common noxious influence, such as an infectious agent or toxin. If the group is exposed over a relatively brief time, so that all cases occur within one incubation period, then the common source outbreak is further classified as a point source outbreak.

Community-based nursing (1): the application of the nursing process in caring for individuals and families in community settings. Community-based nursing emphasizes all levels of prevention (i.e., primary, secondary, and tertiary), but focuses more on secondary and tertiary levels. Home health nursing and nursing in outpatient or ambulatory settings are examples of community-based nursing.

Community health nursing (1): a synthesis of nursing practice and public health practice applied to promoting and preserving the health of populations. Community health nursing practice is continuous and comprehensive and considers the impact of the environment on health. Public health nursing, school nursing, and occupational health nursing are examples of community health nursing.

Conditions of participation (4): regulations that must be met by home health care agencies to be eligible for Medicare reimbursement. Conditions of participation consist of explicit rules and standards that outline requirements for virtually all aspects of home health care and detail such areas as personnel qualifications, notifying patients of their rights, acceptance of patients, plan of care, medical supervision, types of services offered by the agency, and the duties of each service provider.

Contraception (11): actions or interventions to prevent pregnancy. Several methods of contraception are available including abstinence, barriers (e.g., condoms, diaphragm), hormonal methods (e.g., oral contraceptives, Depo-Provera, Norplant), intrauterine devices (IUDs), sterilization, and natural family planning.

Coordination of community resources (4): requires the nurse to be knowledgeable about services offered by his or her own agency and any resources available in the community that would benefit clients. To coordinate care, the nurse must understand the referral process; determine if the client is eligible for the services offered by the agency or organization; have an understanding of how to refer a client for a particular service; know the costs of services and payment mechanism; and be aware of the location, telephone number, hours of operation, and contact person.

Copayment (5): a specified flat fee per unit of service or time that the individual pays and the insurer pays the remaining costs.

Correctional nursing (3): is the provision of primary care and emergency services for inmates in correctional facilities. Correctional nursing typically includes screening activities; direct health care services; analysis of individual health behaviors; and teaching, counseling, and assisting individuals in assuming responsibility for their own health.

Counselor (2): a professional who listens to clients and their families and encourages them to explore issues and options. Counselors assist with identification of problems and possible solutions and provide guidance through the problem-solving process.

Crude mortality rate (6): the mortality rate from all causes of death for a population.

Cultural blindness (8): failure to acknowledge or respect cultural differences and behaving as though they do not exist.

Culture (8): the knowledge, beliefs, art, morals, laws, and other capabilities and habits acquired by man as a member of society. Culture includes nonphysical traits, such as values, attitudes, and customs that are shared by a group of people and passed from one generation to the next. Culture provides the organizational structure or basis for behavior within the group.

Culture shock (8): feelings of bewilderment, confusion, disorganization, frustration, and stupidity, and the inability to adapt to differences in language and word meanings, activities, time, and customs that are part of the new culture.

D

Deductible (5): a sum that must be paid each calendar year before the insurance policy becomes active. Deductible amounts vary greatly, from almost nothing to several thousand dollars.

Depression (15): mental illness that affects almost 19 million people in the United States each year. The most prevalent types of depression are major depression, dysthymia, and bipolar disorder.

Developmental screening (9): monitoring the progression of infants, children, and adolescents through developmental tasks. Assessment of developmental level can be accomplished by using screening tools, a thorough history, physical assessment, and/or direct observation.

Diagnosis-related group (DRG) (5): a classification system that groups patients into categories based on the coding system of the International Classification of Disease, Ninth Revision-Clinical Modification (ICD-9-CM). DRGs are used to establish health care payments under Medicare.

Direct care provider (2): a professional who is involved in the direct delivery of care. This role includes performing tasks or skills for which the nurse has been trained and that are typically associated with nursing practice (e.g., client assessment, taking vital signs, medication administration, changing dressings, and inserting catheters).

Direct transmission (16): transmission of a disease-causing organism through physical contact including biting, kissing, and touching or sexual contact. Airborne transmission through dust and droplet and droplet nuclei may also be direct.

Disability (14): any restriction on or lack of ability to perform an activity in a normal manner or within the normal range, which results from a physical or psychological limitation. Limitations in functional activities, activities of daily living (ADL) and instrumental activities of daily living (IADL) determine disability.

Disaster (14): any event that causes destruction and devastation that cannot be alleviated without assistance. Disasters may be the result of "natural" occurrences (e.g., hurricanes, tornadoes, floods, droughts) or they may be "man-made" (e.g., war, terrorism, civil disasters, accidents).

Discharge planning (4): the process of determining and planning to meet client needs following release from a health care facility. Discharge planning ensures that the client and family needs are identified and evaluated, with responsibility for meeting those needs being transferred to the client, the client's caregiver or significant others, or other health care providers.

Discrimination (8): the differential treatment of individuals because they belong to a minority group; denying equal opportunity by acting on a prejudice.

Disempowerment (14): the loss of power or control over one's circumstances.

Disenfranchisement (14): a feeling of separation from mainstream society in which the individual does not have an emotional connection with any group in particular, or the larger social fabric in general.

Distribution (6): the frequency and pattern of health-related characteristics and events in a population.

Domestic violence (11): pattern of abusive behavior perpetrated by someone who is or was in an intimate relationship with the victim. Domestic violence is the major cause of injury to women.

Dominant value orientation (8): the basic value orientation that is shared by the majority of its members as a result of early common experiences.

E

Early and Periodic Screening, Diagnosis and Treatment Program (EPSDT) (9): a comprehensive and preventive health care program for Medicaid-eligible individuals up to age 21. Services provided by EPSDT include a comprehensive health and developmental history; a comprehensive unclothed physical examination; designated laboratory tests; appropriate immunizations; health education; dental, hearing, and vision services; and any other necessary health care to correct or ameliorate illnesses and conditions found during screenings.

Ecomap (13): a tool that can be used to explain a family's linkages to their suprasystems or the larger environment. The ecomap visually illustrates the dynamic family-environment interactions and shows the connections between the family and the world.

Education for All Handicapped Children Act (PL 94-142) (3): law enacted by Congress in 1975 that gives all students between the ages of 3 and 18 years the right to a free and appropriate public education in the least restrictive environment possible, regardless of physical or mental disabilities. Handicapping conditions covered by this Act include auditory impairment, visually handicapped, mentally retarded, orthopedically impaired, seriously emotionally disturbed (e.g., inability to build interpersonal relationships, inappropriate behavior or feelings, depression), and specific learning disability (e.g., dyslexia).

Educator (2): a nurse who teaches individuals, families, and groups about maintenance of health, threats to health, and relevant lifestyle choices that affect health. The information presented should allow clients to make informed decisions on health matters and to direct self-care to follow treatment regimens.

Elder abuse (12): neglect, physical injury, or exploitation that results in harm to an older adult. Elder abuse can take one of several forms including physical abuse, confinement, psychological or emotional abuse, financial or material abuse, neglect, or abandonment.

Emergency contraception (11): use of high doses of standard birth control pills as postcoital contraception or "morning after pills." Emergency contraception averts pregnancy by prevention of ovulation or prevention of fertilization of the egg or transportation of the egg to the uterus.

Emerging infectious diseases (16): those diseases whose incidence in humans has increased within the past two decades or threatens to increase in the near future. Emerging infections can be new or previously unrecognized infectious diseases, reemerging diseases, or infectious diseases that have developed resistance to previously effective antimicrobial drugs. Examples of emerging infections include New Variant Creutzfeldt-Jakob Disease (nvCJD), virulent strain of influenza, foodborne outbreaks including outbreaks caused by *Cyclospora* parasites, hepatitis A virus, and *Escherichia coli* 0157:H7 bacteria, and multidrug-resistant tuberculosis–strain W.

Enculturation (acculturation) (8): the process of becoming a member of a cultural group; adapting to another culture.

Endemic disease (6): the constant presence of a disease or infectious agent within a given geographical area or population group; it may also refer to the usual prevalence of a given disease within such an area or a group.

Enterostomal care (4): directs nursing interventions specifically related to wound care and specialized care for clients with a colostomy, an ileostomy, or a urostomy. Enterostomal care involves assessment of the wound and evaluation of the efficacy of treatment, cleaning, and debridement and includes obtaining cultures and teaching the patient and/or caregiver how to change the dressing using sterile techniques.

Epidemic disease (6): the occurrence of more cases of disease than expected in a given area or among a specific group of people over a particular period.

Epidemiology (6): the study of the distribution and determinants of health-related states or events in a specified population, and the application of this study to the control of health problems.

Ethnic group (8): designated or basic division of groups of individuals distinguished by customs, characteristics, or language; group of persons who possess common physical and mental traits as a result of heredity, cultural traditions, language, customs, and common history.

Ethnicity (8): a classification of individuals based on a shared culture or affiliation, values, perceptions, feelings, and assumptions.

Ethnocentrism (8): the belief that one's own group is superior to others.

Extended family (13): a family comprised of a nuclear family plus other relatives of one or both spouses; relatives may or may not live with the nuclear family and may include great-grandparents and great-great-grandparents.

F

Family (13): social units or systems comprised of two or more persons in a committed relationship. The family provides protection, nourishment, and socialization for family members.

Family assessment (13): the basic step for promoting the health of a family. A family health assessment may help the nurse identify the health status of individual members of the family and aspects of family composition, function, and process.

Family crisis (13): serious problems experienced in all families. There are two basic types of family crises, the maturational crisis and the situational crisis. A maturational crisis is a normal transition point (e.g., adolescence, marriage, parenthood) when old patterns of communication and old roles must be exchanged for new patterns and roles. A situational crisis can occur when the family experiences an event that is sudden, unexpected, and unpredictable and may lead to disorganization, tension, and severe anxiety. Examples of situational crises include illness, accidents, death, and natural disasters.

Family health tree (13): a method to record pertinent data about a family's medical and health histories. The family health tree typically includes causes of death of deceased family members, genetically linked diseases (i.e., heart disease, cancer, diabetes, hypertension, sickle cell anemia, allergies, asthma), environmental and occupational diseases, psychosocial problems (i.e., mental illness), obesity, and infectious disease.

Family planning services (11): health care and counseling that provides women and men information and care they need to make informed choices about whether and when to become parents. Comprehensive family planning includes consideration of a number of factors regarding childbearing, adoption, use of contraceptives, natural family planning, treatment of infertility, and preconception counseling.

Family roles (13): socially expected behavior patterns that are determined by a person's position or status. In families, roles are the assigned or assumed parts that members play during day-to-day living; they are bestowed and defined by the family.

Federal Emergency Management Agency (FEMA) (14): the federal agency that assesses and responds to disaster events in the United States; responsibilities include emergency planning, preparedness, mitigation, response, and recovery.

Foodborne pathogens (7): microbiological contamination of food that is usually caused by improper storage, handling, and/or preparation of food. Several foodborne pathogens have been cited as being of primary concern with regard to foodborne illnesses. These include *Salmonella, Campylobacter, Escherichia coli* 0157:H7, and *Listeria monocytogenes.*

Functional independence (12): the extent to which the individual is able to complete "normal" and "instrumental" activities of daily living without assistance from others.

G

Gatekeeper (5): The primary care physician within managed care plans is frequently referred to as the "gatekeeper." Usually the gatekeeper is a family practitioner, internist, pediatrician, or gynecologist who is responsible for all primary care for the enrolled patient. To avoid duplication of services and overuse of specialists, the gatekeeper coordinates all care and determines when to refer the client to a specialist.

Genogram (13): a tool that helps the nurse outline or diagram the family's structure to view family patterns. The genogram details births, deaths, divorces, and remarriages and may also identify other characteristics (race, social class), occupations, and places of family residence.

H

Hazardous waste (7): approximately 10% of industrial wastes, which include poisons, inflammable materials, infectious contaminants, explosives, and radionuclides. Some of the most common hazardous wastes include lead, mercury, polychlorinated biphenyls [PCBs], chromium, trichlorolorethane or trichloroethylene, and benzene. Medical waste, including cultures, items contaminated with human blood and blood products, contaminated animal carcasses, wastes from patients isolated with highly communicable diseases, and all used sharps are also hazardous wastes.

Head Start (9): a federally funded, comprehensive preschool program for children who are at risk for academic problems associated with poverty and lack of sufficient social stimulation. Low-income children 3 to 5 years of age are eligible for Head Start programs.

Health maintenance organization (HMO) (5): a managed care organization that contracts with an individual, group, or organization to provide health care for enrollees. The HMO agrees to provide a set of services for a set fee (typically a capitated fee). HMOs attempt to provide services to clients at a cost lower than the fee paid and thereby profit by delivering less costly care and less total services and by minimizing referrals to other providers. HMOs provide care to clients with no or minimal deductibles and copayments.

Health promotion (10): activities or actions related to encouraging individual lifestyles or personal choices that positively influence health (e.g., encouraging physical activity and fitness, good nutrition, substance abuse prevention).

Healthy People 2010 (1): the national prevention initiative of the U.S. Department of Health and Human Services (USDHHS). *Healthy People 2010* has two goals (1) to increase quality and years of healthy life for United States residents and (2) to eliminate health disparities. There are 467 objectives divided among 28 focus areas, and the objectives may be used as framework to guide health-promotion activities in schools, clinics, worksites, and for community-wide initiatives.

Hearing deficit (12): some degree of hearing impairment that may affect up to 33% of individuals aged 65 years and over. The most common types of hearing loss and associated factors are presbycusis (slow decline in hearing ability), tinnitis, conductive hearing loss, and sensorineural hearing loss.

Hearing screening (9): early detection of hearing disorders. Hearing screening includes questioning to determine auditory responsiveness and speech and language development, physical examination to detect abnormalities of the ear canal and tympanic membrane, and pure-tone audiometry testing. Individuals with abnormal results should be referred to a specialist for further testing and treatment.

Herd immunity (6): the resistance of a group to invasion and spread of an infectious agent, based on the resistance to infection of a high proportion of individual members of the group.

Homeless (14): a person who regularly sleeps in a supervised shelter, an institution that provides a temporary residence, or in a public or private place not designated for sleeping.

Home health care (4): that component of health care in which services are provided to individuals and families in their places of residence for the purpose of promoting, maintaining, or restoring health, or maximizing the level of independence, while minimizing the effects of disability and illness.

Home health care nursing (4): integrates medical/surgical, community health, parent-child, gerontological, and psychiatric–mental health nursing into home health care practice. It refers to comprehensive nursing care provided to individuals and families in their place of residence, focusing on the environmental, psychosocial, economic, cultural, and personal health factors affecting health status.

Hospice care (4): palliative care provided to the terminally ill; it is frequently provided in the home. Hospice care focuses on the family and the patient and provides assistance in dealing with emotional, spiritual, and medical problems; coordinating professional and volunteer services; and making the patient as comfortable as possible through pain and symptom management.

Host (6): a person or other living organism that can be infected by an infectious agent under natural conditions.

I

Illness prevention (10): lessening or removal of risk factors for specific diseases and early identification of diseases through screening and prompt remediation.

Immunity (16): protection from infectious disease. There are two basic mechanisms for acquiring immunity—active and passive.

Immunization schedule (16): recommended immunizations for infants and children. Includes a schedule of 11 childhood vaccines by age 18 months including four doses of DTP, three doses of polio vaccine, one dose of MMR, three or four doses of HIB conjugate vaccine, three doses of hepatitis B vaccine, one dose of varicella vaccine and four doses of pneumococcal vaccine. Booster of DTP, polio, and MMR are given to older children.

Impairment (14): an anatomical, mental, or psychological loss or another abnormality that results in an individual experiencing deviation from normal structure, function, or development.

Incidence rate (6): a measure of the frequency with which an event, such as a new case of illness, occurs in a population over a period. The denominator is the population at risk; the numerator is the number of new cases occurring during a given time.

Incontinence (12): the involuntary loss of urine. Incontinence is a significant cause of disability and dependency in older adults contributing to social isolation, embarrassment, feelings of loss of control, and low self-esteem.

Independent practice association (5): a managed care model in which the fiscal agent contracts with a range of physicians who are not associated with each other and work in independent practices to provide services on a capitated basis.

Indirect transmission (16): the transmission of an agent carried from a reservoir to a susceptible host by suspended air particles or by animate (vector) or inanimate (vehicle) intermediaries.

Indoor biological contaminants (7): may result from contaminated central air and heating units that become breeding grounds for mold, mildew, bacteria, viruses, dust mites, and other potential health threats. Biological contaminates can trigger allergic reactions including asthma and spread infectious illnesses (i.e., colds, influenza, and chicken pox).

Infant care (11): information needed by parents related to the care of newborns. Infant care includes feeding, bathing, cord care, stooling and voiding patterns, dressing and diapering, sleeping, and observing for problems.

Infertility (11): the inability to conceive after 1 year of regular sexual intercourse without contraception. In women, the most common causes of infertility are problems in ovulation, blocked or scarred fallopian tubes, and endometriosis. In men, abnormal or too few sperm is the most frequent cause of infertility.

Infusion therapy (4): refers to the delivery of antibiotics, pain medication, total parenteral nutrition, hydration, and chemotherapy in the home.

Instrumental activities of daily living (IADL) (12): the ability to perform necessary functions of life, such as taking transportation, preparing meals, shopping, managing money, routine housework, and using the telephone.

Intentional food additives (7): those substances added to food during processing to enhance the nutritional content, improve flavor, enhance color, improve consistency, or increase the shelf life.

Interdisciplinary collaboration (4): involves initiation and maintenance of a collegial and collaborative relationship with all health care providers working with the client. Professionals involved in interdisciplinary collaboration for health care planning and delivery include nurses, physicians, physical therapists, occupational therapists, speech therapists/speech pathologists, social workers, registered dietitians/nutritionists, home health aides, pharmacists, phlebotomists, laboratory technicians, respiratory therapists, enterostomal therapists, chaplains, and massage therapists.

L

Leader (2): an individual with the ability to influence the behavior of others. Nurse leaders work with others to identify and assess threats to health and to intervene to remove or lessen these threats.

Lead poisoning (7): excessive levels of lead in the blood. Lead poisoning in children can adversely affect intelligence, behavior, and development. Lead-based paint in homes and buildings built before 1960 has been identified as the major source of lead poisoning. Anemia, central nervous system disorders, and renal involvement may result from lead exposure.

M

Managed care (5): the "umbrella," or generic, term that describes a variety of prepaid and managed fee-for-service health care plans. Managed care plans are designed to encourage greater control over the use and cost of health care services through (1) providing incentives to contain costs, (2) providing barriers to inappropriate use of specialists, (3) administrative management of the use of services, and (4) facilitating the paperwork required on the part of consumers.

Manager (2): role that includes planning, organizing, coordinating, marketing, controlling, and evaluating care and care delivery. The role includes management of time, available resources, other personnel, and program organization and coordination, in addition to management of the client's care.

Marginalization (14): persons who are marginalized live on the "margins" or edges of society rather than in the mainstream; marginalization limits control and power.

Medicaid (5): a national and state-sponsored public assistance (welfare) health program. Enacted by Title XIX of the Social Security Act of 1965, Medicaid is financed jointly by the states and federal government, with the federal contributions matching 50% to 77% of state contributions.

Medicare (5): a national health insurance plan begun in 1965 under Title XVIII of the Social Security Act. Those eligible for Medicare are (1) persons 65 years of age and older, (2) disabled individuals who are entitled to Social Security benefits, and (3) end-stage renal disease patients. Medicare uses indirect financing and service delivery administered by the Centers for Medicare and Medicaid Services (CMS) (formerly known as the HCFA) branch of the U.S. Department of Health and Human Services (USDHHS), which contracts with independent providers.

Mental health (15): a state of successful performance of mental function, resulting in productive activities, fulfilling relationships with other people, and the ability to adapt to change and to cope with adversity. Mental health refers not only to the absence of mental disorders but also to the ability of an individual to negotiate daily challenges and social interactions of life without experiencing cognitive, emotional, or behavioral dysfunction.

Mental illness (15): maladaptive responses to distress and an inability to mobilize resources. The mentally ill person is often dependent, has low self-esteem, and has difficulty forming interpersonal relationships.

Migrant health centers (MHCs) (14): health clinics funded by the Migrant Health Act (1962) that serve migrant and agricultural workers and families. MHCs typically offer environmental health services (e.g., rodent control, field sanitation, sewage treatment), infectious and parasitic disease screening and control, and accident prevention programs.

Migrant workers (14): individuals whose principal employment is in agriculture on a seasonal basis and who establish a temporary residence for such employment while traveling from location to location.

Minority group (8): a segment of the population that differs from the majority based on physical or cultural characteristics.

Morbidity rate (6): a measure of the frequency of occurrence of disease in a defined population during a specified time interval.

Mortality rate (6): a measure of the frequency of occurrence of death in a defined population during a specified time interval.

N

Natural history of disease (6): the temporal course of disease from onset (inception) to resolution.

Newborn screening (9): state mandated requirement that all newborns be tested for congenital diseases. Tests are conducted for hypothyroidism, phenylketonuria, galactosemia, hemoglobinopathies (e.g., sickle cell disease, thalassemia), maple syrup urine disease, congenital adrenal hyperplasia, cystic fibrosis, and other conditions.

Norms (8): the rules by which human behavior is governed that are the result of the cultural values held by the group.

Nuclear dyad (13): husband and wife or other couple living alone without children.

Nuclear family (13): mother, father, and child(ren) living together but apart from both sets of the father's and mother's parents; the nuclear family is composed of a married husband and wife and children. The children may be either biological offspring or adopted.

Nursing Interventions Classification (NIC) system (2): a taxonomy of more than 480 nursing interventions that have been defined and developed to include examples of appropriate nursing activities (behaviors or actions that implement the intervention). The identified nursing interventions are divided into seven "domains": (1) physiological: basic (care that supports physical functioning), (2) physiological: complex (care that supports homeostatic regulation), (3) behavioral (care that supports psychosocial functioning and facilitates lifestyle changes), (4) safety (care that supports protection against harm), (5) family (care that supports the family unit), (6) health system (care that supports effective use of the health care delivery system), and (7) community (care that supports the health of the community).

Nutrition guidelines (10): recommendations to help achieve and maintain a healthy weight. General nutrition guidelines for a healthy diet include eating a variety of foods; balancing the food with physical activity to maintain or improve weight; choosing a diet low in fat, saturated fat, and cholesterol; choosing a diet that is moderate in sugars, salt, and sodium; and drinking only in moderation. Also, women should consume adequate calcium and folic acid.

O

Obesity (10): weight 20% or more above desirable weight. Obesity is associated with hypertension, type 2 diabetes, hypercholesterolemia, coronary artery disease, some types of cancer, gallbladder disease, arthritis, sleep apnea, and stroke.

Obsessive-compulsive disorder (15): mental disorder in which an individual is overcome with the urge to engage in some ritual to avoid a persistent frightening thought, idea, image, or event—the obsession. Compulsions are the rituals or behaviors repeatedly performed to prevent, neutralize, or dispel the dreaded obsession. When the individual tries to resist the compulsion, anxiety increases. Common compulsions include handwashing, counting, checking, or touching.

Occupational health nursing (3): the specialty nursing practice that focuses on promotion, prevention, and restoration of health within the context of a safe and healthy work environment. It includes the prevention of adverse health effects from occupational and environmental hazards and provides for and delivers occupational and environmental health and safety services to workers and worker populations.

Occupational health risks (7): workplace risks and hazards related to use of heavy equipment, exposure to chemicals and biohazards, sunlight, cold, and noise, and potential for assault or violence. Occupations with relatively higher rates of occupational risk include mining, logging, agriculture, construction, manufacturing, trucking, and warehousing.

Occupational Safety and Health Act (3): federal legalization passed in 1970 to promote safe and healthful working conditions and to preserve human resources. Among other things, the Occupational Safety and Health Act formed the Occupational Safety and Health Administration (OSHA), which sets and enforces standards of occupational safety and health; formed the National Institute for Occupational Safety and Health (NIOSH), which researches and recommends occupational safety and health standards to OSHA and funds educational centers for the training of occupational health professionals; established federal occupational safety and health standards; and created a mechanism for imposition of fines and other punitive measures for violation of federal occupational safety and health regulations.

Osteoporosis (11): skeletal disease characterized by decreased bone mass, which leads to increased skeletal fragility and subsequent tendency to fracture. Osteoporosis affects about 8 million U.S. residents, including an estimated 18% of women older than 50 years and 90% of women older than 75.

Outbreak (6): synonymous with epidemic. It is sometimes the preferred word because it may escape sensationalism associated with the word epidemic. Alternatively, an epidemic may be referred to as localized as opposed to generalized.

Ozone (7): gas that occurs in two layers in the atmosphere. In the stratosphere, ozone acts to shield the earth from harmful effects of ultraviolet radiation given off by the sun. But, at ground level, high concentrations of ozone are a major health concern because ozone is one of the primary problem gases in air pollution.

Ozone depletion (7): refers to evidence that the Earth's stratospheric ozone layer is being destroyed by chlorofluorocarbons (CFCs). Theoretically, radiation from the sun elicits a chemical reaction between the CFCs and ozone resulting in thinning of the ozone layer.

P

Pandemic (6): an epidemic occurring over a very wide area (several countries or continents) and usually affecting a large proportion of the population.

Panic disorder (15): mental disorder in which individuals progressively experience anxiety attacks. Often the first attack or cluster of attacks follows a variety of life stresses. The initial attack may occur suddenly and unexpectedly while the patient is performing everyday tasks. During an anxiety attack the individual experiences tachycardia; dyspnea; dizziness; chest pain; nausea; numbness or tingling of the hands and feet; trembling or shaking; sweating; choking; or a feeling that he or she is going to die, go crazy, or do something uncontrolled. A diagnosis of panic disorder is made when attacks occur with some degree of frequency or regularity.

Parish nursing (3): nursing care that serves to promote the health of a faith community (churches or synagogues) through working with the pastor and staff to integrate the theological, psychological, sociological, and physiological perspectives of health and healing into the work, sacrament, and services of the congregation. Parish nursing interventions include organization of support groups, provision of referrals to community resources, health education, counseling, and acting as a liaison within the larger health care system.

Passive immunity (16): protection against a communicable disease produced by an animal or human and transferred to another human. Passive immunity often provides effective protection, but this protection wanes over time—usually a few weeks or months. Examples of passive immunity include transplacental transfer of immunity from a mother to her infant and injection of constituents of blood products from human donors (e.g., homologous pooled human antibody, immune globulin).

Perinatal home care (4): care for pregnant and postpartum clients in the home. Perinatal home care includes technologically advanced care for high-risk pregnancies (e.g., uterine monitoring, fetal monitoring, ultrasound, infusion therapy, and hypertension monitoring) and care for neonates with complications (e.g., apnea monitoring). Postpartum care for uncomplicated clients following shortened hospital stays is also a component.

Phobias (15): an irrational fear of something (an object or situation). As many as 8% of Americans are affected by phobias at any given time. Adults with phobias realize their fears are irrational, but facing the feared object or situation might bring on severe anxiety or a panic attack.

Physical activity and fitness (10): regular exercise to promote health. Physical activity helps control blood lipid abnormalities, diabetes, and obesity and can help lower blood pressure. In addition, regular activity helps control weight, increases lean body mass, decreases body fat percentage, produces relief from some symptoms of depression, improves flexibility, increases muscle strength and endurance, and increases bone density.

Polypharmacy (12): the prescribing of multiple drugs for a patient; commonly occurs among older people. Both prescription and nonprescription medications contribute to problems encountered in polypharmacy.

Posttraumatic stress disorder (PTSD) (15): a debilitating condition that follows a terrifying event. Individuals with PTSD have recurring, persistent, frightening thoughts and memories of their ordeal. Traumatic incidents that trigger PTSD may have threatened that individual's life or the life of someone else. Incidents include "shell shock" or "battle fatigue" common to war veterans, violent attack (e.g., kidnapping, rape, mugging), serious accidents, or natural disasters (e.g., earthquake, tornado) or witnessing mass destruction or injury, such as after an airplane crash.

Poverty (14): to have few or no material possessions and to have inadequate access to family and community resources.

Poverty threshold (14): a predetermined index established yearly by the Census Bureau, which provides a set of income thresholds that vary by family size and composition to determine who is poor. If a family's total income is less than the federally defined poverty threshold, then that family is considered poor. In 2000, the poverty threshold for a family of four with two children was $17,463.

Preferred provider organizations (PPOs) (5): business arrangements or contracts between a panel of health care providers, usually hospitals and physicians, and purchasers of health care services (e.g., self-insured employers or health insurance companies). The providers agree to supply services to a defined group of patients on a discounted fee-for-service basis. In PPOs, the organization, usually a health insurer, contracts to provide health services for a set fee using selected physicians. The physician agrees to the fee structure of the PPO in return for the PPO providing patients.

Prejudice (8): a hostile attitude toward individuals because they belong to a particular racial or ethnic group presumed to have objectionable qualities; negative beliefs or preferences that are generalized about a group that leads to "prejudgment."

Prenatal care (11): health care for pregnant women, which reduces complications of pregnancy and promotes a healthy delivery and infant. Prenatal care should include initial and ongoing risk assessment, individualized care based on case management principles, nutritional counseling, education to reduce or eliminate unhealthy habits, stress reduction, social support services, and health education.

Preparedness (14): predicator planning, which is key to effective disaster management. Preparedness includes attempts to forecast events, engineering to reduce risks, public education about potential hazards, and developing a coordinated emergency response plan. Responsibility for disaster planning is shared by the local, state, federal, and voluntary agencies.

Prevalence (prevalence rate) (6): The proportion of persons in a population who have a particular disease or attribute at a specified point in time or over a specified period of time.

Primary health care (1): health promotion and illness prevention activities, such as well child checkups, routine physical examinations, prenatal care, and diagnosis and treatment of common acute or episodic illnesses. Primary health care is traditionally conducted in convenient, community-based settings.

Propagated outbreak (6): an outbreak that does not have a common source but instead spreads from person to person.

Psychiatric home care (4): home care provided for individuals with diagnoses of suspected mental illnesses who need psychiatric services but cannot use traditional outpatient mental health services. Psychiatric home care can prevent hospitalization for clients with diagnoses such as severe depression, schizophrenia, and Alzheimer's disease.

Psychotherapeutic medications (15): are used to treat mental illnesses by controlling symptoms. As with medications for physical health problems, the appropriateness of psychotherapeutic medications and their prescribed regimen depends on the diagnosis, side effects, and patient response. Psychotherapeutic medications include antipsychotics, antimanic medications, anticonvulsants, antidepressants, antianxiety agents, and stimulants.

Psychotherapy (15): treatment for mental disorders that relies primarily on structured conversation aimed at changing a patient's attitudes, feelings, beliefs, defenses, personality, and behavior. In psychotherapy, the therapist's procedures vary across schools of psychotherapy and with the nature of the patient's problem. Various types of psychotherapy include individual or interpersonal therapy, family therapy, couple therapy, group therapy, play therapy, and cognitive therapy.

Public health nursing (3): refers to nursing practice in public health departments. The focus of public health nursing often includes prevention and control of communicable diseases through provision of immunizations; provision of easily accessible (affordable) treatment for sexually transmitted diseases (STDs); and screening, diagnosis, and treatment of certain communicable diseases (e.g., tuberculosis, AIDS, and Hansen's disease). In addition, many public health departments provide prenatal and family planning services, well-baby care, community mental health services, and home health care.

Q

Qualifications for home care (4): Medicare requirements for coverage of home health care services. To qualify for Medicare reimbursement (1) the person to whom the services are provided must be eligible for Medicare; (2) services must be "reasonable and necessary" in relation to the patient's health status and medical needs; (3) the client's care must require intermittent skilled nursing care, physical therapy, or speech therapy; (4) the client must be homebound; (5) the client must be under the care of a physician who develops and monitors a home health plan; and (6) the home health agency must be certified to participate in Medicare.

R

Race (8): classification or grouping of humans primarily based on physical characteristics (e.g., skin color, hair color and texture, eye shape and color, height). Anthropologically, individuals from a given race have a common geographic origin of their ancestors.

Racism (8): excessive belief in the superiority of one's own racial group.

Radon (7): a colorless, odorless, radioactive gas resulting from the natural breakdown (radioactive decay) of uranium. Radon enters buildings through cracks in solid floors, construction joints, and other ways, and dangerously high levels can be found in many homes.

Reportable diseases (16): those communicable diseases that require notification of authorities whenever encountered by a health care professional. There are a large number of reportable diseases and they include AIDS, anthrax, hepatitis A, hepatitis B, most vaccine preventable diseases, STDs, malaria, and Lyme disease.

Researcher (2): a professional who identifies problems or questions for investigation, participates in approved research studies, and disseminates research findings to clients and other professionals. As researchers, nurses should remain informed of developments relative to their individual practice.

Risk (6): the probability that an event will occur (e.g., that an individual will become ill or die within a stated period of time or age).

Risk factor (6): an aspect of personal behavior or lifestyle, an environmental exposure, or an inborn or inherited characteristic associated with an increased occurrence of disease or other health-related event or condition.

Role model (2): a person who demonstrates an action or behavior that is learned by others. Role modeling is both conscious and unconscious and nurses in all settings demonstrate to others both positive and negative actions and attitudes related to health and health care.

Rural nursing (3): nursing care provided to residents in nonurban settings. Rural nursing practice must consider issues and barriers such as distance, isolation, and sparse resources. Rural nurses most often practice in clinic settings, home health, or a combination. Rural nurses must be clinically competent in a very broad number of areas and are typically cross-trained to manage client needs in areas including trauma, routine obstetrical care, care of children and elders, and care of clients with mental health needs.

S

School nursing (3): nursing care provided to students in school settings. Care typically focuses on prevention and control of communicable diseases, care of ill or injured students, administration or oversight of procedures for students with special health needs, administration of screening programs, provision and monitoring for a safe and healthful environment, health promotion, health counseling, and school program management.

Screening (10): interventions to assess the presence of signs of disease in the period of early pathogenesis before symptoms occur. Health screenings should be based on age and risk factors.

Secondary health care (1): refers to relatively serious or complicated care that has historically been provided to patients in hospitals. Recent changes in techniques, procedures, and medical practice have moved much of secondary health care into community settings. Examples of community-based secondary health care include outpatient surgery for complex procedures that would have required hospitalization just a few years ago (e.g., cholecystectomy, hysterectomy, appendectomy, herniorrhaphy), treatment of serious illnesses (e.g., chemotherapy, radiotherapy), and a wide variety of diagnostic testing procedures (e.g., computed tomography, magnetic resonance imaging, angiography).

Secondhand smoke (7): the combination of smoke given off by the burning of a cigarette, pipe, or cigar and the smoke exhaled from the lungs of smokers. The Environmental Protection Agency (EPA) has classified secondhand smoke as a known carcinogen. Secondhand smoke is estimated to cause approximately 3000 lung cancer deaths in nonsmokers each year.

Sexually transmitted diseases (STDs) (16): communicable diseases directly transmitted during sexual contact. The number and type of different STDs has increased dramatically over the last several decades. Of the top 10 infections reported to the CDC in 1998, 5 were STDs (chlamydia, gonorrhea, AIDS, syphilis, and hepatitis B), and it is estimated that more than 15 million cases of STDs occur each year in the United States.

Single-parent family (13): mother or father living with either biological or adopted children; they may be tied emotionally but not legally to a partner.

Skilled nursing services (4): those nursing services that are reimbursable by Medicare. Covered nursing services include observation and assessment of a patient's condition, management and evaluation of a patient care plan, teaching and training activities for the patient and the patient's family or caregivers, tube feedings, tracheotomy aspiration, wound care, ostomy care, rehabilitation care, and venipuncture.

Smoking cessation (10): programs, tools, medications, and various interventions to help tobacco users quit. Interventions include self-help groups, videos and written materials, nicotine chewing gum, nicotine patches, hypnosis, and acupuncture.

Stages of family development (13): evolution of a normal family through a series of several stages. The stages include beginning or establishment, early childbearing, families with young children, families with school-age children, families with adolescents, families as launching centers, middle-age families, and aging families stages.

State Children's Health Insurance Program (SCHIP) (9): created in 1997 to provide health insurance coverage for uninsured children. Most children covered by SCHIP are from working families with incomes too high to qualify for Medicaid but too low to afford private health insurance. Covered services include inpatient and outpatient hospital care, physician's surgical and medical care, laboratory and x-ray services, and well-baby/well-child care including immunizations. Prescription drugs, mental health services, vision care, and hearing-related care may be provided in some states.

Stereotyping (8): the belief or notion that all people from a given group are the same.

Subculture (8): a fairly large aggregate of individuals who share characteristics that are not common to all members of the culture and allow them to be considered a distinguishable subgroup; a group of persons within a culture of the same age, socioeconomic level, ethnic origin, education, or occupation who have an identity of their own but are related to the total culture.

Substance abuse (15): refers to patterns of use of alcohol and/or other drugs that result in health consequences or impairment in social, psychological, and occupational functioning.

Suicide (15): is the most serious potential outcome of mental disorders and a leading cause of death in the United States. Each year, more than 30,000 U.S. residents take their own lives. Depression, schizophrenia, panic disorder, and alcohol and other drug abuse have been implicated in both attempted and completed suicides.

T

Teenage pregnancy (11): pregnancy in young women under the age of 19 years; 95% are unintended. Each year about 10% of teenage girls become pregnant and about 500,000

give birth. Teenage pregnancy is associated with complications of pregnancy (both fetal and maternal), failure of the mother to complete high school, unemployment, poverty, and reliance on government assistance.

Terrorism (14): the unlawful use of force or violence against persons or property to intimidate or coerce a government or civilian population in the furtherance of political or social objectives. In most cases, terrorists use explosives or incendiary devices against their targets, but there is growing concern over the potential for terrorists' use of biologic organisms (i.e., anthrax or smallpox) or chemical agents (i.e., sarin gas, mustard gas).

Tertiary health care (1): management of chronic, complicated, long-term health problems. Tertiary care includes home health care and hospice care and care provided in rehabilitation centers.

Third party reimbursement (5): fiscal payment by an intermediary or "third party" such as an insurance company (e.g., Blue Cross, Aetna), Medicare, or Medicaid. This third party insures beneficiaries against health expenses. The individual pays a premium for coverage, and the insurer then pays health care bills on his or her behalf.

Twelve-step programs (15): mutual help groups that provide supportive interaction to help individuals meet a goal of recovery from use and abuse of drugs, alcohol, or compulsive behavior pattern. Participation in 12-step groups (e.g., Narcotics Anonymous and Alcoholics Anonymous) gives social support and structure that assists in the recovery process.

Transcultural nursing (8): nursing practice focused on the provision of nursing care in a manner that is sensitive to the cultural beliefs and values of individuals, families, and groups. In transcultural nursing, culturally sensitive nursing interventions show an appreciation of and respect for differences and an attempt to decrease the possibility of stress or conflict arising from cultural misunderstanding.

U

Ultraviolet radiation (7): from sun exposure contributes to skin cancer, which is the most common form of cancer in the United States. Exposure to ultraviolet radiation is believed to cause more than 90% of basal and squamous cell carcinomas.

Unintentional food additives (7): those substances that enter and remain in food as a result of their use as pesticides, after being added to animal food, or from packaging.

Universal precautions (6): recommendations issued by the Centers for Disease Control and Prevention to minimize the risk of transmission of bloodborne pathogens, particularly HIV and hepatitis B virus, by health care and public safety workers. Barrier precautions are to be used to prevent exposure to blood and certain body fluids of all patients.

Utilization review (5): a process of monitoring and evaluating the quality of health care, including necessity, appropriateness, and efficiency. The goal of utilization review is to monitor and provide incentives to influence the use of health care services through examination of hospitalization rates, admissions, length of stay, frequency of diagnostic and therapeutic procedures, and appropriateness and efficacy of practice patterns.

V

Vaccine Adverse Event Reporting System (VAERS) (16): developed to provide a single system for the collection and analysis of reports on all adverse events associated with the administration of any U.S. licensed vaccine. The VAERS is operated by the CDC and Food and Drug Administration.

Vaccine-preventable disease (16): those communicable diseases for which effective vaccines are available. The incidence of vaccine-preventable diseases (e.g., measles, mumps, diphtheria, pertussis) has dropped dramatically over the last three to four decades because of active immunization.

Values (8): personal perceptions of what is good or useful; desirable beliefs and standards.

Vector (6): an animate intermediary in the indirect transmission of an agent that carries the agent from a reservoir to a susceptible host.

Vehicle (6): an inanimate intermediary in the indirect transmission of an agent that carries the agent from a reservoir to a susceptible host.

Vision deficit (12): loss of vision in adults increases with age, and it is estimated that more than 90% of older people require the use of corrective lenses and approximately 18% of all older people have significant visual deficits. Cataracts, glaucoma, macular degeneration, and diabetic retinopathy often cause visual problems in the elderly.

Vision screening (9): early detection and referral for treatment of vision disorders. Vision screening includes a careful history, thorough examination, vision testing, and referral of abnormal or asymmetrical results for further testing and treatment.

Vulnerability (14): situation in which a person or group is more likely to develop a health-related problem or problems and to have more serious outcomes stemming from their exposure to multiple risks. Vulnerability is exacerbated by the combined effects of limited resources and contributing factors such as disempowerment, disenfranchisement, and marginalization.

Vulnerable group (14): those people who have an increased risk or susceptibility to adverse health outcomes. Vulnerable groups include disabled persons, homeless persons, migrant workers, persons in extreme poverty, persons who are HIV positive, persons with serious health problems, pregnant adolescents, refugees and recent immigrants, severely mentally ill individuals, substance abusers, very young or very old individuals, victims of disasters, and victims of violence.

W

Women, Infants, and Children Program (WIC) (9): federally funded program that provides food, nutrition counseling, and access to health services for low-income women, infants, and children. Pregnant or postpartum women, infants, and children up to age 5 years who meet income guidelines and residency requirements, and who are determined to be at "nutritional risk" are eligible. Most WIC programs provide vouchers that participants use at authorized stores to purchase nutritious foods.

Workers' compensation (3): a nation-wide, state-operated insurance system, with each state having its own law and program. Workers' compensation benefits are awarded to individuals who sustain physical or mental injuries from their employment, regardless of who or what was the cause of the injury or illness. Workers' compensation generally provides ongoing payment of wages and benefits to the injured or disabled worker or dependent survivor for wages lost, medical care and related costs, funeral and burial costs, and some rehabilitation expenses.

Y

Years of potential life lost (6): a measure of the impact of premature mortality on a population, calculated as the sum of the differences between some predetermined minimum or desired life span and the age of death for individuals who died earlier than that predetermined age.

Z

Zoonoses (6): an infectious disease that is transmissible under normal conditions from animals to humans.

Index

A

Abstinence, sexual, 271, 273t, 274t
Abuse
  of children, 216-219
  of the elderly, 324, 326-328, 326t
Access to health care
  and minority professionals, 95
  and rural health nursing, 39
  and the uninsured, 105-107
Acid rain, 140
Acne, 229t
Acquired immunodeficiency syndrome (AIDS). *See*
    HIV/AIDS
Activities of daily living (ADL), 305, 314, 381
Acupuncture, 175
Acute care facilities. *See also* Hospitals
  and changes in health care delivery, 4
  direct care providers in, 15-16
  nurse counselors in, 17
  nursing interventions in, 22, 25t
  and secondary health care, 92
Adolescents. *See also* Children
  alcohol and drug problems in, 397
  depression in, 401, 403b
  and developmental stages of families, 345-346
  and eating disorders, 406-407
  health of, 188-190
  HIV/AIDS among, 124
  mortality of, 189
  nutritional needs of, 201
  pregnancy, 288-291
  and puberty, 205-206
  and sleep, 203
  smoking and, 123t
  and suicide, 417
Adult day care, 94b
Advanced practice nurses, 96-97
Advocates, nurse, 17-18, 32b
African-Americans, 170, 174, 214
Age
  and depression, 401
  and heart disease, 249
Agoraphobia, 404
AIDS. *See* HIV/AIDS
Air pollution, 137-141, 142b

Figures are indicated by f, tables by t, boxes by b.

Alcohol and drug use
  and breast cancer, 291-292
  and the CAGE questionnaire, 420f
  and children, 206-208
  and correctional institution nursing, 43-44
  facts about, 410b, 411b, 412b
  and mental disorders, 397, 409
  and osteoporosis, 294
  during pregnancy, 278-279
  risk factors for, 410, 412b
  signs and symptoms of, 410, 413-414t
  and stress, 411
  treatment for, 410-412, 415
  and twelve-step programs, 412, 415
Alzheimer's disease, 310-311t, 318-319
Ambulatory care nursing
  defining, 29-30, 50, 91-92
  education of patients in, 16
  education recommendations for nurses in, 31
  interventions, 24t
  practice, 31, 32b, 91-92
  types of providers and, 91
Ambulatory mental health care, 397-398
Ambulatory oncology care, 45-46, 51
Ambulatory surgery nursing
  description of, 46-47
  practice, 47-49, 51
American Academy of Ambulatory Care Nursing
    (AAACN), 31
American Academy of Nursing (AAN), 161
American Academy of Pediatrics (AAP), 200, 283
American Board for Occupational Health Nurses
    (ABOHN), 38
American Cancer Society (ACS), 250, 291-292
American Diabetes Association, 252
American Heart Association (AHA), 238, 239
American Medical Association (AMA), 99
American Nurses' Association (ANA), 5, 36, 44, 57
American Nurses Credentialing Center (ANCC), 31
American Organization of Nurse Executives, 5b
American Red Cross (ARC), 386, 387
American School Health Association (ASHA), 33
Americans with Disabilities Act (ADA), 382
American with Disabilities Act (ADA), 381
Amniocentesis, 281t
Analytical epidemiology, 122, 124-125
Anemia screening, 200
Anorexia nervosa, 407